Adult Nursing Practice

Using Evidence in Care

Edited by

Dr Ian Bullock
National Clinical Guideline Centre, Royal College of Physicians

Professor Dame Jill Macleod Clark
University of Southampton

Professor Jo Rycroft-Malone
University of Bangor

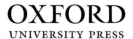

OXFORD
UNIVERSITY PRESS

OXFORD
UNIVERSITY PRESS

Great Clarendon Street, Oxford OX2 6DP,

United Kingdom

Oxford University Press is a department of the University of Oxford.
It furthers the University's objective of excellence in research, scholarship,
and education by publishing worldwide. Oxford is a registered trade mark of
Oxford University Press in the UK and in certain other countries

British Library Cataloguing in Publication Data

Data available

Library of Congress Cataloguing in Publication

Library of Congress Number: 2012938465

ISBN 978-0-19-969741-0

Printed in Italy
on acid-free paper by
L.E.G.O. S.p.A.—Lavis TN

Oxford University press makes no representation, express or implied, that the
drug dosages in this book are correct. Readers must therefore always check
the product information and clinical procedures with the most up-to-date
published product information and data sheets provided by the manufacturers
and the most recent codes of conduct and safety regulations. The authors and
the publishers do not accept responsibility or legal liability for any errors in the
text or for the misuse or misapplication of material in this work. Except where
otherwise stated, drug dosages and recommendations are for the non-pregnant
adult who is not breastfeeding.

Links to third party websites are provided by Oxford in good faith and
for information only. Oxford disclaims any responsibility for the materials
contained in any third party website referenced in this work.

Adult Nursing Practice
Using Evidence in Care

Dedication

During the writing of this book, my mother, Jean Bullock, died of a haemorrhagic stroke. This book is dedicated to her memory and the influence she had on our family life. It is also dedicated to the amazing team of nurses and the wider healthcare team on the Acute Stroke Unit (A4) at Russells Hall Hospital, part of the Dudley Group of Hospitals NHS Foundation Trust. Your commitment to high-quality evidence-based care and compassion was what made the difference to our family.

Ian Bullock

Preface

This book, like any other, started with an idea. This idea germinated for a while and then, through the collective vision of the editors, supported by Oxford University Press and our excellent chapter authors, it developed into what we believe is a unique contribution to the nursing literature. Historically, definitive nursing texts have tended to view their subject and material from a systems-based approach, not dissimilar to the medical model of healthcare. This book is different for a number of reasons. Not least, it celebrates the unique contribution of nursing within the healthcare team and we ask you to plan and deliver nursing interventions from a very different perspective. Our conceptual starting point is characterized by the smart use of evidence and a focus on those areas of care that are a primary nursing responsibility, underpinned by an enquiring approach in day-to-day care.

We are passionate about the use of evidence in nursing and the wider multidisciplinary team, regardless of care setting and patient population. Much has been written over the past two decades about the importance of evidence. This book acknowledges its role, but, more importantly, develops a way of thinking when approaching a common core condition (Part 1), and a commitment to evidence utilization to maximize patient benefit and patient experience. The book also brings together key nursing interventions (Part 2) that illuminate the unique contribution of nursing. By following this conceptual approach to care and highlighting evidence that supports nursing actions and interventions, the chapter authors encourage you to 'think evidence' and be a 'consumer of evidence' when taking a clinical leadership role in these fundamental aspects of care. In a data-rich society, nurses, like other healthcare professionals, can be overwhelmed by 'information overload', with variations in care persisting and potential quality improvement negated by an inability to exploit this information. Through effective signposting to reliable sources of evidence, you are encouraged, in practical ways, to embed relevant and contemporary evidence into your care planning and care delivery.

This approach, whilst incredibly challenging, can be achieved by thinking differently, by being accountable for those aspects of care that are the responsibility of nurses to deliver, and by 'learning' to use evidence, which is the beating heart of this book. We commend it to you and trust that it quickly becomes a trusted resource that helps you to 'make a real difference' to the lives of those for whom you care.

Ian, Jill and Jo

Contents

About the editors

Dr Ian Bullock PhD, MSc, BSc (Hons), RN Ian is currently Chief Operating Officer at the National Clinical Guideline Centre and has developed expertise in evidence-based healthcare, research and development, critical care clinical practice, and clinical and higher education. He is involved in strategic and operational planning at a national and international level with the Royal College of Physicians, and is responsible for a large funded research programme on behalf of the National Institute for Health and Clinical Excellence (NICE), with particular focus on the development of National Clinical Guidelines and Quality Standards. The main focus of this work is evidence translation and utilization, establishing standards for practice, and the interpretation of these into quality markers. Having trained as a nurse in the early 1980s, his career path, whilst not following a typical trajectory, has offered him some amazing opportunities to influence nursing and the wider healthcare community. Ian has established local, national, and international networks within the evidence-based healthcare community, and the cardiorespiratory, resuscitation, and quality improvement fields. He has worked previously for the Royal College of Nursing in a number of senior roles, including Head of Quality Standards. These powerful combinations of clinical practice, education, and research are key drivers in his career commitment to 'make a difference to patient outcomes/experience'.

Professor Dame Jill Macleod Clark DBE, PhD, MSc, BSc (Hons), RN, FRCN Jill is Professor of Nursing in the Faculty of Health Sciences, University of Southampton, and has many years of experience as a clinical nurse, educator, and researcher. She completed her training as a nurse at UCH in London in the 1960s and, since then, her career has focused on enhancing the contribution of nursing interventions to improving patient outcomes. She has an international reputation for her research into health promotion, communication, and interprofessional learning. She has held a number of academic leadership positions, most recently as Dean of Nursing at the University of Southampton. In that role, she championed the move to an all-graduate nursing profession and the provision of the highest quality education programmes for nursing students. She has also led a pioneering clinical academic career pathway scheme in partnership with local healthcare providers. Jill has also been engaged in national policy agendas, acting as Chair of the UK Council of Deans of Health and as a member of the 2008 Research Assessment Panel for Nursing and Midwifery.

Professor Jo Rycroft-Malone PhD, MSc, BSc (Hons), RN Jo was awarded a personal chair in 2008 and is Professor of Implementation Research at Bangor University; she is also the University's Director of Research. She has an international reputation for research that aims to improve service delivery and patient care through the appropriate use of evidence in practice. She is currently a principal and coinvestigator of nationally and internationally competitively funded research grants that explore various aspects of knowledge use in practice, including evaluating different implementation interventions. She has sat on the Chief Medical Officer's Clinical Effectiveness Strategy Group, and is currently a member of the National Institute for Health and Clinical Excellence's (NICE) Implementation Strategy group, the National Institute for Health Research (NIHR) Service Delivery and Organisation Programme's commissioning group, and the Canadian Institutes for Health Research knowledge exchange and transfer funding committee. Jo is also the inaugural editor of the journal *Worldview on Evidence-Based Nursing*, the most cited international journal for evidence-based practice. Jo is Visiting Professor University of Alberta, Canada, and Visiting Professor University of Ulster, Northern Ireland.

About the contributors

Dr John W. Albarran RN, BSc (Hons), PG Dip Ed, MSc, DPhil, NFESC Dr John Albarran is an Associate Professor in Cardiovascular Critical Care Nursing at the Faculty of Health and Life Sciences, University of the West of England, Bristol. John is an experienced educator and researcher with a clinical background in intensive, cardiac, and renal care. He has coauthored/coedited four textbooks linked to cardiovascular critical care, has over 60 peer-reviewed publications, and has presented over 60 papers (36 peer-reviewed conference abstracts) at major national and international conferences across Europe, South America, Australia, and South Africa. Additionally, John leads the Research and Development Committee for the European Federation of Critical Care Nursing Associations (EFCCNA), and has contributed to seven pan-European studies exploring clinical and professional practice issues. He currently coedits *Nursing in Critical Care*, and his research interests include gender issues in cardiac care, cardiac symptom presentations, family-witnessed resuscitation, and end-of-life care.

Nick Allcock Nick is Associate Professor, Director of Postgraduate Studies, and Co-director of the Nottingham Centre for Evidence-Based Nursing and Midwifery (a collaborating centre of the Joanna Briggs Institute) at the University of Nottingham School of Nursing, Midwifery and Physiotherapy.

Anne Baileff RN, RM, BSc (Hons), MSc, Nurse Independent/Supplementary Prescriber Anne is Director of Programmes: Advanced Clinical and Expert Practice in the Faculty of Health Sciences, University of Southampton. She has extensive experience of advanced clinical practice, medicines management, and clinical governance. Anne practised as a consultant nurse in unscheduled care for a number of years, during which time she made a major contribution to the development of innovative nurse-led services. In this role, she was also the non-medical prescribing lead for Southampton City Primary Care Trust and was responsible for the design and governance of patient group directives. As part of her current role, she is the education lead for medicines management and the non-medical prescribing programme in the Faculty of Health Sciences. She has presented at national and international conferences and published in various nursing journals. Her research has explored the experiences of nurse independent supplementary prescribers.

John Baker PhD, MPhil, MSc, BNurs (Hons), RMN, RNT, CPN John Baker is a lecturer in the School of Nursing, Midwifery and Social Work, and is a member of the Mental Health Research Group in the School of Nursing, Midwifery and Social Work. He has worked in a variety of inpatient settings, including acute and low secure rehabilitation. He has published extensively in the mental health field.

Dr Catherine Bryant MA, MB BChir, FRCP Catherine Bryant has been a Consultant Geriatrician at King's College Hospital NHS Foundation Trust in London for more than 10 years. She is committed to excellence in the care of older people in acute hospitals. She established and continues to run a memory clinic within the Clinical Gerontology department at King's. She is widely involved in postgraduate medical education of doctors, and has coauthored a number of articles and book chapters on nursing of older people with dementia and delirium.

Dr Christopher R. Burton PhD, BN, RGN Chris specializes in the development of services that support patients and family members to manage chronic and complex diseases, especially stroke. A key theme of his work is the implementation of evidence of 'what works' to maximize patient and family experience and outcomes. He is a Council Member of the Society for Research in Rehabilitation, a founding steering group member for the National Stroke Nursing Forum, and contributes to the Stroke Association Research Awards Committee and UKSRN Rehabilitation Clinical Studies Group. His current stoke research focuses on the preferences for, and effectiveness of, services for patients and families living with the consequences of stroke (including continence and end of life care), the effectiveness of occupational therapy for stroke in care homes, and vocational rehabilitation. He has delivered clinical leadership programmes for stroke service leads for the Department of Health as part of the English National Stroke Strategy. Within Wales he collaborates with clinicians in the Betsi Cadwaladr University Health Board through the North Wales Stroke Network, and serves as Chair, OPAN Wales Stroke Research Group.

Jessica Callaghan BSc (Hons) Jessica is a Specialist Respiratory Occupational Therapist, Surrey Respiratory Care Team, Surrey Community Health (South West locality). Jessica has worked as an occupational therapist in respiratory care for 8 years, and brings specialist mental health knowledge and experience to the role. She works within a community respiratory team, aiming to maximize patients' functioning in all occupations, especially when anxiety or depression add to the respiratory symptoms and limitations. Jessica has presented at national and international respiratory conferences and has research and education interests. She was a member of two of the subgroups working to develop the Outcomes Strategy for People with Chronic Obstructive Pulmonary Disease (COPD) and Asthma in England (published by the Department of Health in 2011). Her main interest is in the psychological aspects and functional impact of living with lung disease.

Marie Chellingsworth RMN Dip Nursing (MH), BSc (Hons), PGCHE, PG Dip. EBPT, MSc, Marie is a Senior Lecturer in Psychological Therapies and Course Director for Improving Access to Psychological Therapies (IAPT) training for the East Midlands at the University of Nottingham. Marie is a Senior Fellow of the Institute of Mental Health and elected Chair of the East Midlands Branch of the British Association for Behavioural and Cognitive Psychotherapy, a member of the Psychological Wellbeing Practitioner Accreditation Committee, and sits on the IAPT Education and Workforce Group. She is an editor for *CBT Today*, an author of *The Oxford Guide to Low Intensity CBT*, and coauthor of *CBT: A Clinician's Guide to the Five Areas Approach*. She has also written several key documents regarding IAPT and the field of low-intensity working. Marie's research interests include low-intensity psychological interventions, and training nurses and allied health professionals to use CBT-based skills for common mental health problems. She is currently undertaking her PhD.

Michelle Cowen RGN, MSc SpLD (Dyslexia), BEd (Hons), RNT, RCNT, Diploma in Nursing (Lond), ENB 100 Michelle is a Lecturer in Adult Nursing in the Faculty of Health Sciences at the University of Southampton. Her clinical background is predominantly in intensive care and high-dependency surgical nursing, areas about which she now teaches. She has previously been responsible for ENB awards in intensive care nursing, high-dependency nursing, and vascular nursing. Her research interests centre around her other main area of interest, support for students with dyslexia or other known disabilities, on which she regularly presents at international conferences.

Nicola Davey Nicola is a Senior Associate and Programme Manager at the NHS Institute for Innovation and Improvement. She has recently completed a PG Certificate in Advanced Improvement in Quality and Safety and continues to develop her interests in medicines management service improvement through delivery of taught programmes and service improvement. Nicola trained as a pharmacist and worked at London teaching hospitals before moving to primary care where she was Head of Medicines Management for over a decade. Nicola has lectured on risk and medicines management and contributed to chapters on health promotion and clinical roles. She has also undertaken freelance work at national, regional and local level including Commission for Healthcare Improvement reviews and investigations of deaths in custody.

Jan Davis RN, RSCN, RM, BSc (Hons), MBA, Jan is Director of Programmes (Leadership and Health Systems) in the Centre for Innovation and Leadership, Faculty of Health Sciences, University of Southampton, where she has worked for the past 5 years. Her expertise is in advanced practice and she has many years of experience in primary care working as an autonomous practitioner across a range of unscheduled care settings. She has been involved in the development of innovative nurse-led services in which nurses utilize advanced practice skills, including prescribing.

Ruth Day RGN, Lic. Ac, BA (Hons), MA, PhD Ruth Day is the Clinical Nurse Specialist in Acute Pain Management at South Devon Healthcare NHS Trust. She has extensive experience, clinically and educationally, in acute and chronic pain management, having worked in the area for almost two decades. Ruth has established both acute and chronic pain services, has published in peer-reviewed journals, has spoken at local, national, and international conferences, and has edited the British Pain Society newsletter. Her PhD research explored the use of focusing—a psychological technique—in chronic low back pain.

Christine De Laine RN, BN Christine is a Continence Nurse Specialist and team leader for the East Dorset Continence Advisory Service, Dorset HealthCare University Foundation Trust. Working in this specialty since 1984, she has broad clinical and educational expertise. Alongside her clinical role Christine combines a secondment to the University of Southampton, linking with the Continence Technology and Skin Health Group.

Jan Dewing Jan joined Canterbury Christchurch University in 2010 and is also Co-Director of the England Practice Development Centre. A registered nurse, in her current role Jan works in a joint appointment between East Sussex Healthcare NHS Trust and the university, focusing of mutually beneficial ways of working that bring desired outcomes for both organizations and ultimately improve the patient's experience of care and patient safety. Jan has expertise in re-enablement and gerontological practice, including dementia care. Jan has a wide range of clinical and research supervision experience, and her own research interests include knowledge translation, evaluation of services and practices, workplace culture, and patient experience. She publishes regularly and presents at a variety of national and international peer-reviewed conferences. She holds Visiting Professorships with the University of Ulster and with the University of Wollongong in Australia.

Steven J. Ersser PhD, RN Steven has been Professor of Nursing and Dermatology Care and Dean of the Faculty of Health and Social Care at the University of Hull in the UK since 2011, holding the first nursing Chair worldwide in the dermatology field. He was previously Professor of Nursing Development and Skin Care Research and Director of the Centre for Wellbeing and Quality of Life at Bournemouth University. Over the last 20 years, since working as Clinical Lecturer and Senior Nurse in the Oxford Department of Dermatology and National Institute for Nursing, his focus has been to develop research, education, and practice development related to skin and dermatology care within the nursing field nationally and internationally. He founded and then led the International Skin Care Nursing Advisory (ISNG) Board for over a decade, which is recognized by the International Council of Nurses and the International League of Dermatological Societies. As a former Reader in Nursing at the University of Southampton, he worked part-time as a specialist nurse leading a nurse-led clinic supporting patients with chronic skin disease, reflecting his clinical and research interests. In 2006, he was presented with The Stone Award by the British Dermatological Nursing Group for his contribution to the international development of evidence-based dermatology nursing. He is Honorary Professor at the University of Cape Town in South Africa and Adjunct Professor at Memorial University, Newfoundland, Canada. Steven is also co-editor of the evidence-based book *Principles of Skin Care: A Guide for Nurses and Other Health Care Professionals*, published in 2010.

Mandy Fader RN, PhD Mandy is Professor of Continence Technology at the University of Southampton. She has more than 20 years experience in researching continence products and devices and is particularly interested in their effects on skin health and on quality of life. She is an editor for the Cochrane Incontinence group, co-author of the International Consultation on Incontinence section on Management with Continence Products, ex-Trustee of the International Continence Society, and consulting editor for Wound, Ostomy and Continence Nursing.

Roger Gadsby MBE, BSc, MB ChB, DCH, DRCOG, FRCGP Roger Gadsby is an Associate Clinical Professor at Warwick Medical School, University of Warwick. He has been a GP for 31 years and has written four diabetes textbooks, 12 textbook chapters, and over 300 papers and articles, mainly on diabetes topics. At Warwick, he has developed a number of courses in diabetes care. Around 10,000 healthcare professionals, mainly GPs and nurses, have taken the Warwick Certificate in Diabetes Care (CIDC). He is a Diabetes Expert Advisor for theNational Institute for Health and Clinical Excellence (NICE) and was awarded an MBE in 2009 for 'services to medicine and diabetes care'.

Jenny Gordon PhD, BSc, RGN, RSCN, NICE Fellow Jenny is the Programme Manager in the Quality, Standards, Research and Innovation Unit at the Royal College of Nursing, Learning and Development Institute. She has a background in general and paediatric nursing in acute and community settings, having trained at Great Ormond Street Hospitals for Sick Children and University College Hospital, London. Over the past 30 years, Jenny has been involved in nursing in a variety of roles, both clinical and academic. Her current role gives her the opportunity to combine her clinical and academic knowledge and skills to influence, support, and improve outcomes for patients and healthcare professionals. It involves the development of strategies, processes, and resources to facilitate and support the implementation of evidence in healthcare. She is the nursing representative on the Scottish Intercollegiate Guidelines Network (SIGN) Council, was involved in the development of the NICE Guideline for Irritable Bowel Syndrome, and was Chair of the Guideline Development Group of the NICE Guideline on Childhood Constipation. Her team also coordinates the NICE programme within the Royal College of Nursing (RCN), and encourages and supports nurses' involvement with all aspects of NICE work programmes and other national guidance development.

Sue Green RN, BSc, MMedSci, PhD, PGCert Sue is a Senior Lecturer in the Faculty of Health Sciences, University of Southampton. She is currently seconded as Senior Clinical Academic Research Fellow and divides her time between the University and Solent NHS Trust. Her clinical background includes cardiothoracics, medicine, and care of the older adult. Sue's research interest concerns nutritional care by nurses.

Patricia Grocott RGN, DipN (Lon), BSc (Hons), PhD Patricia Grocott is Reader in Palliative Wound Care in the Florence Nightingale School of Nursing and Midwifery, King's College London. Her clinical background is in hospice-based palliative care. Her observations of the lack of suitable wound care products for patients with extensive wounds were the stimulus for her academic research career. Her research has included an in-depth study of patients' experiences of advanced malignant wounds, together with a methodology and patient-recorded outcome measures for palliative wound care. In addition, she has developed a model of user engagement in medical device development, whereby users' needs drive innovation and novel products. This research has involved working with a designer and medical device manufacturers. Patricia has published in various journals and has presented at local, national, and international conferences.

Nicky Hayes RN, BA (Hons), MSc, PGCert (HE) Nicky Hayes is Consultant Nurse for Older People, King's College Hospital NHS Foundation Trust, and is also Older People's Advisor to the Royal College of Nursing. She has carried out research and practice development into a number of areas of care for older people, including falls prevention and the use of hip protectors in hospital and care homes. Nicky has published in a range of journals and specialist textbooks, and is the Consultant Editor of the journal *Nursing Older People*. Her clinical practice focuses on older patients with complex needs and includes a specialism in Parkinsonism in older patients.

Marika Hills RN, MSc Marika Hills works for Macmillan Cancer Support as a Macmillan Development Manager covering the Wolverhampton and Staffordshire areas. Marika has 22 years of experience in cancer and palliative care, her clinical expertise gained from both haematology nursing and specialist palliative care roles. Marika has also worked in cancer management and end-of-life service evaluation and development roles, including national programme implementation with the National Cancer Action Team. Marika has coauthored several publications on end-of-life and after death-care.

Cathy Hughes RN, MSc, DClinPrac Cathy has spent most of her nursing career involved in the care and management of individuals with cancer. After qualifying in 1985, she worked in gynaecology and high-dependency surgery, becoming involved in the specialist management of women with gynaecological cancer. She was a founder member of the National Forum of Gynaecological Oncology Nurses and has been chair of the Women's Health Forum at the Royal College of Nursing. She has held Clinical Nurse Specialist positions at St Mary's Hospital, Paddington (now Imperial Healthcare), and at The Royal Marsden, London. Cathy has also worked in cancer research and completed masters and doctoral degrees in cancer nursing practice. Her most recent post was as Patient Safety Lead for Cancer at the National Patient Safety Agency.

Jane Jackson SRN, MPhil, MCGI Jane is currently Consultant Nurse in Pre-Operative Assessment at West Hertfordshire NHS Trust, where she has introduced pre-operative assessment for all adult patients, and is an Honorary Fellow at the University of Hertfordshire. Jane has been key in the development of patient preparation, incorporating National Institute for Health and Clinical Excellence (NICE), Department of Health, and public health requirements, as well as discharge planning—essential for all patients due for admission, particularly those being admitted on the enhanced recovery programme. Jane qualified as a state registered nurse in 1980 with a degree at University College Hospital, London, since which time she has worked extensively with the surgical patient, including in intensive care and acute and elective surgical wards. In 2000, she attained a masters degree at the University of Luton following research and implementation of preoperative assessment for the elective surgical patient. During 2003, along with seven colleagues across England, Jane was instrumental in setting up the Preoperative Association for Interprofessionals with an interest in patient preparation prior to surgery.

Sarah Kendal BA (Hons), RMN, MHSc, PhD Sarah Kendal lectures on a wide range of nursing courses from basic to postgraduate level in the School of Nursing, Midwifery and Social Work at the University of Manchester. She draws on broad-ranging clinical experience acquired from working in the mental health services for many years. She has a special interest in preventive and early mental health interventions, and her recent research explores mental health support for young people. She has published in peer-reviewed journals and contributed to textbooks on mental health issues. She is a reviewer for several nursing journals.

Martin Kiernan RN, MPH, ONC, Dip N Martin is Nurse Consultant in Infection Prevention and Control at Southport and Ormskirk Hospital NHS Trust. Martin has 21 years of experience in the specialty, and has covered all sectors of healthcare from an infection prevention and control perspective. He is a Former President of the Infection Prevention Society, a former council member of the Tissue Viability Society, and is a member of the Department of Health (England) Advisory Committee on Healthcare-Associated Infection and Antimicrobial Resistance (ARHAI). Martin has published over 50 articles and papers on infection prevention and control in general nursing journals, and is a regular speaker at international and national meetings. His research interests presently centre on the use of indwelling urinary catheters and reducing the prevalence of invasive medical devices.

Vikki Knowles BSc (Hons), RGN Vikki is Respiratory Clinical Lead, SW Locality, Surrey Community Health, and Trainer Education for Health. She has been a respiratory nurse specialist since 1990. She served on the committee of the Association of Respiratory Nurse Specialists, currently serves on the executive committee of the Primary Care Respiratory Society (PCRS), and is a trainer for the Education for Health. She is clinical lead for SW Surrey's community multidisciplinary respiratory care teams. In 2009, Vikki was seconded to Asthma UK to provide clinical leadership for the organization, in which role she was involved in several research projects. Vikki's interests include chronic obstructive pulmonary disease and interstital lung disease, with particular emphasis on palliative care. She was a member of the COPD Clinical Strategy Group looking at end-stage respiratory disease and asthma. She is currently contributing to the development of a good asthma guide and participated in the Lung Improvement Programme looking at chronic disease and self-management for people with COPD.

Andrea Nelson BSc (Hons), RGN, PhD Andrea Nelson is a Professor of Wound Healing and Dean in the School of Healthcare at the University of Leeds. Her clinical interests focus on the care of people with chronic wounds, especially leg, foot, and pressure ulcers. Her academic interests invovle the evaluation of interventions in nursing. She was editor of the *European Wound Management Association Journal*, and associate editor for *Evidence Based Nursing* and *Family Practice*. She is an editor of the Cochrane Wounds Group and contributor to many systematic reviews in wound care. She referees articles for numerous journals and has sat on funding committees for research in Ireland and England. She has made more than 60 invited contributions to conferences and published more than 60 articles in the areas of evidence-based practice, wound care, and nursing.

Christine Norton PhD, MA, RN Christine is nurse consultant (Bowel Control) at St Mark's Hospital in Harrow and Professor of Clinical Nursing and Innovation at Bucks New University and Imperial College Healthcare NHS Trust in London. Christine has worked with incontinent people for over 30 years and has authored seven books and numerous research publications and presentations. She chaired the UK National Institute for Health and Clinical Excellence guidelines on faecal incontinence and the International Consultation on Incontinence Committee on faecal incontinence. Research interests include the role of specialist nurses and conservative management of functional bowel disorders.

Emma Ouldred RGN, MSc, BSc Emma Ouldred has been a dementia nurse specialist at King's College Hospital NHS Foundation Trust since 2002. She first joined King's College Hospital in 1997 as a research nurse. She has always enjoyed caring for older adults and holds a deep respect for these individuals. She has a particular interest in how the hospital environment can impact on patients with dementia, and she is currently leading a team to transform an elderly care ward at King's College Hospital into a dementia-appropriate environment.

Dr Linda Pearce DNursing, MSc, RN, NPdip, OMNC Dr Linda Pearce is a Respiratory Nurse Consultant at West Suffolk Hospital and Clinical Lead for the Suffolk COPD Services, and is an Honorary Lecturer at Essex University. Her interest in respiratory health started as an occupational nurse and progressed through practice nursing. She completed a doctorate in nursing at Essex University and her thesis looked at non-drug management of breathlessness in chronic obstructive pulmonary disease (COPD). Working together with a paediatrician, she also runs an asthma clinic focusing on the complex social and psychological issues that impact on asthma control in children. She is a member of several committees, including the Eastern Region Asthma Mortality & Severe Morbidity Group. Linda has published in various journals and books. She has presented at local, national, and international conferences.

Anne Phillips BSc, MSc, RMN, RGN Anne Phillips is a Senior Teaching Fellow at Warwick Medical School, University of Warwick. Anne has worked in the health service for over 30 years as a nurse in a variety of clinical areas and has spent over 15 years as a diabetes nurse specialist in the acute and community settings. Anne works across the diabetes programme within the medical school and is still actively involved in structured patient education.

Alison Pottle RGN, Dip N, BSc, MSc Alison is a Consultant Nurse in Cardiology, Royal Brompton and Harefield NHS Foundation Trust, Harefield Hospital, Harefield, Middlesex. Alison has extensive clinical experience in cardiology and has worked at Harefield Hospital since 1987. She was one of the first consultant nurses in cardiology in the country when she was appointed in 2000. She has set up a variety of nurse-led services for patients pre and post angioplasty, she runs a rapid access chest pain clinic, and also runs the cholesterol dialysis service at Harefield. Alison has published in various cardiology journals and presents at conferences in the UK and abroad. Her research interests include nurse-led services and the patient experience in cardiology.

Jacqui Prieto RGN, BSc (Hons), BSc, PhD Jacqui Prieto is a Senior Clinical Academic Research Fellow in the Faculty of Health Sciences, University of Southampton. She has worked in the field of infection prevention for over 18 years. This includes 12 years as a clinical nurse specialist, both in acute and community healthcare settings, and 6 years as a lecturer at the University of Southampton. Currently, Jacqui is pioneering a new clinical academic role, combining a senior clinical post in infection prevention and a postdoctoral academic fellowship. As part of her work, Jacqui leads a research and quality improvement programme designed to reduce healthcare-associated infection. Her research interests include implementing interventions to reduce healthcare-associated infection and the patient experience of healthcare-associated infection. She is a reviewer of several peer-reviewed journals and has served on national committees relating to infection prevention.

Samantha Prigmore RGN, MSc, BSc Samantha Prigmore is a Respiratory Nurse Consultant at St Georges Healthcare NHS Trust. Samantha has extensive experience in caring for patients with respiratory conditions in both primary and secondary care. She has a particular interest in the management of asthma in adolescence and during pregnancy, respiratory failure, and palliative care. Her research interests include self-management in both asthma and chronic obstructive pulmonary disease (COPD), and advanced COPD care. She has published in a variety of journals and presented at national and international conferences. She has held an Honorary Lecturer position at Imperial College, and is a trainer for Education for Health.

Jane Scullion RGN, BA (Hons), MSc Jane is Respiratory Nurse Consultant at the University Hospitals of Leicester and Clinical Lead for Respiratory and LTC East Midlands SHA. She has an extensive background in respiratory medicine, with a specific interest in the impact of chronic disease on patients. Jane also chairs the Nurse Advisory Group for the British Thoracic Society, and is a Trustee at both the Primary Care Respiratory Society UK and Respiratory Education UK. She reviews for several peer-reviewed journals and sits on several editorial boards. Jane has published in various journals, and has been involved in and edited respiratory books.

Caroline Smith, née Lawson, MA, BSc (Hons), RGN Caroline is a Consultant Nurse at Yeovil District Hospital NHS Foundation Trust, Somerset. In addition to having a large clinical caseload, responsibilities include working as a peer reviewer for Royal College of Physicians/ British Association of Shoke Physicians (RCP/BASP), local and regional education, and assisting with the local nursing agenda as a senior nurse. Research interests include sitting on the Peninsula Stroke Research Network Management Group and being the principal investigator for several stroke studies. Caroline has published in various nursing journals, nursing textbooks, and presented at numerous conferences for both stroke-specific and general nursing topics.

Anne Sutcliffe BSc (Hons), RN, DN, HV Anne Sutcliffe is Healthcare and Education Officer, Paget's Association, Manchester. Having worked in the field of metabolic bone disease for 20 years, Anne has become an expert practitioner in this area of healthcare. In her current national post, she offers advice and support to those with Paget's disease, develops evidence-based patient information, liaises with health professionals, and is involved in varied educational initiatives with the public and health professions. Prior to this, she worked as an osteoporosis specialist nurse for Newcastle upon Tyne NHS Trust, where she took a lead role in developing, planning, and delivering nursing care and services to patients with osteoporosis and Paget's disease. She has published widely on osteoporosis in medical and nursing journals, has authored one textbook, and has contributed to several others on osteoporosis.

Cameron Swift PhD, FRCP, FRCPI, is Emeritus Professor of Health Care of the Elderly at King's College London School of Medicine. He is a past President of the British Geriatrics Society and former UK Medicines Commissioner. He chaired the Guideline Development Group for the recently launched NICE Clinical Guideline on Hip Fracture.

Debra Ugboma RGN, BN, MPhil Debra Ugboma (née Coupe) is a Lecturer in the Faculty of Health Sciences, University of Southampton. Debra is currently Programme Lead for the Post-Graduate Diploma in Nursing, but has a clinical background in renal nursing and has worked in renal services in Oxford, Cardiff, Birmingham, and Portsmouth. She has presented numerous papers at national and international conferences, and has made chapter contributions to two nursing textbooks. Research interests include long-term conditions and post-registration nurse education.

David Voegeli RGN, BSc (Hons), PGCEA, PhD, FHEA David is a Senior Lecturer in Nursing in the Faculty of Health Sciences, University of Southampton. His clinical background is in critical care nursing and respiratory medicine, and his research interests include inflammation, skin breakdown, and tissue repair. He is a reviewer for several peer-reviewed journals and sits on several editorial boards.

Julie Whitney BSc (Hons), MSc, MCSP Julie is a physiotherapist at Kings College Hospital. She has worked specifically with older people for more than 10 years on acute hospital wards, in the community and day hospital settings. She has an interest in falls prevention and has provided clinical care in falls clinics and now moved on to conducting research into falls prevention. She is now completing her PhD studies investigating falls risk factors in older people with cognitive impairment. She lectures on these subjects and has published in peer-reviewed journals and presented work at national and international conferences.

Helen Willis RGN, BSc (Hons) Helen is a Practice Educator for Wessex Renal and Transplant Service, Portsmouth Hospitals NHS Trust. She has extensive clinical skills and knowledge, and works across the renal specialty. She has worked within the renal service for 24 years, and led the development of a competency-based education programme for renal nursing staff. She also coordinates and facilitates a work-based learning module, which, jointly with the University of Southampton, provides post-registration skills development and academic study for renal nurses. Helen was also part of a research team exploring the provision and facilitation of end-of-life care in high/critical care environments, and has authored journal articles.

Acknowledgements

Jaymeeni Solanki—thanks for your support and help in the final editing stages. Theresa Shaw—CEO Foundation of Nursing Studies—thank you for being a critical friend. Thank you Julie, Matt, Meg, and Sarah, for your love and continued support.

Ian Bullock

A special thank you goes to Brenda for her invaluable contribution in the run-up to the finishing line. I would have been lost without her. I would also to thank the many patients who have taught me so much and influenced my passion for educating future generations of nurses to provide expert, evidence-based care.

Jill Macleod Clark

Figure acknowledgements

1.1 A broad conceptualization of evidence-based practice with shared decision-making. Adapted from Rycroft-Malone *et al.* (2004).

2.4 Reproduced with permission from British Thoracic Society/Scottish Intercollegiate Guidelines Network.

3.2 Reproduced from *Hip Fracture*, Martyn Parker and Antony Johansen, 2006, with permission from BMJ Publishing Group Ltd.

4.1, 4.2, 4.3 Data obtained from the Globocan 2008 database at the International Agency for Research on Cancer (Ferlay *et al.*, 2008).

4.4 National Cancer Institute. Based on artwork originally created for the National Cancer Institute by Jeanne Kelly.

4.5 Reproduced with permission of Cancerhelp UK.

5.1 Reproduced from Thomas and Monaghan, *Oxford Handbook of Clinical Examination and Practical Skills* (2007) by permission of Oxford University Press.

5.2 Reproduced with permission of the European Respiratory Society©.

5.3 Reproduced with permission from the National Institute for Health and Clinical Excellence (2004) Clinical Guideline 101. *Chronic Obstructive Pulmonary Disease: Management of Chronic Obstructive Pulmonary Disease in Adults in Primary and Secondary Care.* NICE: London. Available from **www.nice.org.uk/guidance/CG101.**

5.4 Reproduced with permission from the National Institute for Health and Clinical Excellence (2010) Clinical Guideline 101. *Chronic Obstructive Pulmonary Disease: Management of Chronic Obstructive Pulmonary Disease in Adults in Primary and Secondary Care (Partial Update).* NICE: London. Available from **www.nice.org.uk/guidance/CG101**

6.2, 6.3 Adapted from P. Scarborough, P. Bhatnagar, K. Wickramasinghe *et al.* (2010) *Coronary Heart Disease Statistics 2010.* British Heart Foundation: London. See **www.heartstats.org.**

6.4 Data from P. Scarborough, P. Bhatnagar, K. Wickramasinghe *et al.* (2010) *Coronary Heart Disease Statistics 2010.* British Heart Foundation: London. See **www.heartstats.org.**

6.5 Reproduced by permission of BMJ Publishing Group Ltd and the British Cardiovascular Society.

6.6 Reproduced with permission of the National Heart, Lung and Blood Institute as a part of the National Institutes of Health and the US Department of Health and Human Sciences.

6.11 Reproduced by permission of Oxford University Press and the European Society of Cardiology.

9.1 Diagram © EMIS 2011 as distributed at **http://www.patient.co.uk/diagram/Pancreas.htm**. Reproduced with permission.

10.1 Reproduced by kind permission of John Heseltine.

10.2 Reproduced by kind permission of Dr K. W. Heaton, Reader in Medicine at the University of Bristol. © Norgine Pharmaceuticals Ltd.

11.1 Reproduced from Pocock and Richards, *Human Physiology*, 3rd edn, with permission from Oxford University Press.

12.1 Reproduced from Colbert *et al.* (2009) *Anatomy & Physiology for Nurses and Health Professionals*, 1st revision, by permission of Pearson Education.

12.2a, 12.3, 12.7, 12.8 Reproduced from Saxe *et al.* (2007) *Handbook of Dermatology for Primary Care*, with permission from Oxford University Press.

12.2b, 12.5, 12.6 Reproduced from Mackie (2003) *Clinical Dermatology*, with permission from Oxford University Press.

12.4 Image courtesy of Professor Christine Moffat.

13.2 Reproduced from Fitzgerald O'Connor and Urdang (2008) *Oxford Handbook of Surgical Cross-Cover*, by permission of Oxford University Press.

14.1 Copyright © 2011, Re-used with the permission of the Health and Social Care Information Centre. All rights reserved.

15.4 Reproduced from Monaghan and Thomas, *Oxford Handbook of Clinical Examination and Practical Skills*, with permission from Oxford University Press.

15.5 Reproduced from Crouch *et al. Oxford Handbook of Emergency Nursing*, by permission from Oxford University Press.

16.1 Reproduced from Gut (2002) **50**: 480–4, with permission from BMJ Publishing Group Ltd.

16.2, 16.7, 16.8 Reproduced with permission from Health Publications Ltd.

17.2 National Institute for Health and Clinical Excellence (2010) *Delirium Diagnosis, Prevention and Management.* NICE Clinical Guideline 103. NICE: London. Reproduced with permission.

17.4 National Institute for Health and Clinical Excellence (2010) *Delirium Diagnosis, Prevention and Management.* NICE Clinical Guideline 103. NICE: London. Reproduced with permission.

18.2 Department of Health, 2008 © Crown Copyright.

18.4 Reproduced with permission from G.V. Borg (1982) Psychological basis of perceived exertion. *Medicine and Science in Sports and Exercise* **14**: 377–81.

18.5 Modified from Wood *et al.* © (2007) Management of intractable nausea and vomiting in patients at the end-of-life: 'I was feeling nauseous all of the time . . . nothing was working.' *Journal of the American Medical Association* **298** (10): 1196–207.

20.1 Adapted from Newton and Cameron (2003) *Skin Care in Wound Management.* Medical Communications UK: Holsworthy.

20.3 Reproduced from Soames and Southam, *Oral Pathology,* 4th edn, by permission of Oxford University Press.

22.1 Reproduced from Pendleton, D., Schofield, T., Tate, P., *et al. The Consultation: An Approach to Learning and Teaching* with permission from Oxford University Press.

23.4e Julián Rovagnati—Fotolia.com.

25.1 Adapted from *Rheumatology,* Third edition, Hochberg MC, Silman AJ, Smolen JS, Weinblatt ME, Weisman MH with permission from Elsevier.

25.2 Reproduced from Doherty and McCallum *Foundation Clinical Nursing Skills* by permission of Oxford University Press.

25.3 Reproduced from John D Loeser, Ronald Melzack. Pain (1999): an overview. *Lancet* **353**: 1607–09 by permission of Elsevier.

26.1 Developed by West Hertfordshire NHS Trust. Reproduced with permission.

26.2 Reproduced from *Delivering Enhanced Recovery: Helping Patients to Get Better After Surgery* (Department of Health, 2010).

26.5 Copyright National Obesity Forum.

27.3 Reproduced from Docherty and McCallum, *Foundation Clinical Nursing Skills,* by permission of Oxford University Press.

How to use this book

Adult Nursing Practice: Using Evidence in Care has been specifically designed to help you develop the knowledge and skills that you require for nursing practice. To help you in your learning this book includes:

Chapter 1: Introduction

Follow our expert advice on how to find, assess, and use evidence in adult nursing. As these skills are central to the competencies expected of registered nurses, you will find it very helpful to read Chapter 1 before you begin the book.

Part 1 and Part 2: Cross references

> All of the above examples can result in significant pain (see Chapter 25 Managing Pain ➡). For further examples of the commonest symptoms of cancer, see

Part 1 of this book will help you understand common conditions frequently seen in practice whilst Part 2 will show you how to manage fundamental health needs and symptoms. A condition such as cancer or stroke in Part 1 can cause health needs such as pain, breathlessness or immobility addressed in Part 2. Cross references in the text direct you to relevant chapters and are highlighted by these icons.

Red Flags

> fixed site. The most important alarm features or 'red flag' symptoms 🚩 include:
>
> • signs of rectal or gastrointestinal bleeding (fresh or

Flag icons indicate the warning signs of a worsening condition. These are often accompanied by urgent questions which nurses can use in the assessment and monitoring of the patient.

Nursing Assessment

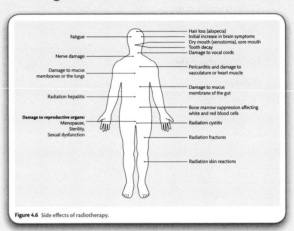

Figure 4.6 Side effects of radiotherapy.

Illustrations outline the health problems and challenges frequently caused by common diseases and health needs, highlighting issues that nurses should assess.

Theory into practice box

> THEORY INTO PRACTICE 6.1
> **Activity: identifying the patient at risk**
>
> Think about your last clinical experience or your current clinical area. Compare the patient groups against the risk factors for CHD. Identify one patient who is at risk or has had an ACS/angina episode.
>
> • How many risk factors does he or she have?
> • How are those risk factors being addressed?
> • What is your role in risk factor management?

Suggested activities take your learning further by exploring key evidence, considering central issues, or by guiding you to apply core knowledge out in your area of practice.

Case studies

CASE STUDY 6.1 *Patient with CHD*

Sarah is a 52-year-old woman who developed angina in her early 40s. She was diagnosed with familial hypercholesterolaemia (a genetic condition affecting cholesterol metabolism) in her 30s following a blood test, which established that she had a significantly raised cholesterol level. Investigation into her family history identified several close family members who had died prematurely from CHD. Sarah does not smoke and has normal blood pressure. She has a BMI of 28.5 and a waist:hip ratio of 1.0. Following the diagnosis with angina, her condition quickly progressed; she was unable to walk more than 100 yards without chest pain and could not work. She underwent a coronary angiogram in 2001, followed by angioplasty and insertion of a stent. Unfortunately, this did not relieve her angina and she went on to have coronary bypass surgery in 2002. Sarah has been free from chest pain since her surgery. She takes several medications to control her cholesterol level and exercises regularly. She has also been able to return to part-time work.

Case studies consider the patient's experience of illness as well as the problems and challenges that they face. Examples of effective evidence based interventions demonstrate the difference that high quality nursing care can make.

Glossary terms

Airway narrowing in asthma is caused by bronchospasm and intrapulmonary inflammation (Figure 2.2). Airway mucosa inflammation leads to **bronchial hyper-responsiveness (BHR)** and damages the small airways. The cellular responses within the immune system cause basement membrane thickening with **oedema** and an infiltrate of inflammatory cells (**eosinophils**, mast cells, **mononuclear cells**, e.g. macrophages and dendritic cells, and **T lymphocytes**), and subepithelial **fibrosis** develops. Bronchial epithelium fragments may shed into the lumen

---

Technical terms in anatomy, pathophysiology as well as medical and nursing treatment are highlighted in blue in the text and are explained in a glossary at the end of the book.

Take your learning further

At the end of each chapter you will be directed to important sources of evidence and references to enable you to explore the literature, clinical guidelines and key issues raised in the chapter. You will also be directed to the Online Resource Centre.

Online resource centre

To help you to develop and apply your knowledge and decision-making skills further, we have provided interactive learning resources on the following site: **www.oxfordtextbooks.co.uk/orc/bullock/**

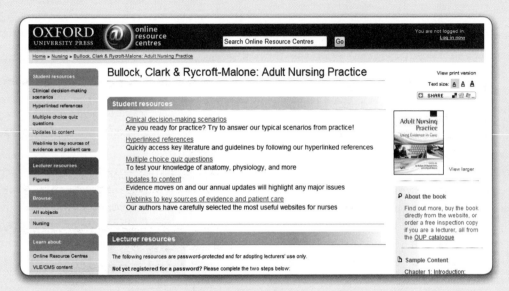

Whilst these are freely available you will need to use the following access codes:

Username: nursingpractice
Password: guidelines

E-learning resources include:

Quiz questions

To test your knowledge of anatomy, physiology and more

Clinical decision-making scenarios

Are you ready for practice? Try to answer our typical scenarios from practice

Updates to content

Evidence moves on and our annual updates will highlight any major issues

Hyperlinked references

Quickly access key literature and guidelines by clicking on our hyperlinked references

Weblinks to key sources of evidence and patient care

Our authors have carefully selected the most useful websites on their topics for nurses

Artwork from the book

For lecturers who recommend the book, illustrations are available for teaching purposes

1 *Introduction* Reframing Adult Nursing Practice

Ian Bullock, Jill Macleod Clark, and Jo Rycroft-Malone

The context of adult nursing

Healthcare delivery has been transformed over the past decades with a rapid expansion in the demand for care driven by demographic changes, technological innovation, and increasing consumer expectations.

This transformation has in turn had a profound impact on the roles of health professionals in general and nurses in particular. The number of patients with multiple pathologies and complex long-term nursing care needs has also escalated, with pressure for rapid throughput in acute hospital care settings resulting in shorter lengths of stay and greater emphasis on care in the community. To meet growing demand, boundaries between the roles of health professional have blurred, with nurses now undertaking activities previously performed by doctors, and unqualified staff undertaking activities previously performed by registered nurses. These changes are all taking place in the context of economic turbulence.

The shift of nursing to an all-graduate profession reflects the recognition that the future role of a registered nurse will carry greater responsibility and autonomy than ever before. The expectations of every student and qualified nurse must therefore also change in relation to the knowledge and skills that they need to deliver expert nursing interventions and clinical leadership. The next generation of nurses will increasingly lead and coordinate the care of a range of patients and clients, supervising and supporting unqualified or lay carers and referring patients to other health professionals when appropriate.

As one of this new generation of qualified nurses, it is important that you are able to demonstrate expertise in the fundamentals of nursing practice. You must be equipped with the knowledge and skills needed to enable you to:

- understand the common health conditions that can affect adults;
- understand the pathophysiology of these common health conditions, and the physical and psychosocial needs and problems that result from them;
- recognize your key role in managing the problems and challenges that patients face;
- ensure that your nursing interventions are evidence-based;
- demonstrate competent assessment skills, critical thinking, and problem-solving skills to make informed clinical nursing decisions in collaboration with the patient and other team members;
- adopt an enquiring and questioning approach, and be confident in accessing and interpreting evidence to inform your choice of nursing interventions.

This book has therefore been designed to support you as you take greater responsibility for clinical decisions around the nursing care of a range of patients. To be an effective, autonomous registered nurse, you must be confident in your knowledge and skills, and be equipped to decide on the best possible nursing interventions for your patients based on up-to-date research evidence. To help students and newly qualified nurses to develop these competencies, this book offers an integrated approach to incorporating research-based evidence, person-centred care, and core nursing knowledge into daily nursing decisions.

Furthermore, the material in this book reframes adult nursing care by placing the fundamental domains of nursing right at the forefront. These domains are those that are indisputably nursing responsibilities and are those that form the essence of nursing practice. They are the activities in which patients expect nursing to have expertise and for which, as a nurse, you should see yourself as the expert. Table 1.1 provides a snapshot of this reframing and shows where you can find each domain in this book.

Box 1.1

It is clear that you will be able to make informed decisions about the best nursing interventions for your patients only when you have a sound knowledge and understanding of the conditions that cause these problems. The first part of this book provides this context, with an overview of some of the commonest high-burden disease conditions that you will encounter when caring for adults in acute or community settings (Table 1.2).

Table 1.1 Key domains of nursing responsibility expertise

Key domain of nursing responsibility expertise	Chapter in which you can find each domain in this book
Managing symptoms, e.g. anxiety and agitation, breathlessness, confusion, pain	14, 15, 17, and 25, respectively
Managing continence	16
Managing end-of-life care	18
Managing hydration	19
Managing hygiene	20
Managing infection prevention	21
Managing medications	22
Managing mobility	23
Managing nutrition	24
Managing perioperative care	26
Managing skin breakdown prevention	27
Managing wounds	28

Table 1.2 Commonly encountered adult health conditions

Commonly encountered adult health conditions	Chapter in which you can find each condition in this book
Understanding asthma	2
Understanding bone conditions	3
Understanding cancers	4
Understanding chronic obstructive pulmonary disorder	5
Understanding coronary heart disease	6
Understanding dementia	7
Understanding depression	8
Understanding diabetes	9
Understanding functional bowel disorders	10
Understanding renal disorders	11
Understanding skin conditions	12
Understanding stroke	13

The material presented in these chapters will help you to develop a sound understanding of the underlying pathophysiology of each condition and the impact it may have on the subsequent development of the health problems outlined in Table 1.1, which all require expert nursing management. Particular attention is given to the principles of evidence-based practice and the knowledge, skills, and tools that will be required by you, as a contemporary nurse, to deliver high-quality, evidence-based, patient-centred care. Throughout each chapter, you are encouraged to recognize clinical signs and to plan appropriate nursing interventions. You are also signposted to the relevant evidence that will inform your choice of interventions. By reframing nursing practice in this way, the integrated conceptual approach to patient care and decision-making skills demonstrated in these chapters can be applied by you to other disease areas not covered by this book. In essence, the book provides a framework for nursing care that translates into any context.

Knowing where to find up-to-date evidence is critical in becoming an active 'consumer' of contemporary evidence.

This evidence for practice is constantly developing. For example, it is possible that an assessment tool or treatment for preventing skin breakdown may change within 6 months of completing a university module on this topic. To remain up to date, you need the following skills and tools.

1. Be able to recognize what clinical information you need—'Do I have the right facts to assess skin vulnerability?'

2. Know where you can find the information needed—'Where should I look for the evidence about skin integrity?'

3. Know how this information is used in the process of care—'How do I go about integrating this knowledge into assessment and interventions for patients with potential skin breakdown?'

4. Understand how this information can be used to measure the effectiveness of care—'How do I assess the impact of the intervention?'

The following section of this chapter provides an overview of evidence-based nursing practice, suggests ways in which you can develop your skills, and guides you through the process of using this approach in day-to-day practice.

Why evidence-based nursing interventions are important

Advances in technology and scientific knowledge have resulted in an exponential increase in consumer participation in, and expectations of, healthcare, as well as an increase in the sources of evidence to inform best practice. This evidence is now largely readily available at the click of a button. At the same time, the health service is under pressure to cope with a growing older population with diverse healthcare needs, the burden of long-term illnesses, and increasing survival rates in critical illness. There have also been a number of high-profile public inquiries regarding the provision of health service (for example, children's heart surgery at Bristol Royal Infirmary between 1984 and 1995, the murder of several older patients by Dr Harold Shipman in 2000, the outbreak of *E. coli* in South Wales in 2005, and the neglect of patients at Mid Stafford-shire Foundation Trust Hospital between 2005 and 2009) that have raised considerable concerns about the quality and safety of patient care and service delivery.

As a nurse, your priority will always be to optimize the patient experience and, where possible, to improve patient outcomes. Traditionally, nursing practice was apprenticeship-based, with care interventions shaped from historical routine and ritual, with a natural reticence to question. Within the contemporary health service context, it is no longer good enough to claim that we know what we are doing because it is the way in which we have always done it. The climate is such that we need to be able to justify not only what we are doing, but also how and why we are doing it. Doing the right thing for patients at the right time is the essence of evidence-based practice.

Trinder and Reynolds (2000) summarized four main reasons why evidence-based practice has emerged strongly across all health disciplines:

1. **Research–practice gap:** a slow and limited use of research in practice, which is highly dependent on the knowledge, skills, and experience of the practitioner, including their biases and arbitrary preferences

2. **Poor quality of research:** a lot of published research can be methodologically weak and/or not applicable to clinical settings

3. **Information overload:** a vast and ever-growing body of research in which it is difficult to distinguish between that which is valid and reliable, and that which is not

4. **Practice is not evidence-based:** practitioners continue to use harmful and ineffective interventions, and there is a slow and often limited uptake of interventions that are known to be useful and effective

Political and professional drivers promote evidence-based practice as the antidote to these problems and as an idea for which the 'time has come'. However, evidence-based practice is not without its critics, including those who state that it is a way of rationalizing healthcare and controlling professionals (see Rycroft-Malone, 2006, for a detailed discussion). Aside from such debates, the most compelling case for evidence-based nursing interventions comes from the unarguable need to take moral and ethical responsibility to practise using the best possible evidence to do more good than harm, and to ensure that scarce resources are used wisely. Evidence-based nursing is not an optional extra. It should be embedded in every nurse's day-to-day practice.

What is evidence-based practice?

There are debates about what evidence-based practice is and therefore the literature is littered with definitions, which often reflect different professional positions. An early and simple definition came from some of the proponents of evidence-based medicine, who described it as the integration of best research evidence within clinical expertise and patient values to facilitate clinical decision-making (Sackett *et al.*, 1996, 2000):

> the conscientious, explicit and judicious use of current best evidence in making decisions about the care of the individual patient. It means integrating individual clinical expertise with the best available external clinical evidence from systematic research.

There are elements of this definition that are worth highlighting, including that decision-making based on evidence needs to be purposeful (*conscientious*), applied in a way that is obvious (*explicit*), and thoughtful (*judicious*); this is relevant to individual patients and includes a mix of experience with research. Since this early definition, the conception and description of evidence-based practice has broadened in scope.

Stetler (1998) opens up the debate on what constitutes evidence for evidence-based practice:

> de-emphasizes ritual, isolated, and unsystematic clinical experiences, ungrounded opinions, and tradition as a basis for nursing practices, and stresses instead the use of research findings and, as appropriate, quality improvement data, the consensus of recognized experts, and affirmed experience to substantiate practice.

Here, the role of other types of evidence, in addition to research, is highlighted. This broader conceptualization of evidence is common to a number of definitions and reflects a recognition that, in the reality of the practice

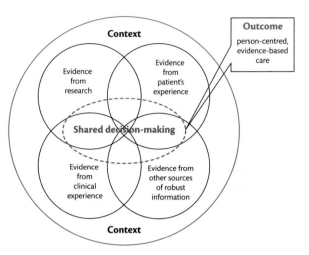

Figure 1.1   A broad conceptualization of evidence-based practice with shared decision-making. Adapted from Rycroft-Malone *et al.* (2004).

setting, both propositional (e.g. research, local data) and non-propositional (e.g. clinical experience, patient experience) are melded together to deliver patient care and to make decisions. For example:

> the process of shared decision making between practitioner, patient and others significant to them based on research evidence, the patient's experiences and preferences, clinical expertise or know how, and other available robust sources of information … which occurs in, and may be influenced by factors in the clinical context. (Rycroft-Malone *et al.*, 2004)

This last definition also brings into play the influence that the context of practice can have on the delivery of evidence-based practice (see Figure 1.1).

In summary, there are a number of features of these definitions that are worth drawing together to illuminate what evidence-based practice is, and how we are using the term within this book.

The delivery of evidence-based nursing interventions involves the following.

- It is a *decision-making process* in which you should engage on an ongoing basis, which is shared with patients and with other members of the multidisciplinary team as appropriate. Evidence-based practice is not a one-off event, but a problem-solving approach to nursing practice and the delivery of patient care.

- It is based on *evidence*, including research evidence, in combination with patients' experiences and preferences, clinical know-how, and other locally collected, robust information. Where available, you should be drawing on robust, good-quality research evidence to inform nursing interventions. The findings from research have to be *particularized* to each patient's situation, which involves wider skills and knowledge.

- Decision-making takes place in a wider *context* of care, which may influence how decisions are made, such as management of available resources. For example, the availability of particular types of pressure-relieving equipment (see Chapter 27 →) may influence the nursing intervention you decide to give to patients at risk of developing pressure ulcers.

What is evidence?

As the previous definitions of evidence-based practice all highlight, research is an important type of evidence that should be informing nursing practice. However, how can you tell which types of research evidence are better than others? There are two answers to this question. The first involves understanding that particular types of research are regarded (by some) as stronger than others, and the second requires you to be able to make a judgement about the quality of the research you are considering. To help you to address these issues, the authors of each chapter in this book have provided an indication of the strength of the evidence underpinning particular nursing interventions and areas of practice.

There are a number of hierarchies of evidence provided in the literature, but they all generally include the following levels, from strongest to weakest.

Level 1: Evidence from a systematic review or meta-analysis of all relevant randomized controlled trials

Level 2: Evidence obtained from well-designed randomized controlled trials

Level 3: Evidence obtained from well-designed controlled trials without randomization

Level 4: Evidence from well-designed case-control and cohort studies

Level 5: Evidence from systematic reviews of descriptive and qualitative studies

Level 6: Evidence from single descriptive or qualitative study

Level 7: Evidence from the opinion of authorities and/or reports of expert committees (e.g. consensus statements)

(Adapted from Guyatt and Rennie, 2002; Polit and Beck, 2008)

There is much debate in the literature about the relevance of evidence hierarchies. It is important to remember that, when undertaking research, the design of the study will be driven by the research question ('horses for courses'). Therefore a question about how effective a nursing intervention is would be appropriately answered by a randomized controlled trial because a trial is an appropriate research design for comparing whether intervention A is better than intervention B. Questions about how a patient experiences a nursing intervention would be better addressed using a qualitative or mixed method study. Therefore, whilst evidence hierarchies provide a level of trust, they do not tell us about the quality of the research and which types of research are more relevant to particular problems. To date, there are few good-quality randomized trials of nursing interventions, and this is fertile ground for future research. Furthermore, we cannot always assume that the findings from a piece of research will necessarily be relevant or applicable to all patients. This is where your critical thinking, reflection, and practical knowledge come into play.

Critical appraisal

One way in which to assess the quality of research, including single studies, systematic reviews, and clinical guidelines, is through critical appraisal. The process of critical appraisal involves addressing three key questions.

1. **Are the results of the study (or review) valid**? Are the findings as close to the truth as possible? Did the researchers use the appropriate study design for the question? Was it rigorously carried out? Can the findings be generalized?

2. **Are the results/findings reliable?** Was the study design executed properly? Were the appropriate numbers of participants involved in the research? Are the findings repeatable?

3. **Are the results applicable?** Are the participants in the research similar to the patients to whom care is being delivered? Are the benefits greater than the risk? Is it feasible to implement the intervention?

The critical appraisal process enables an assessment to be made about the quality of research, and facilitates making a judgement about its relevance to practice change. Usually, the findings from a single study are unlikely, on their own, to change a course of practice about a clinical issue. It takes time for research to accumulate to provide clear direction and recommendations for practice. Being able to appraise research critically, whilst a useful skill for a nurse to possess, does not mean that research will be used in practice on a routine basis.

See the Critical Appraisal Skills Programme (CASP) (full website details given in resources section) for more information, resources, and tools to assist in the critical appraisal process.

Ways of knowing

Research is one source of evidence by which nurses are informed in their practice, Carper (1978) suggests that there are four ways of knowing that form the evidence base upon which nurses should practise (see Box 1.2).

Box 1.2 Four ways of knowing that form the evidence base

Empirical knowledge: knowledge found in textbooks and journal papers that is based on research, and can be proved

Aesthetic knowledge: awareness of the immediate situation, subjective, unique, taking the whole situation into account

Personal knowledge: knowledge and attitudes derived from personal self-understanding and empathy, including imagining one's self in the patient's position

Ethical knowledge: attitudes and knowledge derived from an ethical framework, including an awareness of moral questions and choices

---

THEORY INTO PRACTICE 1.2
Reflection on the use of knowledge and information

Reflect on the way you practise—what sort of information/knowledge do you use when you are making decisions about patient care? What do you do if you are not sure about a particular issue? Have you noticed what sort of information/knowledge other nurses and other professionals, such as doctors, physiotherapists, and occupational therapists, have? If it isn't obvious, ask them.

Information to inform practice and decision-making

Drawing on the findings from single studies is not usually a good basis for decision-making. The best sources of information for practice are systematic reviews (reviews of primary single studies that have been appraised and synthesized) and clinical practice guidelines ('systematically developed statements to assist practitioners and patient decisions about appropriate health care for specific circumstances': Field and Lohr, 1990: 38).

Systematic reviews

There are a number of organizations that facilitate the development and dissemination of systematic reviews.

A well-known publically funded centre for the development and dissemination of systematic reviews is the Cochrane Collaboration: **http://www.cochrane.org/**. The Cochrane Collaboration, established in 1993, is an international network of people helping healthcare providers, policymakers, patients, and their advocates and carers, to make well-informed decisions about human healthcare by preparing, updating, and promoting the accessibility of Cochrane Reviews; over 4,500 have so far been published online in The Cochrane Library. This is a reliable source of information; however, often the findings from the published reviews do not provide clear advice about what to do in practice.

The Joanna Briggs Institute **http://www.joannabriggs.edu.au/**, an international collaboration established in 1996, also conducts and publishes evidence reviews. In contrast to the Cochrane Library, its focus is on providing evidence of direct relevance to practice. Specifically, it aims to:

- develop methods to appraise and synthesize evidence, conducting systematic reviews and analyses of the research literature (evidence translation);
- disseminate information in diverse formats to inform health systems, health professionals, and consumers (evidence transfer);
- facilitate the effective implementation of evidence and the evaluation of its impact on healthcare practice (evidence utilization);
- contribute to clinical cost-effective healthcare through the promotion of evidence-based healthcare practice (evidence utilization).

Some examples of subjects of published reviews include:

- bleeding risks of femoral arterial closure devices compared to compression methods—a systematic review;
- measurement accuracy of non-invasively obtained central systolic blood pressure and central blood pressure—a systematic review;
- impact of rapid infusion rituximab on cancer patients' safety—a systematic review;
- the relationship between error and harm in primary healthcare—a systematic review;
- lateral violence in professional nursing—a comprehensive systematic review;
- a systematic review and meta-analysis on the preventive measures to reduce the incidence of falls among the elderly;
- the effects of life review on the emotional and spiritual well-being of older people—a systematic review.

These reviews can be found online at **http://www.joannabriggs.edu.au/Access%20Evidence/Systematic%20Review%20Registered%20Titles**

A number of nursing journals also publish systematic reviews. These include the following:

- *Worldviews on Evidence-Based Nursing* **http://onlinelibrary.wiley.com/journal/10.1111/%28ISSN%291741-6787**
- *Journal of Advanced Nursing* **http://onlinelibrary.wiley.com/journal/10.1111/%28ISSN%291365-2648**

> **Box 1.3 Tip for recognizing quality evidence**
>
> Being published by a trusted organization or journal does not necessarily mean that a systematic review is of high quality. Critical appraisal of systematic reviews is recommended, see: **http://www.sph.nhs.uk/what-we-do/public-health-workforce/resources/critical-appraisals-skills-programme**

- *International Journal of Nursing Studies* **http://www.elsevier.com/wps/find/journaldescription.cws_home/266/description#description**

Clinical practice guidelines and quality standards

The National Institute for Health and Clinical Excellence (NICE), the national guideline and quality standards development body for England and Wales, defines guidance as being:

- designed to promote good health and to prevent ill-health;
- produced by the people affected by our work, including health and social care professionals, patients, and the public;
- based on the best evidence;
- transparent in its development, consistent, reliable, and based on a rigorous development process;
- good value for money, weighing up the cost and benefits of treatments;
- internationally recognized for its excellence. **http://guidance.nice.org.uk/** (accessed 17 April 2011).

NICE has developed hundreds of guidelines about a wide range of health issues. Topics covered by its guidance range from helping people to stop smoking and encouraging them to be more physically active through to the treatment of cancer, diabetes, musculoskeletal conditions, mental health problems, and the assessment and management of pressure ulcers. Many topics that this book covers have associated NICE clinical guidelines; these should be regarded as trusted sources of information.

Box 1.4 Examples of some recommendations from the NICE clinical guideline on pressure ulcer management

Recommendation for holistic assessment

Patients with pressure ulcers should receive an initial and ongoing holistic assessment. Both intrinsic and extrinsic factors have been identified as important factors for assessment. This assessment should include the following.

- Health status
  - Acute, chronic, and terminal illness
  - Comorbidity, e.g. diabetes and malnutrition
- Mobility status
- Posture (pelvic obliquity and posterior pelvic tilt)
- Sensory impairment
- Level of consciousness
- Systemic signs of infection
- Nutritional status
- Previous pressure damage
- Pain status
- Psychological factors
- Social factors
- Continence status
- Medication

- Cognitive status
- Blood flow

Recommendations for ulcer assessment

Patients with pressure ulcers should receive an initial and ongoing pressure ulcer assessment. Ulcer assessment should include the following.

- Cause of ulcer
- Site/location
- Dimensions of ulcer
- Stage or grade
- Exudate amount and type
- Local signs of infection
- Pain
- Wound appearance
- Surrounding skin
- Undermining/tracking (sinus or fistula)
- Odour

This should be supported by photography and/or tracings (calibrated with a ruler).
**http://www.nice.org.uk/nicemedia/
live/10972/29885/29885.pdf**

NICE commissions the development of guidelines, and these are devised by centres largely run by the professional colleges. The largest of these is hosted by the Royal College of Physicians, the National Clinical Guideline Centre (NCGC), and is a governance partnership between four Royal Colleges (RCGP—general practitioners, RCN—nursing, RCP—physicians, and RCS—surgeons). The NCGC has produced over 75 national clinical guidelines targeted at acute and chronic conditions, mostly for adult care. A full list of these can be found online at **http://www.ncgc.ac.uk/**

The National Collaborating Centres for Cancer (NCC-CC), Mental Health (NCC-MH), and Women's and Children's Health (NCC-WCH) tend to produce targeted specialist clinical guidelines. Full lists for all of these can be found online at **http://www.ncgc.ac.uk/**

This publically funded work programme was recently critically appraised in the *Annals of Internal Medicine*, with the leading editorial stating that these were 'trustworthy' clinical guidelines: **http://www.annals.org/content/154/11/774.full?etoc**

Criteria used are those developed by the Institute of Medicine and can be found online at **http://iom.edu/Reports/2011/Clinical-Practice-Guidelines-We-Can-Trust.aspx**

This assumption was reached in the editorial because it was noted that the guidelines follow high-quality assurance processes and have a real contribution to make in improving both patient outcomes and experience. In addition, this national work programme is one of only few that incorporate cost-effectiveness modelling, which establishes 'best spend' principles for care interventions when planning the delivery of healthcare across large populations.

Methods of development are also published and can be found in Hill *et al.* (2011).

NICE also develops quality standards that are associated with its published guidance and accredited evidence sources in NHS evidence. Standards are defined as 'a set of

Box 1.5 Recommendations for pressure-relieving support surfaces

Decisions about choice of pressure-relieving support surfaces for patients with pressure ulcers should be made by registered healthcare professionals.

Initial choice and subsequent decisions, following reassessments related to the provision of pressure-relieving support surfaces for patients with pressure ulcers, should be based on the following.

- Ulcer assessment (severity)
- Level of risk: from holistic assessment
- Location and cause of the pressure ulcer
- General skin assessment
- General health status
- Acceptability and comfort for the patient
- Lifestyle of the patient
- Ability of the patient to reposition self
- Availability of carer/health professional to reposition the patient
- Cost consideration

specific, concise statements that act as markers of high-quality, cost-effective patient care, covering the treatment and prevention of different diseases and conditions'. They are developed independently by NICE, in collaboration with the NHS and social care professionals, their partners, and service users, and address three dimensions of quality: clinical effectiveness; patient safety; and patient experience. Quality standards are designed to help healthcare professionals to make decisions about care based on the latest evidence and best practice.

The Scottish Intercollegiate Guidelines Network (SIGN) (funded by Healthcare Improvement Scotland) also develops and publishes guidelines: http://www.sign.ac.uk/guidelines/index.html. Like NICE, SIGN guidelines are based on a systematic review of the evidence, undertaken by guideline development group members.

Around the world, there are other guideline development and dissemination centres, including:

- The Agency for Healthcare Quality (AHRQ) in the US: http://www.ahrq.gov/
- The National Institute for Clinical Studies (NICS) in Australia: http://www.nhmrc.gov.au/nics/index.htm

- The Registered Nurses Association of Ontario (RNAO) in Canada, which develops guidelines specifically for issues of relevance to nursing practice, and is also a good source for information for implementation issues: http://ww.rnao.org/Page.asp?PageID=861&SiteNodeID=133

THEORY INTO PRACTICE 1.3
Tip when searching for evidence

Clinical guidelines and quality standards that come from national organizations such as the National Institute for Health and Clinical Excellence (NICE) and Scottish Intercollegiate Guidelines Network (SIGN) should be of high quality. However, not all guidelines that are available to use in practice meet such high standards of development. Therefore critical appraisal of clinical guidelines is recommended. There are a number of tools to assist you in this process. A robustly developed, tried, and evaluated tool is AGREE: **http://www.agreetrust.org/**

This tool considers six areas of the guideline development process: 1) scope and purpose; 2) stakeholder involvement; 3) rigour of development; 4) clarity and presentation; 5) applicability; and 6) editorial independence.

NHS Evidence

NHS Evidence **http://www.evidence.nhs.uk/default.aspx** allows everyone working in health and social care to access a wide range of health information to help them to deliver quality patient care. NHS Evidence:

- has a fast, free, and easy-to-use search to help users search for the information they want;
- ranks search results from credible medical sources according to relevance and quality;
- allows users to personalize a search and register to receive the latest health information.

NHS Evidence is for anyone (e.g. doctors, nurses, allied health professionals, researchers) in health and social care who takes decisions about treatments or the use of resources.

Within NHS Evidence there is also a resource called QIPP (Quality, Innovation, Productivity, and Prevention), which is a collection of evidence, including clinical pathways to support quality and productivity at a local level. A wide range of topics is covered in this database, including many of the topics that are part of this book, such as renal care, end-of-life care, medicines management, cancer care, and diabetes management.

> THEORY INTO PRACTICE 1.4
> **Appraising a practice guideline**
>
> Use the topics covered in this book as a guide to search some of the guideline development organizations' libraries of guidelines. Choose one guideline that is relevant to your clinical practice and undertake an appraisal of it using the AGREE tool: **http://www.agreetrust.org/**

Using evidence in practice and how to use this book

In the reality of the practice context, there are likely to be many circumstances in which you come across practice that is not based on best evidence. There is a growing body of literature identifying some of the challenges that nurses face in routinely using evidence in practice. Some key issues that, as a nurse, you might face and find challenging include the following.

- Access to computers and to online information may not always be possible or readily available.
- The resources you need (e.g. appropriate dressings or equipment) to deliver interventions based on best evidence may not always be available.
- There may be some reluctance amongst other colleagues to practise in an evidence-based way.
- You see other colleagues practising in a way that you know is not in line with current evidence.
- For some issues that you face on a day-to-day basis, there may be an absence of good-quality research evidence for nursing interventions.

If you find yourself in situations in which you are unsure what to do, or do not know where to look for evidence, you should consult with clinical experts such as clinical nurse specialists or consultant nurses, and/or clinical/link tutors. Questions may arise from practice for which university-linked colleagues can help you to develop an appropriate approach to find answers. Many questions may have already been addressed and it will be a case of using appropriate strategies to seek existing systematic reviews or clinical guidelines. In other cases, there may be an absence of reviews or guidelines, in which instance a review may need to be conducted to answer the clinical question.

Registered nurses are taking more responsibility and are more autonomous than ever before. This book can help you to take greater responsibility for clinical decisions about a range of nursing interventions for a range of patients. Critically, these decisions should be informed by up-to-date evidence. The authors of the chapters in this book are encouraging you to take an enquiring and evidence-based approach in the delivery of care to patients. By adopting this approach, you will become an effective, autonomous, and confident nurse ready to play a pivotal role in the health service of the future.

Resources

Critical appraisal
Critical Appraisal Skills Programme (CASP) **http://www.phru.nhs.uk/casp/casp.htm** and **http://www.sph.nhs.uk/what-we-do/public-health-workforce/resources/critical-appraisals-skills-programme**

Databases of systematic reviews
Cochrane Collaboration **http://www.cochrane.org/**
Joanna Briggs Institute **http://www.joannabriggs.edu.au/**

Databases of clinical guidelines
http://guidance.nice.org.uk/
http://www.sign.ac.uk/guidelines/index.html
http://www.ahrq.gov/
http://www.rnao.org/Page.asp?PageID=861&SiteNodeID=133

Conclusion

This chapter sets the context for the rest of this powerful book by indicating how you, as a nurse 'making a difference', can critically utilize reliable sources of evidence to shape your clinical decision-making and practice. As editors, we want you to *think evidence* every time you walk into any care setting. In utilizing reliable sources, as a modern practitioner, you can benefit from high-quality evidence synthesis in promoting high-quality care, underpinned by the care and compassion that has characterized the nursing profession. We are genuinely excited at the significant contribution that nursing has made to improving patient experience and patient outcomes, but the definition of any profession is to continue to add to the knowledge that determines contemporary practice. This challenge is significant, but we believe that this book will provide the roadmap for how to approach the complexity of care in different settings and encourage you to be at the cutting edge of knowledge utilization.

Together, we *can* make a lasting difference.

Online Resource Centre

 To help you to develop and apply your knowledge and decision-making skills further, we have provided interactive learning resources online at **www.oxfordtextbooks.co.uk/orc/bullock**

Whilst these are freely available, you will need to use the access codes at the start of this book.

References

Carper, B.A. (1978) Fundamental patterns of knowing in nursing. *Advances in Nursing Science* **1**(1): 13–23.

Field, J., Lohr, K.N. (1992) *Guidelines for Clinical Practice: From Development to Use*. National Academy Press: Washington.

Guyatt, G., Rennie, D. (2002) *Users' Guide to the Medical Literature*. American Medical Association: Chicago, IL.

Hill, J., Bullock, I., Alderson, P. (2011) A summary of the methods that the National Clinical Guideline Centre uses to produce clinical guidelines for the National Institute for Health and Clinical Excellence. *Annals of Internal Medicine* **154**(11): 752–7.

Polit, D.F., Beck, C.T. (2008) *Nursing Research: Generating and Accessing Evidence for Nursing Practice*, 8th edn. Lippincott, Williams and Wilkins: London.

Rycroft-Malone, J. (2006) The politics of evidence-based practice: legacies and current challenges. *Journal of Research in Nursing* **8**: 15–24.

Rycroft-Malone, J., Seers, K., Titchen, A., *et al.* (2004) What counts as evidence in evidence-based practice. *Journal of Advanced Nursing* **47**(1): 81–90.

Sackett, D.L., Rosenberg, W.M.C., Gray, J.A.M., *et al.* (1996) Evidence-based medicine: what it is and what it isn't (editorial). *British Medical Journal* **312**: 71–2.

Sackett, D.L., Straus, S.E., Richardson, W.S., *et al.* (2000) *Evidence-Based Medicine: How to Practise and Teach EBM*. Churchill Livingstone: London.

Trinder, L., Reynolds, S. (2000) *Evidence-Based Practice: A Critical Appraisal*. Blackwell Science: Oxford.

PART 1
Understanding Common Health Conditions

Using evidence in reframing adult nursing practice

There are 12 chapters in this first part of the book, and they are primarily designed to develop your understanding of some of the commonest health conditions that you will encounter whilst caring for adult patients. It is not designed to be exhaustive, but to prioritize common presentations in an ageing population, resulting in significant burden-of-disease areas.

Each chapter provides an overview of the epidemiology, prevalence, underlying pathophysiological processes, and symptom presentation of the condition. The book is different from traditional texts for undergraduate nursing, as it promotes a different way of thinking about common core conditions, in particular by highlighting the links between pathophysiological processes, symptoms, and the associated health challenges that arise as a result of the condition (e.g. pain, breathlessness, reduced mobility). These health needs provide a definitive focus for nursing care and nursing intervention, highlighting key areas of your responsibility as a nurse and the unique contribution you make to the multidisciplinary healthcare team. In each chapter, you will find guidance on good clinical assessment that should enable you to determine the most appropriate evidence-based nursing interventions for care planning. Chapter authors have emphasized the nursing responsibility to recognize and assess presenting symptoms, as well as the health challenges experienced by the patient. Authors then signpost you to 'trustworthy' sources of evidence upon which to individualize patient care.

Chapter authors specifically guide you to adopt this different way of thinking to traditional medical models of care or systems-based texts, and have illustrated how *every nurse can be an evidence-based practitioner*, a critical consumer of research, optimizing patient experience and patient outcomes.

Symptoms and problems experienced by patients can often reach across any number of conditions. An example is pain, which will be a common problem for patients with cancer, cardiovascular disease, renal disease, functional bowel disorder, and skin conditions. In chapters in Part 1, you will find cross-references to the relevant chapter in Part 2 of the book, which provides comprehensive information to guide your nursing management of a particular symptom or health need such as 'managing pain'. These cross-references are indicated by, for example, (see **Chapter 27** ➡).

Studying these chapters will equip you with a robust understanding of the causes of these common conditions. Once equipped with this knowledge, you will be confident in your ability to reframe your nursing care priorities. This confidence emerges through good clinical assessment and history-taking skills, symptom recognition, and an ability to understand how to retrieve and use evidence. Part 1 purposefully chooses not to cover every disease, but, by exploring the commonest conditions seen in practice, it illustrates how to approach other diseases and apply this conceptual approach to effective nursing care.

2 *Understanding* **Asthma**

Linda Pearce and Samantha Prigmore

Introduction

The aim of this chapter is to provide nurses with the knowledge to be able to assess, manage, and care for people with asthma in an evidence-based and person-centred way. The chapter will provide a comprehensive overview of the causes, risk factors, and impact of asthma, before exploring best practice to deliver care, as well as to prevent or minimize further ill-health. Nursing assessments and priorities are highlighted throughout, and the nursing management of the symptoms and common health problems associated with asthma can be found in **Chapters 15 and 22**, respectively ➡.

Understanding asthma

Definition

In the absence of a standardized definition of asthma, it is accurately described as:

> Airway inflammation and hyper-responsiveness characterised by widespread reversible narrowing of the airways, which varies either spontaneously or in response to treatment. (British Thoracic Society/Scottish Intercollegiate Guidelines Network, 2009)

The clinician diagnosis of asthma is based on symptoms, patient history, lung function testing (including peak expiratory flow rate diary), and the demonstration of an efficacious response to a trial of inhaled therapy.

Prevalence and epidemiology

An estimated 5.4 million people in the UK are receiving treatment for asthma (Lung and Asthma Information Agency, 2006). In 2006–07, there were 67,077 hospital admissions for asthma in England, over 40% of which were for children under the age of 15 (Asthma UK, 2010). Asthma is estimated to cost the NHS £1 billion per year. With one in five households affected, asthma accounts for at least 12.7 million workdays lost each year (Asthma UK, 2005). In 2008, there were 1,071 deaths in England and Wales due to asthma (Office for National Statistics, 2009).

Causes

Atopy is a genetically based condition in which individuals have a tendency to hypersensitivity in their reaction to allergens and other triggers. The reaction is usually immediate and localized, and manifests in diseases such as asthma, hay fever, and contact dermatitis. Genetic studies (Holloway *et al.*, 2010) investigating atopy and asthma have shown linkages to many chromosomal locations indicating genetic heterogeneity (having different characteristics and qualities). There is genetic control over the ability to produce significant quantities of **immunoglobulin E (IgE)**, a blood plasma protein that activates allergic reactions by acting as an antibody, when exposed to environmental allergens. In individuals with atopy, environmental triggers such as house dust mites and pollens cause uncontrolled asthma. A family history of atopy is one of the strongest predictors that a child may develop asthma (particularly maternal history). Coexistent atopy and illnesses such as rhinitis and eczema increase the age-independent risk of developing asthma. Abnormal lung function and increased airway hyperresponsiveness in childhood are both associated with asthma in later life. Respiratory viral infections also have a causative link with the development of non-allergic asthma. Occupational asthma can develop where individuals are exposed to a range of inorganic and organic substances by reason of their employment. Examples of the commonest substances are listed in Table 2.1, and more information can be found online at **http://www.hse.gov.uk/asthma/substances.htm**

The pathophysiology of asthma

To understand asthma, it is helpful if you are already familiar with the normal anatomy and physiology of the respiratory system. Whilst the anatomy of the lower respiratory tract is illustrated in Figure 2.1 as a helpful reminder, we would encourage you to consult a good textbook should you need more detail.

Airway narrowing in asthma is caused by bronchospasm and intrapulmonary inflammation (Figure 2.2). Airway mucosa inflammation leads to **bronchial hyperresponsiveness (BHR)** and damages the small airways. The cellular responses within the immune system cause basement membrane thickening with **oedema** and an infiltrate of inflammatory cells (**eosinophils**, **mast cells**, **mononuclear cells**, e.g. macrophages and dendritic cells, and **T lymphocytes**), and subepithelial **fibrosis** develops. Bronchial epithelium fragments may shed into the lumen of the airway. This increases the likelihood of irreversible hypoxia, which is what may lead to asthma deaths, with mucus consisting of cellular debris (fibrin, epithelial fragments, eosinophils) and extravascular exudates causing airway blockage. Alterations to circadian rhythms may impact on airway calibre (such as reduced circulating adrenaline levels at night in people with asthma) and effectively reduce the individual's natural defence mechanisms. This may result in increased night and morning symptoms.

Undiagnosed, untreated, or inadequately treated, chronic asthma leads to **hypertrophy** of the underlying muscles within the bronchial wall and thickening of the basement membrane, causing airway narrowing that may become irreversible. The extent of these changes seen in asthma reflects the severity of the BHR. There is no difference between the anatomical changes seen in allergic and non-allergic asthma.

Where asthma in individuals is provoked through exposure to an allergen, mast cells in the airway mucosa **degranulate**, producing release of histamine and inflammatory mediators. This leads to **bronchoconstriction**, **vasodilatation**, oedema, and excessive mucus secretion. The acute episode, or '**early response**', usually settles within 1–3 hours, but a '**late response**' may follow with further airway narrowing that may not resolve for some time.

Table 2.1 Occupational causes of asthma

Type of occupation and common substances encountered	Possible exposure to known asthma-inducing agents?
Spray painting, foam moulding using adhesives, surface coatings	Isocyanates, other chemicals
Industrial baking, farm work, and grain transport	Dust from flour and grain
Carpentry, joinery, and sawmilling	Wood dust, particularly from hardwood dusts and western red cedar
Electronics industry— soldering fumes; also in glues and some floor cleaners	Colophony
Any job involving latex, e.g. in which latex-based gloves are worn or latex-based materials are used, such as in car manufacture	Dust from latex rubber
Laboratory work, farm work, work with shellfish	Dust from insects and animals, and from products containing them

This response is thought to be caused by an accumulation of inflammatory cells (mostly eosinophils), which causes further damage to the epithelium and may lead to the release of other inflammatory mediators. The latter can lead to proliferation of fibroblasts; the end result of fibroblast activity is the elaboration of collagens and their deposition below the basement membrane.

Mortality and morbidity

Mortality

Most patient deaths from asthma occur before admission to hospital. The majority of people who die from asthma have severe disease, with the evidence indicating that behavioural and adverse psychosocial factors

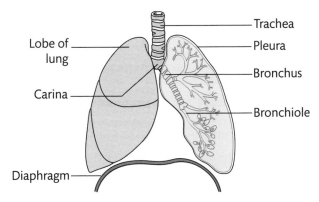

Figure 2.1 Lower respiratory tract.

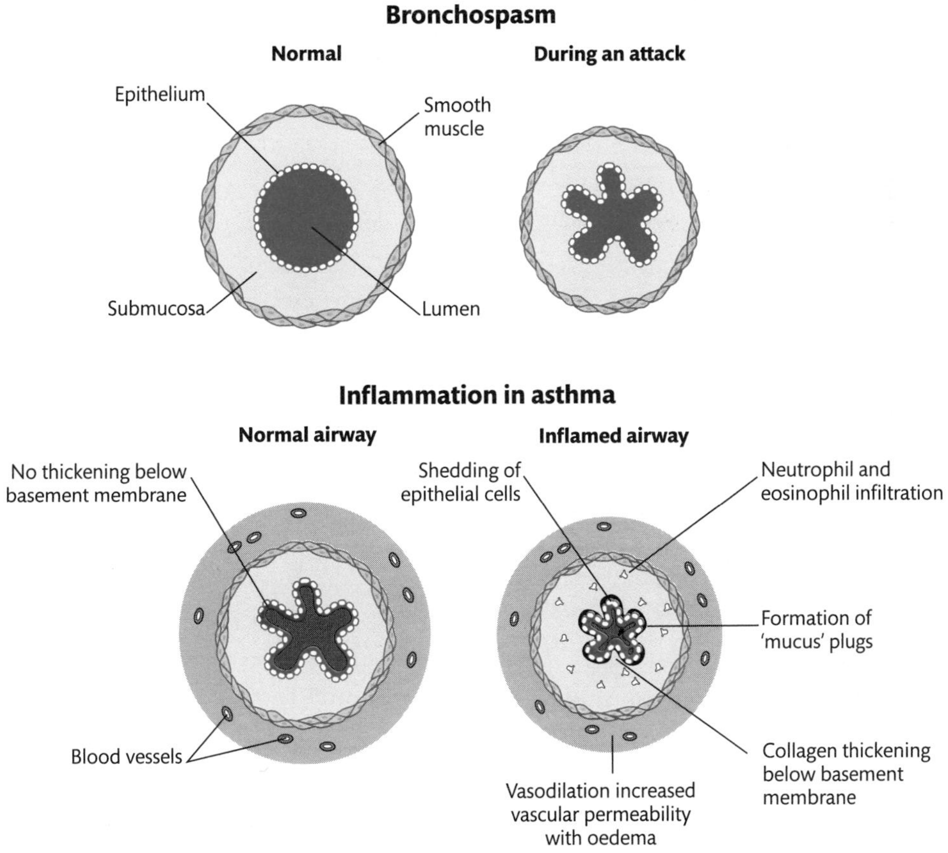

Figure 2.2 Cross-section of the bronchus/bronchioles demonstrating bronchospasm and inflammation in asthma.

increase risk of death (Smith *et al.*, 2005). A minority of asthma deaths occur in those with mild or moderate disease. Enquires have identified a peak of asthma-related deaths in young people occurring in July and August, and in older people during December and January (Harrison *et al.*, 2005).

Studies indicate that these preventable elements are found in most deaths:

- inadequate treatment;
- inadequate objective monitoring;
- poor follow-up review;
- underuse of written management plans;
- heavy reliance on **bronchodilator** therapy;
- failure to recognize the symptoms associated with deteriorating asthma;
- inappropriate prescriptions of ß-blockers or heavy sedation.

(Harrison *et al.*, 2005)

Morbidity

Highest in the 16–24 age group, morbidity decreases in older people, but with a noticeable peak in the 55–64 age group. Some individuals live with symptoms of uncontrolled asthma that may impact on their daily activity. Such restriction of activity is usually as a result of inadequate treatment (Office for National Statistics, 2009).

Assessment of the patient

Nursing clinical assessment

Assessment of the disease is strongly founded on clinical history because clinical examination is often normal between asthma episodes, with history usually eliminating other causes, as described below. Key indicators are:

- a history of atopic disorder (e.g. asthma, rhinitis, hay fever, eczema), either in the patient or the patient's family;
- a history of symptoms on exposure to irritants such as tobacco or airborne pollutants at work (work-related asthma may remit at weekends or when on vacation);

- a history of symptoms, especially if they are worse at night or early morning, arise after exercise, or after being exposed to allergens or to cold air;
- a history of **wheeze**, cough, shortness of breath, or chest tightness after certain medications such as non-steroidal anti-inflammatories or ß-blockers;
- lower-than-predicted **forced expiratory volume (FEV$_1$)** or **peak expiratory flow (PEF).**

If peak flow appears normal, but asthma is suspected, it is important for the patient to measure his or her own PEF accurately twice a day, recording results on a diary card over a period of 2–4 weeks. This may show diurnal variation, with the PEF lower in the morning (a variation of >10–15% around the mean suggests that asthma is the likely diagnosis).

Lung function tests—FEV$_1$, **forced vital capacity (FVC)**, PEF—will differentiate asthma from other lung diseases. Lung function reversibility testing can be carried out with a spirometer or a peak flow meter. The patient's PEF or FEV$_1$ is recorded (best of three efforts). The patient is then given ß$_2$-agonists (e.g. salbutamol) via a pressurized metered dose inhaler and chamber device, and the test is repeated at least 5 minutes later. An increase of >15% is indicative of an asthma diagnosis. Exercise testing is preferred in a patient whose symptoms are exercise-related and who is asymptomatic at the time of testing. Again, the PEF or FEV$_1$ is measured and the patient asked to exercise (usually on a treadmill or after a run of 5 minutes). Five minutes after exercise, the test is repeated; a fall of 15% or greater, with a reversion to the pre-test level after resting or after ß$_2$-agonists, is again indicative of an asthma diagnosis. Normal lung function tests when the patient is symptomatic will exclude asthma.

In assessing patients with suspected asthma, other respiratory conditions such as chronic obstructive pulmonary disease (COPD) must be considered and excluded. The probability of COPD increases with significant smoking history (>20 cigarettes daily). COPD diagnosis is supported by lung function tests showing an obstructive pattern of spirometry with limited or lack of reversibility of FEV$_1$.

Psychosocial assessment

Asthma often has an impact on the patient's life and lifestyle. In children at school, absences can affect peer relationships with classmates and friends and learning progress. Symptoms that are seasonal coincide with spring or summer exams, and can impact on students at school, college, and university.

Asthma also impacts on social life because untreated asthma can restrict activities such as sport, leading to a feeling of isolation from the person's peer group (Ford *et al.*, 2003). Denial of the diagnosis and necessary treatment will demand careful negotiation to ensure concordance with medication (Chapter 22 ➡). The need for regular 'preventative' treatment requires careful explanation and discussion, with particular emphasis on maintaining treatment even though the patient may be completely asymptomatic.

When the trigger factor is work-related, difficulties relating to the removal of the trigger from the work environment are self-evident, especially if the individual cannot be moved from the immediate workplace. This is a big issue at a time of economic instability or when the individual is within 10 years of retirement, as re-employment in a different environment remains challenging.

Symptoms

The symptoms of asthma are:

- wheeze, chest tightness, cough, and/or shortness of breath, especially if they are worse during the night or early morning, or arise after exercise, or being exposed to allergens or cold air;

- a history of:
  - these symptoms after exposure to irritants such as tobacco, or airborne pollutants at work;
  - symptoms after certain medications such as non-steroidal anti-inflammatory drugs or ß2-blockers;
  - widespread wheeze (although it should be remembered that patients are frequently symptom-free between exacerbations).

🚩 **Red flag sign:** In patients *in extremis*, there may be no wheeze and the chest may be silent on auscultation. Such symptoms are indicative of severe, near-fatal asthma, requiring urgent intervention.

Table 2.2 outlines the role of symptoms, signs, and measurements in the initial nursing assessment.

Assessing severity of acute asthma for adults

Several factors, indicated in Table 2.3, should be used to assess the level of severity of acute asthma.

Looking at the patient, understanding pathological causes of symptoms

The differential diagnosis is important, because other severe or life-threatening conditions may also present with wheeze and cough. Features that can help to differentiate other conditions from asthma may accompany the symptoms noted in Table 2.3.

Table 2.2 Initial assessment: the role of symptoms, signs, and measurements

Clinical features	Clinical features, symptoms, and respiratory and cardiovascular signs can identify some patients with severe asthma, e.g. severe breathlessness (including too breathless to complete sentences in one breath), tachypnea, tachycardia, silent chest, cyanosis, or collapse.
	None of these singly or together is specific and their absence does not exclude a severe attack.
PEF or FEV₁	Measurements of airway calibre improve recognition of the degree of severity, the appropriateness or intensity of therapy, and decisions about management in hospital or at home.
	PEF or FEV₁ are both useful and valid measures of airway calibre. PEF is more convenient, can be performed by the patient without aid, and is cheaper.
	PEF expressed as a percentage of the patient's previous best value is most useful clinically. PEF as a percentage of that predicted for sex, height, and age gives a rough guide in the absence of a known previous best value.
Pulse oximetry	Measure oxygen saturation (SpO_2) with a pulse oximeter to determine the adequacy of oxygen therapy.
	The aim of oxygen therapy is to maintain SpO_2 >92%.

Source: Reproduced with permission from British Thoracic Society/Scottish Intercollegiate Guidelines Network www.sign.ac.uk/guidelines/fulltet/101/index.html

CASE STUDY 2.1 *Making the diagnosis*

Caroline is a 23-year-old clerical assistant presenting with history of a nocturnal cough and a feeling of breathlessness for 1 month following a cold. She does not smoke. She describes waking at night coughing; this is not productive. She is breathless on climbing three flights of stairs at work.

There is no significant past medical history. Her younger brother has asthma and multiple allergies. She does not take any medication, has no known allergies, and does not have any pets.

On examination her chest is clear. Her peak flow is reduced at 350 l/min (75% of predicted) and her FEV$_1$ is 2.3 litres (65% of predicted).

Given her symptoms and lung function, you commence her on an inhaled **corticosteroid** (beclometasone 200 mg BD) and bronchodilator (salbutamol 100 mcg as required), requesting that she records her peak flows morning and night for 2 weeks. You demonstrate how to use the metered dose inhaler and advise her to rinse her mouth well after.

She is reviewed 2 weeks later. Her peak flows demonstrate variability, ranging from 300 l/min to 450 l/min, with significant dips in the morning readings. They have improved over the past 4 days. Caroline reports that the cough has resolved and that she is no longer breathless on climbing the stairs at work.

Given her response to treatment and peak flow recordings, firm diagnosis of asthma is made, continuing to step 2 of the Asthma Guidelines **http://www.sign.ac.uk/guidelines/fulltext/101/index.html**. She will require further education relating to asthma and self-management, and regular review.

Chronic cough with the production of sputum

If the cough is generally in the morning and is accompanied by clear or lightly coloured sputum and there is a history of smoking, it may lead to a diagnosis of COPD. Where the sputum is usually coloured and the cough is not mostly restricted to the morning, bronchiectasis may be suggested.

Haemoptysis

The patient should always be asked about **haemoptysis**, as it may be a symptom of serious disease, such as lung cancer or pulmonary embolus.

Sudden dyspnoea

Sudden shortness of breath with no previous history may be indicative of pulmonary embolus, cardiac failure, or pneumothorax.

Fever

Asthma does not cause fever.

Cardiac disease

Cardiac disease with a degree of heart failure may present with wheezing and coughing. These symptoms are often nocturnal and positional, and sputum will be frothy and may be pink or bloodstained. There may also be other symptoms such as peripheral oedema.

Pulmonary fibrosis

This spectrum of diseases may present with wheezing and sometimes coughing, but can be differentiated from asthma by lung function testing, showing a restrictive rather than an obstructive pattern, with a low gas transfer measurement.

Other symptoms

Symptoms of **hyperventilation** such as light-headedness, dizziness, tingling of fingers, or absence of wheeze on

THEORY INTO PRACTICE 2.1
Asthma signs and symptoms

Visit the Asthma UK **www.asthma.org.uk** and the British Thoracic Society **www.brit.thoracic.org.uk** online, and read information on asthma signs and symptoms.

Table 2.3 Assessing severity of asthma exacerbation

Life-threatening asthma	Any one of the following in a patient with severe asthma: • PEF <33% best or predicted • SpO2 ≤92% (will require arterial blood gases) • Silent chest • Cyanosis • Feeble respiratory effort • Bradycardia • Arrhythmia • Hypotension • Exhaustion • Confusion • Coma
Acute severe asthma	Any one of: • PEF 33–50% best or predicted • Respiratory rate =25/min • Heart rate =110/min • Inability to complete sentences in one breath
Moderate asthma exacerbation	• Increasing symptoms • PEF 50–75% best or predicted • No features of acute severe asthma
Brittle asthma	• Type 1: wide PEF variability (>40% diurnal variation for >50% of the time over a period >150 days) despite intense therapy • Type 2: sudden severe attacks on a background of apparently well-controlled asthma

Source: Reproduced with permission from British Thoracic Society/ Scottish Intercollegiate Guidelines Network www.sign.ac.uk/guidelines/fulltet/101/index.html

examination when symptomatic are unlikely to be caused by asthma. These symptoms are commonplace and may coexist in patients with asthma.

Best practice

Clinical guidelines have been described as systematically developed statements that assist in the decision-making about appropriate healthcare for specific clinical conditions (Clinical Resource and Audit Group, 1993).

The consultation document for the clinical strategy for COPD (2010) includes a section on asthma, highlighting the importance of assessment and making the correct diagnosis of asthma, because there are similarities with COPD in presentation of symptoms, and following evidence-based guidelines.

The Scottish Intercollegiate Guidelines Network (SIGN)/British Thoracic Society (BTS) British Guideline on the Management of Asthma (BTS/SIGN, 2009) **www.sign.ac.uk/guidelines/fulltet/101/index.html** will be referred to within this chapter. The Global Initiative for Asthma (GINA) **www.ginasthma.com** is another guideline frequently referenced.

The BTS/SIGN guidelines recommend a stepwise approach to the treatment of asthma, highlighting the importance of commencing treatment at the most appropriate step, and moving up and down the 'treatment ladder' as asthma control and symptoms improve or deteriorate (Figure 2.3).

The clinical goal of asthma management is for the patient to be free of symptoms; this goal may not be shared by the individual. This can be achieved through effective pharmacological interventions and non-pharmacological approaches, using patient self-management strategies, including recognition of known triggers and symptoms of poorly controlled asthma through education, increasing the individual's confidence to adjust treatment independently.

Nursing interventions

Pharmacological interventions

Pharmacological interventions include treatment given via a wide range of delivery modalities. The commonest method of delivery is via the inhaled route, which can be affected by inadequate inhaler technique. Poor/inadequate inhaler technique can significantly reduce the proportion of drugs that reach the lungs and therefore affect the response to treatment. The nurse should be confident that the chosen inhaler device is suitable for the medication selected. Further information regarding devices and drug doses can be obtained from the *British National Formulary* **www.bnf.org**.

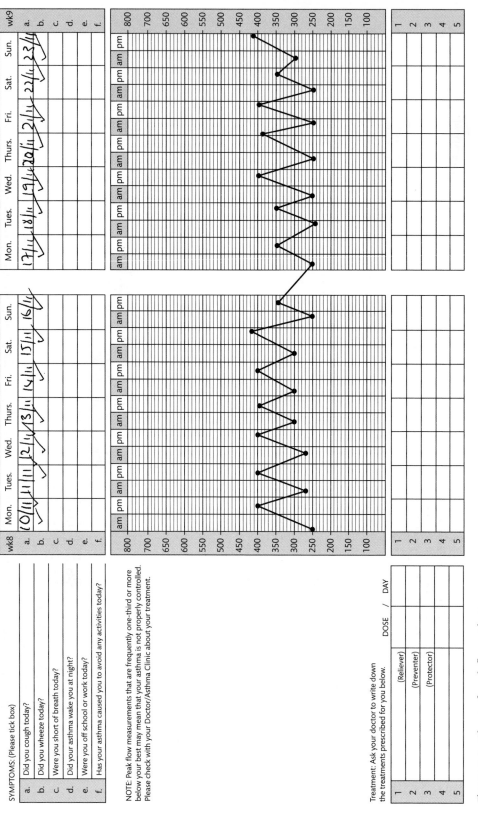

Figure 2.3 Chart of peak flow values.

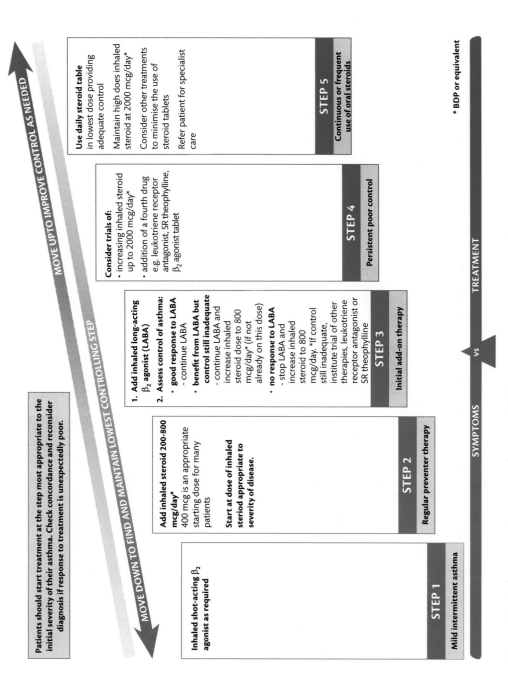

Figure 2.4 Asthma stepwise approach to management.

Reproduced with permission from British Thoracic Society/Scottish Intercollegiate Guidelines Network.

Inhalers

The majority of asthma medication is delivered by inhalation. There is a wide range of inhaler devices available, including pressurized aerosols, dry powder, breath-activated, large and small spacing devices, and nebulization. Nebulized medication is normally reserved for the treatment of acute exacerbations of asthma, which may require admission to hospital.

The wide choice of devices available can make selecting the right device, with the right drug at times, challenging for the healthcare professional. Collaborative working between the patient and the healthcare professional in the selection of the device can improve adherence to treatment.

It is useful for the nurse to consider the following when selecting an inhaler (Robinson and Scullion, 2008):

- the drug required;
- range of available therapies;
- range of available devices and how they work;
- local guidelines and cost-effectiveness of treatment.

The nurse should also consider, from the patient perspective:

- patient preference;
- patient's previous experience with inhalers;
- patient's expectations of treatment;
- patient's ability to use the inhaler;
- lifestyle.

Some practical points to consider include the following.

- Ease of use—consider manual dexterity and level of understanding
- Is it easy to teach how to use the device?
- Situations of use—will it be used solely at home or does it need to be portable?
- Is it going to be used during an acute attack?
- Does the patient require reassurance that the dose has been taken?
- How important is it that the patient knows how many doses have been taken?
- Can the patient tell if the inhaler is running out?
- Can the patient distinguish one inhaler from another?

Further patient information about how to use inhalers can be obtained from Asthma UK **www.asthma.org.uk.**

It is essential that the patient can use the inhaler device selected to deliver the prescribed medication, and this should be checked on a regular basis, especially before 'stepping up' treatment when symptoms are poorly controlled.

Medications

Short-acting ß₂-agonists

Short-acting ß₂-agonists are the first-choice treatment for mild intermittent asthma (Step 1, Figure 2.4) and are normally delivered via the inhaled route. They can also be given orally, intravenously, and subcutaneously.

Predominantly, they are bronchodilators, acting on the ß₂ receptors of the sympathetic nervous system. When stimulated, the ß₂ receptors relax the bronchial smooth muscle, dilating the bronchi and therefore improving the airway calibre. It is also believed that they act at the level of mast cells, inhibiting the release of mediators.

They have a rapid onset of action, usually working within 5–15 minutes, with the bronchodilatory effects lasting a maximum of 4 hours (but not as long in the case of a severe asthma attack).

They do have some side effects, with the commonest being fine tremor, a rapid heartbeat, and palpitations.

It is important to remember that if bronchodilatation occurs through stimulating the ß receptors, then ß-blockers (e.g. atenolol), which have the reverse effect, may potentially cause bronchoconstriction, and therefore ß-blockers should be avoided in individuals with asthma.

Corticosteroids

Corticosteroids influence all aspects of the inflammatory process in asthma, affecting the synthesis of inflammatory proteins and cytokines, and have revolutionized the management of asthma.

As an inhaled therapy, they are used as first-line treatment for patients with persistent asthma symptoms (Step 2, Figure 2.4). They have a wide dose range, with the ability to increase and decrease the dose depending on

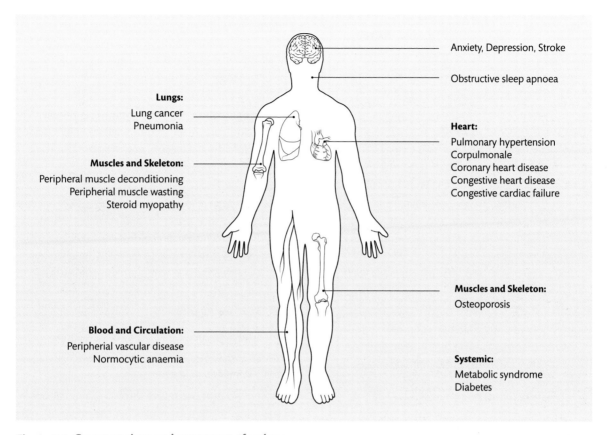

Anxiety, Depression, Stroke

Obstructive sleep apnoea

Lungs:
Lung cancer
Pneumonia

Heart:
Pulmonary hypertension
Corpulmonale
Coronary heart disease
Congestive heart disease
Congestive cardiac failure

Muscles and Skeleton:
Peripheral muscle deconditioning
Peripherial muscle wasting
Steroid myopathy

Muscles and Skeleton:
Osteoporosis

Blood and Circulation:
Peripherial vascular disease
Normocytic anaemia

Systemic:
Metabolic syndrome
Diabetes

Figure 2.5 Common signs and symptoms of asthma.

symptoms. The dose should be reviewed regularly and stepped up or down accordingly.

The common local side effects include oropharyngeal candidiasis and dysphonia, which can be reduced with good oral hygiene following administration. Systematic side effects include adrenal suppression, bruising, osteoporosis, cataracts, glaucoma, adrenal suppression, and other metabolic abnormalities. Side effects can lead to poor adherence.

Regular oral steroids are reserved for patients whose asthma cannot be controlled on other treatment, with the dose titrated to the lowest dose to control the symptoms (Step 5, Figure 2.4). Side effects include fluid retention, increased appetite, weight gain, osteoporosis, thinning of the skin, immunosuppression, gastric irritation, and ulceration, diabetes, hypertension, and cataracts.

However, oral corticosteroids are regularly used in the management of acute asthma attacks, with emergency prescriptions issued to patients as part of their asthma action plan; these are discussed on page 26.

Long-acting ß2-agonists

Long-acting ß2-agonists have bronchodilator action and protect against bronchoconstriction for 12 hours. They are given in an inhaled format and have similar side effects to the short-acting ß2-agonists.

They are usually introduced as an option at Step 3 (Figure 2.4) of the asthma guidelines. They do not have anti-inflammatory properties, and are therefore believed to be dangerous if taken in the absence of inhaled corticosteroids, with evidence supporting an increase in mortality in asthmatic patients taking solely long-acting ß2-agonists as sole therapy (Walters *et al.*, 2007). They should therefore be prescribed to patients already taking inhaled corticosteroids.

Prescribing the two agents in a combination format is encouraged, and is seen as an effective and convenient method of controlling asthma through improved adherence to treatment (British Thoracic Society/Scottish Intercollegiate Guidelines Network, 2009; National Institute for Health and Clinical Excellence, 2008).

They have similar side effects to ß₂-agonists, but can also cause cramps, especially in the legs.

Leukotriene receptor agonists

Leukotriene receptor agonists have a small and variable effect on bronchodilator effect, suggesting that leukotrienes may contribute to baseline bronchoconstriction in asthma. They appear to be most effective in symptoms induced by exercise, cold air, and aspirin. They are also useful in treating patients with atopic asthma presenting with a history of allergic rhinitis.

They are seen as an 'add' treatment at Steps 3/4 (Figure 2.4) of the asthma guidelines, and should be prescribed as a trial in the first instance to see if they are effective in controlling symptoms (Robinson *et al.*, 2001).

They are prepared as an oral preparation, given daily. On the whole, they are well tolerated, but side effects include palpitations, increased bleeding tendencies, abdominal cramps, and nightmares.

Methylxanthines (theophylline)

Methylxanthines (theophylline) have been used to treat asthma for many years. They are an inexpensive class of drug, but have many side effects and potential drug interactions. They act as bronchodilators at a high dose, with growing evidence to suggest that, at a lower dose, anti-inflammatory effects may be present and they may be effective in combination with inhaled corticosteroids (Barnes, 2010).

With the efficacy of inhaled ß₂-agonists and inhaled corticosteroids, methylxanthines are now used at Step 4 (Figure 2.4) of the guidelines, as an oral preparation. They can also be used during acute asthma exacerbations requiring hospitalization and may be given intravenously.

Common side effects include arrhythmias, headaches, gastric symptoms, hypokalaemia, and insomnia.

There are many factors that may influence the plasma concentration of the drug, including smoking, alcohol, drugs (e.g. antibiotics), liver disease, and age. It is therefore important to take these factors into consideration and to ensure that drug plasma levels are monitored to prevent adverse side effects.

Anti-IgE therapy

Anti-IgE monoclonal antibody therapy binds to circulating IgE, and therefore blocks its action through activation of IgE receptors on the mast and other inflammatory cells.

There is currently only one preparation of anti-IgE therapy, omalizumab, which reduces airway inflammation and therefore the incidence of exacerbations of asthma. It is delivered via a subcutaneous injection, every 2–4 weeks, depending on serum IgE level.

It is an expensive treatment, with only 30% of patients responding to the treatment, and therefore a 4-month trial is recommended. A National Institute for Health and Clinical Excellence (NICE) technical appraisal (NICE, 2007) recommends that it should be made available to asthmatics at Steps 4/5 (Figure 2.4) of the guidelines who meet the following criteria:

- confirmed IgE-medicated allergy to a perennial allergen (by measurement of circulating specific IgE levels in blood);
- either two or more severe asthma exacerbations requiring hospitalization, within the previous year, or three or more severe exacerbations within the previous year, with at least one requiring admission to hospital, and a further two requiring treatment in excess of the patient's usual treatment.

For further information for all of the medications discussed, refer to **http://bnf.org/bnf/index.htm**

Non-pharmacological interventions

Although pharmacotherapy forms the basis of care, non-pharmacological strategies complement treatment.

Breathing control

Breathlessness is a very frightening experience and many asthmatics hyperventilate during asthma attacks/exacerbations. Physiotherapy techniques can be taught to patients who frequently experience symptoms secondary to hyperventilation. These involve reproducing the sensation through 'over-breathing' in a controlled setting, and then being taught how to control the respiratory rate and pattern.

The principle of the Buteyko breathing technique is to control hyperventilation by lowering the respiratory rate. Evidence suggests that, although there is no effect on lung function (Holloway and Ram, 2004), a reduction in symptoms and bronchodilator usage can be achieved through using this breathing technique (McHugh *et al.*, 2003; Opat *et al.*, 2000).

Dysfunctional breathing syndrome can often be misdiagnosed as asthma, resulting in an individual being inappropriately treated. Once diagnosed, this syndrome can be managed with the input and expertise of physiotherapists and speech therapists.

Avoidance of trigger factors

Identifying triggers and allergens is key in controlling asthma symptoms, and advice regarding avoidance should be included as part of self-management education.

Measures to reduce numbers of house dust mites have been shown to be successful, but studies suggest that this does not appear to reduce the overall severity of asthma. However, for individuals with a known house dust mite allergy, the following tips may reduce allergic symptoms (British Thoracic Society/Scottish Intercollegiate Guidelines Network, 2009).

- Complete bed covering with hypoallergic covers
- Removal of carpets
- Removal of soft toys from beds
- High temperature washing of bedding
- Acaricides to soft furnishing
- Good ventilation with or without humidification

Management during an acute exacerbation of asthma

Acute exacerbations of asthma need prompt and appropriate treatment, on which the British Thoracic Society/Scottish Intercollegiate Guidelines Network guidelines provide clear information **www.sign.ac.uk/guidelines/fulltet/101/index.html**. Treatment will depend on the severity of the exacerbation, as described in Box 2.1, including the reasons for admission to hospital. Box 2.2 lists the assessment and possible investigations that would take place on admission.

Box 2.1 Severity of asthma exacerbation

Moderate exacerbation (PEF rate 50–75%)
- High-dose ß$_2$-agonists via spacer or nebulized
- Prednisolone 40–50 mg daily for 5 days

Severe exacerbation (PEF rate 33–50%)
- Oxygen 40–60%
- High-dose ß$_2$-agonists via spacer or nebulized
- Prednisolone 40–50 mg daily for 5 days

Life-threatening asthma (PEF rate <33%)
- **Arrange for admission**
- **Oxygen 40–60%**
- **High-dose ß$_2$-agonists via spacer or nebulized**
- **Prednisolone 40–50 mg daily for 5 days**

Box 2.2 Assessment and investigations in hospital

- **Continuing with oxygen therapy**
- **Continuing with high-dose ß$_2$-agonist**
- **Introducing inhaled anticholinergics (ipratropium)**
- **IV magnesium sulphate if poor response to initial treatment**
- **IV aminophylline/ß$_2$-agonists**
- **Consideration for ventilation**

Additional investigations may include:
- Arterial blood gases
- Chest X-ray

Follow-up

Reviewing the patient following an exacerbation is important. It is an ideal opportunity to provide education to highlight events leading up to the attack, to help to identify possible triggers, to provide a basis to discuss potential warning signs, and to review/provide an asthma action plan. Medications can be reviewed and this should include inhaler technique checks.

It is recommended that a patient is reviewed within 2 working days of discharge from hospital by his or her GP/practice nurse, with secondary care-based follow-up with a respiratory specialist (nurse/doctor) within 4 weeks (British Thoracic Society/Scottish Intercollegiate Guidelines Network, 2009).

CASE STUDY 2.2   *Acute asthma management*

Primary care

David is 22 years old and was diagnosed with asthma at the age of 8. He is known to be allergic to cats and tree pollen. His asthma has been well controlled on beclometasone 400 mcg BD and salbutamol 100 mcg as required. He presents to the GP surgery with a history of:

- increased use of his salbutamol over the past 2 days;
- waking at night during the previous night;
- coughing intermittently during the day and night.

On examination, he is speaking in full sentences and appears to be comfortable. However, his peak flow is reduced to 280 l/min, which is 60% of his personal best, and he has a widespread wheeze on auscultation. Observations are: temperature 36.4°C; pulse 92 bpm; respiratory rate 14 bpm; blood pressure (BP) 130\80; and O_2 saturations on air 95%.

Initial treatment would include:

- administration of high-dose inhaled β_2-agonist (salbutamol 100 mcg four puffs) via a metered dose inhaler and large volume spacer;
- oral corticosteroids—prednisolone 40 mcg for 5 days.

Peak flow and chest examination, when repeated 20 minutes later, have improved, with a recording of 480 l/min and good air entry throughout, with no additional chest sounds.

Further questions

It will be necessary to explore David's symptoms to identify possible triggers for this exacerbation and to assess his asthma control.

- How has his asthma been prior to the last few days?

- Has he attended his last asthma review?
- Has he been collecting his prescriptions?
- Is his inhaler technique adequate?
- Has his home or work circumstances altered?
- Has he been exposed to any known triggers (e.g. cats)?
- Has he had signs of a cold?
- Is he taking any additional medication?

Education and review

David should be encouraged to continue with the course of prednisolone for 5 days and to continue with the inhaled corticosteroids, reinforcing the importance of treating the inflammation in his airways. He should use salbutamol 100 mcg two puffs via a large volume spacer as required up to 4-hourly, to ensure optimum bronchodilatation.

He should be given clear instructions on what to do should his symptoms deteriorate further (e.g. should the bronchodilators appear to be less effective), which would include contacting the out-of-hours doctor or attending the emergency department.

He should be reviewed within 1 week to check that he has recovered or is recovering from the exacerbation. This is a good opportunity to review his asthma action plan and to discuss trigger factors, and to ensure he has access to emergency rescue treatment (prednisolone).

Secondary care

David's mother contacts the surgery the following morning and informs the practice that David had been admitted to hospital during the night because he was 'very wheezy' and 'unable to get his breath'.

Nursing care of a patient admitted to hospital would include the following.

- Excellent communication skills will reduce anxiety, providing a calm and confident attitude in providing reassurance.

- Ensuring that the patient is in a comfortable position is essential.
- Regular observations must be made of TPR (temperature, pulse, respirations), BP, O_2 saturations, and PEF monitoring to detect signs of deterioration, because patients with acute asthma can deteriorate quickly and may require ventilatory support. It is also important to observe respiratory effort to detect fatigue.
- Fluid management: intravenous fluids may be prescribed, because patients can become dehydrated secondary to fluid lost during respiration/poor oral intake.
- Administration of drugs: regular nebulized bronchodilators (driven by oxygen) should be given; intravenous corticosteroids if unable to tolerate oral preparations, and antibiotics. Inhaler technique should also be reviewed and corrected when necessary.

- Oxygen should be administered to correct hypoxia, maintaining oxygen saturations between 94% and 98% (British Thoracic Society, 2008).
- Education and self-management strategies should be discussed, and an asthma action plan should be discussed and given prior to discharge (British Thoracic Society/Scottish Intercollegiate Guidelines Network, 2009).
- Follow-up is very important, because it allows for assessment of recovery, as well as reviewing medication and self-management. This review should take place with 2–3 days of discharge by the GP and 2–4 weeks by a respiratory specialist (British Thoracic Society/Scottish Intercollegiate Guidelines Network, 2009).

David was discharged from hospital 3 days later.

Activity

➤ Discuss with a patient what it is like to experience an asthma attack.

➤ Review the content of an asthma action plan.

Management of stable chronic asthma

Asthma reviews

Asthma management requires a patient-centred approach, with nurses playing an important role in the ongoing management of asthma. The majority of asthma management occurring in primary care is by practice nurses. The Quality and Outcomes Framework (QOF) recommend that practices should have an asthma register, with asthmatics being reviewed every 15 months.

The review should include an enquiry into the presence of asthma symptoms, medication usage, inhaler technique, smoking status, and review of an asthma action plan.

There are several validated questionnaires that can be used to measure asthma control, with the most favoured being the Royal College of Physicians (RCP) 3 questions (Pearson, 1999) because it is quick and concise.

The RCP 3 questions are as follows.

1. Have you had difficulties in *sleeping* because of your asthma?
2. Have you had your usual asthma symptoms *during the day*?
3. Has your asthma interfered with your *usual daily activities*?

A positive response to any of the questions suggests a review of treatment, including inhaler technique and concordance with medication.

The Asthma Control test (Juniper *et al.*, 2006) is another tool that can be used independently by patients to assess their asthma: **www.asthmacontroltest.com.**

Achieving concordance

Concordance suggests a negotiated agreement between the healthcare professional and patient. Achieving concordance is likely to result in an improvement in adherence. However, there can be confusion, misunderstandings, and misconceptions around medical treatment and potential side effects, which should be discussed with the patient. It is important to ensure that the consultation is a two-way process, and that the patient is listened to and his or her concerns are discussed. Patients' views about asthma and its management may be different from those of the healthcare professional, and these often need to be explored in greater detail to enable treatment goals to be developed. The use of open-ended questions, asking what the patient would like to improve in his or her asthma management, along with verbal and written instructions, is often beneficial.

Self-management in asthma

For patients to be able to manage their conditions effectively, they need to have a basic understanding of the condition and the treatments available to them.

In asthma, this will include an understanding of the nature of the disease, causes, and treatment, identifying and avoiding trigger factors (i.e. active and passive exposure to tobacco smoke, known allergens, e.g. house dust mite). The patient needs to develop self-monitoring skills and be able to recognize the symptoms of poorly controlled asthma, e.g. breathlessness, cough, wheeze, nocturnal symptoms, and objective assessment, e.g. peak flow recording, as measurements of asthma control. This may involve the provision of ongoing support and guidance to ensure that the patient is confident in recognizing signs of deterioration and thus commencing rescue treatment.

The British Thoracic Society/Scottish Intercollegiate Guidelines Network guidelines recommend that patients with asthma are offered self-management education that is tailored to their individual needs, with a written asthma action plan. As part of an asthma review, self-management strategies should to be discussed with patients and an individualized asthma action plan developed.

Asthma action plans

Written personalized action plans as part of self-management have been shown to improve health outcomes, with reductions in hospital admissions and attendance to emergency departments. The evidence is strongest in those in secondary care with moderate to severe disease, and those who have recently had an exacerbation (Gibson *et al.*, 2002; Osman *et al.*, 2002).

This should include structured education, reinforced with written information, identifying symptoms associated with poor asthma control, including the measurement of

Table 2.4 Generic asthma action plan

Monitoring symptoms	Peak flow (% of best predicted)	Degree of attack	Recommended action
More frequent symptoms, increase in use of reliever inhaler	<80%	Mild to moderate asthma attack	Use reliever inhaler as required
Effects of reliever inhaler lasting <2 hours	<60%	Moderate to severe asthma attack	Contact GP/asthma nurse Commence emergency oral corticosteroids Use reliever inhaler as required
No improvement with reliever or failing to improve with increase in inhaled or oral corticosteroids	<50%	Severe asthma attack	Seek medical help Call emergency services

peak expiratory flow rates, and clear instructions as to what to do should symptoms deteriorate. This might include an increase of the current treatment and commencing emergency oral corticosteroids. Table 2.4 outlines a generic asthma plan.

Useful resources, including asthma action plans and information leaflets, can be obtained from Asthma UK **www.asthma.org.uk** and The British Lung Foundation **www.lunguk.org**.

THEORY INTO PRACTICE 2.2
Observe at an asthma clinic

Arrange to observe asthma education being delivered in an asthma clinic in either primary or secondary care.

Resources

Throughout the chapter and highlighted below is a list of recent sources of the best evidence to inform the nursing care of patients with asthma.

- GINA Report, Global Strategy for Asthma Management and Prevention (2010) **www.ginasthma.com**
- British Thoracic Society, Scottish Intercollegiate Guidelines Network, British Guideline on the Management of Asthma (2009) **www.sign.ac.uk/ guidelines/fulltet/101/index.html**
- National Institute for Health and Clinical Excellence (2007) Omalizumab for severe persistent allergic asthma. NICE technology appraisal guidance 133 **www.nice.org.uk/TA133**
- National Institute for Health and Clinical Excellence (2008) Inhaled corticosteroids for the treatment of chronic asthma in adults and children aged 12 and over. NICE technology appraisal guidance 138 **www. nice.org.uk/TA138**

Because research is always ongoing and best practice evolves, it is important that readers stay up to date and know where to find good-quality sources of evidence. Hence we have provided a list of sources that readers should utilize.

Journals

Primary Care Respiratory Society Journal
Thorax
European Respiratory Journal

Organizations

British Thoracic Society **www.brit-thoracic.org.uk**
Primary Care Respiratory Society **www.PCRS-uk.org**
National Institute for Health and Clinical Excellence (NICE) **http://guidance.nice.org.uk**
The Scottish Intercollegiate Guidelines Network (SIGN) **http://www.sign.ac.uk/guidelines/index.html**
NHS Evidence **http://www.evidence.nhs.uk**
Agency for Healthcare Quality (AHRQ) **http://www. ahrq.gov**
National Institute for Clinical Studies (NICS) **http:// www.nhmrc.gov.au/nics/index.htm**
Registered Nurses Association of Ontario **http://www. rnao.org**

Conclusion

Scientists continue to investigate the complex genetic, immunological, and inflammatory mechanisms that cause asthma. It is recognized that asthma is a common and treatable condition. The provision of personalized care with adequate asthma treatment, minimization of allergen exposure, ensuring good inhaler technique, and concordance might support those with a diagnosis of asthma to be free of symptoms.

Research has demonstrated that the majority of asthma deaths are avoidable. Recognizing the symptoms of asthma and a proactive approach to teaching people self-management skills to recognize deteriorating asthma, providing self-management plans, and targeting high-risk patients should reduce the burden of asthma on the individual, the family, and the health service.

Empowering patients to self-manage their condition is high on the healthcare agenda. People need to receive education and support to ensure that they are confident in increasing/decreasing their medication and/or commencing rescue medication. Nurses, especially those based in primary care, are in an ideal position to provide appropriate and timely education about asthma and treatment options to patients, enabling them to develop skills in self-management.

Asthma UK **www.asthma.uk.org** and the British Lung Foundation **www. lunguk.org** provide patient information that can reinforce information given by healthcare professionals, as well as provide useful tips for those living with asthma. The information is available in a variety of languages. Both charities provide online helpline and support groups.

Online Resource Centre

 To help you to develop and apply your knowledge and decision-making skills further, we have provided interactive learning resources online at **www.oxfordtextbooks.co.uk/orc/bullock**

Whilst these are freely available, you will need to use the access codes at the start of this book.

References

Asthma UK (2005) *Where do we Stand?* **www.asthma.org.uk** (accessed June 2011).

Asthma UK (2010) *New Data Reveals High Cost of Asthma.* **www. asthma.org.uk** (accessed April 2011).

Barnes, P. (2010) Theophylline. *Pharmaceuticals* **3**: 725–47.

British Thoracic Society (2008) Guidelines for the emergency use of oxygen in adults. *Thorax* **63**(Suppl. V1): vi1–vi73.

British Thoracic Society, Scottish Intercollegiate Guidelines Network (2009) *British Guideline on the Management of Asthma.* **www.sign.ac.uk** (accessed 31 March 2010).

Clinical Resource and Audit Group (1993) *Clinical Guidelines.* Scottish Office: Edinburgh.

Ford, E.S., Mannino, D.M., Homa, D.M., *et al.* (2003) Self-reported asthma and health-related quality of life. *Chest* **123**: 119–27.

Gibson, P.G., Powell, H., Wilson, A., *et al.* (2002) Self-management education and regular practitioner review for adults with asthma. *Cochrane Database of Systematic Reviews*, Issue 3. Art. No.: CD001117. DOI: 10.1002/14651858.CD001117.

Harrison, B., Stephenson, P., Mohan, G., *et al.* (2005) An ongoing confidential enquiry into asthma deaths in the Eastern region of the UK, 2001–2003. *Primary Care Respiratory Journal* **14**: 303–13.

Holloway, E., Ram, F.S.F. (2001) Breathing exercises for asthma. Cochrane Database of Systematic Reviews, Issue 1: Art. No. CD001277. DOI: 10.1002/14651858. CD001277. pub2.

Holloway, J.W., Yang, I.A., Holgate, S.T. (2010) Genetics of allergic disease. *Journal of Allergy and Clinical Immunology* **125** (Suppl. 2): S81–S94.

Juniper, E.F., Bousquet, J., Abetz, L., *et al.* (2006) Identifying well controlled and not well controlled asthma using the Asthma Control Questionnaire. *Respiratory Medicine* **100**(4): 616–21.

Lung and Asthma Information Agency (2006) Estimating the prevalence of asthma: QOF v Health Survey for England. **www./aia.ac.uk/QOF. htm** (accessed December 2011)

McHugh, P., Aitchson, F., Duncan, B., *et al.* (2003) Buteyko breathing techniques in asthma: an effective intervention. *New Zealand Medical Journal* **116**(1187): U710.

National Institute for Health and Clinical Excellence (2007) Omalizumab for severe persistent allergic asthma. NICE Technology Appraisal Guidance 133. **www.nice.org.uk/TA133.** (accessed 31 January 2010).

National Institute for Health and Clinical Excellence (2008) Inhaled corticosteroids for the treatment of chronic asthma in adults and children aged 12 and over. NICE Technology Appraisal Guidance 138. **www.nice.org.uk/TA138** (accessed 31 March 2010).

Occupational Asthma **http://www.hse.gov.uk/asthma/substances.htm** (accessed 11 January 2011).

Office for National Statistics (2009) National Statistics on Death Registrations for England and Wales. **http://www. statistics.gov.uk/StatBase/Product.asp?vlnk=618** (accessed January 2010).

Opat, A.J., Cohen, M.M., Bailey, M.J., *et al.* (2000) A clinical trial of the Buteyko breathing technique in asthma as taught by a video. *Journal of Asthma* **37**(7): 557–64.

Osman, L.M., Calder, C., Godden, D.J., *et al.* (2002) A randomised controlled trial of self management planning for adult patients admitted to hospital with acute asthma. *Thorax* **57**(10): 869–74.

Pearson, M.B. (ed.) (1999) *Measuring Clinical Outcomes in Asthma: A Patient-Focused Approach*. Royal College of Physicians: London.

Robinson, D.S., Campbell, D., Barnes, P.J. (2001) Addition of leukotriene antagonists to therapy in chronic persistent asthma: a randomised double blind placebo controlled trial. *Lancet* **357**(9273): 2007–11.

Robinson, T., Scullion, J.E. (2008) *Oxford Handbook of Respiratory Nursing*. Oxford University Press: Oxford.

Smith, J.R., Mildenhall, S., Noble, M.J., *et al.* (2005) Clinician-identified poor compliance is useful in identifying, amongst adults with severe asthma, patients with characteristics likely to put them at risk of adverse outcomes. *Journal of Asthma* **42**(6): 437–45.

Walters, E.H., Gibson, P.G., Lasserson, T.J., *et al.* (2007) Long acting ß2 agonists for chronic asthma in adults and children where background therapy continued varied or no inhaled corticosteroid (review). *Cochrane Database of Systematic Reviews* Issue 1: Art. No. CD001385. DOI: 10.1002/14651858.CD001385.pub2.

3 *Understanding* **Bone Conditions**

Anne Sutcliffe and Cameron Swift

Introduction

The aim of this chapter is to provide nurses with the knowledge to be able to assess, manage, and care for people with bone conditions in an evidence-based and person-centred way. Bone conditions (a major category of musculoskeletal conditions) cover a wide spectrum of diseases, some of which may be considered mild and self-limiting, while others may have a significant impact upon the individual's quality of life and ability to function. It is estimated that up to 30% of all GP consultations are about musculoskeletal complaints; many are age-associated, and population ageing will continue to increase this demand (Oliver, 2009).

The chapter will focus on osteoporosis, hip fracture (perhaps the most serious and costly consequence of osteoporosis or osteopaenia), Paget's disease, and osteoarthritis, respectively. The chapter will provide a broad overview of these common conditions, enabling a proactive approach to patient care within a multidisciplinary context, whether in the primary or secondary care setting. The nursing management of the symptoms and common health problems associated with bone conditions can be found in several Part 2 chapters, and these are highlighted throughout the chapter.

Osteoporosis

Understanding osteoporosis

Definition

Osteoporosis has been defined as:

> A progressive systemic skeletal disease characterised by low bone mass and micro-architectural deterioration of bone tissue, with a consequent increase in bone fragility and susceptibility to fracture. (WHO, 1994)

The World Health Organization (WHO) has recommended a clinical definition of osteoporosis based on a bone mineral density (BMD) measurement of the spine or hip, expressed in standard deviation (SD) units called T scores. Using this definition, an individual is classified as having osteoporosis if his or her T score is ≤−2.5 SD at the spine or hip (WHO, 1994).

Epidemiological profile of osteoporosis and related fractures

It is estimated that osteoporosis occurs in approximately 3 million people in the UK, resulting in more than 230,000 fractures per annum, the most frequent being hip, vertebral body, and forearm fractures. In total, 75,000 hip fractures occur annually (British Orthopaedic Association, 2007), with the average age of incidence being 84 and 83 in men and women, respectively (National Hip Fracture Database, 2010). There is an estimated 30% probability of death during the first year after hip fracture, and approximately half the survivors will suffer from long-term disability and loss of independence (Parker and Johansen, 2006). Accurately quantifying the incidence and prevalence of vertebral fractures is difficult, because many patients with back pain do not seek medical attention and there has also been a lack of a universally recognized definition of vertebral deformity from X-rays. In the UK, it has been estimated that the lifetime risk of a vertebral fracture in a 50-year-old woman is 3.1%, whereas the corresponding figure for a 50-year-old man is 1.2%.

The combined cost of social and hospital care for patients with osteoporotic fracture has been reported to be more than £2.0 billion per year in the UK, with most of these costs being related to hip fracture care in the older person. Fractures in those aged over 60 utilize more than 2 million bed days, and those attributable to hip fracture have been estimated to cost between £5,600 and £12,000 per case (Burge *et al.*, 2001).

The pathophysiology of osteoporosis

Bone is a dynamic tissue that undergoes constant remodelling throughout life; being metabolically active, it is continually formed and resorbed by bone cells known as osteoblasts and osteoclasts, respectively. This remodelling allows the skeleton to increase in size during growth, respond to physical stresses, and repair structural damage due to fatigue or fracture. The control of bone remodelling is complex, and depends on the interaction of mechanical stresses, systemic hormones, and locally produced cytokines, prostaglandins, and growth factors. Provided that the remodelling cycle remains balanced, bone will develop normally, but this process can be overridden by general or local influences, and should resorption exceed formation, this will result in decreased bone mass and potential osteoporosis.

Bone mass and bone loss

Bone mass changes throughout life in three major phases: growth, consolidation, and loss. In both genders, peak bone mass is attained between the ages of 20 and 30, with age-related bone loss starting at around the age of 40 and persisting thereafter throughout life. Changes of bone mass with age are detailed in Figure 3.1.

Genetic factors are the single most significant influence on peak bone mass, with multiple genes being implicated, including the collagen type 1A1, vitamin D receptor, and oestrogen receptor genes. Nutritional factors, particularly adequate dietary calcium intake, sex hormone status, and physical exercise involving weightbearing activity will also affect the peak mass attained.

Oestrogen deficiency is a major factor in the pathogenesis of postmenopausal osteoporosis and also in osteoporosis in men. In older people, vitamin D insufficiency and secondary hyperparathyroidism are significant pathogenetic factors affecting bone loss. Risk factors

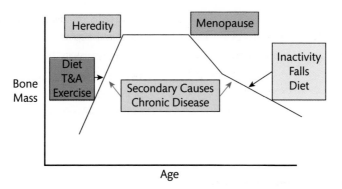

Figure 3.1 Bone mass with age.

associated with increased bone loss may be considered as endogenous or exogenous.

- Endogenous factors include ethnicity, female gender, advancing age, family history of hip fracture.
- Exogenous factors include hypogonadism (male or female), oral glucocorticoid treatment, low body mass index, previous fracture, smoking, immobilization, excess alcohol, and vitamin D insufficiency in the elderly. A number of concomitant diseases may also affect bone mass and bone loss, common examples being rheumatoid arthritis, malabsorption syndromes, hyperthyroidism, and chronic renal and hepatic disease.

Common symptoms and problems

- Osteoporosis itself is asymptomatic and is often recognized after fractures have occurred as a result of skeletal fragility.
- The devastating short- and long-term consequences of hip fracture are considered later in this chapter (and see Chapters 17, 20, 23, and 25 ➡).
- Major consequences of vertebral fractures are acute and chronic back pain (see Chapters 23 and 25 ➡), kyphosis, and height loss, which in turn may result in decreased lung and abdominal volumes (see Chapters 15 and 24 ➡). These fractures may be associated with a decline in both physical and mental function, and may be associated with increased anxiety, depression, and impaired mobility (see Chapters 14 and 23 ➡).

Assessing the patient with osteoporosis

Because the patient with osteoporosis presents across a number of health disciplines, nursing assessment and subsequent intervention will be varied. For example, a patient whose osteoporosis may have been diagnosed through risk assessment and possible DXA (dual-energy X-ray absorptiometry) measurements (patient A) will present to a practice nurse with different needs from the patient who has been admitted to an orthopaedic ward following hip or vertebral fracture associated with reduced bone density (patient B).

Nursing assessment of patient A

Use open and closed questions to clarify a full history, covering

- presenting complaint;
- risk factors for osteoporosis assessment using FRAX®;
- medication history;
- family and social history;
- mobility and functional capacity;
- pain.

Many of these questions have been incorporated into FRAX®, which is an assessment tool validated by WHO. This can be used to predict the 10-year probability of hip fracture alone or other fracture at the spine, forearm, or hip, although there is some concern that in FRAX® and the National Osteoporosis Guideline Group (NOGG) risk in very elderly people might be somewhat underestimated. This is because certain risk factors prevalent in old age (such as falling) are not part of the FRAX® tool (Masud *et al.*, 2011).

> **THEORY INTO PRACTICE 3.1**
> **Activity**
> ---
> Download a copy of FRAX® from **www.sheffield. ac.uk/FRAX**
>
> Consider whether or not this would be a valuable tool in the assessment process.

Nursing assessment of patient B

In addition to the generic questions previously cited, the following should also be addressed:

- spine assessment, including details of height loss, presence of kyphosis, posture;

- more detailed pain assessment relating to specific areas in the spine;
- effect on mobility;
- the patient's concerns about height loss, possible abdominal protrusion, and change in body image and effect on appearance;
- emotional feelings and coping strategies.

Identifying best practice for osteoporosis

Throughout the text, below, and at the end of this chapter, you will find recent sources of the best evidence to inform the nursing care of patients with osteoporosis. Because research is always ongoing and best practice evolves, it is important that readers stay up to date and know where to find good-quality sources of evidence. Hence we have provided a list of resources below that readers should utilize.

CASE STUDY 3.1 *Patient A, who presents to the practice nurse*

Patient profile

- Mrs A, aged 63, generally well
- Osteoporosis, no fracture
- Risk factors: maternal history of hip fracture
- Coeliac disease
- DXA: T score in spine −2.9
- Prescribed alendronic acid 70 mg weekly

Nursing management

- Explain scan results
- Discuss current and future fracture risk, utilizing FRAX®
- Offer lifestyle advice
- Emphasize high dietary calcium intake
- Encourage normal activities
- Reinforce importance of taking bisphosphonate treatment correctly
- Explain reason for long-term adherence

- Promote positive outlook
- Advise about National Osteoporosis Society and its resources

Summary

Mrs A has been diagnosed with osteoporosis and is potentially at risk of fracture, but she is currently asymptomatic and therefore presents with few obvious nursing challenges.

She does require accurate information about osteoporosis, advice on lifestyle issues, and reassurance about her prognosis.

Fracture could be a sign of deterioration in bone mass, but long-term adherence with treatment will help to minimize this risk (Part 2, Chapter 22 ➡).

In view of increased skeletal fragility, falls prevention and mobility issues may need to be addressed in the future (Part 2, Chapter 23 ➡).

CASE STUDY 3.2 *Patient B detailing nurse-led interventions*

Patient profile

- Mrs B, aged 83
- Osteoporosis with vertebral fracture
- Risk factors: intermittent glucocorticoids for asthma
- Spine X-ray: fractures at T11, T12

Nursing management

- Explain X-ray results
- Describe link between steroids and bone loss
- Discuss current and future fracture risk
- Encourage return to normal activities undertaken before fracture
- Advise about National Osteoporosis Society
- Assist with all activities of daily living, if appropriate during 'acute' phase
- Give pressure area care (long-term bed rest not encouraged)
- Reinforce importance of taking bisphosphonate treatment correctly
- Explain reason for long-term adherence
- Reassure that treatment should prevent further fracture
- Check response to analgesia
- Reinforce need to take regularly

- Reassure that pain will subside, but may take 4–6 weeks
- Liaise with physiotherapist regarding breathing exercises, back strengthening exercises, use of hydrotherapy, general mobility, and falls risk

Summary

This patient, with 'acute' vertebral fractures, presents many challenges to nursing, including the following.

- Pain management (Part 2, Chapter 25 ➡), mobility management and falls prevention (Part 2, Chapter 23 ➡), maintenance of hygiene and management of skin care (Part 2, Chapters 20 and 27 ➡)
- She will also require reassurance and encouragement to resume previous activities once the acute pain has subsided.
- Long-term adherence to therapy is essential to maintain bone mass and hopefully to prevent further fracture (Part 2, Chapter 22 ➡).
- Further deterioration could be signified by further fracture; in addition, a kyphotic posture could exacerbate breathing problems associated with pre-existing asthma.

- Currently, the most comprehensive guidance on the management of osteoporosis in the UK is incorporated in The National Osteoporosis Guideline Group (NOGG), which was first produced in 2008 and last updated in July 2010. This provides a clinical guideline for the management of men and women at high risk of fracture **www.shef.ac.uk/NOGG**
- The most recent technology appraisals on drug treatments for primary and secondary prevention of osteoporotic fractures were published in January 2011, with additional reference being made to the use of denosumab in 2010. These are available at **www.nice.org.uk**

- Department of Health (2009) Falls and fractures: effective interventions in health and social care is a series of documents to support the development of services to prevent falls and fractures **www.dh.gov.uk/en/Publicationsandstatistics/dh_103146**

Osteoporosis key points

Because osteoporosis and associated fractures present across a wide domain of specialities, the nursing role needs to be adaptive and flexible according to patient and family needs.

Key features to be addressed include:

- risk factor assessment;
- planning and delivery of practical nursing care with respect to the prevention and management of hip and vertebral fractures, in particular adherence to medication;
- appropriate specific and general lifestyle advice, with a focus on nutritional needs, maintenance of an active lifestyle, and falls prevention;
- liaison with other healthcare professionals;
- psychological support as appropriate.

Hip fracture

Understanding hip fracture

Hip fracture is the most serious of the common fragility fractures. Figure 3.2 illustrates how the types of hip fracture are subdivided into intracapsular and extracapsular depending on their anatomical location in the proximal femur. These fractures are further subdivided depending on whether there is displacement and/or fragmentation (comminution) at the fracture site. Displaced intracapsular fractures disrupt the rather fragile blood supply to the femoral head, and may cause avascular necrosis (when bony tissue in the femoral head dies because of loss of blood supply). Extracapsular fractures often cause substantial blood loss.

Epidemiological profile

About 70,000–75,000 hip fractures occur annually in the UK; this is estimated to rise to 100,000 over the next 10 years (British Orthopaedic Association, 2007). The average age is 83 and at least three-quarters of patients are women. Hip fracture carries a high mortality rate—5–10% at 1 month and 30% at 1 year—and this is higher in men. Two-thirds of the 12-month mortality rate are, however, owing to causes other than the fracture itself. This indicates a high level of comorbidity, and indicates the need for a shared medical and surgical approach to diagnosis and management. The annual UK cost is about £1.4 billion, of which a substantial proportion is caused by hospital bed occupancy. At least one in ten survivors fail to return home, and some degree of residual loss of function is more or less universal.

Presentation and management of hip fracture

Only a small proportion of hip fractures are caused by high-impact trauma or pathologies other than osteoporosis or osteopaenia. The commonest presentation is that of an older person suffering a fall from standing height or lower—a so-called fragility fracture. Pain in the region of the hip and loss of weightbearing ability (particularly in someone previously quite mobile) are key symptoms. Shortening and external rotation of the affected limb are classic signs, but the diagnosis is nevertheless easily missed when these signs are not obvious. Diagnosis with plain radiography is the norm, but this may be difficult when displacement is minimal, and MRI may be required in 2–4% of cases. Delirium is a very common phenomenon with hip fracture, even when there is no prior history of cognitive impairment. The risk of pressure sores is high.

Non-surgical management of hip fracture is now rare. The resulting prolonged pain and immobility, compared with the enhanced safety and effectiveness of modern surgical procedures, regional and general anaesthesia, render it unjustifiable in all but the most exceptional cases (for example, in a clear end-of-life situation). Intracapsular fractures are usually treated either by reduction and fixation or by arthroplasty. Extracapsular fractures are normally fixed either with a sliding hip screw or an intramedullary nail. Delay in operation for other than defined medical reasons is undesirable, and results are worse if surgery takes place later than 48 hours from admission. Regional or general anaesthesia may be used, depending either on an individual's clinical risk status, or on the individual's preference if anaesthetic risk is lower.

Preoperatively, prompt diagnosis, prompt and effective relief of pain, combined surgical, medical, and anaesthetic assessment (including the formulation of a postoperative care and discharge plan) within the framework of a defined orthogeriatric hip fracture programme, and efficient transfer to a trauma ward and subsequently to theatre, are all essential (National Institute for Health and Clinical Excellence, 2011). Pain relief may involve opiates and/or supplementary neural blockade. Adequate rehydration and correction of any electrolyte imbalance are essential.

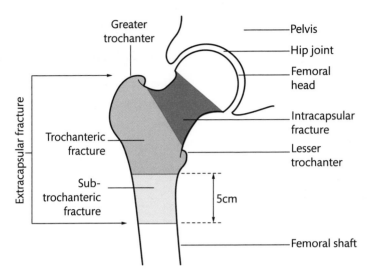

Figure 3.2 Classification of hip fractures.

Reproduced from *Hip Fracture*, Martyn Parker and Antony Johansen, 2006, with permission from BMJ Publishing Group Ltd.

Postoperatively, adequate hydration and nutritional support are required. The use of more specific measures to prevent thromboembolic complications is currently recommended (NICE 2010), although there is surgical debate about the routine use of thromboprophylactic medication in all cases. Weightbearing and mobilization should be initiated the day after surgery, any necessary continued pain relief established, and the organized orthogeriatric team management plan continued. The last may take place entirely within the trauma ward or on an orthogeriatric ward in the acute hospital and may be followed in specific circumstances by further community-based orthogeriatric intervention (such as a short period of supported discharge at home) according to individual need as determined by the orthogeriatric team. This approach includes those admitted from care or nursing homes. Risk of further fracture is high until proved otherwise, and initiation of osteoporosis therapy is more or less routine after hip fracture. Formal falls risk assessment and preventative action should be undertaken as a matter of course.

Assessing the patient with hip fracture and nursing interventions

Nursing assessment is central to the management of hip fracture, both preoperatively and throughout the postoperative period to discharge. In addition to core assessment, close and organized collaboration with other disciplines is required. The appointment of defined orthogeriatric nurse specialists within such a programme has gradually increased. There is considerable overlap of this role with the remit of osteoporosis specialist fracture liaison nurses, and these responsibilities are sometimes combined in a single appointment.

Preoperatively (in accident and emergency)

- Establish all possible rapport with the individual and also with his or her immediate relative(s) and/or carer(s).
- Obtain a full history of the fall, including the immediate circumstances, the background functional status (including cognition), the environment, the medical background (including medication), and in particular any history of previous falls.
- Ensure immediate and subsequent regular assessment and recording of pain (static and dynamic–at least hourly) and response to analgesia (see Part 2, Chapter 25 ➡).
- Facilitate prompt liaison for anaesthetic, surgical, orthogeriatric, and radiological assessment and

decision-making, and for admission to the trauma unit.

- Explore the concerns of the individual and carer(s), and promote understanding of the forward options and plan.
- Undertake an assessment of pressure sore risk and initiate preventative measures (see Part 2, Chapter 27 ➡).
- Achieve adequate hydration status and electrolyte balance (see Part 2, Chapter 19 ➡).
- Assess cognitive status and manage any delirium optimally (see Part 2, Chapter 17 ➡).
- If palliative care only is appropriate, ensure this is managed optimally, including surgery (the best and quickest form of pain relief), except where contraindicated (see Part 2, Chapter 18 ➡).

Postoperatively

- Undertake optimal wound care (see Part 2, Chapter 28 ➡).
- Continue to ensure adequate hydration (see Part 2, Chapter 19 ➡).
- Continue measures to prevent pressure sores (see Part 2, Chapter 27 ➡).
- Collaborate with physiotherapy to establish a mobilization regimen (see Part 2, Chapter 23 ➡) the day after surgery.
- Liaise with all members of the orthogeriatric hip fracture team to clarify and promote the rehabilitation and discharge plan, and ensure regular multidisciplinary review meetings.
- Assist with all activities of daily living as required.
- Review the need for analgesia and assess any ongoing response (see Part 2, Chapter 25 ➡).
- Discuss the forward plan carefully with the individual and carer(s), and encourage all possible avenues of progress.
- Encourage return to normal activity level pre-fracture (or better, where possible).
- Liaise with nursing staff in any additional rehabilitation teams in hospital and/or community.
- Initiate assessment of falls and fracture risk.

Identifying best practice in the management of hip fracture

At the end of the chapter, you will find recent sources of the best evidence to inform the nursing care of patients with hip fractures. To stay up to date and know where to find good-quality sources of evidence, we recommend that readers should utilize the resources listed in the osteoporosis section, as well as journals such as the *International Journal of Trauma and Orthopaedic Nursing*.

Hip fracture key points

Hip fracture is the most serious of the common fragility fractures, with a high mortality rate and a high level of comorbidity. Hence quick and accurate nursing assessment is incredibly important preoperatively. Almost all patients will encounter some degree of residual loss of function, and so postoperative nursing management is very important in reducing potential harm and supporting patients to rehabilitation and discharge.

Key features to be addressed include the following.

Preoperatively

- Prompt assessment and effective management of pain, diagnostic confirmation, cognitive status, pressure sore risk, hydration, and electrolyte balance
- In addition, prompt liaison with the multidisciplinary team for medical and surgical assessment, as well as efficient transfer to a trauma ward and subsequently to theatre

Postoperatively

- Maintain optimal wound care and pain management.
- Ensure hydration and the prevention of pressure sores, and initiate falls assessment.
- From the day after surgery, agree a mobilization strategy with the physiotherapist, and continue multidisciplinary liaison for rehabilitation discharge planning and secondary prevention (to include bone health and falls risk assessments).

- Discuss the forward plan carefully with the individual and carer(s), and encourage return to normal activity level pre-fracture (or better where possible).

Paget's disease

Understanding Paget's disease

Definition

In 1877, Sir James Paget, an eminent British surgeon, described 'osteitis deformans' in an elderly man with progressive skeletal deformities:

> I think we may believe that we have to do with a disease of bones of which the following are the most frequent characteristics:–It begins in middle age or later, is very slow in progress. May continue for many years without influence on the general health and may give no other trouble than those which are due to the changes of shape, size and direction of the diseased bone. (Paget, 1877).

This condition, which subsequently became known as 'Paget's disease' of bone, is characterized by rapid bone remodelling and the formation of bone that is structurally abnormal.

Epidemiological profile of Paget's disease

Paget's disease occurs in 1–2% of white adults over the age of 50, and is more common in men. The prevalence increases substantially with age and, by the eighth decade of life, it has been suggested that it may be present in approximately 8% of men and 5% of women (Van Staa *et al.*, 2002). There is marked ethnic and geographical clustering of the disease, with it being common in some parts of the world, but relatively rare in others. The UK has the greatest prevalence of Paget's disease in the world (Detheridge *et al.*, 1982), with previous research suggesting higher rates of occurrence in Lancashire towns (Barker *et al.*, 1980). Over the past 25 years, the prevalence and severity of disease has reduced substantially in the UK and New Zealand (Poor *et al.*, 2006). This could be explained by modifications of environmental

triggers for the disease and changes in ethnic makeup of the population.

Causation

In Paget's disease, the osteoclasts are greater in size and number and contain many more nuclei than is normal. This causes increased bone resorption during the remodelling cycle, leading to a rapid rate of bone turnover. Increased bone turnover is usually associated with an elevated alkaline phosphatase level shown in blood. The bone subsequently produced is larger than normal, but has disorganized architecture and reduced mechanical strength, thus increasing the risk of fractures and deformities.

Approximately 15–40% of those with Paget's disease have a positive family history, suggesting that genetic factors influence its development. Over recent years, mutations have been identified in four genes that affect the activity of osteoclasts, with the most important one being sequestosome 1 (SQSTM1). This genetic mutation has been reported to account for 20–50% of familial disease resulting in more extensive skeletal involvement (Lucas *et al.*, 2006). It has also been suggested that the disease may result from exposure to a paramyxoviral virus such as measles, respiratory syncytial, or canine distemper virus, but research findings on a viral causation are inconclusive and contradictory (Ralston *et al.*, 2008). Epidemiological studies and observational data have also suggested that other potential environmental triggers may include low dietary calcium intake or vitamin D deficiency in childhood, repetitive mechanical loading, and occupational exposure to toxins.

Common symptoms and problems

Any bone can be affected, but Paget's disease is most commonly found in the spine, skull, pelvis, femur, or tibia (Figure 3.3). The disease may be monostotic, affecting only a single bone or part of a bone, or may be polyostotic, involving two or more bones. Although progression of disease within a given bone may occur, the appearance of new sites after initial diagnosis is uncommon. This information can be very reassuring to patients, who often worry about extension of the disease to new areas of the skeleton as they age.

Frequently, there may be few symptoms associated with Paget's disease and the condition is found by chance if an X-ray or blood test is performed for some other reason.

The commonest features are:

- pain (see Part 2, Chapter 25) (bone pain arising from the affected bone occurs in approximately 80% of symptomatic patients, and is described as 'persistent and nagging', more severe at night, and is not relieved by exercise; there is joint pain when an involved bone is close to a joint, leading to cartilage damage and osteoarthritis);
- deformity (link with Part 2, Chapter 23);
- bowing of long bones;
- skull deformities;

- fracture (link with Part 2, Chapters 23, 25, 26–28);
- fissure fracture;
- complete fracture;
- neurological (link with Part 2, Chapters 23 and 25);
- deafness;
- other cranial nerve palsies;
- spinal cord compressions.

Assessing the patient with Paget's disease

- Establish rapport using listening skills and appropriate non-verbal communication, particularly if the patient has hearing problems.

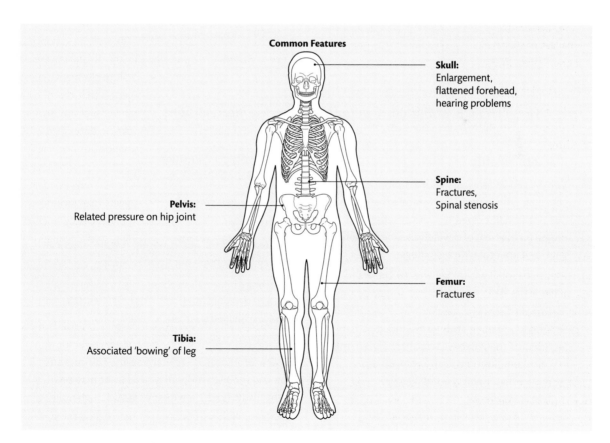

Common Features

Skull:
Enlargement, flattened forehead, hearing problems

Spine:
Fractures, Spinal stenosis

Pelvis:
Related pressure on hip joint

Femur:
Fractures

Tibia:
Associated 'bowing' of leg

Figure 3.3 Common conditions of Paget's disease.

- Clarify full history.
- Access presenting complaint.
- Explore previous medical history.
- Explore medication history.
- Consider family and social history (there is a strong genetic predisposition in Paget's).
- Access mobility and functional capacity.
- Access pain.
- Explore the patient's ideas, concerns, and expectations.

Identifying best practice for Paget's disease

Throughout the text below and at the end of this chapter, you will find recent sources of the best evidence to inform the nursing care of patients with Paget's disease. Because research is always ongoing and best practice evolves, it is important that readers stay up to date and know where to find good-quality sources of evidence. Hence we have provided a list of resources below that readers should utilize.

- Selby, P.L., Davie, M.W.J., Ralston, S.H., Stone, M.D. (2002) Guidelines on the management of Paget's disease of bone. *Bone* **31**(3): 10–19 (On behalf of the Bone and Tooth Society of Great Britain and the Paget's Association)
- Arthritis and Musculoskeletal Alliance (ARMA) (2007) Standards of Care for people with Metabolic Bone Disease. **www.arma.uk.net**

Paget's disease key points

- Whilst Paget's disease is rarely life-threatening, it can be accompanied by some of the classic hallmarks of chronic disease. It is caused by non-reversible pathology, may leave residual disability, and can require a long period of supervision and observation.

CASE STUDY 3.3 *Patient C detailing nurse-led interventions*

Patient profile

Mr C, aged 75, presents with a 3-month history of 'burning' pain in the tibia. He recalls that two paternal uncles had bowed legs. Paget's disease is diagnosed on the basis of elevated alkaline phosphatase level and abnormal X-ray findings.

Nursing management

- Explain disease process
- Discuss meaning of abnormal investigations
- Reassure that effective treatment aims to minimize complications such as bowed legs
- Ensure that mobility is not affected
- Consider falls risk
- Refer to physiotherapist if appropriate
- Explain treatment options
- Discuss analgesia requirements
- Promote positive outlook
- Give written information
- Advise about Paget's Association and its resources

Summary

This patient does not currently require practical nursing intervention but he does need:

- accurate information about Paget's disease;
- treatment guidance;
- advice on lifestyle issues;
- reassurance about his prognosis.

In view of increased skeletal fragility, falls prevention and mobility issues may need to be addressed in the future (Part 2, Chapter 23 ⟶).

Further deterioration could be indicated by increased pain at the pagetic site, pressure on adjacent joints, and deformity.

- Some patients and families may be confused about the nature of the condition, and concerned about the possibility of future complications, including fracture and deformity.

- There are those who are frightened by perceived or actual side effects of medication, and in some cases patients may have unfair expectations of the outcome of therapy.

- Pain is a common feature of Paget's disease, and if this becomes chronic, it may lead to anxiety, depression, social isolation, and failure to cope with everyday activities.

Osteoarthritis

Understanding osteoarthritis

Osteoarthritis is a clinical syndrome of joint pain, variable limitation of function, and reduced quality of life. The joints most commonly involved are the knee, hip (see Figure 3.2), small hand joints (see Figure 3.3), and spine. Structural changes visible on X-ray are, however, commonly found in the absence of symptoms (up to 50% of instances) (Arthritis and Musculoskeletal Alliance, 2004), and this, together with the observation that all joint tissues—cartilage, bone, capsule, ligaments, and muscle—are involved, has supported a concept of the underlying process as one of repair. Symptomatic osteoarthritis occurs when the 'inflammatory' component of the repair process is highly active, or when the extent of joint damage outstrips the capacity of the repair process. The traditional view of osteoarthritis as simple or exclusive 'wear and tear' is no longer tenable, especially when this is linked to an equally fallacious perception of ageing processes. Osteoarthritis is not an element of so-called 'normal' ageing.

Epidemiological profile of osteoarthritis

Estimating the true prevalence of osteoarthritis is difficult because radiographic changes (with or without symptoms) have been used as the basis of diagnosis and grading in most major studies. The difficulty is compounded by the advent of more sensitive imaging techniques. As many as 10% of the UK population over 55 years old, however, are estimated to have painful, disabling knee osteoarthritis (Arthritis Research Campaign, 2002). Less reliable estimates include 3% for the hand and 5–9% for the hip. Pain and its impact on mobility have a profound effect on people's lives, leading in turn to an enormous demand on health and social care systems, and to a negative effect on the national economy from lost work time (Arthritis Research Campaign, 2002). As the population ages, osteoarthritis is expected to become the fourth leading cause of disability worldwide by 2020. About 5% of the UK population aged over 45, and 10% over 75, see their GP annually with osteoarthritis-related complaints. The annual NHS cost of hip and knee replacement surgery is close to £50 million. About 1% of total GNP is lost to the economy by osteoarthritis, if lost work days are included.

Causation

Osteoarthritis is multifactorial in its causation. Contributing factors include:

- genetics (40–60% estimated contribution in peripheral osteoarthritis);
- host factors (in particular, age, female gender, obesity);
- local mechanical stress (for example, from muscle weakness or injury).

At least some of these can be modified by interventions, including changes in lifestyle.

Host factors

- **Age:** There is a simple arithmetic increase in the prevalence of osteoarthritis with age up to about 50–55, after which the age-associated increase rises more steeply and progressively.

- **Gender:** Below the age of 45, trauma-related local osteoarthritis in men is the commonest cause. Above the age of 55, osteoarthritis involving several joints, notably the hand joints and knees, is commoner in women. The effect of gender on hip osteoarthritis in later life is unclear.

- **Race:** Osteoarthritis occurs in all races. Hip osteoarthritis appears, however, to be less common in Asians than in Caucasians, while knee osteoarthritis may be commoner in Asians and Afro-Caribbeans.

- **Obesity:** The proportion of cases of osteoarthritis partly attributable to obesity has been estimated as

63% in the middle-aged and 25% in the older population. The relationship is closest for knee osteoarthritis. It has been found that losing weight may halve the risk of progression.

Diagnosis is typically in an individual aged over 45 with joint pain made worse with use, and morning joint stiffness lasting less than an hour. Investigation to exclude other types of inflammatory arthritis is important where there is any doubt. Exercise, medication to relieve pain, inflammation, or both, weight reduction where necessary, self-management strategies, and joint replacement surgery are the mainstays of treatment. The long-term prognosis for hand osteoarthritis is often good. The likelihood and rate of progression to joint replacement are greatest for hip osteoarthritis, followed by knee.

Assessing the patient with osteoarthritis

The nature of osteoarthritis and its impact on an individual's life dictate the need for a broad and holistic assessment that constitutes a major, but potentially rewarding, challenge to nursing intervention. Key assessment domains include the following.

- Pain—its location, severity, relationship to activity, and response to analgesia
- Mood—the effect of osteoarthritis on mood (especially depression or anxiety)
- Sleep—its quality and quantity
- Understanding—knowledge of osteoarthritis, its nature, prognosis, and options for treatment
- Function—mobility, activities of daily living, need for home space, or other environmental modification
- Lifestyle—employment, leisure, family life
- Support—carer/family relationships, social network
- Exercise—characteristics at presentation and attitudes to possible changes in pattern
- Weight and nutrition—contribution of weight excess (if any) and attitudes to dietary and exercise modification
- Comorbidity—possible implications for medication use and fitness for surgical intervention

---

CASE STUDY 3.4 *Patient D, nursing advice and interventions*

Ms D, aged 56, is a school music teacher (piano and choral), living alone, with normal body mass index, loss of medial joint space, and osteophytes on knee X-ray. She has a maternal history of severe multiple joint osteoarthritis. She has 4 years' progressive typical pain in the right knee, which is worse after standing for teaching sessions, and severe after walking half a mile to the shops. She has had to take several days off work in past 6 months because of pain severity. She is becoming less mobile and active, finds the stairs at home difficult, and has fallen several times over the same period. Her knee joint sometimes 'gels' (locks). She takes occasional oral ibuprofen as necessary, but dislikes taking tablets. She is now developing pain in the distal joints of the right hand.

Nursing interventions

- Discuss pain management. Advise on safe use of paracetamol (regular?) and topical non-steroidal (Part 2, Chapters 22 and 25 ➡).
- Reassure that arthroscopy is not required, but consider fitness for surgery should replacement eventually become necessary.
- Assist with mobility and advise physiotherapy assessment for exercise programme (Part 2, Chapter 23 ➡).
- Initiate falls risk assessment (Part 2, Chapter 23 ➡).
- Assess mood—possible depression, as well as anxiety regarding work and prognosis (in view of maternal history and hand symptoms) (Part 2, Chapter 28 ➡).

CASE STUDY 3.5 *Patient E, nursing strategies*

Mr E, aged 82, is a married retired civil servant. He is obese, hypertensive, does not smoke, and has type 2 diabetes for which he takes insulin. He is becoming progressively immobile and housebound owing to severe left hip OA with advanced X-ray changes. He has a mild right Parkinsonian tremor. He is reluctant to consider surgery.

Nursing interventions

* Reassure regarding feasibility and results of hip replacement, irrespective of age and allowing for diabetes and mild Parkinsonism (Part 1, Chapter 9 →).

* Review home circumstances and mood, and establish contact with wife (Part 2, Chapter 14 →).
* Discuss dietary measures for weight reduction, improved diabetic control, and possible dietitian referral with both (Part 2, Chapters 22 and 24 →).
* Review pain management, including risks/benefits of non-steroidal drugs (Part 2, Chapters 22 and 25 →).
* Assess mobility and advise physiotherapy assessment for mobility and exercise programme (Part 2, Chapter 23 →).

Identifying best practice in the management of osteoarthritis

At the end of the chapter, you will find recent sources of the best evidence to inform the nursing care of patients with osteoarthritis. To stay up to date with best practice, we recommend that you frequently consult these sources.

Osteoarthritis key points

* Osteoarthritis is a clinical syndrome of joint pain (typically the spine, knee, hip, hand, and shoulder joints) with variable limitation of function and reduced quality of life. Nurses play a key role in helping patients to manage the impact of the condition on their lives.
* Key areas for assessment include pain, function (particularly mobility), mood, weight and nutrition, exercise, lifestyle, and medication.
* Liaison with the multidisciplinary team is essential to ensure mobility and good mental health.

Sources of evidence

Osteoporosis

Organizations

National Osteoporosis Society (NOS): patient and public support. Formal network for all healthcare professionals offering education and information **www.nos. org.uk**

Recommended journals

Osteoporosis Review (quarterly journal of NOS) published by Hayward Medical Communications (available free of charge on joining NOS).

Osteoporosis International, a multidisciplinary international journal which is a joint initiative between the International Osteoporosis Foundation and The National Osteoporosis Foundation of USA (subscription) **www. springer.com/medicine/orthop/journal/198**

Hip fracture

National Institute for Health and Clinical Excellence (NICE) Clinical Guideline on Hip Fracture (June 2011)

Scottish Intercollegiate Guidelines Network (SIGN) Guideline 111 (2009) Management of hip fracture in older people **http://www.sign.ac.uk/guidelines/fulltext/111/index.html**

The British Orthopaedic Association/British Geriatrics Society 'Blue Book': Care of patients with fragility fractures **http://www.fractures.com/pdf/BOA-BGS-Blue-Book.pdf**

The National Service Framework for Older People (2001) Standard 6: Falls and Fractures **http://www.dh.gov.uk/en/Publicationsandstatistics/Publications/PublicationsPolicyAndGuidance/DH_4003066**

Recommended journal articles

Ftouh S., Morga A., Swift C. (2011) Management of hip fracture in adults: summary of NICE guidance. *British Medical Journal* **342**(3304).

Parker, M., Johansen, A. (2006) Hip fracture. *British Medical Journal* **333**(7557): 27–30.

Paget's disease

Organizations

Paget's Association: patient and public support. Formal network for all healthcare professionals offering education and information **www.paget.org.uk**

Recommended journal articles

Ralston, S.H., Langston, A.L., Reid, I.R. (2008) Pathogenesis and management of Paget's disease of bone. *Lancet* **372**: 155–63.

Sutcliffe, A. (2009) Paget's disease. 1: Epidemiology, causes and clinical features. *Nursing Times*, February 17–23: **105**(6): 14–15.

Sutcliffe, A. (2009) Paget's disease. 2: Exploring diagnosis, management and support strategies. *Nursing Times*, 24 February–2 March: **105**(7): 14–15.

Sutcliffe, A. (2010) Paget's: the neglected bone disease. *International Journal of Trauma and Orthopaedic Nursing* **14**(3): 142–9.

Osteoarthritis

NICE Clinical Guideline 59 (2008) on osteoarthritis **http://guidance.nice.org.uk/CG59/NICEGuidance/pdf/English**

Arthritis and Musculoskeletal Alliance (2004) *Standards of Care for People with Osteoarthritis*. London: ARMA **http://www.arma.uk.net/pdfs/oa06.pdf**

Arthritis Care **www.arthritiscare.org.uk/AboutArthritis/Conditions/Osteoarthritis**

Arthritis Research UK **http://www.arthritisresearchuk.org/arthritis_information/arthritis_types__symptoms/osteoarthritis.aspx**

Conclusion

Bone conditions are major causes of morbidity, substantially affecting patients' health and quality of life, and are of substantial economic cost to health and society (Oliver, 2009). Whilst bone diseases vary from those that are not life-threatening to those with high morbidity, patients commonly experience loss or limitation of function and disability. Pain is a hallmark feature, and if it becomes chronic, it may lead to anxiety, depression, social isolation, and failure to cope with everyday activities. Nurses play a key role in assessing patients' well-being in both acute and chronic situations, and in turn recognize both potentially dangerous comorbidity and changes in long-term symptoms. Managing conditions proactively to improve functional ability and life expectancy, and the education of patients to enable them to deal with symptoms effectively, are key elements of the nursing role (Oliver, 2009).

Online Resource Centre

 To help you to develop and apply your knowledge and decision-making skills further, we have provided interactive learning resources online at: **www.oxfordtextbooks.co.uk/orc/bullock**.

Whilst these are freely available, you will need to use the access codes at the start of the book.

References

Arthritis and Musculoskeletal Alliance (ARMA) (2007) Standards of care for people with metabolic bone disease. **www.arma. uk.net** (accessed 11 October 2011).

Arthritis Research Campaign (2002) Arthritis: the big picture. **http://www.ipsos-mori.com/Assets/Docs/Archive/Polls/ arthritis.pdf** (accessed 11 October 2011).

Barker, D.J., Chamberlain, A.T., Guyer, P.B., *et al.* (1980) Paget's disease of bone: the Lancashire focus. *British Medical Journal* **280**: 1105–7.

British Orthopaedic Association (2007) The care of patients with fragility fractures. **http://www.fractures.com/pdf/BOA-BGS- Blue-Book.pdf** (accessed 11 October 2011).

Burge, R.T., Worley, D., Johansen, A., *et al.* (2001) The cost of osteoporotic fractures in the UK. *Journal of Medical Economics* **4**: 51–62.

Detheridge, F.M., Guyer, P.B., Barker, D.J. (1982) European distribution of Paget's disease of bone. *British Medical Journal (clinical research edn)* **285**: 1005–8.

Lucas, G.J., Daroszewska, A., Ralston, S.H. (2006) Contribution of genetic factors to the pathogenesis of Paget's disease of bone and related disorders. *Journal of Bone and Mineral Research* **21**(Suppl. 2): 31–7.

Masud, T., Binkley, N., Boonen, S., *et al.* on behalf of the FRAX® Position Development Conference members (2011) Official positions for FRAX® Clinical regarding falls and frailty: can falls and frailty be used in FRAX? *Journal of Clinical Densitometry: Assessment of Skeletal Health* **14**(3): 194–204.

National Hip Fracture Database (2010) *The National Hip Fracture Database Report (Extended Version).* **http://www.nhfd. co.uk/003/hipfractureR.nsf/NHFD_National_Report_ Extended_2010.pdf** (accessed 11 October 2011).

National Institute for Health and Clinical Excellence (2010) Reducing the risk of venous thromboembolism (deep vein thrombosis and pulmonary embolism) in patients admitted to hospital. NICE Clinical Guideline 92 (CG92). **http://guidance. nice.org.uk/CG92**

National Institute for Health and Clinical Excellence (2011) The Management of hip fracture in adults. NICE Clinical Guidance 124 (CG124). **http://guidance.nice.org.uk/CG124** (accessed 11 October 2011).

Oliver, S.M. (2009) *Oxford Handbook of Musculoskeletal Nursing.* Oxford University Press: Oxford.

Paget, J. (1877) A form of chronic inflammation of bones (osteitis deformans). *Medico-Chirurgical Transactions (London)* **60**: 37–64.

Parker, M., Johansen, A. (2006) Hip fracture. *British Medical Journal* **333**(7557): 27–30.

Peat, G., McCarney, R., Croft, P. (2001) Knee pain and osteoarthritis in older adults: a review of community burden and current use of primary health care. *Annals of the Rheumatic Diseases* **60**(2): 91–7.

Poor, G., Donath, J., Fornet, B., *et al.* (2006) Epidemiology of Paget's disease in Europe: the prevalence is decreasing. *Journal of Bone and Mineral Research* **21**: 1545–9.

Ralston, S.H., Langston, A.L., Reid, I.R. (2008) Pathogenesis and management of Paget's disease. *Lancet* **372**: 155–63.

Van Staa, T.P., Selby, P., Leufkens, H.G., *et al.* (2002) Incidence and natural history of Paget's disease of bone in England and Wales. *Journal of Bone and Mineral Research* **17**: 465–71.

World Health Organization (1994) Assessment of fracture risk and its application to screening for postmenopausal osteoporosis. Technical Report Series No. 843. WHO: Geneva.

4 *Understanding* **Cancer**

Cathy Hughes

Introduction

The aim of this chapter is provide an overview of cancer, a biologically similar, but diverse, group of diseases. Understanding the disease process will help the practising nurse to plan nursing care and to seek appropriate specialist advice. Cancer can affect almost any part of the body and has significance for different age groups and within different cultures, so the effect on the individual, the prognosis, and the treatment will significantly differ depending upon cancer site and treatment setting. This chapter will outline symptoms in relation to the site of the body affected to illustrate the effect of cancer on an individual, and consideration will also be given to the wider impact of the disease. This chapter is underpinned by the principles of evidence-based patient-centred care and will focus on the concepts associated with promoting lifestyles that reduce the risk of developing cancer, screening to identify those at risk, detection of early disease, and the care and management of the individual with and beyond cancer.

Understanding cancer

Defining cancer

Cancer refers to a condition in which there is abnormal growth of cells. The characteristics of cancer cells are that they divide uncontrollably, do not require stimulation for growth as do normal cells, and are not restrained by the presence of neighbouring cells. Because cancer is concerned with a failure in the growth control mechanism of the cell at a gene or DNA level and because there are potentially as many different types of cancer as there are types of body cell, no two cancers are exactly alike (Cancer Research UK, 2009).

The site at which a cancer first develops (primary cancer), such as lung or breast, is often used broadly to describe it; however, cancer is generally defined by the origin of the type of cell that has become cancerous. The most frequent sites and types of cancer are as follows.

- Carcinomas—arise in epithelial cells in the skin, gastrointestinal tract, and other internal organs, and make up about 85% of all cancers (Cancer Research UK, 2010a)
- Haematological (blood and lymphatic system) cancers—arise from blood or bone marrow cells; include leukaemia, lymphoma, and myeloma, and make up about 7% of all cancers, but leukaemia is the commonest cancer in children (Cancer Research UK, 2010b)

- Brain and central nervous system cancers—arise from cells in the brain and central nervous system; most brain cancers develop from glial cells that support nerve cells in the brain; they are generally uncommon, less than 2% of all cancers (Ferlay *et al.*, 2008), but are the second commonest cancer type in children (Cancer Research UK, 2011a)
- Sarcomas—arise from cells in the soft tissues (muscles, blood vessels, adipose tissues) and bone; sarcomas are rare and make up about 1% of all cancers, but about 11% of cancers in children (Cancer Research UK, 2010b)

Each cancer site and type will be more accurately named as relevant to the subspecialty, and is significant to understanding treatment and prognosis. Table 4.1 lists some common examples of classifications of cancer.

Prevalence and epidemiological profile of cancer

About half of the countries worldwide collect cancer incidence (the number of people with a new diagnosis

of cancer) and cancer mortality data. Cancer statistics generally include all cancers except non-melanoma skin cancer (NMSC) because they are very common and have been shown to be under-reported in cancer registration data. The World Health Organization's (WHO) International Agency for Research on Cancer (IARC) collects and interprets all of the available data. The Globocan 2008 database currently holds the most up-to-date information at the International Agency for Research on Cancer (IARC) and these data are freely available on its website **www.iarc.fr**.

Incidence

In 2008, the IARC estimated that 12.7 million new cases of cancer were diagnosed across the world. The five most frequently diagnosed cancer sites were lung (1.61 million), breast (1.38 million), colorectum (1.23 million), stomach (0.99 million), and prostate (0.90 million) (Ferlay *et al.*, 2008) (Figure 4.1).

Table 4.1 Examples of different types of cancer and their cellular origin

Types	Cellular origin/description
Squamous cell carcinoma	A cancer that arises from squamous epithelial cells
Adenocarcinoma	A cancer that arises from glandular epithelial cells
Mesothelioma	A cancer that arises from the mesothelial cells, which cover the surface of most of the internal organs. This type of cancer most commonly, but not exclusively, develops in the lungs and is often caused by exposure to asbestos (Cancer Research UK, 2010c)
Ductal breast carcinoma	A cancer that arises in the cells that line the ducts of the breasts
Lobular breast carcinoma	A cancer that arises in the lobules or lobes of the breast
Carcinoid	A cancer that arises in the hormone-producing neuroendocrine cells. Most carcinoid cancers are found in the digestive system, but they can develop in other places such as the lung, pancreas, or kidneys (Cancer Research UK, 2010d)
Leukaemia—includes: - acute and chronic myeloid leukaemia (AML and CML) - acute and chronic lymphoblastic leukaemia (ALL and CLL)	A cancer that arises in the cells of the blood-forming system in the bone marrow AML and CML arise from the myeloid white blood cells ALL and CLL arise from the lymphoid white blood cells
Myeloma	A cancer that arises in plasma cells in the bone marrow
Lymphoma	A cancer that arises in the lymphocyte white blood cells of the lymphatic system
Osteosarcoma	A cancer that arises in bone cells

However, there is significant regional variation in the most commonly diagnosed cancers and marked differences between developing and developed countries. For example, cervical cancer (cervix uteri) is the most frequently diagnosed cancer in India (23 women per 100,000), but it is the 19th most frequently diagnosed cancer in the UK (9 women per 100,000) (World Health Organization/Institut Catala d'Oncologià (WHO/ICO), 2010).

There are also gender differences (Figure 4.2), not just because prostate cancer is found only in men or ovarian cancer in women. For example, men are currently more likely to develop lung cancer and women more likely to develop thyroid cancer (Ferlay *et al.*, 2008).

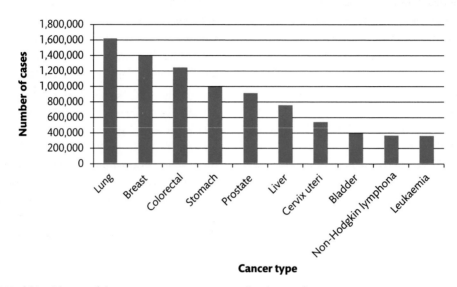

Figure 4.1 **World incidence of the 10 commonest cancers (both sexes).**

Data obtained from the Globocan 2008 database at the International Agency for Research on Cancer (Ferlay *et al.*, 2008).

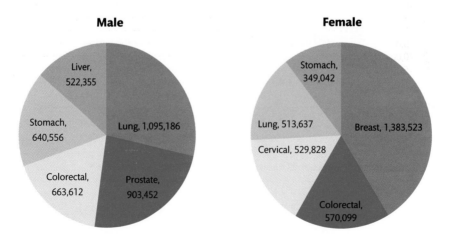

Figure 4.2 **World incidence of male and female cancers.**

Data obtained from the Globocan 2008 database at the International Agency for Research on Cancer (Ferlay *et al.*, 2008).

In the UK, just over 300,000 new cases of cancer were diagnosed in 2008. The commonest cancers were breast, lung, colorectal, and prostate, accounting for over half of all cases (Ferlay *et al.*, 2008) (Figure 4.3).

Mortality

Although advances in detection and treatment have improved mortality rates, cancer remains a significant cause of death. In 2008, around 156,000 patients died of cancer in the UK alone. Worldwide, the most frequent sites causing cancer deaths were lung (1.38 million), stomach (0.74 million), liver (0.69 million), colorectum (0.61 million), and breast (0.46 million). Mortality rates are generally higher in poorer countries and in deprived areas than wealthier ones. Although this difference has not been widely studied, it has often been attributed to accessibility of healthcare (Boyle and Levin, 2008). Factors such as increased exposure to industrial chemicals, poorer nutrition, and lifestyle (including long working hours) could also contribute to mortality differences.

Survival and morbidity

Cancer survivorship is an area of increasing attention and investment. In 2008, an estimated 28 million people were living within 5 years of a cancer diagnosis (Ferlay *et al.*, 2008), and these numbers are increasing because incidence rates are rising while mortality falls (Cancer Research UK, 2011c). Cancer statistics often relate to the first 5 years after diagnosis, but cancer survivorship is concerned with people to and beyond 5 years, with or without active disease (National Coalition for Cancer Survivorship, 2010).

Although morbidity and prevalence are used interchangeably to refer to the presence of disease or illness in an individual or population, morbidity in addition also refers to illness that arises as a result of treatment. Cancer treatments are associated with short- and long-term morbidity and the concept of cancer survivorship includes supporting patients with the after-effects of treatment. In England, the National Cancer Survivorship Initiative (NCSI) aims to 'improve the on-going services and support to those living with, and beyond, cancer' (Macmillan Cancer Support, 2011). The increasing numbers of people who have and have had cancer make it increasingly likely that nurses will be involved with cancer patients during their initial cancer journeys, or long after diagnosis when the consequences of the disease or treatment impact a person's long-term health or well-being. This is especially important in children, among whom survival rates can be higher: in the UK, the overall mortality from cancer was about 51% of the overall incidence, but about 20% in children under 15 years old (Ferlay *et al.*, 2008).

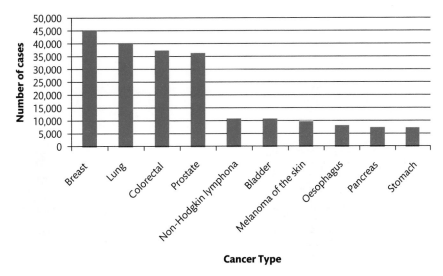

Figure 4.3 **UK incidence of the 10 commonest cancers (both sexes).**

Data obtained from the Globocan 2008 database at the International Agency for Research on Cancer (Ferlay *et al.*, 2008).

Causation

The development of cancer is a multistep process that occurs as a result of changes in critical genes (mutations) that control cell division, growth, and death. In most situations, these changes are acquired over time, but they can also be inherited from parents. Agents that cause damage to genes that ultimately lead to the development of cancer are called carcinogens (American Cancer Society, 2011a). Common carcinogens include tobacco and ultraviolet light (see 'Risk factors').

The aetiology and pathophysiological processes that underlie cancer

Cells are the structural units from which all living organisms are made. The human body consists of trillions of cells, and multicellular life forms depend upon the balance and regulation of cellular functions such as reproduction, growth, development, tissue repair, and regeneration. For all cells, there is a time to die; this may occur because of damage or as part of a natural process of cell death (such as apoptosis) and replication.

The regulation of cell division and cell death is critical to normal tissue structure and function. There are many different genes involved with cell division, DNA repair (to minimize mutations and stop the transmission of any damaged genetic material to subsequent cells), and cell death. Two types of gene are commonly associated with this process: proto-oncogenes and tumour suppressor genes (Box 4.1). Proto-oncogenes encode proteins in a controlled fashion to stimulate cell division and halt cell death, but when they are mutated to become oncogenes, they lead to the uninhibited production of these proteins, leading to the type of abnormality associated with cancer, i.e. uncontrolled growth (Chial, 2008). Tumour suppressor genes are genes that slow down cell division, repair DNA mistakes, and induce cell death. When they become mutated, cells are left to grow out of control, acquire mutations that are not repaired, and are not subject to cell death (American Cancer Society, 2009).

The immune system should also identify any abnormal cells and destroy them, locally or in lymph nodes. However, if errors occur and/or safety mechanisms fail, then the cell has the potential to grow out of control, as discussed above. Individual errors in the control mechanisms of the gene may not be significant, but repeated errors, or certain defects, will result in the formation an uncontrolled, immortal cell (Figure 4.4).

When these uncontrolled cells begin to multiply, they form a mass called a neoplasm, which often (but not always) causes a lump or solid tumour to form. Neoplasms are not necessarily cancers: they may be benign, pre-malignant, or malignant. A neoplasm that is benign does not invade and destroy the tissue in which it originates or to which it spreads; however, it can cause mortality by compressing or obstructing vital structures. A neoplasm that has the ability to invade neighbouring tissues and spread to other organs is malignant or cancerous (Figure 4.5). For example, a tumour in the smooth muscle of the uterus could be a benign neoplasm called a leiomyoma (fibroid); alternatively, it could be a malignant neoplasm called a leiomyosarcoma.

When cancer cells spread from the primary site to other parts of the body (secondary sites), it is called metastasis. This requires invasion of the cancerous cells through the surrounding tissues and penetration of a system for transportation (intravasation), escape from that transport system (extravasation), and growth at a new site with the development of a new blood supply (angiogenesis). The three ways in which cancer cells are transferred to other sites in the body are: via blood vessels; via lymphatic vessels; and within body cavities. Cancer metastasis is not random, and certain cancer cells will grow only in certain receptive environments (the 'seed and soil' concept described in 1889 by Paget). For example, lung, prostate, kidney, and breast cancer commonly spread to bone (Cancer Research UK, 2010e), but brain cancer is more likely to remain in the brain and spinal cord (American Cancer Society, 2011b).

Box 4.1 **Oncogenes and tumour suppressor genes**

Cell growth or proliferation is a normal process that is initiated and discontinued by genes. In general, a mutated gene that promotes abnormal cell proliferation is called an 'oncogene' and a gene that inhibits proliferation is called a 'tumour suppressor gene'.

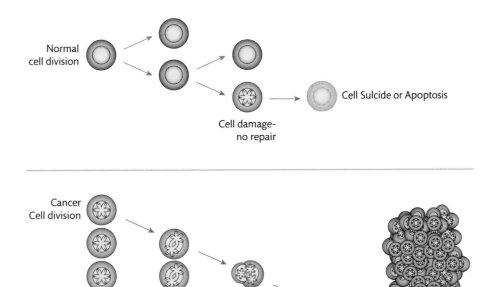

Figure 4.4 Loss of Normal Growth Control.

National Cancer Institute **http://www.cancer.gov/.** Based on artwork originally created for the National Cancer Institute by Jeanne Kelly.

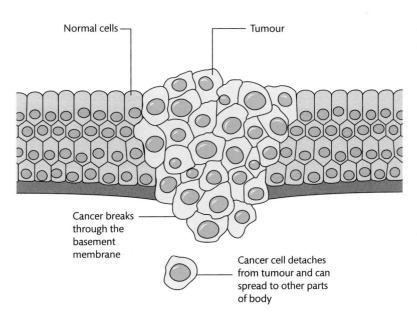

Figure 4.5 The formation of malignant tumours.

Reproduced with permission of Cancerhelp UK.

Risk factors

Age

Cancer is a major condition of old age. It most commonly occurs in older people because the multiple mutations associated with cancer are more likely to have accumulated over time, and the ability of the cell to repair damage becomes less effective with age (WHO, 2011a). In the UK, 65% of the cases are seen in people aged over 65, with less than 1% in children under 15 years old (Ferlay *et al.*, 2008).

Lifestyle and environment

Most of the geographical variation of cancer type and cancer risk is caused by lifestyle and environmental exposure to carcinogens. Tobacco use accounts for about one-third of all cases, and obesity has been associated with an increased incidence of a range of cancers, including breast, bowel, endometrial, oesophageal, pancreatic, and kidney (Boyle and Levin, 2008). The current numbers of people who are overweight and obese in the UK could lead to about 10,000 new cases of cancer each year (Renehan *et al.*, 2010). Other lifestyle factors include exposure to sunlight, alcohol consumption, lack of physical exercise, diet, pollution, and occupational exposure to carcinogens (WHO, 2011b).

Infections

Up to about one-quarter of all cancers are induced by infections such as human papillomavirus (HPV) (associated with oral and genital cancers), *Helicobacter pylori* (associated with stomach cancer), and Epstein–Barr virus (associated with lymphoma) (Boyle and Levin, 2008). Human immunodeficiency virus (HIV) currently affects around 33.4 million people worldwide (United Nations Programme on HIV/AIDS (UNAIDS) and WHO, 2009). Cancers such as Kaposi's sarcoma, non-Hodgkin's lymphoma, and cervical cancer are AIDS-defining conditions. This means that, when an individual who is HIV-positive develops one of these cancers, he or she is then described as having AIDS.

Heredity

Although inherited mutations can contribute to the development of cancer, they make only a minor contribution (5–10%) to the development of most types of the disease (Lichtenstein *et al.*, 2000). Genes have been identified for several of the main inherited cancers, such as the *BRCA* (breast cancer) gene in breast and ovarian cancer, or the genes associated with Lynch syndrome (also referred to as hereditary non-polyposis colorectal cancer) (Arden-Jones *et al.*, 2010; Loud and Hutson, 2010).

Cancer burden

Cancer was traditionally considered to be a disease of Western industrialized nations, but today the major cancer burden is in low- and medium-resource, or developing, countries. The incidence of cancer is increasing globally, partly because of the increases in life expectancy and obesity (Boyle and Levin, 2008). By 2030, it has been estimated that there will be 27 million new cases, 17 million deaths, and 75 million people living with the disease (Boyle and Levin, 2008).

The NHS spends about 5.6% of its budget on cancer, equating to around £4.5 billion per year in England alone (Cancer Research UK, 2008). According to Hospital Episode Statistic (HES) data, the total inpatient Finished Consultant Episodes (FCE) for patients coded as having 'malignant neoplasm' in England in 2009–10 was almost 1.4 million. Cancer site-specific data reflects the variation in disease profile and management. For example, in breast cancer, the mean length of hospital stay was 3.9 days, but in cancers of the digestive tract, this was 10.5 days (The Health and Social Care Information Centre, 2010 **http://www.hesonline.nhs.uk**).

Cancer control

Cancer prevention is a complex concept that is changing with our deeper understanding of the disease and advances in technology. There are essentially four levels of disease prevention (Starfield *et al.*, 2008), and the term that encompasses all of these strategies is cancer control.

- Primary prevention reduces the risk of a healthy individual developing the disease.
- Secondary prevention defines high-risk individuals and concentrates on early detection.
- Tertiary prevention reduces morbidity by preventing complications.
- Quaternary prevention involves avoiding the consequences of excessive medical interventions.

According to the IARC, the four pillars of cancer control are: prevent those cancers that can be prevented; treat those cancers that can be treated; cure those cancers that can be cured; and provide palliation wherever palliation is required (Boyle and Levin, 2008). The World Health Organization has produced a series of publications aimed at population-based strategies for cancer prevention (WHO, 2011c).

Since at least one-third of all cancers can be prevented, strategies to tackle the risks associated with cancer (see 'Risk factors') have a part to play in the reduction of cancer incidence (Boyle and Levin, 2008). Nurses lead many such projects and most nurses have a role to play in promoting healthy lifestyles to patients as part of their everyday practice. Nursing organizations across the world have lobbied governments to improve cancer-related health. For example, the Royal College of Nursing campaigned for and supported a private member's Bill for legislation on the use of sunbeds (Ford, 2009).

Vaccinations can offer prevention for infection-related cancers and are already available for hepatitis B (liver cancer) and human papillomavirus (cervical cancer). In the UK, all schoolgirls aged 12–13 are offered vaccination against the HPV strains that most commonly cause cervical cancer. The vaccination programme is primarily delivered by school nurses and includes giving information for consent. This has been complicated by the moral objection that some parents and schools have expressed about vaccinating children against a sexually transmitted infection (National Cervical Cancer Coalition, 2007).

Screening

Screening for cancer involves the testing of a symptomless population to detect early or pre-malignant disease. In the UK:

- breast screening involves assessing women for the presence of early disease;
- cervical screening involves assessing women for the presence of pre-malignant lesions that may become cancer if left untreated; and
- bowel screening involves assessing individuals for the presence of early cancer or for polyps that can be removed to reduce the risk of developing the disease.

Prostate cancer screening programmes are not currently considered to fulfil the screening criteria. This is because, with available screening techniques, harm potentially outweighs benefit. In England, prostate risk management involves ensuring that men have the information required to make decisions on PSA (prostate-specific antigen) testing and treatment.

The screening programme for prostate cancer could save up to 8,400 lives a year in the UK (Cancer Research UK, 2011d), but it remains a contentious issue, primarily because of the financial cost (an estimated £3.29 billion per year in England alone) (NHS Cancer Screening Programme, 2011), number of lives saved (Autier *et al.*, 2011), harm from overdiagnosis and overtreatment (Duffy *et al.*, 2010; Hakama *et al.*, 2008), selection bias (where those at least risk attend), and understanding of risk (Dillard *et al.*, 2010). Nurses are involved in cancer screening programmes from encouraging individuals to attend through to providing clinical services in which nurses take cervical samples for cytology, work in breast and bowel screening units, and perform colposcopy and colonoscopy, etc. (NHS Cancer Screening Programme, 2011).

Assessing the patient with cancer

Detecting and diagnosing

Cancer can be detected during screening, as an incidental finding during a physical examination or investigation, as the result of a patient presenting to a healthcare practitioner with symptoms, or at post mortem. After prevention, the next most significant method of cancer control is early diagnosis, because cancer diagnosed earlier is more likely to be cured (see 'Stage and grade').

Earlier diagnosis of cancer has been a key strategy in cancer control campaigns in the UK since the European Cancer Registry-based Study on Survival and Care of Cancer Patients project highlighted the poor UK cancer survival rates in relation to comparable European countries (EUROCARE, 2010). Estimates suggest that up to 10,000 lives per year could be saved in England alone if cancers were diagnosed earlier (Richards, 2009), and the National Awareness and Early Diagnosis Initiative (NAEDI) was announced in the Cancer Reform Strategy (Department of Health, 2007) to coordinate and 'provide support to activities and research that promote earlier diagnosis of cancer' (see 'Identifying best practice').

Early changes in the cells or relatively small areas of abnormality may not be significant enough to affect how the tissue or organ functions and therefore do not always cause symptoms. Cancer detected during screening or as an incidental finding is usually asymptomatic. The diagnosis of symptomatic cancer relies on the recognition of the significance of the symptom by the patient and/or the healthcare practitioner (National Patient Safety Agency (NPSA), 2010). The main warning signs for cancer are:

- any unusual lump or swelling—including unusual change in the breast;
- any obvious change in a wart or mole;
- a sore that does not heal, including mouth ulcers;
- persistent cough or croaky voice;
- persistent indigestion or difficulty swallowing;
- unusual bleeding or discharge, including vaginal bleeding between periods or after the menopause;
- change in bowel or bladder habit;
- unexplained weight loss;
- unexplained persistent abdominal pain or discomfort.

(Based on National Institute for Health and Clinical Excellence (NICE), 2005/2011; Vogel, 2011)

These signs and symptoms alone may not always be predictive of cancer. Clusters of symptoms and/or conditions have been shown to increase the likelihood of cancer being present (Hamilton, 2009), but the presence of any of these should alert individuals to seek advice from a healthcare practitioner. It is important for nurses to be able to recognize the warning signs for cancer and know where to access local information on appropriate referral for assessment or reassurance.

Stage and grade

The diagnostic process for a patient with cancer involves defining the grade and stage of cancer. Grading of a cancer refers to the appearance of the cancer cells under the microscope and defines how closely they resemble the original cells. Cancer cells that closely resemble the original normal cells (well differentiated) are usually defined as being of a lower grade, such as grade 1. Cancer cells that look a lot less like the original (poorly differentiated)

are usually defined as grade 3 or 4. Moderately differentiated tumours lie in between and are classified as grade 2. Sometimes, the cancer cells can be so altered that they bear no resemblance to the original cell and it is no longer possible to define the origin, or primary site, of the cancer, and hence these are called carcinoma of unknown primary (CUP), which is a diagnosis in itself. The grade of a cancer can give an indication of how rapidly it may grow (how aggressive the cancer is), which may affect the prognosis (potential outcome of disease).

The next step is to ascertain the site and size of the primary cancer, and to establish the extent of local and distant spread (metastasis). This is called staging. The TNM (tumour, nodes, metastasis) staging system is the most commonly used for a variety of cancers and describes the size of the primary tumour (T), whether there is any spread into the local or regional lymph nodes (N), and if there are any metastases (M) (Vogel, 2011). The TNM information is used to categorize the tumour into stages, which is useful in deciding treatment options and potential outcome (prognosis).

There are generally four categories of staging: the extent of invasion to local tissues (stage I), to adjacent tissues (stage II), within the cavity or region (stage III), or to distant organs or structures (stage IV). For most cancers, the higher the stage, the poorer the likely outcome, or prognosis, will be. For example, 93.2% of people in England with early stage bowel cancer (diagnosed between 1996 and 2002) survived 5 years from diagnosis, compared with only 6.6% of those diagnosed with advanced disease (National Cancer Intelligence Network, 2010a).

The ways in which an accurate diagnosis of cancer site and stage is made include the use of the following.

- **Cytology**—aims to identify the presence and type of abnormal cells in bodily fluids or secretions.
- **Histology**—aims to identify and classify the type of cells that have become cancerous, their specific appearance and features, and the extent of invasion into normal tissue. Samples are obtained as biopsies or surgical specimens.
- **Imaging**—includes X-ray, ultrasound, computerized tomography (CT), magnetic resonance imaging (MRI), and positron emission tomography (PET). These are used to get a 'picture' of the site, size, and spread of cancer, and to help guide sampling for histology or cytology.

- **Tumour markers**—these are proteins produced by some cancers and can be measured in the blood; they help in detection of cancer and in monitoring response to therapy. For example, CA 125 (cancer antigen 125) is produced by ovarian cancer, CEA (carcinoembryonic antigen) by bowel cancer, and PSA (prostate-specific antigen) in prostate cancer.
- **Surgery and scoping**—to visualize the cancer and acquire samples for histology or cytology.

Holistic assessment

Assessment of the patient with cancer should include the physical signs and symptoms experienced by the patient in relation to the site of the cancer, and also the psychological, cognitive, social, and spiritual impact of the disease on the patient and significant others. Other important areas are the actual or potential effects of treatment and the financial impact, something that has been poorly managed, but highlighted in the 2010 Cancer Patient Experience Survey (Department of Health, 2010).

It is important to have structure and rigour in the process of assessment, as described in the *Holistic Needs Assessment for People with Cancer: A Practical Guide for Healthcare Professionals*, produced by the National Cancer Action Team (NCAT, 2011). It is also important to remember that the patient pathway is rarely one straight road, and that appropriate assessments need to be conducted throughout the cancer journey. A review of cancer patient assessment can be found in *The Royal Marsden Manual of Hospital Procedures* (Dougherty and Lister, 2011) and in a report commissioned by the Department of Health and the National Cancer Action Team (NCAT) (Richardson *et al.*, 2005).

Psychological effects of cancer

Cancer has been associated with death, dying, and painful, mutilating treatment for thousands of years: it was first described as a cause of death over 4,500 years ago and the early Egyptians were known to cauterize breast tumours (Lee, 2000). A cancer diagnosis is associated with an increased risk of suicide (Robinson *et al.*, 2009), and almost all patients with a diagnosis of cancer will experience some degree of psychological distress.

Cancer contributes to psychological distress in many ways, including the following.

- **Fear**—although one in three people in the UK will develop some form of cancer, it has been found to be 'our number one fear' (Cancer Research UK, 2007). Fear of cancer has even been associated with the potential to delay diagnosis (Macleod *et al.*, 2009).
- **Uncertainty**—for the individual with cancer, the present and the future become uncertain, and cancer is associated with the concept of *uncertainty in illness* as both an acute and chronic condition (Mishel, 1990).
- **Anxiety**—anxiety associated with cancer has been well documented, but is poorly understood (Cohen and Bankston, 2011). Estimates regarding the levels of anxiety vary considerably between studies.
- **Depression**—depression affects about 15–25% of cancer patients, with many patients and healthcare professions dismissing it as a normal consequence of having cancer rather than referring for treatment (Cohen and Bankston, 2011).
- **Denial**—the model of grief described by Kübler-Ross (1970) sees denial as a healthy way of dealing with a painful situation that can be used by cancer patients as a coping strategy, but denial can adversely affect communication (Dougherty and Lister, 2011) and contribute to delayed diagnosis.
- **Loss and grief**—there is a considerable amount of change associated with a cancer diagnosis: changing physical self, changing perception of self/body, change in role (adopting Parsons', 1951, sick role), change in finances, change in reproductive potential, etc. These changes can be associated with loss and grief, as discussed by Guillaume (2004).
- **Spiritual distress**—individuals may be forced to re-evaluate the meaning of their lives and faith or make decisions that conflict with their ethical/moral beliefs (Taylor, 2004; see Hughes and Kane, 2008, for a discussion on a diagnosis of cancer complicated by pregnancy).
- **Loss of control**—cancer is a disease defined by a loss of cellular control, and patients can also feel out of control and powerless on the cancer journey (Ranchor *et al.*, 2004).

There are a variety of tools for nurses to use when assessing for psychological distress, such as The Distress Thermometer (National Cancer Action Team (NCAT), 2011) and the Hospital Anxiety and Depression Scale (Zigmond and Snaith, 1983). Nurses have been instrumental in ensuring that this aspect of patient care is recognized and appropriately described as a nursing diagnosis (NANDA, 2008). Recognition of psychological distress can facilitate appropriate referral, enhance communication, and allow for care planning that considers ways, however small, to reduce uncertainty, allay fears, and increase perceived control (see Chapter 14 Managing Anxiety →).

Physical effects of cancer

The physical effect of cancer on the individual depends upon the type, site, and the size of the cancer, as well as whether it is primary or metastatic disease. Because cancer is such a large group of diseases, the symptom possibility is vast, complex, and overlapping. The main mechanisms by which cancer has a physical effect are as follows.

- **Infiltration**—the abnormal accumulation of cells can adversely affect the function of the tissues and structures. Loss of function will result in decreased activity or total failure of the organ or structure. For example, a lung mass may reduce lung capacity, resulting in shortness of breath (Moore *et al.*, 2006) (see Chapter 15 Managing Breathlessness →), or loss of normal bone will weaken the structure, making fractures more likely.

- **Compression**—tumours may compress organs or structures, such as nerves and blood vessels, causing loss of normal function. For example, in ovarian cancer, multiple tumour masses can 'sit' on top of the bowel and constrict the abdominal contents, including the lumen of the bowel, causing a blockage or obstruction. This compression may result in symptoms such as feeling full when eating only small amounts of food, persistent abdominal pain, or loss of appetite; it may result in a subacute bowel obstruction in which the symptoms become more pronounced and include nausea and some vomiting; or it may completely block the bowel (acute bowel obstruction), resulting in an inability to retain food or fluids and an absence

of bowel movement, including flatus (Martin, 2011) (see Chapters 19 Managing Hydration and 24 Managing Nutrition →). The increase in abdominal contents may also push against the diaphragm, leading to reduced lung capacity and shortness of breath (see Chapter 15 Managing Breathlessness →).

- **Chemical**—excessive production of hormones can adversely affect body function, for example steroid production by lung cancer can cause weak bones, facial swelling, and muscle weakness. Substances produced by the tumours can directly irritate the lining of the internal organs and encourage excessive fluid production, e.g. the pleura in lung cancer, causing pleural effusion, or the abdomen in ovarian cancer causing ascites.

- **Necrosis**—cancers can also outgrow their own blood supply, resulting in areas of tissue death or necrosis within the tumour. If a cancer breaks through the surface epithelium of the skin, areas of tumour and necrosis may be exposed, resulting in a fungating wound (see Chapter 28 Managing Wounds →).

All of the above examples can result in significant pain (see Chapter 25 Managing Pain →). For further examples of the commonest symptoms of cancer, see Table 4.2.

Best practice in treating cancer

Cancer treatments

Treatments for cancer have traditionally involved the removal or destruction of the cancerous cells and tissues by surgery, radiotherapy, or chemotherapy. They can be used alone or in combination. Newer targeted treatments, often called novel therapies, rely on the modification of the genes and signalling pathways involved in the process of cancer development. For example, these include drugs that block specific growth factor receptors involved in cell proliferation, therapies that induce apoptosis, therapies that block angiogenesis, monoclonal antibodies that deliver toxic molecules specifically to cancer cells, cancer vaccines, and gene therapy (National Cancer Institute, 2011).

Treatments in cancer are used in an attempt to pre- serve life in a life-threatening disease. Treatments can be toxic, mutilating, and debilitating, especially in more advanced disease. As such, they are associated with sig- nificant morbidity and mortality. The risks and benefits of treatments can be finely balanced and should be carefully considered by the multidisciplinary team, together with the patient and his or her family (Hughes and Kane, 2008). Multidisciplinary teams in cancer include specialist nurses (Department of Health, 2008), and evidence suggests that a team approach to cancer care can improve outcomes and quality of life (Hughes and Kane, 2008).

Anti-cancer therapy treatments are used to cure, to reduce the burden of disease (if not curative), and also to control symptoms in a palliative way. Advances in treatments have resulted in patients being alive with the disease for many years, and this has led to the conceptu- alization of cancer as a chronic disease and the challenge of managing cancer as a long-term disorder (Feuerstein and Ganz, 2011). In the chronic setting, cancer can be well controlled with anti-cancer therapy. However, when anti- cancer therapy is no longer effective or appropriate, then cancer symptoms will be managed with best supportive care (see Chapter 18 Managing End-of-Life Care ➡). The point at which palliative care specialists become involved will depend upon the individual service, but early input (not necessarily referral) from a palliative care specialist in the multidisciplinary setting is considered best practice (Department of Health, 2008).

Surgery

Surgery cures more patients with cancer than any other form of treatment (Department of Health, 2007). Surgery is used in the prevention of cancer (for example, mastec- tomy for women with a high risk of developing the dis- ease—(McIntosh *et al.*, 2004)), for diagnosing and staging cancer, in the treatment of cancer (curative, palliative, and for rehabilitation), and in oncological emergencies, for example metastatic spinal cord compression (MSCC) (National Institute for Health and Clinical Excellence (NICE), 2008).

Cancer surgery includes some of the most radical procedures involving removal of whole organs, such as removal of the bladder for bladder cancer, or removal of the penis in penile cancer, or removal of large amounts of tissue and structures such as hindquarter amputation associated with sarcoma, or the radical tissue dissections associated with head and neck cancer. However, mini- mally invasive techniques such as laparoscopic surgery are increasingly being used in cancer treatments to improve patient experience (Hughes *et al.*, 2010). Nurses working in surgical care are routinely involved in the management of patients with cancer and their pre- and post-diagnostic journey.

Radiotherapy

Ionizing radiation involves the use of high-energy X-rays to damage cellular DNA. Almost half of all can- cer patients will receive radiotherapy as part of their treatment and it forms part of the treatment for 40% of all cancer patients who are cured (Royal College of Radiologists, 2008). Radiation is targeted at the tumour and, as such, is a localized treatment. Although normal tissue will be destroyed around the tumour as some of the radiation dose scatters, the normal tissue has the capacity to repair, while the cancerous tissue does not. Radiation therapy can be used alone or as an additional treatment to surgery and/or chemotherapy (adjuvant or neoadjuvant if given prior to the main treatment). It is also a useful tool in the palliative management of patients with advanced cancer, such as bone metasta- sis or MSCC (National Institute for Health and Clinical Excellence (NICE), 2008).

The dose required to destroy the cancer is fraction- ated in an attempt to reduce damage to normal tissue; for example, a 40-Gy dose of external beam radiotherapy to the pelvis for cervical cancer may be fractioned into 20 treatments of 2 Gy. However, significant toxicity is associated with radiotherapy and sensitivity to radiation varies between individuals (Cancer Research UK, 2010f). The side effects are linked to the organs and structures in the field of radiation (Figure 4.6), and patients should be monitored for toxicity during treatment. Side effects may be present in the initial stages of treatment and long after treatment has been completed.

Chemotherapy

Chemotherapy is the broad term used to describe the use of chemicals in disease, but which primarily refers to

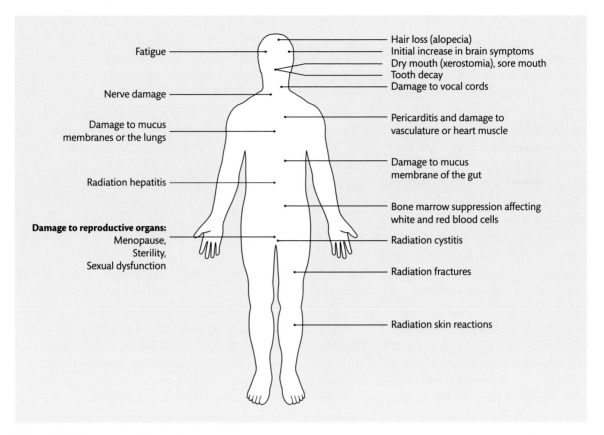

Fatigue

Nerve damage

Damage to mucus
membranes or the lungs

Radiation hepatitis

Damage to reproductive organs:
Menopause,
Sterility,
Sexual dysfunction

Hair loss (alopecia)
Initial increase in brain symptoms
Dry mouth (xerostomia), sore mouth
Tooth decay
Damage to vocal cords

Pericarditis and damage to
vasculature or heart muscle

Damage to mucus
membrane of the gut

Bone marrow suppression affecting
white and red blood cells

Radiation cystitis

Radiation fractures

Radiation skin reactions

Figure 4.6 Side effects of radiotherapy.

the use of agents that are toxic to the cells (cytotoxic) that target and destroy cancer cells (DeVita and Chu, 2008). Chemotherapy is generally given systemically, such as intravenously or orally, but it can be given more directly as in the case of intrathecal or intracavity chemotherapy.

Many different cytotoxic medicines are used in the management of cancer and several drugs are often used in combination. A course of treatment typically consists of several cycles that are given at intervals designed to maximize treatment effect (cancer cell destruction) and minimize side effects (excessive normal cell destruction) by allowing normal cells to recover between treatments. For example, FEC (fluorouracil, epirubicin, and cyclophosphamide) is a treatment regimen used for breast cancer and involves giving about six cycles of the treatment, one every 3–4 weeks. Chemotherapy can be administered as inpatient treatment, but appropriately trained nurses deliver most treatments to outpatients. This has

traditionally been in cancer centres, but there has been a recent trend towards treating patients closer to home in line with the NHS White Paper *Our Health, Our Care, Our Say* (Department of Health, 2006) and also at home (Pattison and MacRae, 2002).

Chemotherapy is associated with many side effects because of the systemic effect of the treatment on normal cells (Figure 4.7), most of which are temporary, but assessment of fitness for chemotherapy and toxicity during treatment ensures that excessive damage to the normal cells does not result in irreversible damage or a fatal consequence. Chemotherapy toxicity can be monitored using an assessment tool based on the National Cancer Institute Common Terminology Criteria for Adverse Events (CTCAE—see 'Finding evidence of best practice'). Even oral chemotherapy should be prescribed and monitored under the supervision of an oncology team (National Patient Safety Agency, 2008).

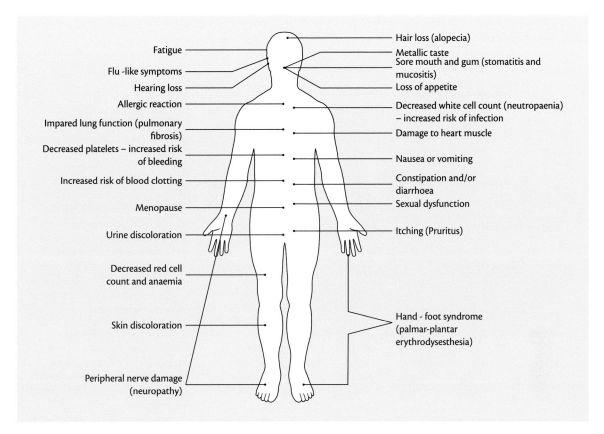

Fatigue

Flu-like symptoms

Hearing loss

Allergic reaction

Impared lung function (pulmonary fibrosis)

Decreased platelets – increased risk of bleeding

Increased risk of blood clotting

Menopause

Urine discoloration

Decreased red cell count and anaemia

Skin discoloration

Peripheral nerve damage (neuropathy)

Hair loss (alopecia)

Metallic taste
Sore mouth and gum (stomatitis and mucositis)

Loss of appetite

Decreased white cell count (neutropaenia) – increased risk of infection

Damage to heart muscle

Nausea or vomiting

Constipation and/or diarrhoea

Sexual dysfunction

Itching (Pruritus)

Hand - foot syndrome (palmar-plantar erythrodysesthesia)

Figure 4.7 **Side effects of chemotherapy.**

Chemotherapy can be used alone or in combination with other treatments, and is also used to control disease that is not curable and to enhance quality of life for significant lengths of time (Cancer Research UK, 2010g). It is less commonly used in the palliation of symptoms in terminal care because the side effects can be severe at the time of treatment and any improvements in quality of life not realized for several weeks.

Management of symptoms

Individuals with cancer can present with no symptoms or present for the first time as an emergency (National Cancer Intelligence Network, 2010b). As the disease progresses, symptoms can become more pronounced and cancer treatments are also associated with symptomatic side effects. Table 4.2 gives examples of nursing interventions for the commonest symptoms associated with cancer and its treatment.

Finding evidence of best practice

Since cancer was identified as one of the five key areas of public health in *The Health of a Nation* (Department of Health, 1992), it has been an important part of UK government health policy. Standardization of best practice has been the focus of improvement in cancer services following publication of the EUROCARE studies and international survivorship data suggesting that the UK lags behind comparable countries in the treatment of cancer (EUROCARE, 2010).

Cancer policy is developed by individual nations and, since devolution in the UK, each of the four countries has been able to address the health priorities of its populations independently. In England, following the publication of what became known as the Calman–Hine Report (Department of Health, 1995), the appointment of the first National Director for Cancer in 1999, and the publication of the NHS Cancer Plan (Department of Health, 2000a),

Table 4.2 Examples of nursing interventions for some of the commonest symptoms associated with cancer and cancer treatments

Symptom	How may this be displayed or described	Causes	Nursing interventions
Alopecia	Mild, pronounced, or total hair loss	Radiotherapy to area affected, such as head or pubis. Many chemotherapy agents can induce hair loss.	Information to prepare the patient for likely hair loss. Discuss the potential use of scalp cooling during chemotherapy. Information on how to protect the newly exposed skin from the sun, etc. Information on how to obtain a wig or other head covering before the hair loss is evident. Recognition of the distress that this side effect causes for patients and understanding of the temporary nature of the side effect. Make use of 'look good feel better' or other offers available to enhance quality of life in relation to appearance.
Altered sexual health	Infertility, loss of sexual organs, decreased/no interest in sex, painful intercourse, relationship stress, poor body image, diminished gender/role identity	Surgical removal of organs and structures associated with sex and sexuality. Damage to organs and structures associated with sex and sexuality from cancer and cancer treatments. Fatigue, anxiety, and depression associated with cancer and cancer treatments may affect sexual health and well-being. Altered self-perception associated with having cancer and as a result of mutilating or debilitating treatments. Pelvic radiotherapy and brachytherapy can cause vaginal stenosis and impotence.	Ensure all potential effects of treatments are discussed and the possibility of fertility-sparing treatments considered. Any sperm or egg collection needs to be completed before treatment commences. Consider referral for specialist fertility advice. Ensure adequate information is given to make informed choices. Formally assess all patients, giving them permission to address sexual concerns. Ensure access to psychosexual counselling and refer as appropriate. Advice regarding vaginal dilators and advice re management of impotence.
Anorexia–cachexia	Weight loss, difficulty in eating, lack of appetite, early satiety, muscle wasting, weakness, fatigue, decreased motor or mental skills, lack of concentration	The exact cause is not fully understood, but results in an imbalance between calorie intake and output. Contributing factors are loss of appetite, changes in taste and smell, nausea, altered bowel function, diarrhoea, chronic blood loss, protein loss, and increased glucose metabolism.	Assess the nutritional status of all patients. Consider the effects of treatments on nutritional status and support pre-treatment if necessary. Consider oral or enteral nutritional support. Consider the use of appetite stimulants. Adequate symptom control. Ensure access to specialist dietetic advice. Understand the psychological impact on the patient and family. See Chapter 24 Managing Nutrition and Chapter 18 Managing End-of-Life Care →

Table 4.2 (*continued*)

Symptom	How may this be displayed or described	Causes	Nursing interventions
Anxiety, depression, grief	Shock, denial, mood changes, restlessness, difficulty retaining information, aggression, feeling of loss of control, feelings of panic, inability to make decisions, suicidal thoughts, loss of interest or pleasure, sleep disturbance, fatigue	Fear associated with having cancer and toxic treatments. Fear of death and concerns about the family and finances. Uncertainty about outcome of treatment. May be due to medications, especially high doses of steroids.	Adequate information and support from named keyworker. Routine use of anxiety and depression measures. Ensure access to counselling for people with cancer. Referral to psychiatrist as appropriate. See Chapter 14 Managing Anxiety
Ascites	Recent weight gain, clothes not fitting, abdominal bloating, feeling full after small meals, indigestion, urinary urgency or frequency, loss of appetite, constipation, difficulty breathing, back or abdominal pain, nausea and vomiting, fatigue	Tumour masses in the abdomen interfering with normal fluid drainage. Irritation of the peritoneum from proteins and chemicals associated with some cancers.	Treatment of the underlying cancer. Fluid may be drained—paracentesis—but the fluid is likely to reform if no anti-cancer treatment ensues. Shunts can be used to drain the fluid back into the vascular system, but are used with limited success. Management of ascites in community and teaching patients to manage drain at home.
Bleeding	Obvious bleeding from the mucous membranes, in the urine, from wounds; signs of anaemia, bruising, pain	Increased risk of bleeding from the cancer, especially haematological cancers. Anti-cancer treatments also affect the risk of bleeding and clotting function.	High-risk patients should be given information on how to prevent and manage bleeding. Monitor haemostasis in high-risk patients and during treatment. Transfuse as necessary.
Breathlessness	Increased respiratory rate and effort, patient may be extremely distressed	May be caused by decreased lung capacity because of tumour mass in the lung(s). May be caused by tumour compression of the bronchus or compression of the diaphragm from abdominal tumour masses or fluid. May be due to fluid in the pleural space, the pericardium or the peritoneum (effusions). May be caused by the use of chemotherapy agents that are toxic to the lungs, causing pulmonary fibrosis. May be as a result of surgery or radiotherapy to the lungs. May be due to anaemia from bleeding caused by the tumour or treatment. May be due to infection associated with chemotherapy-induced neutropaenia. May be caused by pulmonary embolus as a result of immobility and/or being at increased risk of clotting with having active disease.	Adequate assessment of underlying cause and possible treatment. See Chapter 15 Managing Breathlessness

Table 4.2 (*continued*)

Symptom	How may this be displayed or described	Causes	Nursing interventions
Fatigue	Lack of energy, inability to perform usual tasks, excessive tiredness, weakness, dizziness	May be due to anaemia associated with bleeding from the cancer or treatment or reduced red cell count with chemotherapy. May be because of extensive cell destruction associated with cancer treatments. May be due to medications associated with treatments or symptom control. Cancer is also associated with fatigue with no identified cause, and this can be a major side effect of radiotherapy occurring years after completion of treatment.	Adequate assessment of underlying cause and possible treatment. Maintain regular sleeping and rest pattern with an appropriate exercise plan to boost energy. Ensure adequate nutrition and hydration. Encourage the patient to maintain possible functional activity and minimize loss to individual need and ability.
Lymphoedema	Refers to swelling of the limb, which may be associated with warmth or redness, stiffness, or reduced function of the limb	May be caused by reduced lymphatic drainage associated with tumour masses or infiltration. May be caused by treatments that have removed or damaged the lymphatic system, such as surgery or radiotherapy. May be caused or exacerbated by the presence of infection or obesity.	Consider cancer in a patient presenting with lymphoedema. Ensure preventative measures are taken during high-risk treatments. Avoid cannulation or the use of a blood pressure cuff in an affected area. Prevention and early treatment of infection. Ensure patients are given information on prevention. Encourage early and regular mobility post-surgery, especially if lymph nodes have been removed. Ensure access to specialist lymphoedema advice and referral.
Menopausal symptoms	Hot flushes, vaginal dryness, urinary urgency/frequency, stress incontinence, mood changes, bone loss, loss of concentration, irritability, sleeplessness, and restlessness	Early onset of the menopause from surgery to the ovaries, chemotherapy and/or radiotherapy to the pelvis.	Discussion with the multidisciplinary team and/or gynaecologist as to the appropriateness of hormone replacement therapy given the cancer type—it may or may not be contraindicated. Important not to put patient at undue risk, but also not to ignore the seriousness of the symptoms for some women. Consider non-hormonal therapies for various symptoms. (See RCN Complementary approaches to the menopause **www.rcn.org.uk**)
Pain	Direct reporting of pain, emotional distress, mood disorders, reduced social interaction, and depression	Pain may be associated with the cancer as primary or secondary lesions. This may be as a result of constriction, infiltration, necrosis, or loss of function. Anti-cancer treatments can also be associated with pain as tissues are damaged or destroyed. Pain may be acute or chronic.	Adequate assessment of pain and underlying cause. Regular reassessment and measurement. Understand the psychological impact of cancer pain and fear of a painful death. Treat underlying cause where possible. Consider pharmacological and non-pharmacological interventions. See Chapter 25 Managing Pain ➡

Table 4.2 (*continued*)

Symptom	How may this be displayed or described	Causes	Nursing interventions
Skin ulceration	Ulcers, bleeding wounds, wounds slow to heal, redness, and swelling post-treatment	May be caused by the cancer infiltrating the skin. May be as a result of tissue damage from chemotherapy, radiotherapy, or chronic lymphoedema. These types of wound are very different, but delayed healing can be a significant problem in both.	Take appropriate preventative measures for patients having high-risk treatments such as radiotherapy and the administration of vesicant chemotherapy agents. Ensure that malignant ulcers are identified and managed accordingly as a chronic condition that may never heal. See Chapter 28 Managing Wounds ➡
Venous thromboembolism (VTE)	Breathlessness, limb swelling associated with warmth and redness	The risk of clotting is higher with many cancers, especially when associated with surgical or debilitating treatments.	Consider cancer in the presence of a new diagnosis. Risk assess all cancer patients and provide appropriate prophylaxis.
Gastrointestinal disturbances	Soreness or dryness of the mouth, difficulty in swallowing, nausea, vomiting, diarrhoea, constipation, and bowel obstruction	The GI tract may be affected directly by the disease or the treatment, such as a tumour in the oesophagus, or tumour compressing the bowel, or radiotherapy for head and neck, stomach, bowel, or pelvic cancers. The GI tract is particularly sensitive to anti-cancer treatments, and many chemotherapy agents induce profound nausea and vomiting. Many of the medications associated with cancer treatment and pain management are associated with diarrhoea or constipation. Radiotherapy can cause long-term disruptions in bowel habit, resulting in chronic diarrhoea or even faecal incontinence.	Careful assessment of patients for dehydration and malnutrition (see Chapters 19 Managing Hydration and 24 Managing Nutrition ➡). Give appropriate information and advice to prepare patients, and details on how to access specialist advice out of hours, as patients may become very unwell rapidly. Give appropriate information on how to maintain hygiene (see Chapter 20 Managing Hygiene ➡), hydration, and nutrition, including the use of appropriate analgesia, antiemetic, antispasmodic, antidiarrhoeal, or constipation treatment (see Chapter 16 Managing Continence ➡). Monitor patients for secondary infections, such as oral candida (see Chapter 12 Understanding Skin Conditions ➡). Ensure access to dietitian as appropriate, and consider the social and psychological impact of being unable to eat and drink properly. Ensure access to specialist advice and assessment in the event of bowel obstruction (see Chapter 16 Managing Continence ➡).

CASE STUDY 4.1 *Ovarian cancer*

There are a range of cancer patient stories on the NHS Choices website **http://www.nhs.uk/conditions/Cancer/Pages/Introduction.aspx** and on most cancer charity sites. There are stories from people of all ages and all walks of life. Some of the cancers have been successfully treated and others have not. The case study presented here is just one of the many individual stories from the author's own experience.

Marion was 60 years old. She was working part-time as a supply teacher following her recent retirement as head of the PE department at a local secondary school. She had been married to Simon, an accountant, for 35 years. They had one daughter, Claire, who was 26 years old and completing a doctoral degree at university.

Learning points: Most cases of ovarian cancer are sporadic and not inherited. This means that the errors in the cell that cause the abnormal behaviour have occurred over time and are more likely to make the final step to become cancerous as an individual gets older. The average age at which non-hereditary ovarian cancer is diagnosed is 63. The daughters of women with non-hereditary ovarian cancer are at no greater risk of developing the disease than other women. Women who have had continuous ovarian ovulation cycles (those with few or no children who have not been on the oral contraceptive pill) are more at risk from developing ovarian cancer. Cancer treatments can last for many weeks and will impact physically, psychologically, and socially; there will also be a financial impact, even in retirement when additional income can be less formally obtained and a patient could lose his or her pension with long periods of hospitalization. Older children in higher education may still be financially dependent upon their parents.

Marion had been feeling increasingly tired and had some mild abdominal discomfort and bloating. She had also noticed that she seemed to be putting on weight around her abdomen despite eating less and not feeling like eating very much.

Learning points: Ovarian cancer is a solid tumour that spreads through the coelomic epithelium lining the abdomen, leaving deposits of tumour 'seeded' all over the abdomen. As the tumour masses enlarge, they begin to constrict other organs by taking up space and effectively 'squashing' the abdominal contents, including the bowel and stomach. A second feature that contributes to abdominal distension, commonly seen in ovarian cancer, is the development of ascites (advanced disease).

Marion visited her GP several times, but her GP failed to recognize her symptoms as ovarian cancer, and suggested that she diet and take more exercise. Marion was reassured that putting on weight at her age was to be expected.

Learning points: On average, a GP will see only eight cases of cancer a year and one woman with ovarian cancer every 5 years. Ovarian cancer was traditionally considered to be the 'silent killer' because of the lack of symptoms associated with early disease. Recent research has challenged this view and led to the development of Department of Health 'Key Messages' in the recognition of symptoms, and the National Institute for Health and Clinical Excellence (NICE, 2011) Ovarian Cancer Guideline includes symptom recognition.

Marion became acutely ill, with abdominal distension, nausea, and vomiting. She became breathless, and went to her local accident and emergency department. Her abdominal distension was obvious and a pelvic examination revealed a large pelvic mass. Her condition was stabilized and she had a pelvic ultrasound and CA 125 performed.

Learning points: 23% of patients with cancer in the UK continue to be diagnosed as emergencies. Delayed diagnosis is thought to contribute to the relatively poor survival rates for cancer in the UK against comparable countries. The tumour and fluid in the abdomen push up against the diaphragm, making breathing more difficult, but ovarian cancer may also spread outside the pelvis and lead to malignant pleural effusions. Ovarian cancer is associated with the increased production of a protein, CA 125, which is used as a tumour marker for the diagnosis of primary disease and recurrence.

Marion was transferred to the gynaecological oncology team. Her ultrasound showed a significant pelvic mass and her CA 125 was 6000 U/ml. She was booked for a CT scan and debulking surgery.

Learning points: In England in the NHS, gynaecological oncology teams in designated peer-reviewed cancer centres should manage women with ovarian cancer. The specialist multidisciplinary team (MDT) should have at least one specialist gynaecological oncology nurse as a core member of the team. CA 125 can be raised in benign conditions; values over 35 U/ml are considered abnormal. The age of a patient and the presence of a complex mass increase the risk of malignancy as a diagnosis. CT scanning allows for the assessment of abdominal disease and 'operability' of the tumour.

Marion was diagnosed as having stage III ovarian cancer and, although almost all of the cancer had been removed surgically, she had a 6-week course of chemotherapy using two agents: carboplatin and paclitaxel. She lost her hair and had mild nausea around the time of each chemotherapy infusion, but otherwise tolerated the treatment reasonably well. Following surgery, her CA 125 returned to normal.

Learning points: Ovarian cancer is staged according to the FIGO staging system (International Federation of Gynaecology and Obstetrics). Stage III indicates that the cancer has spread outside the pelvis to the abdominal cavity, but not beyond, and most ovarian cancer is diagnosed at stage III. Surgery alone would not be sufficient to cure the cancer, and chemotherapy is used as an adjunctive treatment to increase the chance of cure, but also to lengthen the time to relapse. Ovarian cancer control is more likely in women in whom the CA 125 returns to normal postoperatively. The main side effect of carboplatin is nausea, which is controlled with antiemetics, and the main side effect of paclitaxel is alopecia.

Marion was well for 13 months. She returned to work and saw her daughter graduate. She was seen for follow-up every 3 months, and her progress monitored with clinical examination and a serum CA 125 test. Her CA 125 began to rise and a CT scan was performed to assess for the presence of recurrent disease. Several tumour masses were identified in the abdomen and a second course of chemotherapy was commenced to control or palliate the disease. Carboplatin as a single agent was given. She remained disease-free for another 9 months, but again the disease recurred. She was given a further course of chemotherapy with a new agent, but developed bowel obstruction during the treatment.

Learning points: Most women with stage III ovarian cancer will have recurrences. Once the disease recurs, it is no longer considered possible to achieve a cure. Cancer treatments may not always offer a cure, but can significantly improve quality and quantity of life. Chemotherapy can be repeated several times; the same agents can be used, if successful, for a long period of time or different agents can be used. Bowel obstruction in ovarian cancer primarily results from the 'squashing' effect of the tumour masses on the lumen of the bowel rather than infiltration of the bowel.

Chemotherapy was discontinued, and the palliative care team took over the primary management of Marion and the support of her family. She suffered from ascites, recurrent bouts of bowel obstruction, nausea, and cachexia. She passed away at home in the company of her husband and daughter, with the support of the community specialist palliative care team and Marie Curie nursing care.

Learning points: Involvement of the palliative care team early in the MDT management allows for appropriate referral for terminal care. End-of-life care includes preferred place of care and the use of other agencies helps to keep a family together at home if they wish. Good palliative care includes bereavement care for relatives.

efforts have concentrated on access to high levels of expertise and the reconfiguration of cancer services into cancer units and cancer centres. These are monitored by a system of peer review against measures in a series of tumour site-specific 'Improving Outcomes Guidance' (for example, breast, colorectal, lung, and gynaecological) and *The Manual for Cancer Services Standards* (Department of Health, 2000b, 2004, 2008) with the individual measures for specialist services (see **www.cquins. nhs.uk**). The *Cancer Reform Strategy* (Department of Health, 2007) and associated reviews have set the direction for cancer services to 2012. Searching for 'cancer' on the Department of Health website **http://www.dh.gov. uk/** gives access to the relevant documents relating to the structure of cancer services and specific publications relating to cancer practice. Other governmental sites include the following.

- The National Cancer Action Team **http://www.ncat. nhs.uk/** coordinates high-quality cancer care through the 28 local cancer networks

- NHS Improvements **http://www.improvement.nhs. uk/cancer/**

- The National Institute for Health and Clinical Excellence (NICE) has a section dedicated to publications regarding cancer **http://guidance.nice.org.uk/Topic/ Cancer**, including a series of site-specific clinical guidelines

- The National Cancer Intelligence Network (NCIN) analyses information collected about cancer patients in the UK **http://www.ncin.org.uk/home.aspx**

- The National Cancer Research Network (NCRN) provides the NHS with an infrastructure to support high-quality cancer studies and has an extensive portfolio of clinical trials **http://www.ncrn.org.uk/**

It is beyond the scope of this chapter to discuss the key policy documents and priorities for each of the four countries, but further cancer information can be found at:

- Wales—**http://wales.gov.uk/topics/health/ nhswales/majorhealth/cancer/?lang=en**

- Scotland—**http://www.scotland.gov.uk/Topics/ Health/health/cancer**

- Northern Ireland—**http://www.dhsspsni.gov.uk/ sqsd_service_frameworks_cancer**

EVIDENCE BOX 4.1
Evidence-based tips

Searching for cancer information on the Internet can be time-consuming because the demand for information from the public means that there are a lot of sites, many with poor-quality, even misleading, information. It can be more useful to enter a trusted site, such as a government agency, international agency, leading charity, professional college, etc., and then search for the cancer information required or use general terms such as 'cancer', 'oncology', 'cancer services', or 'cancer research'. This will often give you the source information rather than articles reviewing the policy or simply referencing it. There are organizations for just about everything; have a guess at an organization dedicated to what you want to know and you will probably find one. If you do need to search the Internet or large databases, then be as specific as possible, preferably after using the trusted sites, seminal publications, or leading clinicians' names to refine your searching terminology.

International information on cancer can be obtained from the World Health Organization **http://www. who.int/topics/cancer/en/**, International Agency for Research on Cancer (IARC) **http://www.iarc.fr/** (including the Globocan international cancer database), and also from cancer-specific organizations in other countries, such as the American National Cancer Institute (NCI) **http://www.cancer.gov/**, which has details of the Common Terminology Criteria for Adverse Events (CTCAE) **http://www.acrin.org/Portals/0/Administration/Regulatory/CTCAE_4.02_2009-09-15_QuickReference_5x7. pdf**

In the UK, Cancer Research UK is one of the largest cancer charities **http://www.cancerresearchuk.org/**, together with Macmillan Cancer Support **http://www.macmillan. org.uk/Home.aspx**. A full list of UK sources of information and support regarding cancer is available at **http://www. patient.co.uk/showdoc/171/**. Information on UK cancer screening can be found at:

- England—http://www.cancerscreening.nhs.uk/index.html
- Wales—http://www.screeningservices.org.uk/
- Scotland—http://www.nsd.scot.nhs.uk/services/screening/index.html
- Northern Ireland—http://www.cancerscreening.n-i.nhs.uk/

The National Cancer Intelligence Network is a UK-wide network using information about cancer to improve clinical outcomes and details of the statistical services for each of the four countries, and can be found at http://www.ncin.org.uk/collecting_and_using_data/otherdatasources.aspx

Nursing organizations supporting nurses in cancer care include:

- The Royal College of Nursing (Cancer and Breast Care Forum) http://www.rcn.org.uk/
- The United Kingdom Oncology Nurses Society http://www.ukons.org/
- The European Oncology Nursing Society (EONS) http://www.cancernurse.eu/index.php
- Various site-specific groups such as the National Forum of Gynaecological Oncology Nurses

Conclusion

Cancer is a major health issue for all countries across the world. Nurses are involved in cancer control at all levels: preventing cancers with health promotion; leading screening and early detection programmes; providing treatments and care in chemotherapy, radiotherapy, and surgical services; helping patients to adjust and live with or beyond cancer; and providing palliative care in the community and in inpatient settings.

Cancer is a complex disease with an enormous range of physical, psychological, and social challenges faced by the patient and the family. Cancer treatment and care is best coordinated by a multidisciplinary team that includes a dedicated nurse. This chapter has attempted to provide an overview of the area for nurses to consider the condition, and a direction to further information about specific cancers, treatments, and support.

Online Resource Centre

 To help you to develop and apply your knowledge and decision-making skills further, we have provided interactive learning resources online at www.oxfordtextbooks.co.uk/orc/bullock/

Whilst these are freely available, you will need to use the access codes at the start of the book.

References

American Cancer Society (2009) *Oncogenes, Tumour Suppressor Genes and Cancer.* American Cancer Society web-based information. http://www.cancer.org/Cancer/CancerCauses/GeneticsandCancer/OncogenesandTumorSuppressorGenes/oncogenes-tumor-suppressor-genes-and-cancer-mutations-and-cancer (accessed 29 July 2011).

American Cancer Society (2011a) *Known and Probable Human Carcinogens.* American Cancer Society web-based information. http://www.cancer.org/Cancer/CancerCauses/OtherCarcinogens/GeneralInformationaboutCarcinogens/known-and-probable-human-carcinogens (accessed 29 July 2011).

American Cancer Society (2011b) *Brain and Spinal Cord Tumours in Adults.* American Cancer Society web-based information. http://www.cancer.org/cancer/braincnstumorsinadults/detailedguide/brain-and-spinal-cord-tumors-in-adults-what-are-brain-spinal-tumors (accessed 29 July 2011).

Arden-Jones, A., Thomas, S., Doherty, R., *et al.* (2010) Hereditary cancer. In J. Corner, S. Bailey (eds) *Nursing Care in Context,* 2nd edn. Blackwell Publishing: Oxford, pp. 427–45.

Autier, P., Boniol, M., Gavin, A., *et al.* (2011) Breast cancer mortality in neighbouring European countries with different levels of screening but similar access to treatment: trend analysis of WHO mortality database. *British Medical Journal* 343: d4111. http://www.bmj.com/content/343/bmj.d4411.full?sid=0e7647ef-2f07-4738-b3d8-449acc212dde (accessed 29 July 2011).

Boyle, P., Levin, B. (eds) (2008) *World Cancer Report 2008.* World Health Organization, International Agency for Research on Cancer: Lyon.

Cancer Research UK (CRUK) (2007) *Cancer is our Number One Fear but Most People do not Understand how Many Cases can be Prevented.* Cancer Research UK press release archive. http://info.cancerresearchuk.org/news/archive/pressrelease/2007-04-25-cancer-is-our-number-one-fear-but-most-dont-understand-how-many-cases-can-be-prevented (accessed 29 July 2011).

Cancer Research UK (CRUK) (2008) *NCRI Session: The Cost of Cancer Care.* Cancer Research UK web report. http://scienceblog.cancerresearchuk.org/2008/10/21/ncri-session-the-cost-of-cancer-care/ (accessed 29 July 2010).

Cancer Research UK (CRUK) (2009) *How Many Different Types of Cancer are There?* Cancer Research UK web-based information. http://info.cancerresearchuk.org/cancerandresearch/all-about-cancer/what-is-cancer/different-types-of-cancer/ (accessed 29 July 2011).

Cancer Research UK (CRUK) (2010a) *Types of Cells and Cancer.* Cancer Research UK web-based information. http://cancerhelp.cancerresearchuk.org/about-cancer/what-is-cancer/cells/types-of-cells-and-cancer (accessed 29 July 2011).

Cancer Research UK (CRUK) (2010b) *Childhood Cancer Statistics: Incidence.* Cancer Research UK web-based information. http://info.cancerresearchuk.org/cancerstats/childhoodcancer/incidence/ (accessed 29 July 2011).

Cancer Research UK (CRUK) (2010c) *Mesothelioma.* Cancer Research UK web-based information. http://cancerhelp.cancerresearchuk.org/type/mesothelioma/ (accessed 29 July 2011).

Cancer Research UK (CRUK) (2010d) *Carcinoid.* Cancer Research UK web-based information. http://cancerhelp.cancerresearchuk.org/type/carcinoid/ (accessed 29 July 2011).

Cancer Research UK (CRUK) (2010e) *Prognosis of Secondary Bone Cancer.* Cancer Research UK web-based information. http://cancerhelp.cancerresearchuk.org/about-cancer/cancer-questions/prognosis-of-secondary-bone-cancer (accessed 29 July 2011).

Cancer Research UK (CRUK) (2010f) *Radiotherapy.* Cancer Research UK web-based information. http://cancerhelp.cancerresearchuk.org/about-cancer/treatment/radiotherapy/ (accessed 29 July 2011).

Cancer Research UK (CRUK) (2010g) *Chemotherapy.* Cancer Research UK web-based information. http://cancerhelp.cancerresearchuk.org/about-cancer/treatment/chemotherapy/ (accessed 29 July 2011).

Cancer Research UK (CRUK) (2011a) *Brain Tumour Risks and Causes.* Cancer Research UK web-based information. http://cancerhelp.cancerresearchuk.org/type/brain-tumour/about/brain-tumour-risks-and-causes (accessed 29 July 2011).

Cancer Research UK (CRUK) (2011b) *Prevalence (Number of Cancer Survivors): UK.* Cancer Research UK web-based information. http://info.cancerresearchuk.org/cancerstats/incidence/prevalence/ (accessed 29 July 2011).

Cancer Research UK (CRUK) (2011c) *Skin Cancer: UK Incidence Statistics.* Cancer Research UK web-based information. http://info.cancerresearchuk.org/cancerstats/types/skin/incidence/ (accessed 29 July 2011).

Cancer Research UK (CRUK) (2011d) *Cancer Screening Saves Lives.* Cancer Research UK web-based information. http://info.cancerresearchuk.org/spotcancerearly/screening/how-do-we-know/ (accessed 29 July 2011).

Chial, H. (2008) Proto-oncogenes to oncogenes to cancer. *Nature Education* 1: 1. http://www.nature.com/scitable/topicpage/proto-oncogenes-to-oncogenes-to-cancer-883 (accessed 29 July 2011).

Cohen, M.Z., Bankston, S. (2011) Cancer-related distress. In C.H. Yarbro, D. Wujcik, B. Holmes Gobel (eds) *Cancer Nursing: Principles and Practice,* 7th edn. Jones and Bartlett Sudbury, MA pp. 677–85.

Department of Health (1992) *The Health of a Nation: A Strategy for Health in England.* HMSO: London.

Department of Health (1995) *A Policy Framework for Commissioning Cancer Services.* HMSO: London.

Department of Health (2000a) *The NHS Cancer Plan.* HMSO: London.

Department of Health (2000b, 2004, 2008) *The Manual for Cancer Services Standards* HMSO: London.

Department of Health (2006) *Our Health, Our Care, Our Say: A New Direction for Community Services.* HMSO: London.

Department of Health (2007) *Cancer Reform Strategy.* Department of Health: London.

Department of Health (2010) *National Cancer Patient Experience Survey Programme: 2010 National Survey Report.* Department of Health: London.

DeVita, V.T., Jr, Chu, E. (2008) A history of cancer chemotherapy. *Cancer Research* **68**(21): 8643–53.

Dillard, A.J., Couper, M.P., Zikmund-Fisher, B.J. (2010) Perceived risk of cancer and patient reports of participation in decisions about screening: the DECISIONS study. *Medical Decision Making* **30**(5S): 96S–105S.

Dougherty, L., Lister, S. (2011) *The Royal Marsden Hospital Manual of Clinical Nursing Procedures Student Edition,* 8th edn. The Royal Marsden Hospital: London.

Duffy, S.W., Tabar, L., Olsen, A.H., *et al.* (2010) Absolute numbers of lives saved and overdiagnosis in breast cancer screening, from a randomized trial and from the Breast Screening Programme in England. *Journal of Medical Screening* **17**(1): 25–30.

EUROCARE (2010) *Survival of Cancer Patients in Europe.* Details and publications of the European Cancer Registry-based study on survival and care of cancer patients are available from: **http://www.eurocare.it/** (accessed 29 July 2011).

Ferlay, J., Shin, H.R., Bray, F., *et al.* (2008) *GLOBOCAN 2008, Cancer Incidence and Mortality Worldwide: IARC CancerBase No. 10* [Internet]. International Agency for Research on Cancer: Lyon. **http://globocan.iarc.fr** (accessed 29 July 2011).

Feuerstein, M., Ganz, P.A. (2011) Quality healthcare for cancer survivors. In M. Feuerstein, P.A. Ganz (eds) *Health Services for Cancer Survivors.* Springer: New York, pp. 373–85.

Ford, S. (2009) MP proposes sunbed ban for under 18s. *Nursing Times.net.* **http://www.nursingtimes.net/mp-proposes-sunbed-ban-for-under-18s.5009778.article** (accessed 29 July 2011).

Guillaume, C. (2004) Loss and grief. In C.H. Yarbro, M.H. Hansen, M. Goodman (eds) *Cancer Symptom Management,* 3rd edn. Jones and Bartlett: Sudbury, MA, pp. 706–19.

Hakama, M., Coleman, M., Alexe, D.M., *et al.* (2008) Cancer screening: evidence and practice in Europe 2008. *European Journal of Cancer* **44**(10): 1404–13.

Hamilton, W. (2009) The CAPER studies: five case-control studies aimed at identifying and quantifying the risk of cancer in symptomatic primary care patients. *British Journal of Cancer* **101**(S2): S80–6.

Health and Social Care Information Centre (2010) HES online hospital episode statistics. Primary diagnosis summary. **http://www.hesonline.nhs.uk/Ease/servlet/ContentServer?siteID=1937&categoryID=889** (accessed 27 July 2011).

Hughes, C., Kane, N. (2008) Multidisciplinary care. In S. Kehoe, E. Jauniaux, R. Martin-Hirsch, *et al.* (eds) *Cancer and Reproductive Health.* RCOG Press: London, pp. 268–78.

Hughes, C., Knibb, K., Allan, H. (2010) Laparoscopic surgery for endometrial cancer: a phenomenological study. *Journal of Advanced Nursing* **66**(11): 2500–9.

Kübler-Ross, E. (1970) *On Death and Dying.* Routledge: London.

Lee, H.S.J. (2000) *Dates in Oncology: A Chronological Record of Progress in Oncology over the Last Millennium.* Parthenon Publishing: London.

Lichtenstein, P., Niels V., Holm, M.D., *et al.* (2000) Environmental and heritable factors in the causation of cancer: analysis of cohorts of twins from Sweden, Denmark, and Finland. *New England Journal of Medicine* **434**(2): 78–85.

Loud, J.T., Hutson, S.P. (2011) Genetic risk and hereditary cancer syndromes. In C.H. Yarbro, D. Wujcik, B. Holmes Gobel (eds) *Cancer Nursing: Principles and Practice,* 7th edn. Jones and Bartlett: Sudbury, MA, pp. 135–66.

Macleod, U., Mitchell, E.D., Burgess, C., *et al.* (2009) Risk factors for delayed presentation and referral of symptomatic cancer: evidence of common cancers. *British Journal of Cancer* **101**(S2): S92–S101.

Macmillan Cancer Support (2011) *National Cancer Survivorship Initiative: Mission Statement.* Macmillan Cancer Support: London. **http://www.ncsi.org.uk/** (accessed 29 July 2011).

Martin, V. (2011) Ovarian cancer. In C.H. Yarbro, D. Wujcik, B. Holmes Gobel (eds). *Cancer Nursing: Principles and Practice,* 7th edn. Jones and Bartlett: Sudbury, MA, pp. 1546–80.

McIntosh, A., Shaw, C., Evans, G., *et al.* (2004) (update 2006) *Clinical Guidelines and Evidence Review for the Classification and Care of Women at Risk of Familial Breast Cancer.* National Collaborating Centre for Primary Care/University of Sheffield: London.

Mishel, M.H. (1990) Reconceptualization of the uncertainty in illness theory. *Image: the Journal of Nursing Scholarship* **22**(4): 256–62.

Moore, S., Plant, H., Bredin, M. (2006) Breathlessness. In N. Kearney, A. Richardson (eds) *Nursing Patients with Cancer: Principles and Practice.* Elsevier: Oxford, pp. 507–27.

NANDA International (2008) *Nursing Diagnoses: Classification and Definitions 2009–2011 Edition.,* Wiley-Blackwell: Indianapolis, IN .

National Cancer Action Team (NCAT) (2011) *Holistic Needs Assessment for People with Cancer: A Practical Guide for Healthcare Professionals.* National Cancer Action Team: London. **http://www.ncat.nhs.uk/our-work/living-with-beyond-cancer/holistic-needs-assessment** (accessed 29 July 2011).

National Cancer Institute (2011) *Targeted Cancer Therapies.* National Cancer Institute web-based cancer information. **http://www.cancer.gov/cancertopics/factsheet/Therapy/targeted** (accessed 29 July 2011).

National Cancer Intelligence Network (2010a) Colorectal cancer survival by stage: NCIN data briefing. **http://www.ncin.org.uk/publications/data_briefings/colorectal_cancer_survival_by_stage.aspx** (accessed 29 July 2011).

National Cancer Intelligence Network (2010b) Routes to diagnosis: NCIN data briefing, **http://www.ncin.org.uk/publications/data_briefings/routes_to_diagnosis.aspx** (accessed 29 July 2011).

National Cervical Cancer Coalition (2007) *Controversial Issues: College States Position on HPV Vaccine.* National Cervical Cancer Coalition: WoodLand Hills, CA. **http://www.nccc-online.org/health_news/topics/controversial/college_states.html** (accessed 29 July 2011).

National Coalition for Cancer Survivorship (2010) *Definition of Cancer Survivor.* National Coalition for Cancer Survivorship: Silver Spring, MA. **http://www.canceradvocacy.org/about/org/** (accessed 29 July 2011).

National Collaborating Centre for Cancer (NCCC) (2010) *Diagnosis and Management of Metastatic Disease of Unknown Primary.* National Collaborating Centre for Cancer: Cardiff.

National Collaborating Centre for Cancer (NCCC) (2011a) *Ovarian Cancer: The Recognition and Initial Management of Ovarian Cancer*. National Collaborating Centre for Cancer: Cardiff.

National Collaborating Centre for Cancer (NCCC) (2011b) *The Diagnosis and Treatment of Lung Cancer (update)*. National Collaborating Centre for Cancer: Cardiff.

National Institute for Health and Clinical Excellence (NICE) (2005, update 2011) *Referral Guidelines for Suspected Cancer*. NICE Clinical Guideline 27 (CG27). National Institute for Health and Clinical Excellence: London. http://guidance.nice.org.uk/CG27 (accessed 29 July 2011).

National Institute for Health and Clinical Excellence (NICE) (2008) *Metastatic Spinal Cord Compression: Diagnosis and Management of Adults at Risk of and with Metastatic Spinal Cord Compression*. NICE Clinical Guideline 75 (CG175). National Institute for Health and Clinical Excellence: London. http://guidance.nice.org.uk/CG75 (accessed 29 July 2011).

National Institute for Health and Clinical Excellence (NICE) (2010) *Metastatic Malignant Disease of Unknown Primary Origin*. NICE Clinical Guideline 107 (CG107). National Institute for Health and Clinical Excellence: London. http://www.nice.org.uk/CG104 (accessed 11 October 2011).

National Patient Safety Agency (2008) *Oral Anti-Cancer Medicine: Risks of Incorrect Dosing*. Rapid Response Report, NPSA/2008/RRR01. National Patient Safety Agency: London. http://www.nrls.npsa.nhs.uk/resources/?entryid45=59880 (accessed 29 July 2011).

National Patient Safety Agency (2010) *Delayed Diagnosis of Cancer: Thematic Review*. National Patient Safety Agency: London. http://www.nrls.npsa.nhs.uk/resources/?EntryId45=69894 (accessed 29 July 2011).

NHS Cancer Screening Programme (2011) Details and guidelines for the screening programmes (breast, bowel and cervical) and prostate cancer risk management. NHS Cancer Screening Programme: London. http://www.cancerscreening.nhs.uk/ (accessed 29 July 2011).

Paget, S. (1889) The distribution of secondary growths in cancer of the breast. *Lancet* **133**(3421): 571–3.

Parsons, T. (1951) *The Social System*, 2nd edn. Free Press. Chicago IL.

Pattison, J., MacRae, K. (2002) Home chemotherapy: NHS and independent sector collaboration. *Nursing Times* **95**(35): 34–5.

Ranchor, A., Wardle, J., Steptoe, A., *et al.* (2004) The adaptive role of perceived control before and after diagnosis: a prospective study. *Social Science and Medicine* **70**(11): 1825–31.

Renehan, A.G, Soerjomataram, I., Tyson, M., *et al.* (2010) Incident cancer burden attributable to excess body mass index in 30 European countries. *International Journal of Cancer* **1**(126): 692–702.

Richards, M.A. (2009) The size of the prize for earlier diagnosis in England. *British Journal of Cancer* **101**(S2): S125–9.

Richardson, A., Sitzia, J., Brown, V., *et al.* (2005) *Patients' Needs Assessment Tools in Cancer Care: Principles and Practice*. King's College London: London.

Robinson, D., Renshaw, C., Okello, C., *et al.* (2009) Suicide in cancer patients in South East England from 1996 to 2005: a population based study. *British Journal of Cancer* **101**(1): 198–201.

Royal College of Radiologists, Society and College of Radiographers, Institute of Physics and Engineering in Medicine, *et al.* (2008) *Towards Safer Radiotherapy*. Royal College of Radiologists: London.

Starfield B., Hyde J., Gérvais J., *et al.* (2008) The concept of prevention: a good idea gone astray? *Journal of Epidemiology and Community Health* **62**(7): 508–83.

Taylor, E.J. (2004) Spiritual distress. In C.H. Yarbro, M.H. Hansen, M. Goodman. (eds) *Cancer Symptom Management*, 3rd edn. Jones and Bartlett: Sudbury, MA, 693–706.

United Nations Programme on HIV/AIDS (UNAIDS), World Health Organization (WHO) (2009) *09 AIDS Epidemic Update*. UNAIDS and WHO report. http://www.unaids.org/en/media/unaids/contentassets/dataimport/pub/report/2009/jc1700_epi_update_2009_en.pdf (accessed 29 July 2011).

Vogel, W. (2011) Diagnostic evaluation, classification and staging. In C.H. Yarbro, D. Wujcik, B. Holmes Gobel (eds) *Cancer Nursing: Principles and Practice*, 7th edn. Jones and Bartlett: Sudbury, MA, pp. 166–99.

World Health Organization (WHO)(2011a) *Cancer*. World Health Organization: Geneva. http://www.who.int/mediacentre/factsheets/fs297/en/ (accessed 29 July 2011).

World Health Organization (WHO)(2011b) *Cancer Prevention*. World Health Organization: Geneva. http://www.who.int/cancer/prevention/en/ (accessed 29 July 2011).

World Health Organization (WHO)(2011c) *Cancer Control: Knowledge into Action*. World Health Organization: Geneva. http://www.who.int/cancer/modules/en/index.html (accessed 29 July 2011).

World Health Organization/Institut Catala d'Oncologià (WHO/ICO) Information Centre on HPV and Cervical Cancer (HPV Information Centre) (2010) *Human Papillomavirus and Related Cancers in India: Human Papillomavirus and Related Cancers in United Kingdom*. Summary reports. http://www.who.int/hpvcentre (accessed 29 July 2011).

Zigmond, A.S., Snaith, P.R (1983) The Hospital Anxiety and Depression Scale. *Acta Psychiatrica Scandinavica* **67**(6): 361–70.

5 *Understanding* Chronic Obstructive Pulmonary Disease

Samantha Prigmore and Jane Scullion

Introduction

The aim of this chapter is to provide nurses with the knowledge to be able to assess, manage, and care for people with chronic obstructive pulmonary disease (COPD) in an evidence-based and person-centred way. The chapter will provide a comprehensive overview of the causes, risk factors, and impact of COPD, before exploring best practice to deliver care, as well as to prevent or minimize further ill-health. Nursing assessments and priorities are highlighted throughout, and the nursing management of the symptoms and common health problems associated with COPD can be found in Chapters 2, 15, 18, and 22, respectively ➡.

Understanding COPD

Defining COPD

Chronic obstructive pulmonary disease (COPD) is predominantly caused by smoking and is characterized by airflow obstruction that is not fully reversible (National Institute for Health and Clinical Excellence (NICE), 2010). This broad definition embraces previously used definitions such as chronic bronchitis, emphysema, and chronic asthma. Historically, perceptions of the treatment for and care of the patient with COPD were negative, because of the chronic nature of this progressive disease, which was often viewed as self-inflicted through its links with smoking. Current emphasis, regardless of

aetiology, is that it is both preventable and treatable (National Institute for Health and Clinical Excellence (NICE), 2010).

Epidemiology

Currently around 1 million UK citizens are diagnosed with COPD; prevalence data are higher, at 1.7 million (Britton, 2003). This appears to be underreported because it is thought that there could be as many as another 2 million people currently undiagnosed (British Lung Foundation, 2006). COPD is already a significant burden of disease area, with expectations that, by 2020, it will be the third largest cause of mortality (Murray and Lopez, 1997).

Reasons for increasing prevalence include that:

- an ageing population increases the likelihood of chronic disease development;

- diagnosis of COPD is better guided by both national and international COPD guidelines, with inclusion in the Quality and Outcomes Framework (QOF) in general practice bringing financial incentives for maintaining COPD registers and improving COPD care;

- increasing public awareness leads to more people seeking help on symptom presentation;
- more women being diagnosed, correlating to more women smoking, perhaps owing to greater social acceptability;
- other as yet unknown causes.

THEORY INTO PRACTICE 5.1

Activity

Look at prevalence rates and the burden of COPD by analysing:

- primary care data **www.gpcontract.co.uk**
- secondary care data (Hospitals Episodes Statistics—HES—data) **www.hesonline.nhs.uk**

QOF data indicate general practice prevalence for COPD and HES data provide hospital admissions for COPD.

Causes of COPD

Tobacco smoking is the most documented causative agent for the development of COPD, with an estimated 90% of those diagnosed with the disease being current or ex-smokers (Kumar and Clark, 2005). Despite stringent anti-smoking legislation, incidence rates of COPD are continuing to grow.

This leaves around 10% of those diagnosed with COPD due to other causes.

- Occupational exposure is difficult to establish, especially if it is compounded by smoking. Currently, only coal workers with emphysema and chronic bronchitis receive compensation under the UK industrial injuries legislation 1993 (see UK industrial injuries legislation in the 'Resources' section).
- Environmental factors such as low socio-economic status lead to higher prevalence. This may be because of higher cigarette consumption, poor diet, type of occupation, exposure to passive smoking, or hereditary/genetic factors. Indoor pollutants also contribute to an increased prevalence of COPD, especially for those cooking over biomass (animal waste/plant material) fires.

- Alpha-1 antitrypsin deficiency is a hereditary form of early onset emphysema with rapid progression, and should be suspected in any individual presenting with rapidly deteriorating lung function and a familial history. Early diagnosis, smoking cessation (if relevant), and immediate treatment are important.
- In 2002, the British Lung Foundation (BLF) published *Cannabis: A Smoking Gun*, showing that cannabis is up to 50 times more carcinogenic than cigarettes and that just three cannabis joints a day (equivalent to 20 cigarettes) could damage lung tissue, leading to both acute and chronic bronchitis. Unfortunately, cannabis users often feel that this is a safer substance to smoke than tobacco products.

THEORY INTO PRACTICE 5.2

Activity

Look at the reasons other than smoking for the development of COPD, and decide which ones you think may be amenable to changes in legislation similar to those being enforced to address smoking rates? Which ones require a change in public attitudes?

The pathophysiology of COPD

To understand COPD, it is helpful if you are already familiar with the normal anatomy and physiology of the respiratory system. Should you require a reminder, please consult a good anatomy and physiology textbook.

COPD results in two basic pathological processes, chronic bronchitis and emphysema, with patients presenting with a wide spectrum of combinations of these two phenotypes. COPD is also described as an 'umbrella' term, covering chronic asthma; it is debatable whether this is about individuals continuing to smoke or being continually exposed to noxious substances. Lung tissue damage resulting from under treatment or medication non-compliance is also contributory. Fixed obstruction may simply be a consequence of having asthma for many years.

The lung's function is to deliver oxygen to the body and to remove carbon dioxide. Reduced ability to do this obviously has a consequent impact on multiple organ systems.

Emphysema describes a pathological process by which there is inflammation and destruction of the walls of the

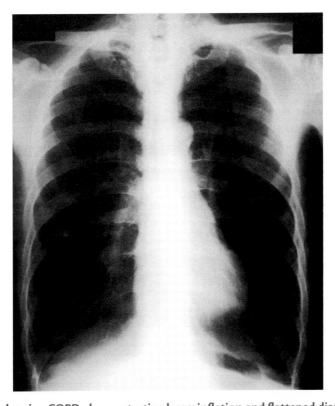

Figure 5.1 **Radiograph showing COPD, demonstrating hyperinflation and flattened diaphragm.**

Reproduced from Thomas and Monaghan, *Oxford Handbook of Clinical Examination and Practical Skills* (2007) by permission of Oxford University Press.

air sacs or alveoli, causing incomplete gas transfer (oxygen transfer and removal of carbon dioxide), airway narrowing, and loss of elasticity. This leads to air trapping in the alveoli, subsequent increased residual volume, and hyperinflation of the lungs.

Chronic bronchitis is the body's response to irritants (noxious substances) that cause inflammation and narrowing in the airways. Production of large amounts of thick sticky mucus is a consequence, leading to the recognizable 'smokers cough'.

> **Box 5.1** **Common symptoms of COPD**
>
> - Breathlessness
> - Cough
> - Sputum production—'smokers cough'
> - Frequent winter bronchitis
> - Wheeze
> - Pain
> - Dehydration
> - Fatigue

Common symptoms

The combination of emphysema and chronic bronchitis gives rise to the symptoms of COPD. Figure 5.1 shows a radiograph of COPD, demonstrating hyperinflation and flattened diaphragm.

Lung tissue damage makes individuals more prone to infections (known as 'exacerbations'). Although the pathological changes causing symptoms in COPD are related to the lung, it is recognized that COPD is a systemic disease and, in addition to the common symptoms in Box 5.1, there are additional changes (Box 5.2). Figure 5.2 illustrates the systemic side effects of COPD.

It is estimated that the direct cost of providing care in the NHS for people with COPD is almost £500 million a year (National Institute for Health and Clinical Excellence (NICE),

2010). More than half this cost relates to the provision of care in hospital. *Clearing the Air: A national study of COPD* concluded that the cost difference between treating mild and severe COPD is £1,150 per person. The total annual cost for the NHS for missing the 2.8 million cases of undiagnosed COPD will reach £3.2 billion (Commission for Healthcare Audit and Inspection, 2006).

> ### Box 5.2   Additional systemic changes
>
> - Muscle wasting
> - Weight loss
> - Pulmonary hypertension
> - Cor pulmonale—right-sided heart failure secondary to pulmonary hypertension
> - Anxiety and depression
> - Hypogonadism

Mortality and morbidity

Whilst mortality is high, morbidity impacts heavily on individuals, their carers, and also on society. Increasingly, those with COPD are unable to work, with associated economic impact, and typically they are high users of healthcare resources in both primary and secondary care settings. It is the combined physical and psychosocial impact of this chronic condition that has multiple societal impacts, with the challenge focused on primary and secondary prevention, promoting awareness, early diagnosis, and optimal treatment (Department of Health, 2010).

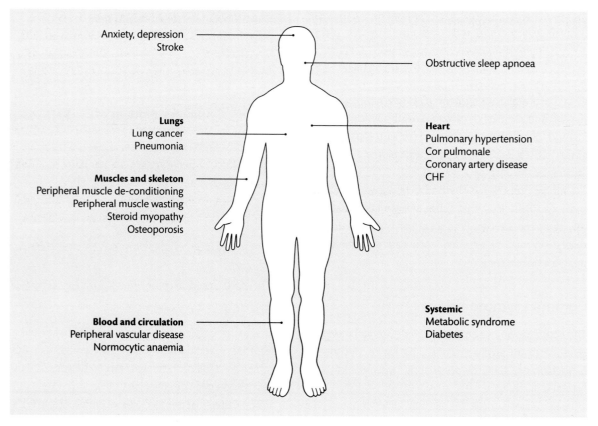

Figure 5.2 Systematic side effects of COPD.
Reproduced with permission of the European Respiratory Society©.

Assessment of the patient with COPD

Clinical nursing assessment

Good history-taking is important. Guidelines indicate that COPD should be considered in patients over the age of 35, who have a risk factor (generally smoking), and who present with one of the following symptoms:

- exertional breathlessness;
- chronic cough;
- regular sputum production;
- frequent winter 'bronchitis';
- wheeze.

> (National Institute for Health and Clinical Excellence (NICE) 2010; Department of Health, 2010)

If these factors are present, COPD screening should be considered.

Patients often present for diagnosis at a late stage; this may be because they do not wish to consider smoking cessation or to be told to stop smoking, or they have mistakenly attributed their symptoms to the ageing process. This is a serious problem, because COPD treatment is difficult when it has progressed, highlighted by the COPD National Strategy, which advocates prevention, early diagnosis, and treatment (Department of Health, 2010).

A diagnosis of COPD relies on clinical judgement based on a combination of the patient's history, physical examination, and confirmation of the presence of irreversible airflow obstruction using spirometry (Department of Health, 2010). Although a peak flow meter will show obstruction, it is not a conclusive diagnostic tool for COPD.

Spirometry

Spirometry is recognized as the gold standard for the diagnosis of COPD (National Institute for Health and Clinical Excellence (NICE), 2010; Department of Health, 2010). Spirometry measures:

- the amount of air that can be forced out of the lungs in 1 second—known as the forced expiratory volume in 1 second (FEV1);
- the total amount of air that can be expired—known as the forced vital capacity or (FVC).

Values for FVC and FEV_1 that are over 80% of the predicted values are defined as within the normal range. This is based on averages for people of a similar gender, age, and height.

The FEV_1 FVC ratio is expressed as a percentage. A normal adult is able to expire at least 80% of his or her vital capacity forcibly in 1 second. A ratio under 70% suggests underlying obstructive physiology (Scullion and Holmes, 2010). Usually, we take the post-bronchodilator measures of FEV_1 and FVC, so readings after a bronchodilator, nebulizer, or inhaler has been given. This is because COPD is by definition irreversible, and although some patients may have some reversibility, they will never be able to get normal readings even if given bronchodilator medications.

When looking at spirometry, asthma is a differential diagnosis that should be considered. Asthma is a reversible condition, so, by definition, if treated, normal readings should be achieved on spirometry (see **Chapter 2 Understanding Asthma** ⟶).

National Institute for Health and Clinical Excellence (NICE) (2010) and GOLD (2009) guidelines classify the severity of obstruction as:

Stage 1/Mild	FEV_1/FVC <70% FEV_1 >80%
Stage 2/Moderate	FEV_1/FVC <70% FEV_1 50–79%
Stage 3/Severe	FEV_1/FVC <70% FEV_1 30–49%
Stage 4/Very severe	FEV_1/FVC <70% FEV_1 <30%

Assessing breathlessness

The Medical Research Council (MRC) dyspnoea scale is a good measure of breathlessness and in primary care is one of the requirements in the QOF standards for COPD (Fletcher *et al.*, 1959).

The Medical Research Council dyspnoea scale for grading the degree of a patient's breathlessness is as follows.

1. Not troubled by breathlessness except on strenuous exercise
2. Short of breath when hurrying or walking up a slight hill
3. Walks slower than contemporaries on the level because of breathlessness, or has to stop for breath when walking at own pace
4. Stops for breath after about 100 m or after a few minutes on the level
5. Too breathless to leave the house, or breathless when dressing or undressing

> (**www.gp-training.net/protocol/respiratory/copd/ dyspnoea_scale.htm** (accessed May 2011))

Body mass index

Record the COPD patient's body mass index (BMI) as a type of cachexia can develop (more familiar in patients with cancer). Monitoring any change is vital because weight loss has a positive correlation with a poorer prognosis. Address the nutritional status, because patients can become malnourished. Obesity-related diabetes adds obvious complexity, reducing activity levels, and further complications arise when treating exacerbations with oral corticosteroids.

Explore reasons for poor dietary intake, including assessment of social and financial circumstances, and the related impact that symptoms associated with COPD have on individuals, limiting their ability to access and prepare fresh food because of breathlessness, depression, and fatigue.

Note that patients who have a low body mass index (BMI) of <20 are at a greater risk of complications and increased mortality, resulting in:

- more frequent exacerbations and admissions to hospital;
- reduction in physical activity;
- reduction in quality of life.

For patients with a low BMI, basic advice should be given, e.g. eating small meals, regular snacks. The National Institute for Health and Clinical Excellence (NICE, 2010) recommends the introduction of dietary supplements, along with exercise. Referral for dietary advice should be considered.

Obesity will also contribute to symptoms such as breathlessness. Obesity can occur due to inactivity, increased appetite secondary to corticosteroid use, or poor diet. It can have significant effects on patients with COPD, causing:

- increased breathlessness and symptoms;
- reduced mobility;
- development of comorbidities—diabetes, sleep apnoea, and hypoventilation.

For many, weight gain is a sensitive subject and losing weight is difficult. Therefore, sensitive questioning regarding food intake, including portion size and snacks, should be undertaken, whilst addressing the importance of a healthy balanced diet.

Psychosocial assessment

Early recognition of the potential social, emotional, and psychological impact of COPD will inform planning focused on improvement of the patient's quality of life.

COPD is not purely a disease of old age, so for younger people with COPD there are important societal issues around work, maintaining fitness, and independence. Some people with COPD will be eligible for disabled 'blue' badges and benefits, so you can advise them to apply for these.

Emotionally and psychologically it is recognized that there is a higher prevalence of anxiety and depression in people diagnosed with COPD (Maurer *et al.*, 2008). Because COPD is a progressive chronic disease, consider the impact of deteriorating physical function. COPD is a palliative condition, as treatment focuses on alleviating symptoms with no cure. End-of-life care is an important consideration (see Chapter 18 Managing End-of-Life Care ➡).

Assessing the effects of symptoms on patients

Breathlessness is the commonest feature of COPD and is a major cause of disability, leading to many physical problems, including reduced physical activities around the house as well as being unable to work (Robinson and Scullion, 2009). Principally breathlessness is caused by hyperinflation of the lungs and is a very uncomfortable and, at times, frightening sensation. As a result of breathlessness, patients may reduce their activity levels to avoid experiencing this. As a consequence of this, they are prone to deconditioning, which causes further loss of physical functioning and increased levels of breathlessness at a lower level of intensity or activity (see Chapter 15 Managing Breathlessness ➡).

Fatigue as a symptom is difficult to treat. This may result from muscle fatigue and deconditioning; this, however, is not relieved by increased sleep or rest and often has high impact, seeming to the patient to be 'overwhelming'.

Symptoms such as cough and producing sputum mean that the patient is more prone to chest infections (exacerbations). The patient may also be embarrassed in public because of coughing and sputum production. There is the additional problem of related stress incontinence.

Pain is a difficult symptom to understand and also to treat in COPD. It may be caused by muscular pain or

---

CASE STUDY 5.1 *Diagnosing COPD*

Sarah, a 57-year-old woman, presents with a history of increasing breathlessness and productive cough for several months. She is a smoker (10–20 cigarettes daily for past 30 years). On questioning, she has noticed that she cannot walk very far, having to stop after about ½ mile. She has also noticed that, over the past few years, she has found carrying shopping difficult and is unable to climb the stairs at home without becoming breathless.

Her mood is low because she is worried that she will not be able to look after her grandchildren.

Your clinical diagnosis is COPD and you arrange for spirometric tests. Her spirometry reveals the following measurements.

- FEV_1 1.58 (52% predicted) (normal ≥80%)
- FVC 2.78 (78% predicted) (normal ≥80%)
- FEV_1/FVC 56% (normal >70%)

These results confirm moderate COPD.

List the interventions/treatments you would want Sarah to commence. Answers are provided at the end of the chapter.

---

comorbid conditions such as arthritis or osteoporosis (see Chapter 25 Managing Pain ➡).

Additional problems for the patient are dehydration owing to related impact of mouth breathing, or through self-restriction of fluids to avoid mobilizing to the bathroom and possible breathlessness.

Identifying best practice

The main evidence-based guidelines used in the management of COPD are the National Institute for Health and Clinical Excellence (NICE, 2010) **www.nice.org.uk/guidance/CG101** and the Global Initiative for Obstructive Lung Disease (GOLD) (2009) **www.copd.com/**.

Both guidelines accept that COPD is a progressive disorder that requires a multidisciplinary approach (Figure 5.3) to manage and improve the symptoms experienced by those individuals diagnosed with the condition.

Nursing management of COPD

Nursing patients with COPD is hugely rewarding, providing opportunity for holistic care involving the multidisciplinary team. Long-term management is often nurse-led, with service modelling delivered within the community

setting. Nursing expertise is demonstrated by diagnosis, regular review, symptom management, education and support, management of exacerbations, and palliative and end-of-life care planning. These skills are not setting-specific (community, primary, or secondary care) and span the disease spectrum. Promoting self-management is optimal, with acute nursing skills available when required in caring for patients requiring ventilatory support.

Smoking cessation

COPD is predominantly caused by smoking, and therefore smoking cessation is essential. Once the lung damage has occurred, it is not reversible, but stopping smoking will slow decline in lung function.

Quitting can be difficult owing to nicotine dependence and habitual behaviours. Every effort should be made to support smoking cessation and this should be offered routinely to all people who smoke (West *et al.*, 2000; National Institute for Health and Clinical Excellence (NICE), 2006). Opportunistic and brief interventions are beneficial and can be successful. You should aim to discuss individuals' smoking status and establish their desire to stop smoking with every contact (during a review, hospital admission, or visits to the pharmacist). It is estimated that the annual quit rate for smoking cessation in COPD patients is around 15%, therefore ongoing support and encouragement is required.

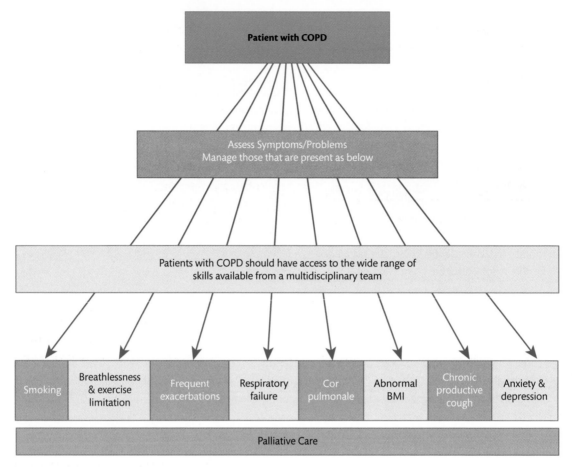

Figure 5.3   Management of stable COPD.

Reproduced with permission from the National Institute for Health and Clinical Excellence (2004) Clinical Guideline 101: *Chronic Obstructive Pulmonary Disease: Management of Chronic Obstructive Pulmonary Disease in Adults in Primary and Secondary Care*, NICE: London. Available from **www.nice.org.uk/guidance/CG101**.

Several effective interventions for smoking cessation are available. Nicotine replacement therapy is available in a variety of preparations, i.e. patches and lozenges along with oral preparations, such as as bupropion and vareni-cline, which have been demonstrated to be cost-effective interventions (National Institute for Health and Clinical Excellence (NICE), 2007).

National Institute for Health and Clinical Excellence (NICE) guidelines support the stop smoking services and these are often available in the community setting, i.e. local pharmacists. Other resources include QUIT, an independent charity offering support from experienced counsellors **www.quit.org.uk**, and NHS Choices can help to identify smoking cessation services by postcode **www.smoke free.nhs.uk**

Pulmonary rehabilitation

Pulmonary rehabilitation is defined as 'an evidence-based multidisciplinary and comprehensive intervention for patients with chronic respiratory disease who are symptomatic and often have decreased daily activities'. Integrated into the individualized treatment for the patient, pulmonary rehabilitation is designed to reduce symptoms, optimize functional status, increase participation, and reduce healthcare costs through stabilizing or reversing systematic manifestations of the disease (Nici *et al.*, 2006).

A Cochrane review of pulmonary rehabilitation (Lacasse *et al.*, 2006) confirms the improvements as the relief of dyspnoea and fatigue, improved emotional functioning, and enhancing the patient's sense of control over

> **Box 5.3 The aims of pulmonary rehabilitation (adapted from Garrod, 2004)**
>
> - Reduce dyspnoea
> - Increase exercise tolerance
> - Improve functional performance
> - Increase muscle endurance (peripheral and respiratory)
> - Improve muscle strength (peripheral and respiratory)
> - Ensure long-term commitment to exercise
> - Help allay patient fear and anxiety
> - Increase knowledge of lung condition and promote self-management

> **Box 5.4 Target educational content of pulmonary rehabilitation programmes**
>
> - Disease management
> - Smoking cessation
> - Medication
> - Nutrition
> - Self-management
> - Living with COPD
> - Energy conservation
> - Personal relationships
> - Benefits advice
> - Relaxation
> - Travel

his or her condition. The aims of pulmonary rehabilitation are outlined in Box 5.3.

Pulmonary rehabilitation should be available and offered to all patients with COPD, with benefits being maintained for up to 2 years. Exercise should be continued to maintain the optimum benefits, with evidence to support early intervention during and after exacerbation (Puhan *et al.*, 2005). Pulmonary rehabilitation programmes can be delivered in both primary and secondary care, with similar beneficial outcomes. The course should include both exercise and education elements (see Box 5.4).

Physical training is the major component to the programme and should include exercise endurance and strength training, including both upper and lower limb exercises and breathing control. The programme should run over a minimum of 6 weeks, with two supervised exercise sessions a week, with home training encouraged.

Anxiety and depression

Patients with COPD often become socially isolated; because of symptoms experienced, they have to give up activities that they enjoy. This can result in anxiety and depression. Owing to the similarities in COPD, anxiety, and depression, the latter are often overlooked and may not be diagnosed in patients with COPD, with the National Institute for Health and Clinical Excellence (NICE, 2004a) estimating the prevalence of depression at 40% in patients with COPD. It is suggested that people with moderate to severe COPD are 2.5 times more likely to suffer with depression (Van Manen *et al.*, 2002), particularly those who are hypoxic and severely breathless and who have been admitted to hospital with an exacerbation (NICE, 2004a), and therefore screening using validated tools in this high risk group may be useful.

Once diagnosed, treatment should be initiated, either by therapy or antidepressant medications.

Cognitive behavioural therapy (CBT) is an established psychological approach that is recommended as first-line treatment for depression and mild to moderate anxiety in the UK (NICE, 2004a; 2004b).

CBT has been shown to be of benefit for patients with COPD (Heslop *et al.*, 2009) because it focuses on problems and their solutions, encourages self-management, and specifically addresses misconceptions, unhelpful beliefs, and maladaptive patterns of behaviour. The last are common in patients with COPD. They include beliefs that mild breathlessness on exertion is harmful and that supplemental oxygen is needed for breathlessness even when oxygen saturations are normal, as well as the overuse of inhalers and emergency admission to hospital because of an inappropriate fear of dying when breathless.

Pharmacological interventions

Pharmacological treatment plays a central role in the management of COPD, and should be used in conjunction with smoking cessation and pulmonary rehabilitation, with the aim of improving symptoms and quality of life and preventing exacerbations.

Whilst the asthma guidelines use a stepwise approach to symptom control, early COPD guidelines used an 'escalator', moving up the treatment options to control symptoms (British Thoracic Society, 1997), with the current National Institute for Health and Clinical Excellence (NICE, 2010) guidelines recommending increasing treatment according to symptoms.

Figure 5.4 highlights the recommended approach to introducing inhaled treatment (National Institute for Health and Clinical Excellence (NICE), 2010).

Many of the medications used in COPD are inhaled. These can be difficult to use and it is important to allow

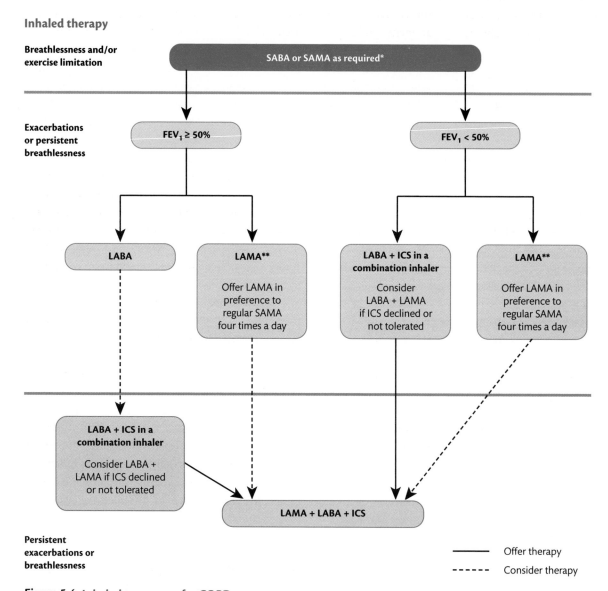

Figure 5.4 Inhaled treatment for COPD.

Reproduced with permission from the National Institute for Health and Clinical Excellence (2010) Clinical Guideline 101: *Chronic Obstructive Pulmonary Disease: Management of Chronic Obstructive Pulmonary Disease in Adults in Primary and Secondary Care (Partial Update)*, NICE: London. Available from **www.nice.org.uk/guidance/CG101.**
SABA, short-acting beta agonists; SAMA, short-acting muscarinic antagonists; LABA, long-acting β_2 agonists; LAMA, long-acting muscarinic antagonists; ICS, inhaled corticosteroids .

time to select the most appropriate device to ensure effective use and adequate drug delivery. Inhalers are available in aerosol or dry powder format. On selecting an inhaler device, consideration should be given to the inspiratory flow required to ensure adequate lung deposition, because dry powder devices require a fast in-breath, whilst aerosol devices require a slow and steady in-breath.

Patients with COPD may have the added difficulties of poor dexterity secondary to arthritis, loss of muscle power (e.g. post cerebrovascular accident), and memory loss. By allowing the patient to handle the device and be involved in the prescribing decisions, adherence and response to treatment may improve (see Chapter 22 Managing Medicines ➡). Response to bronchodilator therapy should not be assessed by lung function alone; consider other measures such as improvement in symptoms, activities of daily living, exercise capacity, and rapidity of symptom relief. Assessment following commencement of treatment is necessary.

National Institute for Health and Clinical Excellence guidelines (NICE, 2010) recommend regular **short-acting β_2 agonists** (SABA, e.g. salbutamol/terbutaline), which have been discussed in Chapter 2 (Understanding Asthma ➡), and/or a **short-acting muscarinic antagonist** (SAMA, e.g. ipratropium) as an initial treatment for breathlessness.

If breathlessness persists, a SAMA should be introduced, if not already commenced. Muscarinic antagonists work on the muscarinic receptors in the lungs, causing the smooth muscle in the bronchioles to relax, resulting in bronchodilatation. They last for approximately 4–6 hours. Common side effects include a dry mouth, glaucoma, and prostatism. SAMA are available in a metered dose aerosol.

Long-acting β_2 agonists (LABA, e.g. salmeterol/formoterol/indacaterol) should be considered if breathlessness persists despite regular short-acting β_2 agonists and short-acting muscarinic antagonists. They are available as a dry powder and metered dose preparation and are taken twice a day (salmeterol and formoterol) or once a day (indacaterol).

Long-acting muscarinic antagonists (LAMA, e.g. tiotropium) have a similar profile to the short-acting preparation. It is believed that they can reduce hyperinflation, which results in an increased exercise tolerance and an improvement in breathlessness. Outcomes from studies reveal a reduction in exacerbation rates, and lung function (FEV$_1$) may be maintained (Tashkin *et al.*, 2008). Tiotropium has the added benefit of lasting for 24 hours, which can improve symptom control and adherence to treatment. This medication is available as a dry powder and soft mist preparation.

Inhaled corticosteroids

Inhaled corticosteroids (ICS) as a monotherapy are not licensed for the treatment of COPD. Studies have demonstrated that, in patients with moderate to severe disease (FEV$_1$ <50% predicted), the introduction of ICS (fluticasone or budesonide) and a LABA result in a reduction in exacerbations and improve health-related quality of life (Calverley *et al.*, 2007; Szafranski *et al.*, 2003). National Institute for Health and Clinical Excellence guidelines (NICE, 2010) recommend that they should be commenced in individuals with moderate obstruction and a history of two or more exacerbations a year. However, patients should be informed that there is evidence that there is an increase in the incidence of non-fatal pneumonia when taking high-dose inhaled corticosteroids (Crim *et al.*, 2009), although this evidence was found only when using fluticasone.

To improve adherence with treatment, they can be prescribed as a combination inhaler, including a LABA. Currently Seretide® and Symbicort® are the two combination inhalers licensed for patients with COPD, and are available for use in COPD as a dry powder preparation.

Methylxanthines

Methylxanthines are used for their bronchodilatory effects at a higher dose, which is often accompanied by side effects, including headaches, nausea and vomiting, and ventricular tachycardia. The benefit versus the impact of contraindications needs to be considered when prescribing these.

Mucolytics

For many patients with COPD, expectorating sputum can be tiring and difficult, despite effective sputum clearance techniques. The introduction of mucolytic agents provides some relief and will ease the discomfort. Currently the National Institute for Health and Clinical Excellence (NICE, 2010) recommends a trial of mucolytics (carbocisteine or mecysteine), emphasizing the importance of evaluating the effectiveness of treatment.

Phosphodiesterase 4 (PD4) inhibitors

Phosphodiesterase 4 (PD4) inhibitors (e.g. roflumilast) are believed to exhibit a broad range of anti-inflammatory effects resulting in an improvement in lung function and reduction in exacerbation rate (Fabbri *et al.*, 2009). It is available as an oral preparation, with side effects including gastrointestinal disturbances, significant weight loss, and psychiatric disturbances. Therefore, it is not suitable for all patients with COPD.

Oxygen therapy

Many patients with COPD become hypoxaemic, which can be corrected with supplementary oxygen therapy. There is strong evidence that long-term oxygen therapy (LTOT) can reduce mortality (Medical Research Council, 1981; Nocturnal Oxygen Therapy Trial Group, 1980). Patient monitoring for chronic hypoxaemia is essential and home oxygen considered. Chronic hypoxaemia leads to increased pulmonary arterial pressure, polycythaemia, and neuropsychological changes. The benefits of LTOT are indicated in Box 5.5.

Oxygen assessment should include maximization of pharmacological treatment and confirmation of hypoxaemia, with correct oxygen flow rate determined to correct the hypoxaemia.

Encourage smoking cessation and assess risks associated to safe installation and use of home oxygen support.

Concordance with LTOT oxygen therapy is essential. Normally, it is prescribed for a minimum of 15 hours in a 24-hour period, with patients encouraged to wear it at night, when there is an increased risk of worsening respiratory failure. Portable or ambulatory oxygen systems are available to allow continuous oxygen therapy.

It is important to explain the reasons for LTOT in understandable language for the patient, including the basic principles of oxygen therapy and how it will help his or her condition. The selection of the most appropriate delivery device (mask or nasal cannula) is important. For some people, a nasal cannula causes discomfort, sore ears, and facial markings, whilst others find a mask claustrophobic. The financial implications may also affect concordance to treatment. The concentrator (see Figure 5.5) runs off electricity and, although the cost of the electricity used is reimbursed, it will increase household expenditure. The concentrator itself can be offputting because it is large and produces noise and heat.

Patients who comply with treatment do significantly better. This includes both pharmacological and non-pharmacological interventions. Working closely and fostering a genuine relationship with patients to alleviate anxieties and fears of the condition and treatment can improve concordance.

Surgery

Whilst COPD is predominantly treated with pharmacological interventions and lifestyle changes, in a small minority of patients with emphysema, surgical interventions may be of benefit to reduce dynamic hyperinflammation in the form of lung volume reduction surgery and bullectomy. Lung transplantation may also be an option in some patients with COPD.

Identifying and managing acute exacerbations

A COPD exacerbation is defined as 'a sustained worsening of the patient's symptoms from his or her usual stable state that is beyond normal day to day variations and is acute in onset' (National Institute for Health and Clinical Excellence (NICE), 2010). The causes of exacerbations

---

Box 5.5 The benefits of long-term oxygen therapy

- Increased survival
- Increased quality of life
- Prevention of deterioration of pulmonary haemodynamics
- Reduction in secondary polycythaemia
- Neuropsychological benefits with reduction in symptoms of anxiety and depression
- Improved sleep quality
- Reduction in cardiac arrhythmias
- Increase in renal blood flow

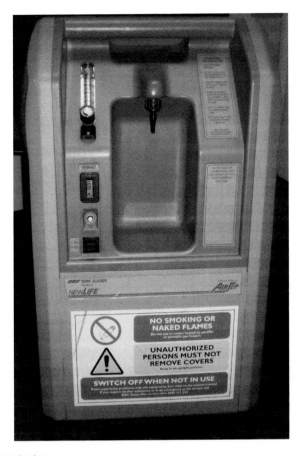

Figure 5.5 **An oxygen concentrator.**

include viral and bacterial infections, air pollutions, and environmental irritants.

Exacerbations are an important event for patients with COPD. They cause a significant impact on quality of life and increase the rate of lung function decline. Worsening disability with slow recovery rate can leave patients incapacitated for several weeks.

For many, they can be self-limited and managed effectively by the patient, but for more severe exacerbations, admission to hospital may be necessary. 'Hospital at home' and early supported discharge schemes are often employed to support and monitor patients, and have been evaluated as being safe and cost-effective in selected patients (Ram *et al.*, 2004). Such schemes are often nurse-led and enable working across care settings.

Initial treatment includes bronchodilators, antibiotics, and oral corticosteroids. Oxygen should be given with care to correct hypoxia, because potential for type 2 respiratory failure is present. For patients with a history of type 2 respiratory failure, target oxygen saturations should be between 88% and 92%, and patients should be issued with oxygen alert cards, highlighting that they are at risk if given too much oxygen (British Thoracic Society, 2008).

Non-invasive ventilation

Non-invasive ventilation (NIV) should be considered, and bi-level positive pressure ventilation should be available as a treatment option in all patients presenting with acute acidosis type 2 respiratory failure (British Thoracic Society, 2002; National Institute for Health and Clinical Excellence (NICE), 2010).

Bi-level positive ventilation improves tidal volume, reduces the work of breathing, and improves gas exchange through 'splinting' open of the alveoli. This in turn corrects acidosis, hypercapnia, and hypoxia.

Not all patients are suitable for NIV, but the success rate is good for those who are able to have and tolerate it. Success is determined by the correction of the blood gas imbalance, with pH being the best marker reflecting alveolar ventilation (Plant and Elliott, 2003).

Criteria include two of the following:

- Moderate to severe acidosis (pH 7.35)
- Hypercapnia $PaCO_2$ 6.0–8.0 kPa
- Respiratory rate >25 breaths per minute
- Moderate to severe dyspnoea, with use of accessory muscles and paradoxical abdominal movement

Exclusion criteria include:

- respiratory arrest;
- cardiovascular instability;
- gag reflex absent;
- recent facial or gastrointestinal surgery;
- craniofacial trauma, nasopharyngeal abnormalities;
- facial burns;
- undrained pneumothorax.

Good communication and interpersonal skills are essential when initiating NIV, because patients are often scared and frightened, and may be confused/agitated due to hypoxia and hypercapnia. This method of ventilatory support is delivered via a snugly fitted mask with a good seal between the face and mask. Synchronization of the respiratory rate of the patient and the ventilator, along with adequate inspiratory and expiratory ventilator pressures being selected, will help the patient to tolerate NIV.

Invasive ventilation

The decision to ventilate a patient invasively will depend on his or her quality of life, severity of disease, and wishes, and therefore may be an option for some patients for whom NIV has failed

It is important to discuss treatment options with patients when they are in a stable condition, because often the decision to escalate treatment is made during an acute episode.

Follow-up care

Reviewing patients following an exacerbation is an important part of their ongoing management. Recovery time can be lengthy and readmission to hospital is common.

The Clinical Strategy for COPD (2010) recommends that all patients are reviewed by a specialist within 2 weeks if admitted to hospital and all others within a 6–8-week period. The purpose of the review is to assess their clinical state, including spirometry and oxygen saturations/blood gases, review medications and inhaler technique, and interventions, and to discuss lifestyle adjustments, e.g. smoking cessation, and self-management strategies.

For all patients with COPD, ongoing monitoring of symptoms and disease severity is an important aspect of care and allows adjustment to treatment, further investigation, and timely referrals to the multidisciplinary team.

Managing advanced disease and palliative care

An acute exacerbation can be a very frightening experience for patients and an admission to hospital increases the risk of mortality. Symptom management should be reviewed and, for patients with more severe airflow obstruction, involvement of the palliative care team may be appropriate. Advance care planning should also be considered in this group of patients.

However, such discussions are often difficult and avoided by healthcare professionals owing to the sensitivity of the subject and the difficulties in predicting mortality in patients with COPD (see also Chapter 18 Managing End-of-Life Care ➡).

Patient education and self-management

The following areas need to be included when educating the patient with COPD:

- understanding and living with COPD;
- non-pharmacological treatment—smoking cessation, pulmonary rehabilitation, and NIV;
- pharmacological interventions, including oxygen therapy;
- knowing symptoms of an exacerbation, when to start additional treatment, and when to seek advice;
- local support (e.g. breathe-easy clubs run by the British Lung Foundation, **www.lung.org.uk**).

Self-management plans for patients with COPD have shown appropriate interventions for exacerbations (Wood-Baker *et al.*, 2006), with an increased use of antibiotics

CASE STUDY 5.2 *Management of the acute exacerbation of COPD*

Mr White is 69 years old and has COPD. He presents to the GP surgery with a 2-day history of feeling more breathless, expectorating more sputum, and needing to use his inhaler more frequently. The GP diagnoses a chest infection or exacerbation of COPD and contacts the community respiratory nurse, requesting an assessment and management at home. The community respiratory nurse visits Mr White and undertakes an assessment.

Assessment

Physical assessment: Temperature 37.3°C, pulse rate 84 bpm, respiratory rate 18 breaths/min, BP 140/70, oxygen saturations on air of 93%, and chest examination revealed widespread inspiratory and expiratory wheeze.

Psychosocial assessment: Mr White lives alone in a two-bedroomed house, with an upstairs toilet. He is usually independent and is able to do his own shopping and housework. However, he is finding it difficult to climb stairs to use the bathroom and has not felt able to go to the shops for the past few days, and has little fresh food in the house. He smokes 20 cigarettes a day.

Management plan

Mr White has been prescribed antibiotics and corticosteroids by the GP. The nurse ensures that he understands the treatment and also explains that he may use his short-acting β_2 agonists every 2–4 hours to help his breathlessness. She checks that he is able to use his inhaler effectively.

She discusses the importance of smoking cessation, but Mr White does not wish to stop smoking at present.

She refers him to social services for emergency home care and the delivery of a commode. She arranges for the district nurses to visit him in the evening to ensure that he has not deteriorated, and ensures that he has the contact number for the district nurses and the out-of-hours services. She arranges to visit him the following morning.

The following morning, Mr White is more breathless, appears cyanosed, and a little confused. His observations reveal temperature 38.2°C, pulse 98 bpm, respirations 18 breaths/min, and oxygen saturations 87% on air. The respiratory nurse is concerned that Mr White may be in type 2 respiratory failure and may benefit from non-invasive ventilation. She arranges for him to be admitted to hospital.

Mr White is taken to the local hospital and it is confirmed that he has developed type 2 respiratory failure, secondary to a severe exacerbation of COPD. He is admitted for non-invasive ventilation.

Nursing care of a patient requiring NIV

When nursing a patient requiring non-invasive ventilation, basic nursing care is vital to ensure adherence with treatment. This should include the following.

- Explain the treatment to alleviate anxieties. The patient should have the call bell accessible at all times.
- The patient should be closely monitored, including oximetry and general observations being documented.
- Careful administration of supplementary oxygen is essential to prevent further deterioration in blood gases.
- Correctly fit the face mask, ensuring that it is not too tight, which could result in pressure sores, especially across the bridge of the nose, or too loose, resulting in irritation of the eyes and inadequate ventilation.
- Hydration and nutrition needs should be assessed, and patients should be offered regular oral fluids and may require intravenous fluids.

Mr White responded well to NIV and, prior to discharge, he was seen by the smoking cessation team and felt that he would like to stop smoking. He was commenced on appropriate nicotine replacement therapy and ongoing support via his community pharmacist was arranged.

He was referred for early pulmonary rehabilitation and back to the community respiratory team for ongoing management of this exacerbation and long-term care in the community.

and oral corticosteroids (Effing *et al.*, 2007). Therefore the Consultation Document for the Clinical Strategy for COPD (Department of Health, 2010) encourages the implementation of self-management/action plans for all patients with COPD.

However, it should be acknowledged that individuals need to address issues on a number of different levels, including symptoms, behavioural, cognitive and social/environmental factors, which are addressed within pulmonary rehabilitation programmes, for self-management to be effective.

Self-management strategies should incorporate five core skills to increase confidence in the management of any long-term condition (Department of Health, 2001):

- problem-solving;
- decision-making;
- resource utilization;
- developing effective partnership with health providers;
- taking action.

Supporting written information about living with COPD is available from the British Lung Foundation **www.lung.org.uk.**

Identifying best practice

Throughout the chapter and below are a list of recent sources of the best evidence to inform the nursing care of patients with COPD. Because research is always ongoing and best practice evolves, it is important that readers stay up to date and know where to find good-quality sources of evidence. Hence we have provided a list of resources that readers should utilize.

- National Institute for Health and Clinical Excellence (2010) **www.nice.org.uk/guidance/CG101**
- Global Initiative for Obstructive Lung Disease (GOLD) Global strategy for the diagnosis, management and prevention of COPD (2009 update) **www.copd.com/**

- British Thoracic Society (2002) Non invasive ventilation in acute respiratory failure: British Thoracic Society Standards of Care Committee. *Thorax* **57**: 192–211
- British Thoracic Society (2008) Emergency oxygen guidelines for adult patients. *Thorax* **63** (Suppl. VI): vi1–vi73
- Effing, T.W., Monninkhof, E.M., van der Valk, P.D.L. (2007) Self-management education for patients with chronic obstructive pulmonary disease. Cochrane Database Systematic Reviews Issue 4 Art No.:CD002990
- National Institute for Health and Clinical Excellence (NICE) (2006) Brief interventions and referral for smoking cessation in primary care and other settings. Public Health Intervention Guidance **http://www.nice.org.uk/nicemedia/live/11375/31864/31864.pdf**
- National Institute for Health and Clinical Excellence (NICE) (2007) Varenicline for smoking cessation. Technical Appraisal 123 **www.nice.org.uk/TA123**

Resources

Organizations

British Thoracic Society
Primary Care Respiratory Society
National Institute for Health and Clinical Excellence (NICE) **http://guidance.nice.org.uk/**
The Scottish Intercollegiate Guidelines Network (SIGN) **http://www.sign.ac.uk/guidelines/index.html**
NHS Evidence **http://www.evidence.nhs.uk/**
Agency for Healthcare Quality (AHRQ) **http://www.ahrq.gov/**
National Institute for Clinical Studies (NICS) **http://www.nhmrc.gov.au/nics/index.htm**
Registered Nurses Association of Ontario **http://www.rnao.org**

Journals

Primary Care Respiratory Society Journal
Thorax
European Respiratory Journal

Conclusion

Without effective prevention and treatment, COPD can be a life-limiting disease, with significant impact on both morbidity and mortality. The importance of early diagnosis is crucial to commencing interventions, with the goals of treatment being to minimize the progression of the disease, to reduce symptoms experienced, and to maximize physical function, resulting in an overall improvement in quality of life.

The emphasis on the importance of managing all long-term conditions and reflecting on the Consultation Document for the Clinical Strategy for COPD (2010) will hopefully drive forward the importance of prevention, identification, and treatment to improve the burden of disease. Nurses in both the acute and primary care settings are in an ideal position to support, educate, and care for patients with COPD throughout the entire disease trajectory.

Answer to Case study 5.1

The following should be encouraged: smoking cessation, pulmonary rehabilitation, and influenza/pneumonia vaccinations. Commence on a short-acting beta agonist (SABA) initially, then review, support, and monitor her mood.

Online Resource Centre

 To help you to develop and apply your knowledge and decision-making skills further, we have provided interactive learning resources online at **www.oxfordtextbooks.co.uk/orc/bullock/**

Whilst these are freely available you will need to use the access codes at the start of the book.

References

British Lung Foundation (2002) *Cannabis: A Smoking Gun*. British Lung Foundation: London.

British Lung Foundation (2006) *Missing Millions*. British Lung Foundation: London.

British Thoracic Society (1997) Guidelines on the management of chronic obstructive pulmonory disease. *Thorax* **52** (Suppl. 5): S1–S28.

British Thoracic Society (2002) Non invasive ventilation in acute respiratory failure: British Thoracic Society Standards of Care Committee. *Thorax* **57**: 192–211.

British Thoracic Society (2008) Emergency oxygen guidelines for adult patients. *Thorax* **63** (Suppl. VI): vi1–vi73.

Britton, M. (2003) The burden of COPD in the UK: results from the Confronting COPD survey. *Respiratory Medicine* **97**(Suppl. C): S71–9.

Calverley, P.M.A., Anderson, J.A., Celli, B., *et al.*, for the TORCH Investigators (2007) Salmeterol and fluticasone propionate and survival in chronic obstructive pulmonary disease. *New England Journal of Medicine* **356**: 775–89.

Commission for Healthcare Audit and Inspection (2006) *Clearing the Air*. HMSO: London.

Crim, C., Calverley, P.M.A., Anderson, A., *et al.* (2009) Pneumonia risk in COPD patients receiving inhaled corticosteroids alone or in combination. *European Respiratory Journal* **34**(3): 641–7.

Department of Health (2001) *The Expert Patient. A New Approach to Chronic Disease Management for the 21st Century*. HMSO London.

Department of Health (2010) *Consultation on a Strategy for Services for Chronic Obstructive Pulmonary Disease* (COPD). HMSO London.

Effing, T.W., Monninkhof, E.M., van der Valk, P.D.L. (2007) Self-management education for patients with chronic obstructive pulmonary disease. *Cochrane Database of Systematic Reviews* Issue 4: Art No. CD002990. DOI: 10. 1002/14651858. CD003793. Pub2.

Fabbri, L.M., Calverley, P.M.A., Izquierdo–Alonso, J., *et al.* (2009) Roflumilast in moderate-to-severe chronic obstructive pulmonary disease treated with longacting bronchodilators: two randomised clinical trials. *Lancet* **374**: 695–703.

Fletcher, C.M., Elmes, P.C., Fairbairn, M.B., *et al.* (1959) The significance of respiratory symptoms and the diagnosis of chronic bronchitis in a working population. *British Medical Journal* ii: 257–66.

Garrod, R. (2004) *Pulmonary Rehabilitation: An Interdisciplinary Approach.* Whurr Publishers: London.

Global Initiative for Chronic Obstructive Lung Disease (GOLD) (2009 update). *Global Strategy for the Diagnosis, Management and Prevention of COPD.* **www goldcopd com/** (accessed May 2011).

Heslop, K., De Soyza, A., Baker, C.R. (2009) Using individualised cognitive behavioural therapy as a treatment for people with COPD. *Nursing Times* **105**: 14–17.

Kumar, P., Clark, M. (2005) *Clinical Medicine*, 6 edn. Elsevier Saunders: London, pp. 900–1.

Lacasse, Y., Goldstein, R., Lasserson, T.J., *et al.* (2006) Pulmonary rehabilitation for chronic obstructive pulmonary disease. *Cochrane Database of Systematic Reviews* Issue 4: Art. No. CD00379. D01: 10.1002 | 14651858. CD003793. pub2.

Maurer, J., Rebbapragada, V., Borson, S., *et al.* (2008) Anxiety and depression in COPD: current understanding, unanswered questions and research needs. *Chest* **134**: 43S–56S.

Medical Research Council Working Party (1981) Long term domiciliary oxygen therapy in chronic hypoxic cor pulmonale complicating chronic bronchitis and emphysema. *Lancet* i: 681–6.

Murray, C.J.L., Lopez, A.D. (1997) Alternative projections of mortality and disability by cause 1990–2020: Global Burden of Disease Study. *Lancet* **349**: 1498–504.

National Institute for Health and Clinical Excellence (NICE) (2004a) *Depression: Management of Depression in Primary and Secondary Care.* National Institute for Health and Clinical Excellence (NICE): London.

National Institute for Health and Clinical Excellence (NICE) (2004b) *Anxiety: Management of Anxiety (Panic Disorder, with or without Agoraphobia, and Generalised Anxiety Disorder) in Adults in Primary, Secondary and Community Care.* National Institute for Health and Clinical Excellence (NICE): London.

National Institute for Health and Clinical Excellence (NICE) (2006) Brief interventions and referral for smoking cessation in primary care and other settings. Public Health Intervention Guidance 1. **http://www.nice.org.uk/nicemedia/live/11375/31864/31864. pdf** (accessed 4 April 2010).

National Institute for Health and Clinical Excellence (NICE) (2007) Varenicline for smoking cessation. Technical Appraisal 123. **www.nice.org.uk/TA123** (accessed 4 April 2010).

National Institute for Health and Clinical Excellence (NICE) (2010). The management of chronic obstructive pulmonary disease in adults in primary and secondary care. NICE Clinical Guideline 102 (CG102). National Institute for Health and Clinical Excellence (NICE): London.

Nici, L., Donner, C., Wouters, E., *et al.* (2006) American Thoracic Society/European Society statement on pulmonary rehabilitation. *American Journal of Respiratory and Critical Care Medicine* **12**: 1390–413.

Nocturnal Oxygen Therapy Trial Group (1980) Continuous or nocturnal oxygen therapy in hypoxaemic chronic obstructive lung disease. *Annals of Internal Medicine* **93**: 391–8.

Plant, P., Elliott, M. (2003) Chronic obstructive pulmonary disease 9: management of ventilator failure in COPD. *Thorax* **58**: 537–42.

Puhan, M.A., Scharplatz, M., Troosters, T., *et al.* (2005) Respiratory rehabilitation after acute exacerbation of COPD may reduce risk for readmission and mortality: a systematic review. *Respiratory Medicine* **6**: 54.

Ram, F., Wedzicha, J., Wright Greenstone, M. (2004) Hospital at home for patients with acute exacerbations of COPD: systematic review of the evidence. *British Medical Journal* **329**: 315–19.

Robinson, T., Scullion, J. (2009) *Oxford Handbook of Respiratory Nursing.* Oxford University Press: Oxford.

Scullion, J., Holmes, S. (2010) The importance of primary care spirometry. *Independent Nurse* 15 February: 33–4.

Szafranski, W., Cukier, A., Ramirez, A., *et al.* (2003) Efficacy and safety of budesonide/formoterol in the management of chronic obstructive pulmonary disease. *European Respiratory Journal* **21**(1): 74–81.

Tashkin, D.P., Celli, B., Senn, S., *et al.* (2008) A 4-year trial of tiotropium in chronic obstructive pulmonary disease. *New England Journal of Medicine* **359**(15): 1543–54.

Van Manen, J.G., Bindels, P.J.E., Dekker, F.W., *et al.* (2002) Risk of depression in patients with chronic obstructive pulmonary disease. *Thorax* **57**: 412–16.

West, R., McNeill, A., Raw, M. (2000) Smoking cessation guidelines for health professionals: an update: Health Education Authority. *Thorax* **55**(12): 987–99.

Wood-Baker, R., McGlone, S., Venn, A., *et al.* (2006) Written action plans in chronic obstructive pulmonary disease increase appropriate treatment for exacerbations. *Respirology* **11**: 619–26.

6 *Understanding* Coronary Heart Disease

Alison Pottle

> ## Introduction
>
> The aim of this chapter is to provide nurses with the knowledge to be able to assess, manage, and care for people with coronary heart disease (CHD) in an evidence-based and person-centred way. The chapter will provide a comprehensive overview of the causes, risk factors, and impact of CHD. In guiding you through patient assessment, the differences between acute coronary syndromes (ACS) and angina are established before exploring best practice to deliver care, as well as to prevent or to minimize further ill-health. Nursing assessments and priorities are highlighted throughout, and the nursing management of the symptoms and common health problems associated with coronary heart disease can be found in Chapters 15, 22, 24, and 25, respectively. →

Understanding coronary heart disease

Definitions

CHD is defined as the failure of the coronary arteries to deliver adequate oxygen for myocardial work. It is almost always caused by atherosclerosis—a gradual build-up of fatty plaques within the artery wall that reduces blood flow. This failure to meet metabolic demands results in a range of clinical conditions sharing common pathological process (Baxendale, 1992), including ACS and angina.

Chest pain is the symptom that informs clinical decision-making. It is classified based on history-taking and investigations such as the electrocardiogram (ECG).

Angina

Angina was first described by Heberden in 1772 as a 'painful and disagreeable sensation in the breast, which seems as if it would take their life away if it were to increase or continue.' (cited by Fox *et al.*, 2006). Stable angina is described as a clinical syndrome that is characterized by discomfort in the chest, jaw, shoulder, back, and arms, typically elicited by exertional emotional stress and relieved by rest or nitroglycerine (Fox *et al.*, 2006).

Acute coronary syndrome

ACS is an umbrella term for several clinical presentations, including unstable angina, non-ST elevation myocardial infarction (NSTEMI), and ST elevation myocardial infarction

(STEMI). The European Society of Cardiology defines ACS as '. . . a life threatening manifestation of atherosclerosis . . . caused by a ruptured atherosclerotic plaque . . . causing sudden complete or critical reduction in blood flow' (Bassand *et al.*, 2007). Patients with ACS present with acute chest pain. The differentiation between STEMI, NSTEMI, and unstable angina is made on the ECG findings and on the measurement of biochemical markers (Bassand *et al.*, 2007).

ST elevation myocardial infarction

STEMI is defined as typical acute chest pain and persistent (>20 minutes) ST segment elevation on the ECG. The great majority of these patients will show a typical rise of the biochemical markers of **myocardial necrosis** (Van de Werf *et al.*, 2008).

ST elevation on the ECG represents acute injury to the myocardium. Figure 6.1 shows the changes to the ST segment that occur with STEMI and NSTEMI.

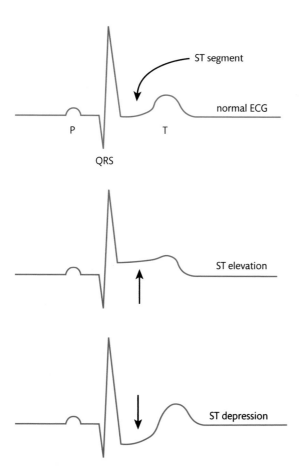

Figure 6.1   Changes to the ST segment that occur with STEMI and NSTEMI.

There are two theories as to why this change to the ECG happens. The 'current of injury' theory suggests that, during myocardial injury, the damaged cells lose their membrane integrity, which results in K^+ leakage. The outside of the cells become more electrically negative, which decreases the charge of the baseline. If the damage is near to the positive electrode of the ECG, the baseline decreases in voltage and the ST segment is then elevated from the baseline. The 'incomplete depolarization' theory is based on the belief that damaged cells do not completely depolarize, with electrodes placed in close proximity to the damaged cells showing a more positive ST segment (Smith *et al.*, 2002). ST segment elevation may not occur instantly when the patient suffers the STEMI; however, ST elevation has to occur to make the diagnosis of STEMI. The area of infarction can be determined by examining which ECG leads show ST elevation. Figure 6.7 shows a common ST elevation pattern. Figure 6.8 shows left bundle branch block, which can be an alternative ECG presentation of an acute **myocardial infarction**. The priority is for the patient to receive treatment (angioplasty or thrombolysis) to minimize myocardial damage. Further ECG changes will occur, such as inversion of the T wave, indicating ischaemia, and development of Q waves, indicating myocardial necrosis. The aim of prompt treatment for patients with ACS is prevention or minimization of permanent myocardial damage.

For ACS, it is useful to consider the symptoms that patients will experience, for example sweating, pain in the arms/jaw, and shortness of breath (SOB). This is discussed later.

Prevalence and epidemiological profile

Diseases of the heart and circulatory system (cardiovascular disease or CVD) are the number one cause of death globally: more people die annually from CVD than from any other cause. By 2030, it is estimated that almost 23.6 million people will die from CVD, mainly from heart disease and stroke. The largest percentage increase is predicted to occur in the Eastern Mediterranean region, and the largest increase in number of deaths is expected to be in the South East Asia region (World Health Organization, 2009). In the UK, CVD accounts for almost 191,000 deaths each year—one in three of all deaths. Almost half (46%) of all deaths from CVD are from CHD (Scarborough *et al.*, 2010). Figure 6.2 shows the deaths by cause in men in the

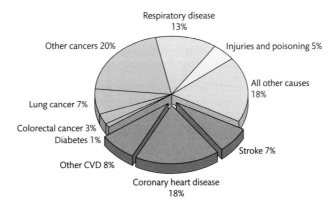

Figure 6.2 Deaths by cause in men in the UK in 2008.

Adapted from Scarborough, P., Bhatnagar, P., Wickramasinghe, K. *et al.* (2010) *Coronary Heart Disease Statistics 2010*, British Heart Foundation: London. See **www.heartstats.org**.

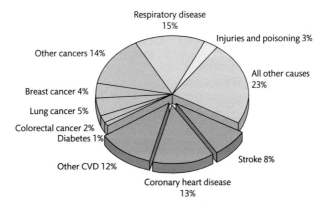

Figure 6.3 Deaths by cause in women in the UK in 2008.

Adapted from Scarborough, P., Bhatnagar, P., Wickramasinghe, K. *et al.* (2010) *Coronary Heart Disease Statistics 2010*, British Heart Foundation: London. See **www.heartstats.org**.

UK in 2008 and Figure 6.3 shows the deaths by cause in women in the UK in 2008.

The incidence of myocardial infarction (MI) has decreased in a number of developed countries, including the UK, during the past three decades. This is thought to have been driven by favourable changes in risk factors. Recent estimates of incidence of MI in the UK, based on national-level data from hospital and mortality statistics, suggest that, in Scotland, the incidence rate of MI has decreased by about 25% between 2000 and 2009 in both men and women (Scarborough *et al.*, 2010). The incidence of MI increases sharply with age. Incidence is higher in men than in women, but the difference between the sexes decreases with increasing age. There is a consider-

able north–south gradient in the UK. Figures comparing 2005 with 2007 suggest that the incidence of MI appears to be 20% and 35% higher in Scotland compared to England for both men and women, respectively (Scarborough *et al.*, 2010).

Latest figures from England and Scotland suggest that there are an estimated 62,000 MIs in English men and 39,000 in English women every year, and 8,000 MIs in Scottish men and 5,000 in Scottish women annually. If the rates for Northern Ireland and Wales were comparable to those in England, there would be approximately 124,000 MIs in the UK every year (Scarborough *et al.*, 2010).

There are various estimates of the incidence of angina. Data from samples of GP registries suggest that, in 2009, the incidence of angina was highest in Scotland and lowest in England for both men and women. Overall in the UK, incidence rates were 75% higher in men than women, with the highest incidence rates being in the 65–74 age group in both sexes. Using these incidence rates, it is suggested that there are approximately 28,000 new cases of angina in the UK every year (Scarborough *et al.*, 2010).

Data from the 2006 Health Survey for England suggest that the prevalence of CHD in England was 6.5% in men and 4.0% in women. Overall, it is estimated that there are 970,000 men and 439,000 women aged 35 and over living in the UK who have had an MI. In addition, there are just over 1.1 million men and 850 000 women aged over 35 living in the UK who have angina (Joint Health Surveys Unit, 2008).

Management of this problem in primary care

The Quality Outcomes Framework (QOF) was implemented into general practice in 2004 and provides information on the number of patients in each practice with certain conditions. Data from 2008–09 suggest that there were around 2.3 million people in the UK with CHD. The prevalence of CHD was higher in Scotland (4.4%), Wales (4.2%), and Northern Ireland (4.1%) than in England (3.5%) (Scarborough *et al.*, 2010).

Mortality

CHD is the commonest cause of death in the UK. In 2008, around one in five men and one in eight women died from the disease, a total of around 88,000 deaths (Scarborough *et al.*, 2010). CHD is the commonest cause of premature death in the UK, with about one-fifth of

premature deaths in men and one in ten premature deaths in women being due to CHD. However, death rates for CHD have declined in the UK over the past three decades, falling by 44% in the past 10 years (under 75 age group). This trend is not repeated in younger age groups, with some evidence suggesting that rates are beginning to plateau in this age range (Allender *et al.*, 2008).

As well as human costs, CHD has major economic consequences for the UK, costing the healthcare system around £3.2 billion in 2006. The cost of hospital care for people who have CHD accounts for about 73% of these costs. However, the total cost of CHD to the UK is much higher when production losses from those of working age and from informal care of those with the disease are added. In 2006, estimated production losses due to mortality and morbidity associated with CHD cost the UK over £3.9 billion, with around 65% of this cost due to death and 35% due to illness in those of working age. The cost of informal care for those with CHD was estimated to be around £1.8 billion in the same year (Scarborough *et al.*, 2010) (Figure 6.4). In 2008–09, 2.9% of all outpatient attendances were for a cardiology condition and there were over 420,000 finished consultant inpatient episodes for ischaemic heart disease (Hospital Episode Statistics, 2009).

Risk factors

The cause of atherosclerosis is unknown, although epidemiological evidence points to a complex interaction of genetic and environmental influences. A number of 'risk factors' have been identified that appear to have a positive association with the occurrence of CHD. Evidence

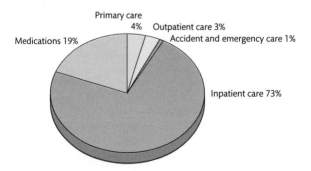

Figure 6.4 Healthcare costs of CHD in the UK in 2006.

Data from Scarborough, P., Bhatnagar, P., Wickramasinghe, K. *et al.* (2010) *Coronary Heart Disease Statistics 2010*, British Heart Foundation: London. See **www.heartstats.org**.

suggests that CHD is largely preventable by adopting a healthy lifestyle and avoidance or correction of risk factors. Risk factors that can be altered are termed 'modifiable', while those that can not be changed are 'non-modifiable'. These are listed in Box 6.1.

Modifiable risk factors are very common in the UK. Smoking causes CHD because it:

- decreases oxygen to the heart;
- increases blood pressure and heart rate;
- increases blood clotting;
- damages cells that line coronary arteries and other blood vessels.

The long-term risk of smoking to individuals is quantified in a 50-year cohort study of British doctors, which found that the mortality from CHD was around 60% higher in smokers (80% higher in heavy smokers—25 or more cigarettes per day) than in non-smokers (Doll *et al.*, 2004). In Great Britain, 21% of adults smoke cigarettes, with men aged 20–34 and women aged 16–24 having the highest prevalence. Data from the World Health Organization (WHO) Global Burden of Disease study show that smoking prevalence in men in the UK is considerably lower than the average for the European region—26% compared to 45%. The prevalence is comparable for women (World Health Organization **http://apps.who.int/ghodata/#**, accessed 16 October 2011).

The risk of CHD is directly related to blood cholesterol. The World Health Report 2002 estimates that around 8% of all disease burden in developed countries is caused by raised blood cholesterol, and that over 60% of CHD is due to total cholesterol levels in excess of 3.8 mmol/l (World Health Organization, 2002). The INTERHEART case-control study estimated that 45% of MIs in western Europe are caused by abnormal blood lipids and that those with raised lipids have a threefold risk of MI compared with those with normal levels (Yusuf *et al.*, 2004). Raised cholesterol levels increase the deposition (laying down) of cholesterol within the artery wall, forming atheroma and narrowing the lumen of the vessel.

Increases in both systolic and diastolic blood pressure directly affect the risk of CHD. Meta-analysis of prospective data on over 1 million adults has shown that, for those aged 40–69, each 20 mmHg increase in systolic blood pressure or 10 mmHg increase in diastolic blood pressure doubles the risk of death from CHD (Lewington *et al.*, 2002). In 2011, the National Institute for Health and Clinical Excellence (NICE) produced guidelines on the clinical management of patients with hypertension. The guidelines encourage the use of ambulatory blood pressure monitoring or home blood pressure monitoring to make the diagnosis rather than single measurements in a clinic. Hypertension is defined in three stages.

1. Stage 1 hypertension—clinic blood pressure of 140/90 mmHg or higher and subsequent ambulatory blood pressure monitoring daytime average, or home blood pressure monitoring average, blood pressure of 135/85 mmHg or higher
2. Stage 2 hypertension—clinic blood pressure of 160/100 mmHg or higher and subsequent ambulatory daytime average, or home blood pressure average of 150/95 mmHg or higher
3. Stage 3 hypertension—clinic systolic blood pressure of 180 mmHg or higher, or clinic diastolic blood pressure of 110 mmHg or higher

Treatment involves lifestyle changes, including advice on diet, exercise, salt intake, smoking, caffeine consumption, and alcohol intake. Antihypertensive medication is recommended for all patients with stage 2 or stage 3 hypertension. For those with stage 1 hypertension, the decision on whether to initiate drug therapy includes consideration of

---

Box 6.1 Risk factors for CHD

Modifiable:
- Smoking
- Hypercholesterolaemia
- Hypertension
- Obesity
- Physical inactivity
- Risk of developing diabetes (lifestyle changes)

Non-modifiable:
- Male gender
- Increasing age
- Ethnic origin
- Pre-existing diabetes
- Family history of premature CHD

the patient's age, other medical conditions (such as renal disease and diabetes), and the 10-year cardiovascular risk (NICE, 2011).

The British Hypertension Society guidelines in 2004 define optimal blood pressure as <120/<80 mmHg (Williams *et al.*, 2004). Constant high blood pressure hardens and thickens the artery walls, causing atherosclerosis. Arteries may also become more susceptible to plaque build-up.

As well as being an independent risk factor for CHD, obesity is also a major risk factor for hypertension, raised blood cholesterol, and diabetes (World Health Organization, 2000). The adverse effects of excess weight are increased when fat is concentrated in the abdomen—the so-called 'apple shape'—rather than around the hips—the 'pear shape'. It is therefore important to measure the waist:hip ratio rather than body mass index (BMI) as a very fit, muscular athlete may have a BMI within the obese range, but have very little body fat (Lindfield and Lemic, 2007). The INTERHEART study estimated that 63% of MIs in western Europe and 28% of MIs in central and eastern Europe were caused by abdominal obesity, and that those with abdominal obesity were at over twice the risk of MI compared to those without (Yusuf *et al.*, 2004). Physical activity levels for the UK are low, with only 39% of men and 29% of women reporting that they meet the current physical activity levels recommended by the government (Joint Health Surveys Unit, 2008). However, data from a subgroup of the study showed that only 6% of men and 4% of women actually met the government recommendations, suggesting overreporting of physical activity levels. European levels of regular physical activity (exercising at least five times a week) in 2009 range from 3% in Bulgaria to 23% in Ireland. The UK is among the highest in Europe (14%) at meeting the five times a week exercise target, and is above the EU average of 9% (Scarborough *et al.*, 2010).

The risk of CHD is higher in men than in women and increases with age. The risk of CHD for men living in the UK, but born in South Asia and Eastern Europe, and among women living in the UK, but born in South Asia, is also much higher than average. It is unclear whether this variation is because of environmental or genetic factors.

Diabetes substantially increases the risk of CHD. Raised blood glucose levels can cause damage to the artery walls, increasing the risk of atherosclerosis. Men with type 2 diabetes have a twofold to fourfold greater annual risk of CHD, and in women the risk is increased threefold to fivefold (Garcia *et al.*, 1974). Diabetes not only increases the risk of CHD, but also magnifies the effect of other risk factors such as raised cholesterol, hypertension, smoking, and obesity.

The presence of multiple risk factors has a synergistic effect. The Multiple Risk Factor Intervention Trial (MRFIT) confirmed that individuals are more at risk of CHD if they have multiple mild risk factors rather than if they have one severe risk factor (Neaton and Wentworth, 1992).

It is particularly important to assess the overall risk of CHD in primary prevention because asymptomatic individuals with a number of slightly abnormal risk factors will not usually attract medical attention. A large number of scoring systems have been produced to help in the assessment of CHD risk. Most of these are based on the American Framingham Study, which was a large population-based study in the 1970s (Dawber *et al.*, 1951; Beswick and Brindle, 2006). This study is now 40 years old and Framingham-based risk scores have been shown to overestimate the risk of CHD in some populations and to underestimate the risk in others. This has prompted the development of newer risk assessment tools. The Joint British Societies guidelines (JBS 2) have been developed to promote a consistent approach to the management of those with established CHD and those at high risk of developing the condition. The joint societies have produced tables (Figure 6.5) and a computer program **http://www.patient.co.uk/doctor/Primary-Prevention-of-Cardiovascular-Disease-(CVD).htm** that calculates the risk of an individual developing cardiovascular disease (CVD) in the next 10 years. The aim is to target preventative measures on those with the highest risk, which is defined as those with any established form of CVD, diabetics, and asymptomatic people with an estimated risk of CVD of ≥20% over 10 years (British Cardiac Society *et al.*, 2005).

In addition to modifiable and non-modifiable risk factors, there may be other factors that increase risk, but receive less attention. Patients often refer to 'stress' as a cause of CHD. There is some evidence that depression, social isolation, and lack of social support are significant risk factors for CHD and are independent of the 'conventional' risk factors (Bunker *et al.*, 2003). Also, aspects of

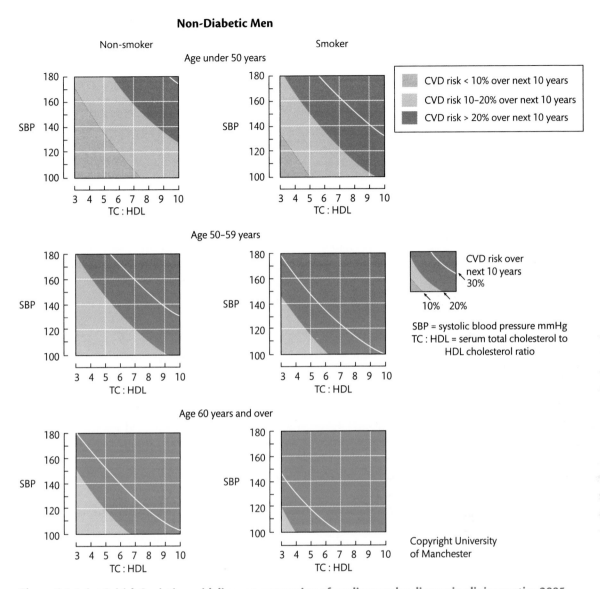

Figure 6.5 Joint British Societies guidelines on prevention of cardiovascular disease in clinic practice 2005.

Reproduced by permission of BMJ Publishing Group Ltd and the British Cardiovascular Society.

work-related stress may be associated with an increased risk (Kuper *et al.*, 2002).

The decline in mortality from CHD in the UK over the past 10 years is explained by changes in prevention and treatment, because alterations in the genetic profile of the population would not account for this degree of change. It is clear that genetic factors are important in the aetiology of CHD because it often aggregates in families, especially those with a maternal history of the disease (Rissanen and Nikkilä, 1979). The occurrence of CHD in a first-degree relative before the age of 50 in men or 55 in women is also a strong independent risk factor.

THEORY INTO PRACTICE 6.1

Activity: identifying the patient at risk

Think about your last clinical experience or your current clinical area. Compare the patient groups against the risk factors for CHD. Identify one patient who is at risk or has had an ACS/angina episode.

- How many risk factors does he or she have?
- How are those risk factors being addressed?
- What is your role in risk factor management?

The pathophysiology of CHD

In the majority of cases, CHD is caused by atherosclerosis. Other causes are rare, and some of these are listed in Box 6.2.

Atherosclerosis is a complex disorder that is not fully understood. It is characterized by progressive accumulation of lipids, complex carbohydrates, blood and its products, and calcific deposits within the intimal layer of the artery wall, with infiltration and increased production of vascular smooth muscle cells. These processes result in atheroma. It was originally thought that atherosclerosis was a slowly progressing degenerative disease affecting the elderly, but the development and progression is an inflammatory process that is dynamic and readily modifiable (Weissberg, 2000). Atheroma tends to be distributed within focal areas of the artery in plaques, which frequently occur around branching vessels or areas of arterial curvature. This would suggest that haemodynamic stressors may play a part in initiating the process. Repeated endothelial injury from toxins such as smoking, vasospasm, and other haemodynamic stressors is thought to be important in the initiation and progression of these plaques. There are three types of atherosclerotic plaque:

Box 6.2   Rare causes of CHD

Arteritis
- Systemic lupus erythematosus
- Polyarteritis nodosa
- Ankylosing spondylitis
- Syphilis
- Takayasu disease

Embolism
- Infective endocarditis
- Left atrial/ventricular thrombus
- Left atrial/ventricular tumour
- Prosthetic valve thrombus
- Complication of cardiac catheterization

Coronary mural thickening
- Amyloidosis
- Radiation therapy

Congenital coronary artery disease
- Anomalous origin from pulmonary artery
- Arteriovenous fistula

---

fatty streaks; fibrous plaques; and advanced (complicated) lesions.

Fatty streaks

Fatty streaks are flat, lipid-rich lesions that have been observed in the arteries of children as young as 2 years old (Berenson *et al.*, 1998). **Monocytes** penetrate the vessel wall and transform into fat-laden foam cells within the intima by absorbing low-density lipoprotein cholesterol. These lesions are thought to be benign and cause little or no obstruction to the coronary artery, but they are the precursor to advanced atheromatous lesions. Conversion of fatty streaks to atheroma is dependent on proliferation of vascular smooth muscle cells to **fibroblasts**.

Fibrous plaques

As the fatty streaks become more fibrous, white plaques are produced that protrude into the lumen of the artery. Further proliferation of vascular smooth muscle cells results in formation of a tough fibrous cap. Beneath this, a 'lipid pool', composed of lipids that are released when foam cells die, develops. The fibrous plaque may progress and further narrow the lumen of the vessel or it may degenerate.

Advanced lesions

Advanced lesions are composed of fibrous tissue, **fibrin**, lipids, and blood products. The lipid-rich core may increase in size and become calcified. Figure 6.6 shows the difference between a normal coronary artery and an atheromatous one.

Atherosclerotic plaques have been described as either concentric, in which the plaque is distributed equally around the circumference of the artery, or eccentric, in which the plaque does not involve the entire circumference of the vessel, resulting in areas of normal or near normal wall (Waller *et al.*, 1992).

The majority of fatal CHD events (70%) are thought to be caused by the eccentric type (Waller, 1989). Atherosclerosis is a disease with periods of stability and instability, and is often asymptomatic. The development of symptoms is closely related to the pathology of the plaque.

Stable angina

Stable angina is caused by smooth endothelialized plaques, which cause luminal stenosis. A stenosis of more than 70%

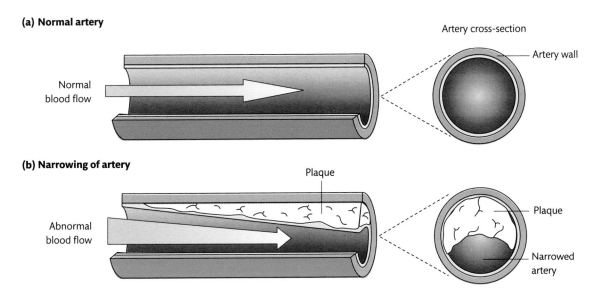

Figure 6.6 (a) Normal coronary artery; (b) coronary artery with plaque build-up.

Reproduced with permission of the National Heart, Lung and Blood Institute as a part of the National Institutes of Health and the US Department of Health and Human Sciences.

of the luminal diameter is likely to cause an imbalance between the myocardial demand for oxygen and the ability of the coronary artery to supply it. This produces myocardial ischaemia, which the patient experiences as angina. In stable angina, this typically occurs on exertion, especially when walking up a hill, on a cold day, after a heavy meal. Angina can also occur as a result of emotional stress. Periods of physical or emotional stress cause release of catecholamines, causing an increase in heart rate, an increase in the velocity and force of myocardial contraction, an elevation in blood pressure, and an increase in myocardial oxygen demand. When there is significant coronary artery stenosis, an oxygen deficit results. Myocardial ischaemia increases the catecholamine release, resulting in further increases in heart rate and blood pressure, further oxygen lack, and a vicious cycle ensues. Tachycardia also causes a reduction in diastole, which is when the coronary arteries fill. The pain with angina is typically described as a retrosternal discomfort, which disappears quickly on stopping the precipitating activity, thus supporting the concept of oxygen supply versus oxygen demand. The discomfort may start in the lower, middle, or upper sternal area, the lower jaw, or the arm. It is usually described as a tightness, constriction, pressure, heaviness, strangulation, or indigestion-like feeling that comes on gradually and disappears with rest. Occasionally, the discomfort is replaced by breathlessness on exertion, the so-called 'angina equivalent'. The area of pain is usually

at least the size of a clenched fist and may cover most of the central chest area. Dyspnoea, diaphoresis, and nausea may occur owing to the activation of the sympathetic and parasympathetic nervous systems (Klein, 1988). Patients will frequently restrict their activities to reduce the symptoms. This may result in anxiety, depression, insomnia, fatigue, and decreased self-esteem (Riegal and Dracup, 1992).

Acute coronary syndrome

ACS is caused by either plaque erosion or plaque rupture. Plaque erosion tends to occur at the site of a pre-existing severe stenosis. The erosion causes the underlying connective tissue matrix to be exposed, which provides a focus for platelet deposition and thrombosis. Plaque rupture is the initiator of most ACSs and sudden cardiac death. Fissuring of a plaque is a random and unpredictable event, which may occur in response to mechanical stress, inflammation, or coronary artery spasm. The risk of plaque rupture appears to be related more to morphology than plaque size or severity of stenosis (Falk *et al.*, 1995). Factors that increase the vulnerability of plaques include:

- a lipid pool of more than 40% of the overall plaque volume;
- a thin fibrous cap;
- a high number of macrophages; or
- a low number of vascular smooth muscle cells in the cap.

Plaque rupture exposes the cholesterol pool and the highly thrombogenic matrix to the circulation, encouraging platelet aggregation. This results in deposition of fibrin and formation of thrombus. In ACS, the thrombus is platelet-rich and causes partial vessel occlusion. This platelet-rich thrombus may release vasoconstrictor agents, such as thromboxane A_2, and **serotonin**, which may cause vasospasm. The duration of vessel occlusion results in varying effects on the myocardium. In unstable angina, the occlusion tends to be transient and episodic and there is usually no damage to the myocardium, whereas in NSTEMI, an increase in the level of biochemical markers such as troponin indicates areas of myocardial necrosis.

ST elevation myocardial infarction

In STEMI, there is total vessel occlusion at the site of the plaque rupture. The coronary artery is occluded by thrombus and myocardial necrosis results. Occlusive thrombi are found in 90% of patients immediately following STEMI in the infarct-related artery; however, the frequency diminishes with time owing to spontaneous thrombolysis. There may be a delay of up to 2 weeks between the plaque rupture and its clinical consequences (Van de Werf *et al.*, 2008). The incidence of STEMI is related to circadian rhythm and is highest in the early morning. This is because of the combination of ß-adrenergic stimulation, hypercoagulability of the blood, and hyperreactivity of platelets at this time. Activities associated with an increase in sympathetic stimulation and vasoconstriction, such as physical and emotional stress, may also trigger plaque disruption and coronary thrombosis (Van de Werf *et al.*, 2008).

Assessment of the patient with CHD

The nursing assessment of a patient with CHD will vary depending on the initial presentation. Rapid diagnosis and early risk stratification of patients presenting with acute chest pain is important to identify patients in whom early intervention can improve outcome. Nurses are frequently the first point of contact for the patient and are therefore in a unique position to use their clinical skills to identify those patients who are in need of immediate treatment (Albarran and Kapeluch, 1994).

All patients presenting with chest pain are likely to be anxious, which may affect their ability to answer questions (Teasdale, 1993). Good nursing care involves assessing both the physical and psychological effect of chest pain on the patient.

The following section will first examine the assessment of a patient with suspected ACS and then describe the assessment of the patient with angina.

Acute coronary syndrome

A diagnosis of ACS is usually based on the history of chest pain lasting for more than 20 minutes or not responding fully to nitroglycerine. The patient must be made as comfortable as possible and must receive adequate pain relief. An ECG should be obtained as soon as possible. Although this may not show ST elevation immediately, it is rarely normal. The diagnosis of STEMI is based on clinical assessment and the results of tests, and is described in Box 6.3 (Van de Werf *et al.*, 2008).

Figures 6.7 and 6.8 show the typical ECG presentations of ST-segment elevation and left bundle branch block. ACS due to NSTEMI or unstable angina presents with either ST-segment depression or T wave inversion on the ECG (Figure 6.9). The ECG must also be assessed with regard to the patient's heart rate and rhythm.

Investigations

There are various biochemical markers that can be tested to confirm the diagnosis of STEMI/NSTEMI or unstable angina. These markers are released into the bloodstream following myocardial damage. Until the

---

Box 6.3 The diagnosis of STEMI

- History of chest pain/discomfort
- Persistent ST segment elevation or presumed new left bundle branch block (repeat ECGs may be needed)
- Elevated markers of myocardial necrosis (troponin, CK-MB)
- Echocardiography to determine the extent of major acute myocardial ischaemia and rule out other causes of chest pain/discomfort

(adapted from Werf *et al.*, 2008)

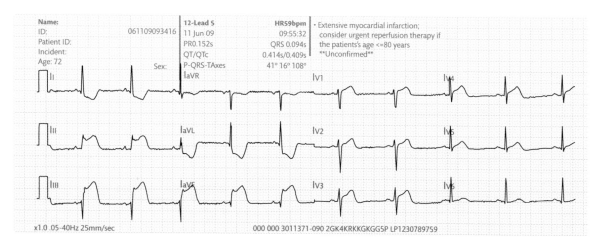

Figure 6.7 ECG of STEMI showing ST elevation in leads II, III, and AVF.

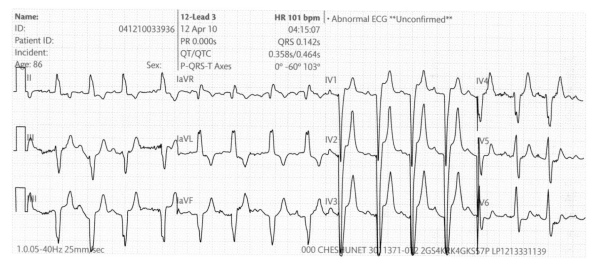

Figure 6.8 ECG of left bundle branch block.

1990s, creatine kinase (CK) was the main biochemical marker used to detect myocardial damage. CK is present in large quantities in tissues that consume energy rapidly (such as skeletal, smooth, and cardiac muscle). It is also found in other tissues (such as the brain, intestines, lung, and bladder) and therefore the level may increase following damage to any of these tissues. An isoenzyme of CK, CK-MB, is more sensitive to myocardial damage and has been measured more recently. However, elevations in CK-MB can also be due to skeletal muscle injury. Cardiac troponin T and troponin I have replaced CK testing in clinical practice for

the diagnosis of myocardial damage because they are highly specific and more sensitive to detect myocardial necrosis (Saenger and Jaffe, 2008). Table 6.1 shows the time course of CK-MB and troponin elevation following myocardial infarction.

It is important that serial measurements of troponin levels are taken. Blood samples should be taken immediately and then repeated at 12 hours because the initial results may be too early to show a rise in the level, even though the patient has started to have an ACS. Individual laboratories have their own normal ranges; however, generally a rise in CK-MB should be

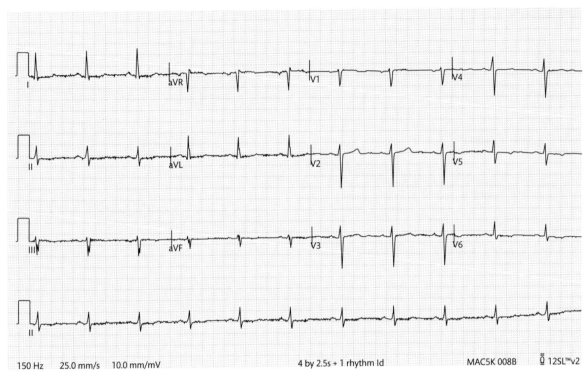

150 Hz   25.0 mm/s   10.0 mm/mV   4 by 2.5s + 1 rhythm ld   MAC5K 008B   Q̄ 12SL™v2

Figure 6.9 ECG of NSTEMI showing T wave inversion in V3–6 and flat T waves in II, III, and AVF.

THEORY INTO PRACTICE 6.2

Activity: reviewing the ECG

Compare the ECGs in Figures 6.7, 6.8, and 6.9 with a normal ECG.

- What are the differences?
- What is the significance of the changes you see in the figures?

Table 6.1 Time course of CK-MB and troponin elevation following myocardial infarction

	CK-MB	Troponin
Onset (hours)	3–12	3–12
Peak (hours)	18–24	18–24
Duration (days)	2–4	5–10

Source: Korff *et al.* (2006).

---

more than twice the upper limit of normal to diagnose myocardial damage. Any rise of troponin above the normal range would suggest myocardial injury. In addition to the above biochemical markers, blood should also be sent to check renal and liver function, markers of infection, and anaemia to exclude other causes of chest pain.

Signs and symptoms

Unstable angina presents with a change in the pattern of angina with an increase in frequency, severity, and/or duration of pain. In STEMI and NSTEMI, chest pain usually lasts for more than 20 minutes and often persists for several hours. The pain is typically retrosternal and across the whole chest, and is described as 'crushing', 'vice-like', or a 'heavy weight on the chest' and may radiate to the throat, jaw, neck, shoulders, and arms. Symptoms of breathlessness, nausea, vomiting, dizziness, diaphoresis, and apprehension often coexist. Presyncope and occasionally syncope may occur due to bradyarrhythmias. Painless infarcts may present in about 10% of patients, especially those with diabetes and the elderly. Associated symptoms may be more prominent in these patients and 50% are likely to have a

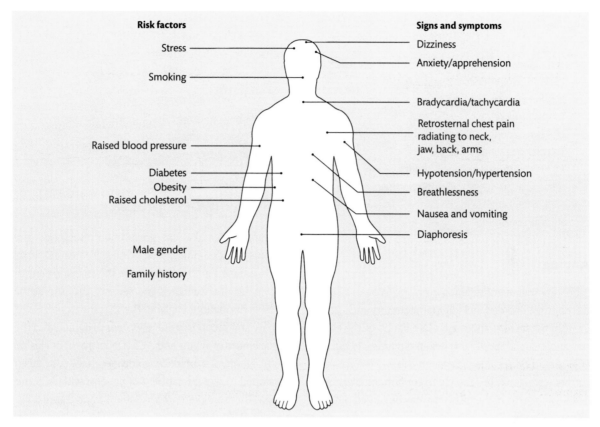

Risk factors

Stress

Smoking

Raised blood pressure

Diabetes
Obesity
Raised cholesterol

Male gender

Family history

Signs and symptoms

Dizziness

Anxiety/apprehension

Bradycardia/tachycardia

Retrosternal chest pain radiating to neck, jaw, back, arms

Hypotension/hypertension

Breathlessness

Nausea and vomiting

Diaphoresis

Figure 6.10 Typical signs and symptoms of a patient with ACS.

history of angina or previous infarction. It is important to remember that men and women may experience different symptoms. The absence of chest pain or discomfort with ACS is more common in women than in men (Canto *et al.*, 2007).

Women may also complain of pain in the back or neck rather than in the chest or may have dizziness, shortness of breath, or unusual fatigue.

In assessing the patient with a suspected ACS, the nurse needs to consider the physical, psychological, and social effects of the condition. Physical examination of the patient is frequently normal, and must include detailed examination of the heart sounds and chest wall. The nursing assessment starts with the general appearance of the patient, including colour, signs of cyanosis, skin temperature, evidence of sweating, and anxiety or apprehension. Explanation of all of the assessment and reasons for tests is vital. ECG monitoring should be initiated as soon as possible to facilitate detection of life-threatening arrhythmias.

Heart and respiratory rate, blood pressure, and oxygen saturation levels should be recorded as dictated by the patient's condition. Patients suffering from ACS will often find it difficult to accept what is happening to them. Identification of risk factors is essential and patients should be informed that this will be discussed with them prior to discharge from hospital. It is important that adequate information is given to patients, but that this is done in stages to allow them time to assimilate what is being said. Patients will require a short period of bed rest and will then need to follow a mobilization plan. Explanation from the nurse regarding the importance of this will aid compliance.

Figure 6.10 shows the typical signs and symptoms of a patient with an acute MI. The condition of the patient with an MI can change quickly. The nurse must be aware of signs of deterioration and inform medical staff promptly. Signs of a worsening condition can be recognized by asking the red flag questions listed in Box 6.4.

Box 6.4 Red flag questions

- Is the patient complaining of further chest pain?
- Has the patient become acutely breathless?
- Is there any change in heart rate—either bradycardia or tachycardia?
- Has the patient had any arrhythmias—especially ventricular arrhythmias, heart block?
- Has the patient developed hypotension?
- Is there any reduction in urine output?
- Is there any change in the patient's mental state, such as confusion?

Box 6.5 Tests used to confirm the diagnosis of angina

- Exercise ECG
- Stress echocardiogram
- Perfusion scan (either CT or MRI)
- CT coronary angiography
- Angiography

Angina

Patients suspected of suffering from angina need a complete history recorded, including family history and assessment of risk factors. Thorough examination of the chest wall and heart sounds is also required (Hutter, 1995). An ECG should be recorded, although this is often normal. Further testing may be required to confirm the diagnosis. Box 6.5 lists some of the tests that may be carried out.

Identifying best practice

In March 2000, the UK government published the National Service Framework for Coronary Heart Disease, which outlined a 10-year plan for the management of CHD. It set out standards and services that should be available throughout England. The 12 standards included primary and secondary prevention of CHD, and also the management of angina and ACS (Department of Health, 2000). Numerous practice guidelines have also been developed to direct treatment of patients with ACS and angina. These are presented in Table 6.2 and Figure 6.11.

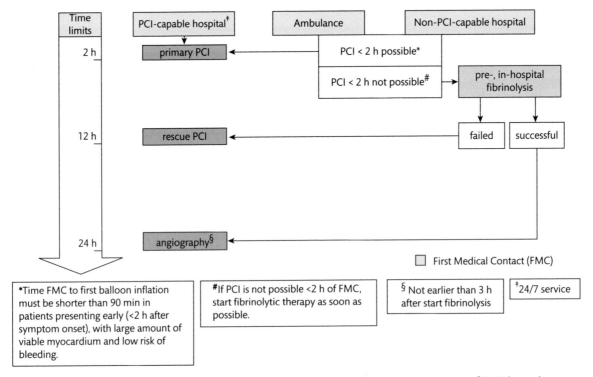

Figure 6.11 European Society of Cardiology reperfusion strategies for the management of AMI in patients presenting with persistent ST segment elevation.

Reproduced by permission of Oxford University Press and the European Society of Cardiology.

Table 6.2 Best practice guidelines for patients with ACS and angina

Condition	Aim of treatment	Treatment options	Evidence
ACS—STEMI	Restoring coronary flow and myocardial tissue perfusion as early as possible	Primary percutaneous coronary intervention (primary PCI)—performed within 90 minutes of first medical contact with patient provided that there are no contraindications to the procedure If above not possible—pre-hospital thrombolysis given as soon as possible Rescue PCI within 12 hours in those patients for whom thrombolysis fails (Figure 6.11) Delayed angiography and PCI (24–72 hours after presentation) for patients who have had successful thrombolysis Coronary artery bypass surgery for patients with unfavourable anatomy for PCI or failed PCI. Emergency surgery should be considered only for patients in whom there is a large area of myocardium in jeopardy. Where possible, surgery should be delayed for 3–7 days.	European Society of Cardiology, Van de Werf *et al.*, 2008 Scottish Intercollegiate Guideline Network clinical guideline (SIGN) 2007 European Society of Cardiology, Wijns *et al.*, 2010
ACS—unstable angina and NSTEMI	Diagnosis and treatment	Risk stratification of patients is vital Patients at medium to high risk due to ongoing chest pain and dynamic ECG changes should undergo early coronary angiography and revascularization, with PCI or coronary artery bypass grafting as appropriate Stable patients should undergo angiography within 72 hours	European Society of Cardiology, Bassand *et al.*, 2007 Scottish Intercollegiate Guideline Network clinical guideline (SIGN) 2007 National Institute for Health and Clinical Excellence, 2010
Drug therapy after ACS Prasugrel Glycoprotein IIb/IIIa inhibitors Clopidogrel	Prevention of thrombotic events in patients with ACS treated with PCI Prevention of thrombotic events post ACS—platelets have an important role in the pathology of ACS Prevention of thrombotic events post ACS	Prasugrel in combination with aspirin should be used in patients post primary PCI Glycoprotein IIb/IIIa inhibitors should be used in the management of unstable angina and ACS, because there is a reduction in death and MI Clopidogrel in combination with aspirin should be used in high-risk patients post ACS	National Institute for Health and Clinical Excellence, 2009 National Institute for Health and Clinical Excellence, 2002 National Institute for Health and Clinical Excellence, 2004
Stable angina	Assessment and appropriate treatment	Patients with stable angina should be appropriately assessed and investigated to determine the appropriate treatment required Investigation includes history-taking, the use of non-invasive testing such as ECG stress testing, echocardiography, and myocardial perfusion scintigraphy, and invasive testing with angiography Treatment for stable angina may include medical therapy, PCI, or CABG	European Society of Cardiology, Fox *et al.*, 2006 National Institute for Health and Clinical Excellence, 2003 National Institute for Health and Clinical Excellence, 2010a Scottish Intercollegiate Guideline Network clinical guideline (SIGN) 2007a

> EVIDENCE BOX 6.1
> ## Update on NICE guidance
>
> - The National Institute for Health and Clinical Excellence (NICE) guidance on IIb/IIIa inhibitors and that on clopidogrel have not been updated since their publication in 2002 and 2004, respectively. The current validity of these pieces of guidance could therefore be questioned.
> - There is also National Institute for Health and Clinical Excellence (NICE) guidance expected on the use of ticagrelor, another anti-platelet agent, published in 2011: http://guidance.nice.org.uk/TA/Wave20/70
> - A guideline on stable angina was published in 2011 (NICE, 2011a): http://guidance.nice.org.uk/CG/Wave17/25
> - There is also guidance available on risk assessment and prevention, both in primary care and post MI/ACS, which is shown in Table 6.3.

Because research is always ongoing and best practice evolves, as outlined in Evidence box 6.1, it is important that readers stay up to date and know where to find good-quality sources of evidence. Hence we have provided a list of sources that readers should utilize.

Sources of evidence

Journals

European Heart Journal

European Journal of Cardiovascular Prevention and Rehabilitation

Circulation

Heart

Organizations

National Institute for Health and Clinical Excellence (NICE) **http://guidance.nice.org.uk/**

The Scottish Intercollegiate Guidelines Network (SIGN) **http://www.sign.ac.uk/guidelines/index.html**

NHS Evidence **http://www.evidence.nhs.uk/**

Agency for Healthcare Quality (AHRQ) **http://www.ahrq.gov/**

National Institute for Clinical Studies (NICS) **http://www.nhmrc.gov.au/nics/index.htm**

Registered Nurses Association of Ontario **http://www.rnao.org**

World Health Organization **http://www.who.int/en/**

Table 6.3 **CHD prevention**

Prevention advice	Evidence
<ul><li>Give advice and support on stopping smoking</li><li>Give advice and support on losing weight</li><li>Give advice on increasing physical activity—30 minutes of cardiovascular exercise daily</li><li>Give advice on a healthy diet—reduce fat and salt intake, five portions of fruit and vegetables daily, two portions of oily fish per week</li><li>Give advice on light to moderate alcohol intake—less than 21 units per week for men and less than 14 units per week for women</li><li>Reduce cholesterol levels</li><li>Reduce blood pressure levels</li><li>Maintain control of glucose levels for those with diabetes</li></ul>	<ul><li>European Society of Cardiology, Graham *et al.* (2007)</li><li>Scottish Intercollegiate Guideline Network clinical guideline (SIGN) (2007b)</li></ul>
Secondary prevention post MI/ACS—advice on all risk factors for CHD as above	European Society of Cardiology; Van de Werf *et al.* (2008) Scottish Intercollegiate Guideline Network clinical guideline (SIGN) (2007) National Institute for Health and Clinical Excellence (2007)

CASE STUDY 6.1 *Patient with CHD*

Sarah is a 52-year-old woman who developed angina in her early 40s. She was diagnosed with familial hypercholesterolaemia (a genetic condition affecting cholesterol metabolism) in her 30s following a blood test, which established that she had a significantly raised cholesterol level. Investigation into her family history identified several close family members who had died prematurely from CHD. Sarah does not smoke and has normal blood pressure. She has a BMI of 28.5 and a waist:hip ratio of 1.0. Following the diagnosis with angina, her condition quickly progressed; she was unable to walk more than 100 yards without chest pain and could not work. She underwent a coronary angiogram in 2001, followed by angioplasty and insertion of a stent. Unfortunately, this did not relieve her angina and she went on to have coronary bypass surgery in 2002. Sarah has been free from chest pain since her surgery. She takes several medications to control her cholesterol level and exercises regularly. She has also been able to return to part-time work.

Conclusion

CHD continues to be an important health problem that is unlikely to go away. New treatments will continue to help to improve survival from events such as STEMI and NSTE-MI. However, focus needs to be directed to prevention because CHD is largely avoidable if lifestyles are modified and risk factors addressed. Nurses have an important role in education and therefore are in an ideal role to assist with prevention of CHD.

Online Resource Centre

 To help you to develop and apply your knowledge and decision-making skills further, we have provided interactive learning resources online at **www.oxfordtextbooks.co.uk/orc/bullock/**

Whilst these are freely available you will need to use the access codes at the start of the book.

References

Albarran, J., Kapeluch, H. (1994) Role of the nurse in thrombolytic therapy. *British Journal of Nursing* **3**(3): 104–9.

Allender, S., Scarborough, P., O'Flaherty, M., *et al.* (2008) 20th century CHD mortality in England and Wales: population trends in CHD risk factors and coronary death. *BMC Public Health* **8**: 148.

Bassand, J.P., Hamm, C.W., Ardissino, D., *et al.* (2007) Task force for the diagnosis and treatment of non-ST-segment elevation acute coronary syndromes of the European Society of Cardiology: Guidelines for the diagnosis and treatment of non-ST-segment elevation acute coronary syndromes. *European Heart Journal* **28**(13): 1598–660.

Baxendale, L.M. (1992) Pathophysiology of coronary artery disease. *Nursing Clinics of North America* **27**(1): 143–52 (Review).

Berenson, G.S., Srinivasan, S.R., Bao, W., *et al.* (1998) Association between multiple cardiovascular risk factors and atherosclerosis in children and young adults: the Bogalusa Heart Study. *New England Journal of Medicine* **338**(23): 1650–6.

Beswick, A., Brindle, P. (2006) Risk scoring in the assessment of cardiovascular risk. *Current Opinion in Lipidology* **17**(4): 375–86.

British Cardiac Society, British Hypertension Society, Diabetes UK, HEART UK (2005) JBS 2. Joint British Societies' guidelines on prevention of cardiovascular disease in clinical practice. *Heart* **91**(Suppl. 5): v1–v52.

Bunker, S.J., Colquhoun, D.M., Esler, M.D., *et al.* (2003). 'Stress' and coronary heart disease: psychosocial risk factors. *Medical Journal of Australia* **178**(6): 272–6.

Canto, J.G., Goldberg, R.J., Hand, M.M., *et al.* (2007) Symptom presentation of women with acute coronary syndromes: myth vs reality. *Archives of Internal Medicine* **167**(22): 2405–13.

Dawber, T.R., Meadors, G.F., Moore, F.E. (1951) Epidemiological approaches to heart disease: the Framingham Study. *American Journal of Public Health* **41**: 279–86.

Department of Health (2000) National Service Framework for Coronary Heart Disease. **http://www.dh.gov.uk/en/Publicationsandstatistics/Publications/PublicationsPolicyAndGuidance/DH_4094275** (accessed 16 October 2011).

Doll, R., Peto, R., Boreham, J., *et al.* (2004) Mortality in relation to smoking: 50 years' observations on male British doctors. *British Medical Journal* **328**(7455): 1519–27.

Falk, E., Shah, P.K., Fuster, V. (1995) Coronary plaque disruption. *Circulation* **92**(3): 657–71.

Fox, K., Garcia, M.A., Ardissino, D., *et al.* (2006) Task force on the management of stable angina pectoris of the European Society of Cardiology: ESC Committee for Practice Guidelines (CPG)—Guidelines on the management of stable angina pectoris. *European Heart Journal* **27**(11): 1341–81.

Garcia, M.J., McNamara, P.M., Gordon, T., *et al.* (1974) Morbidity and mortality in diabetics in the Framingham population: sixteen year follow-up. *Diabetes* **23**(2): 105–11.

Graham, I., Atar, D., Borch-Johnson, K., *et al.* (2007) Fourth task force of the European Society of Cardiology and other societies on cardiovascular disease prevention in clinical practice. *European Journal of Cardiovascular Prevention and Rehabilitation* **14**(Suppl. 2): S1–S113.

HES online (2009) Hospital Episode Statistics. The Health and Social Care Information Centre: London. **www.hesonline.nhs.uk**.

Hutter, A.M. (1995) Chest pain: how to distinguish between cardiac and non-cardiac causes. Interview by Eric R. Leibovitch. *Geriatrics* **50**(9): 32–6, 39–40.

Joint Health Surveys Unit (2008) *Health Survey for England 2006. Cardiovascular Disease and Risk Factors.* The Information Centre: Leeds.

Klein, D.M. (1988). Angina: pathophysiology–and the resulting signs and symptoms. *Nursing* **18**(7): 44–6.

Korff, S., Katus, H.A., Giannitis, E. (2006) Differential diagnosis of elevated troponins. *Heart* **92**: 987–93.

Kuper, H., Marmot, M., Hemingway, H. (2002) Systematic review of prospective cohort studies of psychological factors in the aetiology and prognosis of coronary heart disease. *Seminars in Vascular Medicine* **2**(3): 267–314.

Lewington, S., Clarke, R., Qizilbash, N., *et al.* Prospective Studies Collaboration (2002) Age-specific relevance of usual blood pressure to vascular mortality: a meta analysis of individual data for one million adults in 61 prospective studies. *Lancet* **360**(9349): 1903–13.

Lindfield, R., Lemic, N. (2007) Obesity and cardiovascular disease: a population perspective. *British Journal of Cardiac Nursing* **2**: 8–16.

National Institute for Health and Clinical Excellence (NICE) (2002) Guidance on the use of glycoprotein IIb/IIIa inhibitors in the treatment of acute coronary syndromes. NICE Technology Appraisal Guidance 47. **http://guidance.nice.org.uk/TA47/Guidance/pdf/English** (accessed 16 October 2011).

National Institute for Health and Clinical Excellence (NICE) (2003) Myocardial perfusion scintigraphy for the diagnosis and management of angina and myocardial infarction. NICE Technology Appraisal 73. **http://guidance.nice.org.uk/TA73/Guidance/pdf/English** (accessed 16 October 2011).

National Institute for Health and Clinical Excellence (NICE) (2004) Clopidogrel in the treatment of non-ST-elevation acute coronary syndrome. NICE Technology Appraisal 80. **http://guidance.nice.org.uk/TA80/NICEGuidance/pdf/English** (accessed 16 October 2011).

National Institute for Health and Clinical Excellence (NICE) (2007) Post myocardial infarction secondary prevention in primary and secondary care for patients following a myocardial infarction. NICE Clinical Guideline 48(CG48) **http://guidance.nice.org.uk/CG48/NICEGuidance/pdf/English** (accessed 16 October 2011).

National Institute for Health and Clinical Excellence (NICE) (2009) Prasugrel for the treatment of acute coronary syndromes with percutaneous coronary intervention. NICE Technology Appraisal Guidance 182. **http://guidance.nice.org.uk/TA182/NICEGuidance/pdf/English** (accessed 16 October 2011).

National Institute for Health and Clinical Excellence (NICE) (2010) Unstable angina and NSTEMI. NICE Clinical Guideline 94(CG94) **http://guidance.nice.org.uk/CG94/NICEGuidance/pdf/English** (accessed 16 October 2011).

National Institute for Health and Clinical Excellence (NICE) (2010a) Chest pain of recent onset. Nice Clinical Guideline 95(CG95). **http://guidance.nice.org.uk/CG95/NICEGuidance/pdf/English** (accessed 16 October 2011).

National Institute for Health and Clinical Excellence (NICE) (2011) Hypertension. Clinical management of primary hypertension in adults. NICE clinical guideline 127. **http://guidance.nice.org.uk/CG127** (accessed 16 October 2011).

National Institute for Health and Clinical Excellence (NICE) (2011a) Management of stable angina. NICE clinical guideline 126. **http://guidance.nice.org.uk/CG126** (accessed 16 October 2011).

Neaton, J.D., Wentworth, D. (1992) Serum cholesterol, blood pressure, cigarette smoking and death from coronary heart disease: overall findings and differences by age for 316,099 white men—Multiple Risk Factor Intervention Trial Research Group. *Archives of Internal Medicine* **152**(1): 56–64.

Riegel, B.J., Dracup, K.A. (1992) Does overprotection cause cardiac invalidism after acute myocardial infarction? *Heart Lung* **21**(6): 529–35.

Rissanen, A.M., Nikkilä, E.A. (1979). Aggregation of coronary risk factors in families of men with fatal and non-fatal coronary heart disease. *British Heart Journal* **42**(4): 373–80.

Saenger, A.K., Jaffe, A.S. (2008) Requiem for a heavyweight: the demise of creatine kinase-MB. *Circulation* **118**: 2200.

Scarborough, P., Bhatnagar, P., Wickramasinghe, K., *et al.* (2010) *Coronary Heart Disease Statistics,* 2010 edn. British Heart Foundation: London. **www.heartstats.org** (accessed 16 October 2011).

Scottish Intercollegiate Guidelines Network (SIGN) (2007) Acute coronary syndromes–93. **http://www.sign.ac.uk/guidelines/fulltext/93/index.html**

Scottish Intercollegiate Guidelines Network (SIGN) (2007a) Management of stable angina–96. **http://www.sign.ac.uk/guidelines/fulltext/96/index.html**

Scottish Intercollegiate Guidelines Network (SIGN) (2007b) Risk estimation and the prevention of cardiovascular disease–97. **http://www.sign.ac.uk/guidelines/fulltext/97/index.html**

Smith, W.S., Zvosec, D.L., Sharkey, S.W., *et al.* (2002) *The ECG in Acute MI: An Evidence-Based Manual of Reperfusion Therapy.* Lippincott Williams and Wilkins: Philadelphia, PA.

Teasdale, K. (1993) Information and anxiety: a critical appraisal. *Journal of Advanced Nursing* **18**(7): 1125–32.

Van de Werf, F., Bax, J., Betriu, A., *et al.* (2008) Management of acute myocardial infarction in patients presenting with persistent ST-segment elevation: the task force on the management of ST-elevation acute myocardial infarction of the European Society of Cardiology. *European Heart Journal* **29**(23): 2909–45.

Waller, B.F. (1989) The eccentric coronary atherosclerotic plaque: morphologic observations and clinical relevance. *Clinical Cardiology***12**(1): 14–20.

Waller, B.F., Orr, C.M., Slack, J.D., *et al.* (1992) Anatomy, histology and pathology of coronary arteries: a review relevant to new interventional and imaging techniques–Part III. *Clinical Cardiology* **15**(8): 607–15.

Weissberg, P.L. (2000) Atherogenesis: current understanding of the causes of atheroma. *Heart* **83**(2): 247–52.

Wijns, W., Kolh, P., Danchin, N., *et al.* (2010) Guidelines on myocardial revascularization: the task force on myocardial revascularization of the European Society of Cardiology (ESC) and the European Association for Cardio-Thoracic Surgery (EACTS). European Heart Journal **31**: 2501–55.

Williams, B., Poulter, N.R., Brown, M.J., *et al.* (BHS Guidelines Working Party for the British Hypertension Society) (2004) British Hypertension Society guidelines for hypertension management 2004 (BHS-IV): summary. *British Medical Journal* **328**(7440): 634–40.

World Health Organization (2000) *Obesity: Preventing and Managing the Global Epidemic—Report of a WHO Consultation on Obesity.* World Health Organization: Geneva.

World Health Organization (2002) *The World Health Report 2002: Reducing Risks, Promoting Healthy Life.* World Health Organization: Geneva.

World Health Organization Global Health Observatory (2006) **http://apps.who.int/ghodata/#** (accessed 16 October 2011).

World Health Organization (2009) Cardiovascular disease. **www.who.int/cardiovascular_disease/resource/atlas/en/** (accessed 16 October 2011).

Yusuf, S., Hawken, S., Ounpuu, S., *et al.* (INTERHEART Study Investigators) (2004) Effect of potentially modifiable risk factors associated with myocardial infarction in 52 countries (the INTERHEART Study): case-control study. *Lancet* **364**(9438): 937–52.

7 *Understanding* **Dementia**

Jan Dewing

Introduction

This chapter presents a comprehensive understanding of dementia as a commonly encountered condition/syndrome in the nursing care of older adults and offers insights into the health challenges faced by people living with dementia. It will provide nurses with the knowledge to be able to assess, manage, and care for people with dementia in an evidence-based and person-centred way. After a comprehensive overview of the causes, risk factors, and impact of dementia, it will outline best practice to deliver care, as well as to prevent or minimize further ill-health. Nursing assessments and priorities are highlighted throughout, and the nursing management of the symptoms and common health problems associated with dementia can be found in **Chapters 14** and **17**, respectively ➡.

Understanding dementia

In the past, dementia was most often described in terms of mental disability. However, it is now more often described in terms of neurological disability (i.e. changes in the brain). For example, the Mental Health Foundation describes dementia as:

> A decline in mental ability which affects memory, thinking, problem-solving, concentration and perception.

The NHS Choices website states:

> Dementia describes the effects of certain conditions and diseases on a person's mental ability, personality and behaviour.

Definitions

Dementia is generally classified according to two international classification systems: the American Psychiatric Association Diagnostic and Statistical Manual of Mental Disorders fourth edition (DSM-IV); and the International Classification of Diseases tenth edition (ICD-10). Dementia can be defined as a syndrome whereby there is gradual death of brain cells, resulting in a loss of brain ability that is severe enough to interfere with normal activities of living for more than 6 months. Problems with brain function should not have been present at birth and it is not associated with a loss or alteration of consciousness. This latter point distinguishes dementia from delirium, which is a state of mental disorientation that can happen if you become medically unwell, also known as an 'acute confusional state' (Royal College of Psychiatrists, 2009). (See Chapter 11 ➡).

It is vital that nurses hold central what dementia means for people living with it. For example, people will commonly experience changes to their perception, senses, memory, and the range of skills they need to carry out everyday activities. Crucially, dementia is not just about memory loss.

The majority of people with dementia are older people (aged over 65), although dementia is not an inevitable part of the ageing process. A small number of people can develop dementia in their fourth or fifth decade, and this is known as early onset dementia. It is important that nurses working with older people do not assume that all forgetfulness or short-term memory impairment means that the person has dementia. For example, anaemia or some thyroid gland problems can present like a dementia.

Types of dementia

Dementia is a syndrome rather than one specific disease. Some forms of dementia, such as Alzheimer's disease, which is the most frequently occurring type, are degenerative (i.e. they get worse over time). Other forms of dementia, such as vascular dementia, may be non-degenerative (i.e. they may not get worse over time—however, vascular dementia may also be degenerative). Thus, there are different types of dementia, depending on what happens in the brain, including the development of abnormal pathology. The most commonly occurring types of dementia (in medical terms) are Alzheimer's, vascular, Lewy body dementia, and frontotemporal dementia.

Many textbooks show biomedical typologies as a way of organizing dementia into categories and sub categories such as the following.

- **Neurodegenerative:** Alzheimer's, frontotemporal degeneration, dementia with Lewy bodies (DLB), Pick's disease, and progressive supranuclear palsy (PSP)
- **Vascular:** infarction, haemorrhage, vasculitis (e.g. syphilis), Binswanger disease, or systemic lupus erythematosus, subdural haematoma, and subarachnoid haemorrhage
- **Endocrine:** thyroid disease, diabetes, Cushing's disease, Addison's disease, parathyroid disease

- **Vitamin deficiency:** B_{12}, thiamine, nicotinic acid
- **Systemic diseases:** anaemia, respiratory disease, renal disease, hepatic disease
- **Neurological disorders:** head injury, neoplasms, normal pressure hydrocephalus, multiple sclerosis, Parkinson's disease, Huntington's disease
- **Infection:** syphilis, HIV, CJD (Creutzfeldt–Jakob disease), Lyme disease

Prevalence and epidemiological profile of dementia

The Dementia UK Report (2007) reveals how great the social and economic impact of caring for dementia patients could become. It states that, within 20 years, nearly 1 million people will be living with dementia, rising to 1.7 million by 2050, creating a medical and social care crisis. Even if this is not the case, there is evidence to suggest that services for people with dementia are underdeveloped.

Dementia is a global concern. Ferri *et al.* (2005) estimate that, worldwide, there are 24.3 million people living with dementia. The World Alzheimer Report (Wimo *et al.*, 2010: 2) puts this figure higher, at 35.6 million people, increasing to 65.7 million by 2030 and 115.4 million by 2050. Nearly two-thirds of these people live in low- and middle-income countries, where the sharpest increases in numbers are set to occur. Facts and figures relevant to the UK are highlighted in Box 7.1.

A recent Department of Health publication (2009) suggests that around 700,000 people in the UK have some form of dementia, costing our society an estimated £17 billion a year. The real cost is more, because this does not include the cost of care provided by families and carers; this may add around another 30%. In the absence of any breakthrough in curative treatments, the costs of care are likely to rise exponentially.

THEORY INTO PRACTICE 7.1
Reflective activity

How would a clinical setting for adults in which you are currently or have recently been working cope if it had at least twice as many people with dementia?

Box 7.1 The Alzheimer's Society summary

- There are currently 750,000 people with dementia in the UK; 16,000 of these are younger people.
- There are over 11,500 people with dementia from black and minority ethnic groups in the UK.
- Two-thirds of people with dementia are women.
- One-third of people aged over 95 have dementia.
- In all, 60,000 deaths a year are directly attributable to dementia.
- Delaying the onset of dementia by 5 years would reduce deaths directly attributable to dementia by 30,000 a year.
- Two-thirds of people with dementia live in the community, while one-third live in a care home. Of all people living in care homes, 64% have a form of dementia.
- There will be over 1 million people with dementia by 2025.

(from http://alzheimers.org.uk, 2010)

The pathophysiology of dementia

Dementia is usually caused by degeneration and gradual, yet excessive, death of brain cells in the cerebral cortex; this is the part of the brain responsible for thoughts, memories, actions, and personality (Adams, 1997: 185). Death of brain cells in this region leads to the cognitive impairment that generally characterizes what we know as dementia. In Alzheimer's disease, the brain becomes blocked by two abnormal structures, called neurofibrillary tangles and senile plaques (Nelson *et al.*, 2009). Neurofibrillary tangles are twisted masses of protein fibres inside nerve cells, or neurons. Senile plaques are composed of parts of neurons surrounding a group of proteins called β-amyloid deposits (Tanzi, 2005; Gyure *et al.*, 2001). Why these structures develop is as yet not understood (Nelson *et al.*, 2009). Additionally, in Alzheimer's, there is an unusually high level of depletion in the neurotransmitter acetylcholine and the enzymes that ensure its metabolism.

Risk factors

Current research (NICE, 2006) indicates a number of possible risk factors across the lifespan that may contribute to the development of dementia. These include:

- ageing;
- family history (Huang *et al.*, 2004);
- learning disability (Holland, 1994);
- lifestyle (especially smoking, poor diet, and exercise);
- poor educational status;
- emotional health (Kitwood, 1987; 1988; 1989; 1990a; b);
- physical health (especially inflammatory processes and bloodflow restriction).

You can find out more about how risk factors are classified in dementia from NICE (2011: 135–42) **http://www.nice.org.uk/nicemedia/live/10998/30320/30320.pdf.**

Some rare kinds of Alzheimer's disease affecting people of working age can be inherited. It has been established that faulty genes may cause the build-up of the amyloid protein found in dementia in some rare cases. Recent research seems to show that there may also be a genetic risk factor in other cases of Alzheimer's disease. However, this does not mean that someone whose parent had Alzheimer's will automatically develop the disease. For example, apolipoprotein E (ApoE) is a class of lipoprotein that plays a role in how cholesterol is metabolized. ApoE 4 is one of several variants of the protein. People who have the *ApoE 4* gene are between three and eight times more likely to develop Alzheimer's disease than those who do not carry the gene. The level of risk partially depends on whether the person inherits one or two copies of the gene. In regard to risk factors in general, NICE (2006) advises that risk factors should be reviewed and, if appropriate, treated.

Psychosocial models of dementia

Psychosocial explanations or models propose alternative causes of dementia. The most well-known model, apart from the general social disability model, is the dialectical dementia model (Kitwood, 1987; 1988; 1989; 1990a; b; 1993a; b; 1997). Kitwood argues that dementia (D) is a result of a combination of factors—biography (B), personality (P), general health (GH), neurological impairment (NI), and social psychology (SP)—represented as:

$$D = B + P + GH + NI + SP$$

In refining the model through case studies, Kitwood (1993a, b) put forward a number of biographical life events that he said could contribute to a dementia process developing, including:

- retirement, redundancy, and major role changes or losses;
- bereavement;
- rejection;
- prolonged or intense conflict;
- accident;
- assault or burglary;
- major physical illness or surgery;
- geographical change.

In regard to nursing practice, this model, amongst others in contemporary dementia literature (Dewing, 2008a), opens up a number of philosophical principles that are cornerstones to nursing practice. For example, people living with dementia:

- are people no matter how advanced their dementia is;
- have the same value as other people;
- perceive and experience what is going on around them;
- are capable of a feeling and emotionally based life;
- have residual capacity for making choices and exercising preferences even after formal or legal capacity has ceased.

This means that there are multiple options for planning positive nursing interventions. At this point in time, the evidence base on which nurses can draw in regard to specific nursing interventions is relatively new and therefore still limited. However, nurses need to think beyond the standard medical portrayal of dementia and be aware of other possible perspectives on dementia. This means that continuous professional and interprofessional discussion is needed to establish locally what is to be best practice. Of central concern is an appreciation that capacity and ability can vary even in the same person according to the environment they are in and how others communicate with them. Being respectful and compassionate, patient, and kind are vital aspects of nursing care.

Assessing the person with dementia

Common features present in individuals with dementia and, whilst the number and frequency of these vary from individual to individual, their presence guides you and other healthcare professionals to make a full assessment and a diagnosis of the condition. These often appear as subtle changes to normal activity, with memory, poor execution of familiar tasks, low mood or changes in mood, disorientation (even in familiar settings), numeric or language difficulties, and passivity being frequently present. In noting these, a comprehensive assessment of the individual should include:

Assessment of:

- the person's physical health
- depression
- possible undetected pain or discomfort
- side effects of medication
- individual biography, including religious beliefs and spiritual and cultural identity
- psychosocial factors
- physical environmental factors
- behavioural and functional analysis conducted by professionals with specific skills, in conjunction with carers and care workers.

(From NICE CG42, 2011, Supporting people with dementia and their carers in health and social care)

In some types of dementia, other specific features can present. For example, with vascular dementia, sudden onset and stroke-like symptoms can present. Generally, most people with dementia do not hallucinate early on in the condition (they may do so later); however, in DLB, there is a tendency for individuals to experience visual hallucinations (seeing things that are not there) early, typically saying that they can see people or animals. In frontotemporal dementia, there can be a change in emotion, personality, and behaviour, which can be accompanied by a loss of inhibitions leading to unusual behaviour. Examples are making sexually suggestive gestures in a public place, being rude to others, or making tactless comments. Compulsive and/or aggressive behaviour may also be present.

Table 7.1 Diagnostic criteria for dementia

Type of dementia	Diagnostic criteria
Alzheimer's disease	Preferred criteria: NINCDS/ADRDA Alternatives include ICD-10 and DSM-IV
Vascular dementia	Preferred criteria: NINDS-AIREN Alternatives include ICD-10 and DSM-IV
Dementia with Lewy bodies	International Consensus criteria for dementia with Lewy bodies
Frontotemporal dementia	Lund-Manchester criteria, NINDS criteria for frontotemporal dementia

Source: DSM-IV, Diagnostic and Statistical Manual of Mental Disorders, fourth edition; ICD-10, International Classification of Diseases, 10th revision; NINCDS/ADRDA, National Institute of Neurological and Communicative Diseases and Stroke/Alzheimer's Disease and Related Disorders Association; NINDS–AIREN, Neuroepidemiology Branch of the National Institute of Neurological Disorders and Stroke–Association Internationale pour la Recherche et l'Enseignement en Neurosciences. NICE Clinical Guideline 42 (2011) Supporting people with dementia and their carers in health and social care **http://guidance.nice.org.uk/CG42**.

Box 7.2 The mini-mental state examination (MMSE)

The mini-mental state examination (MMSE), or Folstein test, is a 30-point questionnaire test that is used to screen for cognitive impairment. It is commonly used to screen for dementia. It is also used to estimate the severity of cognitive impairment at a given point in time and to follow the course of cognitive changes in an individual over time. A score of 23–25 or less out of 30 is considered impaired. Low to very low scores correlate closely with the presence of dementia, although other mental disorders can also lead to abnormal findings on MMSE testing. The presence of physical problems can also interfere with taking the test. As with many psychological tests, the MMSE is subject to copyright and is now under licence. You will need to check if your clinical area has access to it.

The diagnosis of dementia

Diagnosis of dementia is facilitated by a number of diagnostic tools widely in use. These are detailed in Table 7.1 relative to the type of dementia.

NHS Choices provides useful information on the diagnosis process; this is found online at **http://www.nhs.uk/conditions/Dementia/pages/Diagnosis.aspx**. Diagnosis of dementia should be made only following specialist assessment, incorporating cognitive and mental state examination, physical examination, and any other relevant investigations. Review of medication is important to identify and possibly withdraw any drugs that adversely affect cognitive functioning. People assessed for dementia should be asked if they wish to know the diagnosis and with whom this should be shared.

Formal cognitive testing should use standardized instruments, with the mini-mental state examination (MMSE) being the preferred tool (Box 7.2). A number of alternatives are available; examples are the abbreviated mental test, the 6-item cognitive impairment test (6-CIT), the general practitioner assessment of cognition (GPCOG), and the 7-minute screen. Those interpreting the scores of such tests should take full account of factors affecting performance, such as cultural issues, educational level, prior level of functioning, language, sensory impairment, psychiatric illness, or physical/neurological problems.

Timing of diagnosis

The focus on early diagnosis and intervention is to enhance quality of life and to delay the progression of the disease. Whilst healthcare professionals can be reluctant to diagnose dementia in its early stages, the vast majority of people with dementia (and their carers) report the importance of early diagnosis (Carpenter *et al.*, 2008; Robinson *et al.*, 2005). The numbers of people diagnosed with dementia and the percentage of those reviewed by their GP are now recorded as part of the Quality and Outcomes Framework (QOF). A consequence of this is that it is likely that detection rates may increase in the coming years.

Memory clinics

Memory clinics provide a structure for a service in which specialist investigations and diagnosis can be offered and a referral point to access other services. Not all people attending a memory assessment service or memory clinic will have dementia (Banerjee *et al.*, 2007).

Further information on planning memory clinic services can be found online at **http://www.nice.org.uk/ usingguidance/commissioningguides/memoryassess mentservice/assumptions.jsp**.

Once diagnosed and as dementia progresses, symptom progression may include difficulties with normal activities of living, such as continence, personal hygiene, nutritional status, and mobility. For further information about specialist assessment of clinical cognitive assessment, and specialist services available for dementia assessment, visit **http://guidance.nice.org.uk/CG42**.

Nursing responsibilities

At the time of diagnosis of dementia, and at regular intervals subsequently, assessment should be made for medical comorbidities and key psychiatric features associated with dementia, including depression, to ensure optimal management for the patient. You need to feel confident and be competent in using cognitive tools to screen people and support early referral to relevant healthcare practitioners for specialist assessment. Your responsibility is also in interpreting the meaning of formal specialist assessments, using this and other evidence to inform care planning and discussion with people with dementia and their families/carers.

Progression of dementia

When caring for individuals with dementia, a number of useful tools are available when establishing the progression of the condition. These are used formally and informally by healthcare professionals in determining adjustments necessary to care plans, including care decisions about different pharmacological and non-pharmacological interventions, care setting, and the level of support required. An example of how dementia can progress is found at **http:// helpguide.org/elder/alzheimersdiseasesymptomsstages. htm**.

Tools are available to determine probable progression of dementia, such as the Clinical Dementia Rating (CDR). Whilst progression can vary, it is usually gradual. Sudden changes in severity are unusual, even in vascular dementia, in which you are more likely to witness multiple tiny steps

of change (Pace *et al.*, 2011). Key to the nursing role is not necessarily to focus on what the person is now unable to do, but, through careful assessment and adjustment, to work with the individual, the family, and/or carers to help him or her to achieve what he or she still can.

Definitions of advanced dementia

Advanced dementia follows disease progression and often presents with total dependence, requiring high levels of care. If the family or other caregivers cannot cope, long-term care may become inevitable. Advanced dementia is demonstrated by:

- a score of less than 10 on the mini mental state examination;
- the individual matching stage 3 on the Clinical Dementia Rating (CDR) scale.

(Pace *et al.*, 2011)

Many of the changes seen with advanced dementia are included in Figure 7.1.

Best practice interventions

There is much that can and should be done to promote and sustain physical well-being for people with dementia. In the early to mid stages of dementia, there are many older people who will also have an undiagnosed depression or related anxiety problems. Nurses need to identify the signs and differences between dementia and depression, and initiate screening and, if needed, a medical referral for assessment and investigation (see Chapters 14 and 17 ➡). People with dementia in the middle stages and their families need a range of advice and support to manage the consequences of dementia in their homes. Often, environmental modifications need to be considered. Regular drug review and prevention of malnutrition, dehydration, constipation, and infection, as well as pain and discomfort, are major issues for people with advanced dementia.

Many areas of nursing care for people with dementia still need better evidence. Where a good evidence base exists, this should be drawn upon. For example, Fick and Mion (2008) provide guidelines on pain assessment and delirium to help nurses to promote and sustain optimal

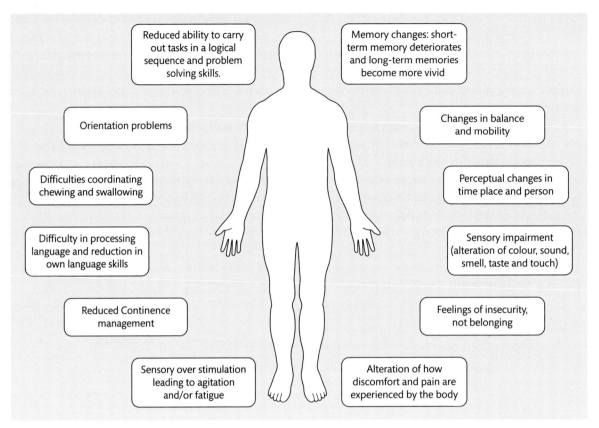

Reduced ability to carry out tasks in a logical sequence and problem solving skills.

Memory changes: short-term memory deteriorates and long-term memories become more vivid

Orientation problems

Changes in balance and mobility

Difficulties coordinating chewing and swallowing

Perceptual changes in time place and person

Difficulty in processing language and reduction in own language skills

Sensory impairment (alteration of colour, sound, smell, taste and touch)

Reduced Continence management

Feelings of insecurity, not belonging

Sensory over stimulation leading to agitation and/or fatigue

Alteration of how discomfort and pain are experienced by the body

Figure 7.1 **Some of the main effects of a dementia syndrome (Note this is later in the syndrome when there are likely to be widespread brain/body changes.)**

health and physical well-being for people with moderate or advanced dementia.

General guidelines on nursing care

For a general guideline on nursing care for people with delirium, dementia, and depression, see the following.

- Registered Nurses Association of Ontario (2003) *Screening for Delirium, Dementia and Depression in Older Adults*. Registered Nurses Association of Ontario: Toronto, Canada **http://www.rnao.org/best-practices/PDF/BPG_DDD.pdf**
- A publication by Age UK (2008) in which older people talk about their experiences with pain **http://www.britishpainsociety.org/book_pain_in_older_age_ID7826.pdf**

- British Pain Society Assessment of Pain in Older People: National Guidelines (2007) **http://www.britishpainsociety.org/bookpain older people.pdf**

Overarching principles for nursing interventions

In 2009, the National Dementia Strategy for England was launched. The Scottish Strategy is being developed following the *Remember I'm Still Me* report issued by Scotland's Care Commission and Mental Welfare Commission (2010). The report focused on care of people living with dementia in care homes and found many serious concerns, including widespread evidence of deprivation

CASE STUDY 7.1 *An example of living with dementia*

Tommy Harland is a retired postman living in a village to which he and his wife retired. His wife died after a long illness about 2 years ago and there was no other family. Neighbours have noticed Tommy behaving strangely. He has been seen going out in the garden, day and night, with no clothes on and digging holes. His household rubbish has been piling up outside his back door. One morning, his neighbour was alarmed when she could smell smoke in his house. On checking what was happening, she could see that something was on fire on the cooker top. She called the fire brigade. The fire brigade staff found Tommy asleep on a mattress on the living room floor. The room was in a very poor state. They called an ambulance. Tommy was taken to hospital to be checked over for the effects of smoke inhalation. This led to a medical assessment of his health and Tommy being admitted to a dementia assessment unit.

Six weeks later

Tommy had been diagnosed with Alzheimer's and frontotemporal lobe dementia. He had been started on a course of antidepressants, because he was found to be clinically depressed after the death of his wife. Plans were in place for Tommy to return home with a care package. His neighbour agreed to keep an overview of him and to contact social services if she was worried. Assistive technology was used to control the gas cooker and fire. Carers assisted Tommy with his personal care, meals, and house management. Tommy also joined a day centre to which he went once a week on a day that other men attended.

Two years later

Tommy had his care package increased and otherwise had continued to live at home. His neighbour then noticed he was up and active during the nights. Then another neighbour reported that she had seen Tommy out walking through the village early in the mornings. A case review took place and it was felt that Tommy had deteriorated; however, his wandering was reasonably safe and neighbours were willing to keep an eye on him. Shortly after this, Tommy started leaving the house even earlier and was partially undressed. He seemed distressed and anxious as he was walking about the village. His neighbour contacted social services.

Questions

➤ Tommy wants to carry on living at home—what can you do to see if this is possible?

➤ If it is not possible, what needs to happen next and what is your role in that process?

➤ How do you think Tommy might feel and react? What can you do to support him through this process?

 Further case studies are available on the Online Resource Centre.

You are advised also to consider the following.

1. Listen to what people with dementia and families/carers tell you is useful.

2. Refer to the NICE clinical guideline on dementia: the treatment and care of people with dementia in health and social care **http://www.nice.org.uk/guidance/index. jsp?action=byID&r=true&o=10997**

3. Search the web to find sources you feel are user-friendly.

of liberty and the use of antipsychotics to control residents' behaviour. Wales also has a National Dementia Plan and Northern Ireland is looking at developing a similar plan.

The English strategy contains a wide range of objectives based around three central themes.

1. Raising public and professional awareness
2. Ensuring an early and accurate diagnosis with appropriate initial support and information
3. Delivering high-quality care for people with dementia throughout their life course

It has 17 objectives, including the following.

- Improving public and professional awareness
- Good quality early diagnosis and intervention for all
- Good quality information post diagnosis
- Improved community personal support services
- Considering the potential for housing and telecare support
- Living well with dementia in care homes
- Improved end-of-life care
- An informed and effective workforce

The chapter will now focus on overarching principles for nursing care: consent and choice; improving public and professional awareness; and good-quality information post diagnosis.

Consent and choice

People with dementia should have the opportunity to make informed decisions and then, when capacity no longer exists, to exercise choices about their care and treatment in partnership with their health and social care professionals and families/care partners. Where capacity to make decisions no longer exists, health and social care professionals should follow guidance from the Department of Health: 'Seeking consent: working with older people' (2001a) and 'Seeking consent: working with people with learning disabilities' (2001b) (**www.dh.gov.uk**). Even at an advanced point, many people living with dementia retain capacity to make choices about specific day-to-day aspects of their care and life (Dewing, 2002; 2008b). All health and social care professionals should follow the code of practice accompanying the Mental Capacity Act 2005 (**www.dca.gov.uk/menincap/bill-summary.htm**).

It is recommended that you look this up at the Office of Public Service Information (2005).

When working with people who have dementia, ensuring consent and choice can become more of a challenge. For example, nurses can mistakenly feel that people with dementia do not know what they want or are unsafe to make and exercise choices. There can also be a tension between doing what is in the best interest of the person with dementia and what the family/care partner wants done. Families/care partners can offer valuable insights and help with assessment and caring, and should not be excluded from decision-making processes. However, not everyone knows the 'patient' well or can think and act in a way that enables his or her best interests to be put first. Nurses must be mindful that doing something or not doing something because of family wishes may not be evidence-based, especially when the person with dementia is expressing an alternative preference.

Improving public and professional awareness

Although public awareness about dementia is growing, it is still common for people to assume that Alzheimer's is the only type of dementia. Nurses have a responsibility to understand what dementia is, and to know how they would describe it to members of the public and how they would help people to gain an accurate understanding of dementia. Knowing what resources are available for the public to access is core to being able to suggest this to them when it is timely to do so. What three websites would you suggest families/carers use for the following?

- Finding out about different types of dementia
- How to obtain a specialist assessment and diagnosis
- What happens after a diagnosis
- Acute hospital care for people with dementia
- Getting community support established or increased
- Carers' support
- Finding suitable care homes
- Palliative and then end-of-life care planning

You are advised to take the following actions.

1. Make use of the sources of evidence at the end of this chapter to guide you to further resources in relation to the above.

2. Listen to what people with dementia and families/carers tell you is useful.
3. Search the web to find sources you feel are user-friendly.

Good-quality information post diagnosis

Good communication between care providers and people with dementia and their families and carers is essential, so that people with dementia receive the information and support they require. Evidence-based information should be offered in a form that is suited to the needs of the individual. Treatment, care, and information provided should be culturally appropriate and in a form that is accessible to people who have additional needs, such as physical, cognitive, or sensory disabilities, or who do not speak or read English.

Following a diagnosis of dementia, unless the person with dementia clearly indicates to the contrary, information should be provided about:

- the signs and symptoms of dementia;
- the course and prognosis of the condition;
- treatments;
- local care and support services;
- support groups;
- sources of financial and legal advice, and advocacy;
- medicolegal issues, including driving and advance care planning;
- local information sources, including libraries and voluntary organizations.

Carers and relatives should also be provided with the information and support they need, and carers should be offered an assessment of their own needs. There is a growing evidence base about different types of therapy and intervention, such as cognitive behavioural therapy (CBT), music therapy, alternative therapies, walking, and exercise.

Identifying best practice

NICE clinical guideline on dementia: the treatment and care of people with dementia in health and social care http://www.nice.org.uk/guidance/index.jsp?action=byID&r=true&o=10997

NICE has also produced a clinical guideline on Parkinson's disease. People with this condition often develop dementia www.nice.org.uk/CG035

You can search for specific aspects of best practice in dementia care online at http://www.thecochranelibrary.com/view/0/index.html

Sources of evidence

Organizations

Dementias and Neurodegenerative Diseases Research Network (DeNDRoN) http://www.dendron.org.uk/ The NIHR Dementias & Neurodegenerative Diseases Research Network (NIHR DeNDRoN) is one of six topic-specific clinical research networks funded by the Department of Health in England. DeNDRoN supports the development and delivery of clinical research in the NHS in the dementias, Parkinson's disease, motor neurone disease, Huntington's disease, and other neurodegenerative diseases.

The Dementia Information Portal is a website that follows the implementation of the National Dementia Strategy. It offers information and support to anyone with an interest in improving services for people with dementia http://www.dementia.dh.gov.uk

Department of Health (2001c) National Service Framework for Older People. Department of Health: London.

A dementia gateway is provided by Social Care Centre for Excellence (SCIE) http://www.scie.org.uk/publications/dementia/usefulresources.asp

Working Group for the Faculty of the Psychiatry of Old Age of the Royal College of Psychiatrists, Royal College of General Practitioners, British Geriatric Society & Alzheimer's Society (2004) Summary: guidance for the management of behavioural and psychological symptoms in dementia and the treatment of psychosis in people with history of stroke/TIA http://www.rcpsych.ac.uk/specialties/faculties/oldage/bgscasig.aspx

National Institute for Health and Clinical Excellence (NICE) http://guidance.nice.org.uk/

The Scottish Intercollegiate Guidelines Network (SIGN) http://www.sign.ac.uk/guidelines/index.html

NHS Evidence http://www.evidence.nhs.uk/

Agency for Healthcare Quality (AHRQ) http://www.ahrq.gov/

National Institute for Clinical Studies (NICS) http://www.nhmrc.gov.au/nics/index.htm

Registered Nurses Association of Ontario **http://www.rnao.org**

World Health Organization **http://www.who.int/en/**

Journals

Age and Ageing

Aging and Society

Dementia: The International Journal of Social Research and Practice

International Journal of Older People Nursing

International Journal of Geriatric Psychiatry

Journal of the American Geriatrics Society.

Recommended journal articles

Fick, D., Hodo, D. (2004) A retrospective study of delirium superimposed in dementia. *The Gerontologist* **44**(1): 59–68.

Conclusion

People can and do live with, rather than 'suffer' from, dementia. Accordingly, nurses and all healthcare workers need to be optimistic about their contribution and interventions. Good practice begins with attending to consent and choice.

Early screening and diagnosis is an increasing priority. Introducing information, support, and treatment/therapies as early as possible can help to enhance quality of life for the person with dementia and the family/care partner(s).

Online Resource Centre

 To help you to develop and apply your knowledge and decision-making skills further, we have provided interactive learning resources online at **www.oxfordtextbooks.co.uk/orc/bullock/**

Whilst these are freely available, you will need to use the access codes at the start of the book.

References

Adams, T. (1997) Dementia. In I. J. Norman, S. J. Redfern (eds) *Mental Health Care for Elderly People.* Churchill Livingstone: Edinburgh, pp. 183–204.

Alzheimer's Disease International **http://www.alz.co.uk/info/early-symptoms** (accessed 10 May 2011).

American Psychiatric Association (2000) *Diagnostic and Statistical Manual of Mental Disorders (DSM-IV),* 4th edn, text revised. American Psychiatric Association: Washington DC.

Banerjee, S., Willis, R., Matthews, D. (2007) Improving the quality of care for mild to moderate dementia: an evaluation of the Croydon memory service model. *International Journal of Geriatric Psychiatry* **22**: 782–8.

Carpenter, B.D., Xiong, C., Porensky, E.K., *et al.* (2008) Reaction to a dementia diagnosis in individuals with Alzheimer's disease and mild cognitive impairment. *Journal of the American Geriatrics Society* **56**(3): 405–12.

Department of Health (2001a) *Seeking Consent: Working with Older People;* **http://www.dh.gov.uk/en/Publicationsandstatistics/Publications/Publications-PolicyAndGuidance/DH_4009325** (accessed 10 May 2011).

Department of Health (2001b) *Seeking Consent: Working with People with Learning Disabilities.* **http://www.dh.gov.uk/en/Publicationsandstatistics/Publications/PublicationsPolicy-AndGuidance/DH_4007861** (accessed 10 May 2011).

Department of Health (2001c) *National Service Framework for Older People.* Department of Health: London.

Department of Health (2009) *Living Well With Dementia: A National Dementia Strategy Implementation Plan.* Department of Health: London. **http://www.dh.gov.uk/publications** (accessed 10 May 2011).

Dewing, J. (2002) From ritual to relationship: a person centred approach to consent in qualitative research with older people who have a dementia. *Dementia: The International Journal of Social Research and Practice* **1**(2): 156–71.

Dewing, J. (2007) Participatory research: a method for process consent with persons who have dementia. *Dementia: The International Journal of Social Research & Practice* **6**(1): 11–25.

Dewing, J. (2008a) Personhood and dementia: revisiting Tom Kitwood's ideas. *International Journal of Older People Nursing* **3**: 3–13.

Dewing, J. (2008b) Process consent and research with older persons living with dementia. *Association of Research Ethics Journal* **4**(2): 59–64.

Ferri, C., Prince, M., Brayne, H., *et al.* (2005) Global prevalence of dementia: a Delphi consensus study. *Lancet* **366**: 2112–17.

Fick, D., Hodo, D. (2004) A retrospective study of delirium superimposed in dementia. *The Gerontologist* **44**(1): 59–68.

Fick, D., Mion, L. (2008) Delirium superimposed on dementia. *American Journal of Nursing* **108**(1): 52–60.

Gyure, K.A., Durham, R., Stewart, W.F., *et al.* (2001) Intraneuronal Aβ-amyloid precedes development of amyloid plaques in Down syndrome. *Archives of Pathology & Laboratory Medicine* **125**(4): 489–92.

Holland, A.J. (1994) Down's syndrome and dementia of the Alzheimer's type. In A. Burns, R. Levy (eds) *Dementia.* Chapman and Hall Medical: London, pp. 695–707.

Huang, W., Qiu, C., von Strauss, E., *et al.* (2004) APOE genotype, family history of dementia, and Alzheimer disease risk: a 6-year follow-up study. *Archives of Neurology* **61**: 1930–4.

Kitwood, T. (1987) Dementia and its pathology: in brain, mind or society? *Free Associations* **8**: 81–93.

Kitwood, T. (1988) The technical, the personal, and the framing of dementia. *Social Behaviour* **3**: 161–79.

Kitwood, T. (1989) Brain, mind and dementia: with particular reference to Alzheimer's disease. *Ageing and Society* **9**(1): 1–15.

Kitwood, T. (1990a) The dialectics of dementia: with particular reference to Alzheimer's disease. *Aging and Society* **10**(2): 177–96.

Kitwood, T. (1990b) Understanding senile dementia: a psychobiographical approach. *Free Associations* **19**: 60–76.

Kitwood, T. (1993a) Person and process in dementia. *International Journal of Psychiatry* **8**: 541–5.

Kitwood, T. (1993b) Towards a theory of dementia care: the interpersonal process. *Ageing and Society* **13**: 51–67.

Kitwood, T. (1997) *Dementia Reconsidered: The Person Comes First.* Open University Press: Buckingham.

National Institute for Health and Clinical Excellence (NICE) (2011) *Dementia [JD17]: The NICE Guideline on Supporting People with Dementia and their Carers in Health and Social Care.* (This clinical guideline has been amended to incorporate the updated NICE technology appraisal of drugs for Alzheimer's disease, published in March 2011). www.nice.org.uk/guidance/TA217 http://www.nice.org.uk/nicemedia/live/10998/30320/30320.pdf (accessed 14 October 2011).

Nelson, P.T., Braak, H., Markesbery, W.R. (2009) Neuropathology and cognitive impairment in Alzheimer disease: a complex but coherent relationship. *Journal of Neuropathological Experimental Neurology* **68**(1): 1–14.

Oborne, C.A., Hooper, R., Li, K.C., *et al.* (2002) An indicator of appropriate neuroleptic prescribing in nursing homes. *Age and Ageing* **31**: 435–9.

Office of Public Service Information (2005) *The Mental Capacity Act 2005.* HMSO: London.

Pace, V., Treloar, A., Scott, S. (2011) *Dementia: from Advanced Disease to Bereavement.* Oxford University Press: Oxford.

Robinson, L., Clare, L., Evans, K. (2005) Making sense of dementia and adjusting to loss: psychological reactions to a diagnosis of dementia in couples. *Aging & Mental Health* **4**: 337–47.

Royal College of Psychiatrists (2009) Delirium leaflet. http://www.rcpsych.ac.uk; (last accessed 10 May 2011).

Scotland's Care Commission and Mental Welfare Commission (2010) *Remember I'm Still Me.* http://www.carecommission.com/images/stories/documents/publications/reviewsofquali tycare/remember_im_still_me_-_may_09.pdf (accessed 12 October 2011).

Tanzi, R. (2005) Tangles and neurodegenerative disease–a surprising twist. *New England Journal of Medicine* **353**(17): 1853–5.

van der Flier, W.M., Scheltens, P. (2005) Epidemiology and risk factors of dementia. *Journal of Neurology, Neurosurgery and Psychiatry* **76**(Suppl. 5): v2–v7.

Wimo, A., Prince, M., Alzheimer's Disease International (2010) *World Alzheimer Report: The Global Economic Impact of Dementia. Executive Summary.* Alzheimer's Disease International http://www.alz.co.uk/research/world-report (accessed 10 May 2011).

World Health Organization (2007) *International Statistical Classification of Diseases and Related Health Problems,* 10th edn (ICD-10). World Health Organization: Geneva.

8 *Understanding* Depression

Marie Chellingsworth

Introduction

The aim of this chapter is to provide you with the knowledge to be able to recognize, assess, manage, and care for people with depression in an evidence-based and person-centred way. Depression is disabling and causes significant impact upon many areas of the person's day-to-day functioning; it is therefore important that nurses have the knowledge and skills to recognize whether someone might be depressed and know how to take the appropriate course of action. This chapter will provide a comprehensive overview of the causes and impact of depression, before exploring best practice to deliver care, as well as to prevent or to minimize further ill-health. Nursing assessments and priorities are highlighted throughout, and the nursing management of the symptoms and common health problems associated with depression can be found in Chapter 14. →

Understanding depression

I lost my balance. I fell flat on my face and I couldn't get up again. And if that implies a certain grace, a slow and easy free-fall, then you have me wrong. It was violent and painful and, above all humiliating . . . I came to understand that we are not simply fighting an illness, but the attitudes that surround it. Imagine saying to someone that you have a life-threatening illness such as cancer, and being told to pull yourself together or get over it. Imagine being terribly ill and too afraid to tell anyone lest it destroy your career. Imagine being admitted into hospital because you are too ill to function and being too ashamed to tell anyone, because it is a psychiatric hospital. Imagine telling someone that you have recently been discharged and watching them turn away, in embarrassment or disgust or fear. Bad enough to be ill, but to feel compelled to deny the very thing that, in its worst and most active state, defines you is agony indeed. (Sally Brampton (2008) in *Shoot The Damn Dog.*)

Sally's experience of her depressive episode from her memoir sets the scene of just what people with depression can experience and how big an impact it can have upon their lives. We may all feel low and 'fed up' at times, and often we use the term 'depressed' as an adjective to describe how we are feeling in general conversation. These fluctuations in mood are usually short-lived and are a natural phenomena, but this is not defined as a 'depressive episode'.

Defining depression

Depression is considered to be a heterogeneous group of conditions rather than a single condition. Unipolar depression, the focus of this chapter, is a high prevalence disorder and is characterized by anhedonia (an inability to experience pleasure from activities that are usually enjoyable) and a range of associated emotional, cognitive, physical, and behavioural symptoms (National Institute for Health and Clinical Excellence (NICE), 2009a). Symptoms of depression and low mood can persist over several weeks, months, and, in some cases, even years.

Depression symptoms can be best considered as occurring on a continuum of severity (Lewinsohn *et al.*, 2000). This may be categorized from sub-threshold symptoms (not meeting the criteria for a full depressive episode) to mild, moderate, or severe, as illustrated in Figure 8.1. The severity is based upon the number of symptoms with which a patient presents, their duration, and their impact upon the person's daily functioning. We may all be at varying places on the continuum at various times in our lives and our moods can fluctuate on a daily basis.

According to the *Diagnostic and Statistical Manual of Mental Disorders* (DSM-IV; American Psychiatric Association, 2000), the diagnostic tool used to categorize mental health conditions and to improve recognition of disorders, if symptoms of depression have been present for 2 weeks or more, this can be defined as a depressive episode. This would then be categorized as mild, moderate, or severe based on the presentation. Healthcare practitioners need to be alert to the symptoms of depression, because individuals can present in any care setting. Often, GPs and routine practice settings play a major role in the detection and management of depression.

Up to 10% of people with depression subsequently go on to experience **hypomanic/manic episodes** (Kovacs, 1996), fitting the criteria for bipolar affective disorder (also referred to as manic depression), which emphasizes the need to question patients about a history of elevated mood and to be alert to new episodes occurring. This condition is different from the more commonly encountered unipolar depression. Bipolar affective disorder sufferers have periods of moods at two extremes (two poles). Patients with this condition have episodes of significantly elevated raised mood, and also have periods during which mood is very depressed. Whilst outside the scope of this chapter, more information can be found in the clinical guideline 'The management of bipolar disorder in adults, children and adolescents, in primary and secondary care' (National Institute for Health and Clinical Excellence (NICE), 2011 **www.nice.org.uk**).

Of considerable note is that only one-third of depression sufferers are found to be suffering from unipolar depression alone (Zimmerman *et al.*, 2008). Many have comorbid anxiety-based mental health problems such as **panic disorder** (with or without agoraphobia), **social phobia**, **post-traumatic stress disorder**, **generalized anxiety disorder**, or **obsessive compulsive disorder** (Scott, 2007). In these circumstances, one of three diagnoses can be made depending on the symptoms that dominate the clinical picture, as follows.

1. Depression
2. Anxiety disorder
3. Mixed depression and anxiety when both are below the threshold for either disorder
   (National Institute for Health and Clinical Excellence
   (NICE), 2009a)

For more detailed information about anxiety-based disorders, see **Chapter 14** .

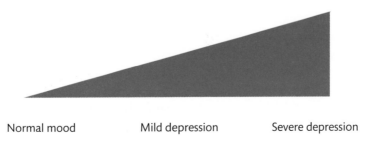

Normal mood   Mild depression   Severe depression

Figure 8.1 Depression symptoms can be best considered as occurring on a continuum of severity.

Prevalence of depression

Depression is often defined as a 'common mental health problem' (National Institute for Health and Clinical Excellence (NICE), 2009a; Richards and Whyte, 2009) owing to its high prevalence. However, this term should not mistakenly lead one to underestimate the seriousness, significance, or impact that even milder episodes of depressed mood can have upon the sufferer.

Mental illness accounts for over one-third of the burden of illness in Britain, with some 40% of all physical and mental disability being due to mental illness. Similarly, roughly 40% of people on incapacity benefits suffer from mental illness (and mental illness is a secondary factor for at least another 10%). At the GP surgery, one-third of those who seek consultation each year have mental health problems, taking up at least one-third of GPs' time. According to the Depression Report (2006), published by the London School of Economics, one in six are diagnosed as having depression or chronic anxiety disorder, which means that one family in three is affected at any one time (Layard, 2006). It is known that patients with physical health conditions are at greater risk of becoming depressed (NICE, 2009b) and that, once a second episode of depression is encountered, the risk of subsequent episodes increase (NICE, 2009a).

World estimates of the proportion of people likely to experience depression in their lifetime vary between studies and areas, but are between approximately 4% and 10% for major depression, and between 2.5% and 5% for dysthymia (low-grade chronic depressive symptoms) (National Institute for Health and Clinical Excellence (NICE), 2009a). Depression affects 9% of individuals over the age of 18 in any given year, and approximately 16% of adults will experience depression in their lifetime (Kessler *et al.*, 2003). Prevalence is said to be between 1.5 and 2.5 times higher in women than in men (National Institute for Health and Clinical Excellence (NICE), 2009a).

Depression can cause a significant impact on working and employment, with lost work days due to the condition and the condition itself causing difficulties in finding or maintaining employment. The cost of depression has been analysed by the London School of Economics (2006) to be some £12 billion per year. This equates to 1% of the total national income, with a cost to the taxpayer of £7 billion per year.

Mortality and morbidity

Depression leads to over a fourfold higher risk of suicide compared with the general population (National Institute for Health and Clinical Excellence (NICE), 2009a). In 2009, there were 5,765 cases recorded of death by suicide in the UK (Office of National Statistics, 2011). Approximately 1 in 333 of those prescribed antidepressants in primary care make a suicide attempt in a 9-month period, with a corresponding figure of 1 in 129 for those starting psychotherapy (Simon and Savarino, 2006). With a long-term physical health condition, these figures rise further.

Large population-based epidemiological studies have reported higher suicide risk linked with various major physical diseases, including cancer, diabetes, end-stage renal disease, epilepsy, multiple sclerosis, stroke, and traumatic brain injury (National Institute for Health and Clinical Excellence (NICE), 2009b). These findings indicate the importance of detecting and treating depressive disorder in people with chronic physical health problems, who may often not present in mental health services, but in adult healthcare settings. This reinforces the need for the adult nurse to be aware of depression and its impact, and to be able to recognize symptoms and presentations consistent with the condition.

When mood is depressed, thoughts of suicide are often reported, however, the majority of patients, even those with more severe depression, or depression in the context of chronic health problems, do not want to commit suicide or act on these thoughts. However, risk status can change regularly with the nature of the condition and some patients do go on to attempt suicide or self harm. Checking that the patient knows where to get appropriate help if the situation deteriorates and ensuring that this information is given is important. Assessment of risk is therefore required for each patient at regular routine intervals, rather than any assumptions being made. The practising nurse or student nurse should always consult a mentor, appropriate multidisciplinary team member, or supervisor for guidance and support in undertaking any risk assessment, or upon disclosure of suicidal thoughts from a patient. Referral onto specialist mental health services and ensuring collaborative care planning is likely to be required if there is intent or plans in place. Comprehensive risk assessments carried out by a mental health workers will assess current and previous history of thoughts, plans, actions, risk to self or others, neglect of self or others and preventative factors in the person's life that would stop them commiting suicide (Farrand *et al.*, 2010).

Causes of depression

The Cartesian split between mind and body tends to make us think of 'mental illnesses' like depression as not having a physical component (Goodwin, 2004). This is far from accurate, and advances in genetics and biochemistry are helping us to understand in more detail what role they may play. Environmental and social factors also seem to play a part. What is less understood, however, is why some people go on to experience depression and others do not when faced with similar situations and biological or genetic predispositions. The extent to which factors may be causal to each other also needs further understanding: for example, does depressed mood cause negative thinking due to biological changes, or can negative thinking itself cause depression? Many theories attempt to explain the phenomena of depressed mood, but there is no singularly agreed causal factor. The cause of depression therefore should not be viewed as related to a single factor, but rather as caused by a range of biological, physiological, and environmental factors. They do not offer mutually exclusive alternatives; they demand some form iof unification (Goodwin, 2004).

Cognitive

Thoughts can have an influencing effect upon mood. An often-cited theory for the cause of depression is the role of the person's cognitions (thoughts). We give meaning to our experiences partly by interpreting the mood states that they provoke or recall (Goodwin, 2004). When down, negative interpretations to events and experiences can be made, which then in turn have further impact on how we feel and what we do. We hold beliefs and assumptions that can be 'distorted'. Thoughts are often negative about the self, others, and the future. This is referred to as 'Beck's cognitive triad' (Beck, 1976) and places 'cognitive distortions' as central. However, we may be more genetically predisposed to seeing things in a more pessimistic way. Biochemical tone may determine unconscious biases at various levels of neuro-psychological functioning, such as attention, encoding, stimulus evaluation, and recall (Goodwin, 2004). So whether the cognitions themselves

are the cause of depression or the biological aspects of depressed mood induce such thought patterns is not yet fully understood.

Environmental

Adverse childhood experiences such as poor parental relationships, neglect, physical abuse, sexual abuse, and bereavement are considered to increase a person's chance of developing depression. Such experiences may lead to negative thought patterns and low self-esteem, and poor coping and problem-solving abilities, which can then be triggers for depression later in life when combined with stressful events such as loss of a job or of a close relationship (NICE, 2009a).

Similarly, individual depressive episodes often have some noticeable antecedents (significant life event or difficulty) that occurs before the episode, such as marriage and relationship difficulties, divorce bereavements, retirement, or loss of job. However, many people have these environmental factors without getting depressed, and therefore it may be that some people are more genetically or biologically predisposed to these triggering factors.

Genetic

One theory of depression is that of genetic predisposition. Some types of depression, such as major depression, are more common in the relatives of people who also have the disorder. This suggests that some element of depression may be inherited or genetic. No single gene has been found that causes depression and what exactly is inherited is not known. It may be changes in brain structures or brain function, including alterations to the physiological responses to stress, which are genetic. An alternative explanation may be that the family situation can increase the risk through environmental factors and nurturing. Again, these factors are not an isolated cause and genetics are likely affected also by environmental factors; any explanation of the causes of depression that ignores either would be limited (Goodwin, 2004). One way to counteract this is to look to twin studies as a marker.

Twin studies seek to find a discrepancy between the concordance between monozygotic twins (genetically identical) and dizygotic twins (non-identical). If rates are higher in genetically identical twins than in non-identical twins, it gives stronger weight to a genetic origin. Twin studies have been conducted in depressive disorders. In twin studies for unipolar depression, 46% of monozygotic twins developed the same depressive illness and 20% of dizygotic twins (McGuffin *et al.*, 1996). This finding has been replicated similarly in other twin studies (Goodwin, 2004) and allows conclusion that depression is markedly, but by no means overwhelmingly, a genetic condition (Goodwin, 2004).

Biological/biochemical

People experiencing depression can have neurotransmitter imbalances. When an imbalance occurs, it is believed that depression can result. However, of course, it is also possible that the chemical change is the result of depression. Antidepressant medications reverse depressive symptoms by altering these chemical levels, and given that antidepressants are effective treatments, this adds significant weight to the role that they play. The monoamine hypothesis states that reserpine, which depletes monoamines, can induce a depressed mood. The monoamines involved in mood regulation are noradrenaline, dopamine, and 5-hydroxytryptaime (5-HT, serotonin), and acetylcholine. Monoamines appear to be regulators of key behavioural states and physical functions such as sleep and wakening, appetite, motivation, motor activity, aggressiveness, sexual responsiveness, and aspects of learning and memory (Goodwin, 2004). We know that these are the physical and behavioural symptoms sufferers of depression often report. We know that certain drugs that release monoamines, such as ecstasy and amphetamines, can induce excitement, overactivity, and euphoria (Goodwin, 2004). Therefore, the role of monoamines in mood regulation appears important, and indeed antidepressants work by having primary action on monoamines.

Assessing the patient with depression

When assessing the patient with depression, it can be useful to consider the symptoms as affecting three main domains: a person's physical well-being; his or her behaviours or activities; and his or her thinking.

All of these can be impacted as a result of depression and therefore all require assessment to ensure a holistic approach.

The ABC model of emotion is used widely to understand and assess depression (Richards and Whyte, 2009), focusing on the following factors.

- Autonomic (physical symptoms such as appetite, sleep, pain, and concentration that are affected as a result of the difficulties)
- Behaviours (what the person is doing or not doing as a result of his or her difficulties)
- Cognitions (the content of his or her thoughts and how these are affected)

The model is a useful tool because it facilitates the identification of where interventions are required and where symptoms or comorbidities may be impacting on each other. These three domains interact with each other, as summarized in Figure 8.2, making the problem worse. This is called a 'vicious cycle' in that they can serve to make other areas worse and have a knock-on negative effect, and can maintain the depression. For example, a depressed diabetic may think: 'What is the point? I can't be bothered' (C). This may lead to him or her not taking insulin as prescribed (B), which can worsen his or her physical health (A). However, intervention into one of these areas can have a helpful impact upon the others, improving mood, and breaking the vicious cycle. It is also used within **cognitive behavioural therapy (CBT)**, which is an evidence-based form of psychological treatment for depression (see later in the chapter for details of CBT and other evidence-based treatments).

Physical signs of depression

Depression and low mood can have a significant impact upon the person physically. Physical symptoms such as tearfulness, irritability, sleep problems (such as early morning wakening or difficulty falling or staying asleep), diurnal mood variation (feeling better or worse in mornings compared to later in the day), concentration problems, exacerbation of current pain, or increased pains secondary to muscle tension are all common. Appetite changes are also common, with suffers often reporting losing weight. They may eat more (comfort eating), or eat foods that are quick and easy to prepare ('junk' foods), which may cause weight gain. More subtle symptoms may be noticeable, such as difficulties concentrating, increased pain, headaches, or constipation being signs of a depressed mood. Care must be taken to ensure which symptoms are related to any physical health problem that the patient may already have, or which may be caused or worsened by the depression or vice versa. For example, many of these physical symptoms of depression may also be present in the physical health condition itself, which may mimic these symptoms.

A patient with chronic lower back pain may think: 'I cannot exercise or walk far, or my back will hurt more' (C). This leads him or her to avoid activities that may exert him or her and to sitting or lying down for long periods (B). This in turn causes stiffness and muscle wastage (A), and reinforces a further reduction of activity and impacts further on mood deterioration.

Behavioural signs of depression

Behavioural changes, such as changes in activity levels, can affect the person. When the person has symptoms of depression, everyday activities or those previously enjoyed can seem overwhelming, and motivation to carry them out may be lowered; thus an avoidance of these activities takes place. This avoidance then leads to symptom relief in the short term and so,

understandably, further avoidance of activities then takes place. Avoidance of these activities, however, can lead to further problems and further deterioration of mood in the long term. Similarly, the person may adopt other unhelpful behaviours, such as drinking more alcohol, not eating well, or taking non-prescribed or street drugs in an attempt to feel better. Other behaviours, including spending money, gambling, or self-harm (such as cutting), may be evident. It is best to think of behavioural changes to be assessed in two main categories: things the person is avoiding or has reduced as a result of his or her symptoms of depression; and things he or she may be doing more as a result to try to feel better.

For example, a patient with cancer may have physical symptoms of increased pain (A). He or she may think: 'What is the point? I will die anyway and I do not want to be a burden' (C). This leads to him or her not seeing his or her friends or answering the phone (B), leading to further deterioration in mood.

Cognitive signs of depression

Cognitive changes occur including pessimistic and recurrently negative thoughts about oneself, one's past, and the future, mental slowing, and rumination (Cassano and Fava, 2002). When someone is depressed, negative thoughts are harder to dismiss. These thoughts can worsen how the person feels and

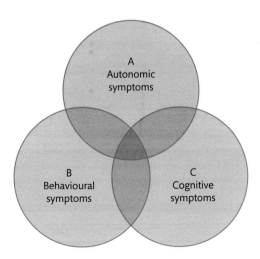

A Autonomic:
How the person is affected physically

B Behavioural:
How the person's behaviour or activities are affected

C Cognitive:
How the person's thinking is affected

Figure 8.2 ABC model of depression.

impact on what he or she does. (Williams and Chellingsworth, 2010). He or she may spend time ruminating (going over and over negative thoughts). Beck (1976), one of the key authors in the field of cognitive behavioural therapy (CBT), states that the thoughts of a patient when depressed centre around loss. This may be an *actual* loss (for example, a bereavement, a loss of employment, a relationship breakdown or divorce), but may also be a *perceived loss* whereby the person feels that he or she has lost something important to his or her sense of self, such as his or her role in life or how he or she views his or herself.

A patient with a physical healthcare problem may experience a muscle weakness and pain (A in Figure 8.2), leading to a reduction in previously enjoyed activities (B in Figure 8.2). This can lead to negative thoughts, such as 'I am a failure as a parent because I can no longer play football with my son' (C in Figure 8.2), which can lead to further avoidance and negative mood. The loss here is both an actual loss in terms of mobility, but also a perceived loss of his or her role as a good parent.

CASE STUDY 8.1 *Andrew*

Gemma was a student adult nurse on branch placement on her local dialysis unit at the teaching hospital. She had been there for 4 months and was able to spend time with patients in various stages of their renal care pathway under the supervision of her mentor.

Andrew was a 31-year-old renal patient whom Gemma had met previously in the outpatient clinic. He had recently been told that he now required dialysis treatment and that this should begin as soon as possible; however, he had missed an appointment last week and had to be contacted to reschedule. At his next appointment at the dialysis unit, Gemma's mentor had arranged for her to spend some time with Andrew, discussing how he felt about the move to dialysis and going through the information leaflet that he had been given at his previous appointment to see if he had any questions about the treatment.

Gemma noticed that Andrew was not his usual self: usually, he was really well presented and wearing smart clothes; today, he did not seem to have taken as much care over his appearance, was unshaven, and was not making much eye contact. Gemma asked Andrew how his mood had been since his last appointment. He stated that he had been feeling down and tearful, and that today was the first day that he had got dressed or left his house in over a week. He had been feeling this way for about 2 months and had little pleasure or interest in anything, but it had got a lot worse since he was told he needed dialysis. Gemma passed her concerns onto her mentor, and together they spoke to Andrew. After the appointment, they summarized this further using the ABC structure as a reflective activity for Gemma's portfolio. Andrew's symptoms are summarized in Figure 8.3.

It was clear that all of these areas were impacting on each other for Andrew. He had headaches and felt tired all of the time so did not want to go out—it all seemed too much effort. He was not sleeping properly, so was drinking alcohol to get to sleep even though he knew he should not be doing this because of his health condition. His thoughts were negative about his future and about his treatment, which led to him missing an appointment and feeling worse. Since he had missed the appointment, he had not spoken to any of his colleagues and had stopped answering the phone. He felt a burden to his family. He had had some thoughts that his family would be better off without him, but had no plans to act on the thoughts and they were fleeting. Gemma and her mentor discussed the above sensitively with Andrew and referred him to see Dr Paulo, the renal unit health psychologist, who worked as part of the multidisciplinary team and who could provide further psychological management and support.

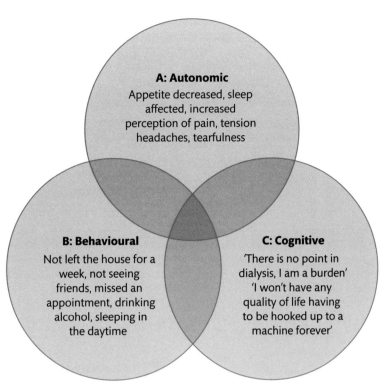

A: Autonomic
Appetite decreased, sleep affected, increased perception of pain, tension headaches, tearfulness

B: Behavioural
Not left the house for a week, not seeing friends, missed an appointment, drinking alcohol, sleeping in the daytime

C: Cognitive
'There is no point in dialysis, I am a burden' 'I won't have any quality of life having to be hooked up to a machine forever'

Figure 8.3 **Andrew's symptoms.**

Nursing management

Best practice

The National Institute for Clinical Excellence (NICE) clinical guidelines for depression (2009a) use a stepped care model of service delivery. The adult nurse can play an important role in the identification of the patient with depression. The accurate identification of the condition is seen as the essential first step in its management. This includes people who have sought treatment because of depressive symptoms and those being treated for other conditions, including physical health conditions (National Institute for Clinical Excellence (NICE), 2009a). Therefore, whichever setting you find yourself in, an understanding of depression and how to assess the patient accurately is a key priority. This is especially true given the high rates of depression in those with physical ill-health as outlined previously.

The adult nurse is likely to see patients who may be depressed as part of routine care delivery for physical health conditions, or in routine general practice. As such, the skills required for the adult nurse are recognition of depression. Depending upon the severity of the symptoms, the nurse would coordinate support for the patient,

and ensure appropriate liaison and referral to appropriate members of the wider multidisciplinary team or mental health specialists, if appropriate, for further assessment and treatment.

Studies indicate that up to 50% of patients suffering from depression are not recognized when they attend primary care (Williams *et al.*, 1995; Mitchell *et al.*, 2009). The National Institute for Clinical Excellence (NICE) (2009a) recommends that all clinicians are alert to possible depression (particularly in people with a past history of depression or a chronic physical health problem with associated functional impairment) and consider asking the two following key questions.

- During the past month, have you often been bothered by feeling down, depressed, or hopeless?
- During the past month, have you often been bothered by having little interest or pleasure in doing things?

If an affirmative response is given by the patient to either or both questions, then an assessment of depression should be made by a practitioner competent to carry out a mental health assessment.

If the person also has a chronic physical health problem, NICE (2009a) advises asking three further questions to improve accuracy.

- During the last month, have you often been bothered by feelings of worthlessness?
- During the last month, have you often been bothered by poor concentration?
- During the last month, have you often been bothered by thoughts of death?

If an affirmative response is given by the patient to either or both questions, then an assessment of depression should be made by a practitioner competent to carry out a mental health assessment. For a student nurse, this will require liaison with the practice mentor and other members of the multidisciplinary team to ensure that the patient's needs are met and that the nurse is working within his or her own competency levels.

The nurse's role in recognition and assessment

Accurate recognition and assessment of the patient with suspected depression requires a biopsychosocial approach, with accurate information gathering of the ways in which low mood has affected the following:

- Autonomic symptoms—how the problem is affecting the patient physically;
- Behaviour—what he or she is and is not doing since feeling this way;
- Cognitions—how his or her thinking has been affected.

The impact of these ABC symptoms on the person's daily life should be assessed in terms of his or her relationships with family and social contacts, work life, and activities of daily living such as maintaining self-care, and also any hobbies and interests. Clear consideration and assessment should be made of any comorbidity issues, such as any acute physical condition or chronic long-term health condition, because symptoms may mirror those of depression, e.g. tiredness, pain, and sleep disturbances.

An assessment of the depressed patient should take place in a therapeutic way, viewing the patient as the expert on his or her own experience of depression and recovery. Recommendations for working with a patient

> **Box 8.1 Recommendations for working with a patient with depression**
>
> - Build a trusting relationship and work in an open, engaging, and non-judgemental manner.
> - Explore treatment options in an atmosphere of hope and optimism.
> - Be aware that stigma and discrimination can be associated with a diagnosis of depression.
> - Ensure that discussions take place in settings in which confidentiality, privacy, and dignity are respected.
>
> (National Institute for Health and Clinical Excellence (NICE), 2009a)

with depression have been published as part of the National Institute for Health and Clinical Excellence Guideline for Depression (NICE, 2009a). The guidelines recommend the following key points when working with patients with depression, their families, and carers.

Managing an acute and severe episode of depression

The management of a patient with severe depressed mood or suicidal thoughts and intent requires specialist input from mental health services. For student nurses, decision-making and care planning should always be led by, and delivered in conjunction with, senior colleagues and staff.

Management of a severe depressive episode (when patients are at significant risk, e.g. they may have suicidal intent and plans to carry this out, or an inability to look after themselves safely) may require inpatient treatment on an acute mental health ward. There are also community mental health services, called Crisis Resolution and Home Treatment (CRHT), which work with people to manage the crisis out of hospital if possible. It is recommended that all efforts are made to ensure that a person with depression can give meaningful and informed consent before treatment starts, especially those with severe depression requiring inpatient treatment or those who are subject to the Mental Health Act 2007 (National Institute for Health and Clinical Excellence (NICE), 2009a).

Evidence-based pharmalogical interventions

Antidepressant medication is a widely available efficacious treatment that can help with depressive symptoms. The adult nurse may need to administer these and so knowledge of this group of medications is important. It must be considered that antidepressant medication is also used to treat anxiety disorders, premenstrual dysphoric disorder, and pain (Wasserman, 2011). Therefore it is important to understand why an individual patient has been prescribed an antidepressant.

Antidepressants act primarily to block active transport of neurotransmitters back into neurons or to increase the availability of monoamines such as 5-HT and noradrenaline (Goodwin, 2004).

Antidepressants and the way in which they work are often misunderstood. Antidepressants are not addictive and have minimal withdrawal symptoms at most. Newer types of antidepressant also do not cause significant weight gain. To make an informed choice about pharmacological options for depression, the person should be given information about the choice of medications available, what common side effects may occur, for how long he or she will be expected to take it, how long it may be until it starts working, and what other treatment options, such as psychological interventions, are available when it is prescribed. Obviously, in some cases in which treatment involves detainment under the Mental Health Act 2007, or capacity to consent is affected, then medications may be need to be given without the consent of the person. However, these instances occur as part of specialist mental health services care provision.

Routine assessment of the patient should include gathering information on any medication he or she may have been prescribed for his or her mood currently or previously, its name and dose, if the patient took this (or not) as prescribed, his or her thoughts regarding the medication, and if it was/is helpful.

Not all patients respond to the same antidepressant medication and there are different categories of antidepressant. The effects of antidepressants do not begin immediately and the patient may have to take them for several weeks before starting to feel the benefit. Similarly, they should not be discontinued immediately as the person begins to feel better, because over the course of days and weeks the medication may leave the person's system and symptoms may return. Patients should be encouraged to discontinue antidepressants with supervision and liaison from their GP or mental health professional. SSRIs and other antidepressants may interact with medications prescribed for chronic physical health problems, and this should be considered and relevant advice sought (NICE, 2009a). Approximately, one-fifth of all people who receive antidepressant medication are troubled by side effects. These are often temporary. After a few weeks, most people have become accustomed to their medication. One way of minimizing the risk of side effects is by gradually raising the dosage (Wasserman, 2011).

For further more detailed information regarding antidepressants, see NICE (2009a, 2009b) and Wasserman (2011).

Selective serotonin reuptake inhibitors (SSRIs)

SSRIs are the first-line pharmacological treatment in NICE Guidelines (NICE, 2009a). They have fewer side effects than other types of antidepressant and the risk of a deliberate overdose being lethal is smaller than with other antidepressant types. The fact that they have fewer side effects on the heart and the digestive system makes SSRIs suitable for long-term preventive treatment of depression, and also in care of the elderly. Another advantage of the SSRIs is their effectiveness against compulsive disorders, panic attacks, and premenstrual syndromes (Wasserman, 2011). SSRIs work on a single receptor. Among the SSRIs available in the UK are fluoxetine, paroxetine, sertraline, and citalopram.

Side effects of SSRIs include sexual dysfunction, insomnia, nausea, diarrhoea, headache, and weight loss. It has also been reported that SSRIs may induce restlessness, disquiet, brooding, and suicidal thoughts in adolescents and young people (Wasserman, 2011). Most side effects are transient and last a short time after starting treatment, but the patient should be advised to seek help if these continue for longer than a few weeks. It should be explained to the patient that it can take several weeks for the medication to reach a therapeutic level and that he or she might not feel an improvement straight away. This can vary from person to person.

Tricyclic and tetracyclic antidepressants (TCAs)

TCAs are also sometimes called the older type of anti-depressant. They have been used in treating depressions since 1950 (Wasserman, 2011). They are well documented to help with long-term and preventive treatment of depression. TCAs benefit severely depressed people. They are also prescribed to treat compulsive disorders. Types of TCA available in the UK are amitriptyline, imipramine, and clomipramine. They are still prescribed and are particularly useful for severe depression.

TCAs cause a range of side effects. They can reduce digestive activity and cause constipation, palpitations, dry mouth and associated dental cavities, urinary retention, and dry membranes, especially in the eyes, and reduced libido. Weight gain, fatigue, sleep problems, dizziness and low blood pressure and reduced attentiveness can also occur. Elderly people may sometimes become confused (Wasserman, 2011). Dietary changes, such as the addition of fibre-rich foods, can assist with digestive problems and constipation As with all medications, if side effects persist, the patient should be encouraged to speak to his or her GP or mental health professional.

Monoamine oxidase inhibitors (MAOIs) and reversible inhibitors of monoamine oxidase (RIMAs)

RIMAs have a much lower likelihood of causing a hypertensive crisis than MAOIs and dietary restrictions are usually not required. Moclobemide is the only RIMA licensed in the UK. MAOI inhibitors are a long-standing group of antidepressants. They are less commonly prescribed since SSRIs have become available due to their side effects and the dietary requirements that they impose upon the patient. However, if other types of antidepressant have been tried unsuccessfully, then MAOIs can be prescribed. As well as treating low mood and depression, MAOIs are used to treat symptoms of anxiety and a number of other symptoms.

The side effects that occur are dizziness, nausea, and insomnia. They may also produce postural hypertension at relatively low doses. An important consideration is that MAOIs have the potential to induce hypertensive crisis if foods containing tyramine are eaten (the so-called 'cheese effect') or drugs that increase monoamine

neurotransmission are co-prescribed. These foods and drugs must be strictly avoided when taking an MAOI, and for at least 14 days after discontinuination.

Serotonin and noradrenaline reuptake inhibitors (SNRIs)

SNRIs are used to treat major depression, especially in cases that fail to respond to selective serotonin reuptake inhibitors (SSRIs). They do not cause many of the side effects of TCAs. At low doses, nausea, sexual disturbances, and insomnia may occur. At higher doses, increased blood pressure has been observed (Wasserman, 2011).

There are other antidepressants available and the reader's attention is drawn to the work of Wasserman (2011) for a brief further reading section and to NICE (2009a) for more specific information.

Electroconvulsive Therapy (ECT)

ECT consists of sending an electric current through the brain to trigger a seizure, or fit, with the aim of relieving severe depression. The treatment is given under a general anaesthetic and uses muscle relaxants, so that the muscles do not contract and the body does not convulse during the fit. ECT is viewed as controversial by some, and exactly why and how it works is not fully understood. It was discovered when it was noted that depressed patients with epilepsy felt better after a seizure in the 1930s. It is a recommended treatment to be considered for depression that is severe and life-threatening, and when a rapid response is required or other evidence-based treatments have failed (NICE, 2009a). It is not used routinely for people with moderate depression, but can be considered if the patient's depression has not responded to multiple treatments. The patient, wherever possible, should be fully informed of the risks and benefits associated with having ECT, including:

- the risks associated with a general anaesthetic;
- medical comorbidities;
- potential adverse events—notably cognitive impairment;
- the risks associated with not receiving ECT.

The decision to use ECT should be made jointly with the patient, if possible, However, treatment may be given under the Mental Health Act 2007.

Evidence-based psychological interventions

There are a number of psychological therapies for depression. NICE (2009a) reviews the evidence of these treatments, as well as medications, and recommends the following as evidence-based psychological therapies that patients with depression should be able to access. Evidence-based psychological interventions are now more widely available than ever before due to government investment in the Increasing Access to Psychological Therapies (IAPT) initiative (Department of Health, 2007; IAPT, 2009). IAPT services use the stepped care model to deliver psychological interventions. This initiative is the single biggest change in the provision of effective treatments for depression in primary and secondary care (NICE, 2009). IAPT services based in primary care should be available within each area of England, and in many areas take self-referrals from the person with low mood or depression, or they can be referred by his or her GP or another healthcare practitioner. Psychological therapies are also often available via secondary and specialist mental health services, and via self-funding treatment from a private practitioner. Care should be taken to ensure that the therapist is appropriately accredited or registered to provide the treatment and receives supervision.

Cognitive behavioural therapy (CBT)

Cognitive behavioural therapy (CBT) is the psychological treatment of choice for depression due to its large evidence base. It is a short-term active form of therapy based in the here and now. CBT looks at the patterns in how a person feels, and his or her thinking, physical symptoms, and behaviours. Patients are given work to complete between sessions (homework) and the aim of CBT is to break into the 'vicious cycle' of depressed mood by working on either negative thinking or avoided activities, or a combination of these. CBT can be delivered in face-to-face sessions or by using telephone contact and the use of guided CBT self-help materials.

At present, registered nurses can undertake further post-qualification training in CBT and it is anticipated that elements of basic CBT training may be delivered to pre-registration nurses in the future. Some self-help strategies outlining the condition using a CBT approach may be a useful addition to the area in which the adult nurse works to support his or her role. There are some excellent

resources on CBT outlined at the end of the chapter on pages 138–39 pages 138–39 and we suggest that you access these if you want further information or are interested in learning more about these approaches.

There is also useful information regarding CBT as a treatment for depression on the Improving Access to Psychological Therapies (Department of Health) website **http://www.iapt.nhs.uk/workforce/high-intensity/** or from the British Association of Behavioural and Cognitive Psychotherapy (BABCP) **www.babcp.com.**

Behavioural activation

Behavioural activation is often seen as a treatment under the CBT family umbrella, but which uses a purely behavioural approach to treat depressed mood. It is not a first step in CBT, but rather an effective treatment in its own right (Richards, 2010) and is recommended in NICE Guidelines for Depression (2009a). Behavioural activation is as effective as CBT and more effective than other psychological therapies (Richards, 2010). It is said to be a treatment in which it is easy to train practitioners to use to support patients. Behavioural activation is based upon the role of avoided behaviours in depression and how, when depressed, a patient's avoidance of activities as a coping strategy gives symptom relief in the short term and so is negatively reinforced. In further avoiding activities, the patient is, however, removed from activities that give positive reinforcement and mood can deteriorate further. The activities to which a patient is supported to return are routine, necessary, and pleasurable activities in a graded way (Richards *et al.* 2010). For a useful guide to behavioural activation, see Lovell and Richards (2008) available online at **www.rethink.org/document.rm?id=6617.**

Interpersonal therapy (IPT)

Interpersonal therapy (IPT) focuses on current relationships and interpersonal processes. It is time-limited, and focused on difficulties arising in the daily experience of maintaining relationships and resolving difficulties during an episode of major depression (NICE, 2009a). The patient and therapist agree to work on a particular focal area selected from the following: interpersonal role transitions; interpersonal roles/conflicts; grief; and/or interpersonal deficits. IPT is therefore appropriate when a person has a key area of difficulty that is specified by the treatment (for example, grief or interpersonal conflicts). The main aims of the therapy are to help patients to make links between their moods and their interpersonal contacts and to recognize that, by appropriately addressing interpersonal situations, they may simultaneously improve both their relationships and their depressive state. Further reading on IPT can also be found on the IAPT website, which is owned by the Department of Health **http://www. iapt.nhs.uk/workforce/high-intensity/interpersonal-psychotherapy-for-depression/** and in the NICE Guideline for Depression (NICE, 2009a), or from IPT-UK **www. interpersonalpsychotherapy.org.uk.**

Behavioural couples therapy

Behavioural couples therapy for depression aims to help couples to understand the ways in which difficulties in their relationship can contribute to depression, in one (or sometimes both) partners. Couples can find it hard to talk openly and honestly with each other about depression, and so meeting with a couples therapist aims to help the couple with better communication. Behavioural couples therapy is indicated for people who have a regular partner and whose relationship may contribute to the development or maintenance of depression, or in cases in which involving the partner is considered to be of potential therapeutic benefit. Behavioural couples therapy for depression should normally be based on behavioural principles, and an adequate course of therapy should be 15–20 sessions over 5–6 months. Further information regarding behavioural couples therapy can be found at **http://www.iapt. nhs.uk/workforce/high-intensity/couple-therapy-for-depression/**.

For people with depression who decline an antidepressant, CBT, IPT, behavioural activation, and behavioural couples therapy, NICE (2009a) recommends considering counselling for people with persistent subthreshold depressive symptoms or mild to moderate depression, or short-term psychodynamic interpersonal psychotherapy (DIT) for people with mild to moderate depression.

Counselling for depression

Counselling can be defined as 'a systematic process which gives individuals an opportunity to explore, discover and clarify ways of living more resourcefully, with

a greater sense of well-being' (NICE, 2009a). Counselling has been a widely used treatment for depression over the years, particularly in primary care over the past decade. Counselling has many different forms, but involves talking through difficulties with the counsellor in a non-directive way. It usually comprises 6–10 sessions over 8–2 weeks (NICE, 2009). Its effects are not currently well supported in research and therefore NICE recommends that counselling for depression should be offered if the patient has not benefited from medication or other psychological therapies, or if he or she declines these other therapies. Treatment should be short term and the uncertainty of the effectiveness of the therapy should be discussed with the patient (NICE, 2009a). Useful information on counselling for depression can be found online at **http://www. iapt.nhs.uk/workforce/high-intensity/counselling-for-depression/** and in the NICE Guideline for Depression (NICE, 2009a), or from the British Association of Counselling (BACP) **www.bacp.co.uk.**

Short-term dynamic psychotherapy: brief dynamic interpersonal therapy (DIT)

DIT is a form of brief psychodynamic psychotherapy developed for treating depression. It is a time-limited (16 sessions) psychodynamic intervention. DIT assumes that: behaviour is unconsciously determined; internal and external influences shape thoughts and feelings, and therefore inform our perceptions of ourselves in relationships with others; adult interpersonal strategies and ways of relating are generated by childhood experience, particularly within the family; unconscious processes, including defences and identifications (projective and introjective processes), underpin the subjective experience of relationships; and thinking about behaviour and emotional experience in terms of mental states has significant therapeutic effects. The therapy focuses on the patient's current relationships, including the relationship with the therapist. It can help people with emotional and relationship problems. It explores difficult things in the past that continue to affect the way people feel and behave in the present. It is also referred to as 'psychoanalytic psychotherapy'. Like counselling, currently its effects are not well supported in research, so other evidence-based therapies should be offered first and the uncertainty of the treatment should be

CASE STUDY 8.2 *John*

John is a 45-year-old man under the care of a practice nurse for his angina. He reports that he has been feeling increasingly down since his wife left him for another man 6 months ago. He has also changed jobs and had to find a new house to rent, because he could not afford the rent on the property he had shared with his wife by himself. John has two children from a previous relationship who live abroad in Australia with their mother and her current partner. He does not see them as often as he would like–usually only once per year, although on some years this has proved difficult because the costs of flights have been prohibitive. He has been to his GP on three separate occasions complaining of headaches and difficulty sleeping, with various aches and pains. On his last visit the GP completed with John a measure of depression called a Patient Health Questionnaire 9 (PHQ-9). On this measure, he scored 12, which is indicative of moderate depression.

Questions

➤ What would be an evidence-based pharmacological treatment option for John's depression and why?

➤ What would be an evidence-based psychological treatment option for John's depression and why?

➤ What routine screening questions recommended by NICE (2009a) would you ask John?

➤ What useful information might the practice nurse be able to give to John about depression or treatment options?

➤ What actual losses can you identify in the case study?

➤ What perceived losses can you identify in the case study?

➤ What 'vicious cycles' are evidenced that may be maintaining his problems?

John's difficulties can be illustrated as in Figure 8.4.

---

discussed with the patient (NICE, 2009a). Further information on DIT is available at **http://www.iapt.nhs.uk/ workforce/high-intensity/brief-dynamic-interpersonal-therapy-dit/or** in the NICE Guideline for Depression (NICE, 2009a).

Identifying best practice

Throughout the text, you will find recent sources of the best evidence to inform the nursing care of patients with depression. Because research is always ongoing and best practice evolves, it is important that readers stay up to date and know where to find good-quality sources of evidence. Hence we have provided a list of resources below that readers should utilize.

• NICE guidance CG90. Depression in adults. **http:// guidance.nice.org.uk/CG90**

• NICE guidance CG91. Depression with a chronic physical health problem. **http://guidance.nice.org.uk/ CG91**

Sources of evidence

Organizations

British Association of Behavioural and Cognitive Psychotherapy (BABCP) **www.babcp.com**

British Association of Counselling and Psychotherapy (BACP) **www.bacp.co.uk**

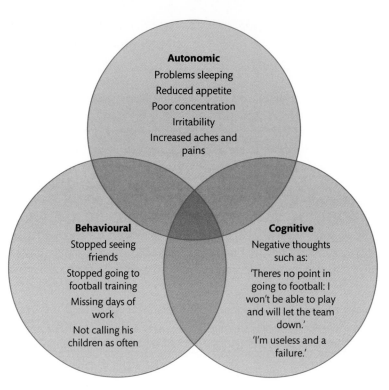

Figure 8.4   John's difficulties.

Department of Health Improving Access to Psychological Therapies Programme **www.iapt.nhs.uk**
Royal College of Psychiatry
MIND
National Institute for Health and Clinical Excellence (NICE) **http://guidance.nice.org.uk/**
The Scottish Intercollegiate Guidelines Network (SIGN) **http://www.sign.ac.uk/guidelines/index.html**
NHS Evidence **http://www.evidence.nhs.uk/**

Journals

American Journal of Psychiatry
British Journal of Psychiatry
British Medical Journal
Evidence Based Mental Health
Journal of Clinical Psychiatry
Journal of Psychiatric Research
The Lancet

Useful resources for depression

Lovell, K., Richards, D. (2008) A Recovery Programme for Depression. Rethink **www.rethink.org/document.rm?id=6617**

This CBT self-help guide uses behavioural activation and CBT techniques, and is a valuable resource for patients with depression. It explains the CBT model in a user-friendly format, and is widely used within the IAPT programme in the UK. It can be purchased at low cost or worksheets downloaded for free as pdf files.

Northumberland Self Help Guides, **http://www.ntw.nhs.uk/pic/selfhelp**

The Northumberland CBT self-help guides provide a good overview of CBT and its approaches to depression.

Royal College of Psychiatry Depression Leaflet **http://www.rcpsych.ac.uk/mentalhealthinformation/mentalhealthproblems/depression/depression.aspx**

An excellent free information sheet about depression, available in a number of languages.

Royal College of Psychiatry Cognitive Behavioural Therapy Leaflet **http://www.rcpsych.ac.uk/mentalhealthinfoforall/treatments/cbt.aspx**

An excellent information sheet about CBT, available in a number of languages.

Williams, C., Chellingsworth, M. (2010) *A Clinician's Guide to CBT: The Five Areas Model*. Hodder Arnold: London.
A clinician's guide for health practitioners wanting to learn more about CBT self-help techniques, and how to integrate these into their practice and support patients to use them.

Williams, C. (2009) *Overcoming Depression and Low Mood: A Five Areas Approach*. Hodder Arnold: London.
A patient modular CBT self-help book that has won several awards.

Conclusion

As a practising adult nurse, you have a responsibility to have a theoretical and practical understanding of depression and its effects. This includes knowledge of evidence-based treatment options, both pharmacological and psychological. Knowledge of appropriate referral pathways, and also of common side effects of medications, is important. Using the ABC approach is a structured and useful approach to recognizing and assessing a person's mood, and being able to consider appropri-

ate interventions. Often, the responsibility of the adult nurse, particularly student nurses, will be to consult with relevant colleagues about assessment and management issues in depression after recognizing symptoms consistent with depressed mood in a patient, or after asking the two recommended screening questions (NICE, 2009). There are a number of useful evidence-based resources that are available to assist you in delivering best practice for people with depression.

Online Resource Centre

 To help you to develop and apply your knowledge and decision-making skills further, we have provided interactive learning resources online at **www.oxfordtextbooks.co.uk/orc/bullock/**

Whilst these are freely available, you will need to use the access codes at the start of the book.

References

American Psychiatric Association (2000) *Diagnostic and Statistical Manual of Mental Disorders*, 4th edn, text revision, DSM-IV-TR. American Psychiatric Association: Washington, DC.

Beck, A.T. (1976) *Cognitive Therapy and the Emotional Disorders*. Penguin Group: London.

Brampton, S. (2008) *Shoot the Damn Dog: A Memoir of Depression*. Bloomsbury Publishing: London.

Cassano, P., Fava, M. (2002) Depression and public health: an overview. *Journal of Psychosomatic Research* **53**: 849–57.

Department of Health (2007) *Improving Access to Psychological Therapies: Specification for the Commissioner-Led Pathfinder Programme*. Department of Health: London.

Farrand, P., Ritterband, L., Bennett-Levy, J. (2010) Introducing and Supporting guided CBT. In J. Bennett-Levy, H. Christensen, P. Farrand *et al.* (eds) *The Oxford Guide to Low Intensity CBT Interventions*. Oxford University Press: Oxford, pp. 87–9.

Goodwin, G. (2004) Mood disorder. In E. Johnstone, D.G. Cunningham-Owens, S.M. Lawrie *et al.* (eds) *Companion to Psychiatric Studies*, 7th edn. Churchill Livingstone: London, pp.

Increasing Access to Psychological Therapies (IAPT) (2009) IAPT *Workforce Capacity Tool: Guidance for Use*. http://www.iapt.nhs.uk/2008/01/17/workforce-capacity-tool/.

Kessler, R.C., Berglund, P., Demler, O., *et al.* (2003) The epidemiology of major depressive disorder: results from the National Comorbidity Survey Replication (NCS-R). *Journal of the American Medical Association* **289**: 3095–105.

Kovacs, M. (1996) Presentation and course of major depressive disorder during childhood and later years of the life span. *Journal of the American Academy of Child and Adolescent Psychiatry* **35**: 705–15.

Layard, R. (2006) *The Depression Report.* London School of Economics: London.

Lewinsohn, P.M., Solomon, A., Seeley, J.R., *et al.* (2000) Clinical implications of 'subthreshold' depressive symptoms. *Journal of Abnormal Psychology* **109**: 345–51.

McGuffin, P., Katz, R., Watkins, S., *et al.* (1996) A hospital based twin register of the heritability of DSM-IV unipolar depression. *Archives of General Psychiatry* **53**:129-36.

Mitchell, A.J., Vaze, A., Rao, S. (2009) Clinical diagnosis of depression in primary care: a meta-analysis. *Lancet* **374**: 609–19.

National Institute for Clinical Excellence (NICE) (2009a) *Depression in Adults (update): Depression the Treatment and Management of Depression in Adults.* NICE: London.

National Institute for Clinical Excellence (NICE) (2009b) *Depression in Adults with a Chronic Physical Health Problem: Treatment and Management.* NICE: London.

Office of National Statistics (2010) *Suicide rates in the UK 2000–09.* http://www.statistics.gov.uk/pdfdir/sui0111.pdf (accessed 1 December 2011).

Richards, D. (2010) Behavioural activation. In J. Bennett-Levy, H. Christensen, P. Farrand *et al.* (eds) *The Oxford Guide to Low Intensity CBT Interventions.* Oxford University Press: Oxford, pp. 141–50.

Richards, D., Whyte, M. (2009) *Reach Out: National Programme Student Materials to Support the Delivery of Training for Practitioners Delivering Low Intensity Interventions.* Rethink: London.

Scott, K.M., Bruffaerts, R., Simon, G.E., *et al.* (2007) Obesity and mental disorders in the general population: results from the World Mental Health Surveys. *International Journal of Obesity* **32**: 192–200.

Simon, G.E., Savarino, J. (2007) Suicide attempts among patients starting depression treatment with medications or psychotherapy. *American Journal of Psychiatry* **164**: 1029–34.

Wasserman, D. (2011) *Depression:The Facts*, 2nd edn. Oxford University Press: Oxford.

Williams, C., Chellingsworth, M. (2010) *A Clinician's Guide to CBT: The Five Areas Model.* Hodder Arnold: London.

Williams, Jr, J.W., Kerber, C.A., Mulrow, C.D., *et al.* (1995) Depressive disorders in primary care: prevalence, functional disability, and identification. *Journal of General Internal Medicine* **10**: 7–12.

Zimmerman, M., McGlinchey, J.B., Posternak, M.A., *et al.* (2008) Remission in depressed outpatients: more than just symptom resolution? *Journal of Psychiatric Research* **42**: 797–801.

9 *Understanding* Diabetes Mellitus

Anne Phillips and Roger Gadsby

> ## Introduction
>
> The aim of this chapter is to provide nurses with the knowledge to be able to assess, manage, and care for people with type 1 and type 2 diabetes mellitus in an evidence-based and person-centred way. Diabetes mellitus is a long-term condition that can affect people of all ages; consequently, people with diabetes mellitus can be found in every healthcare environment, from hospitals to care homes. The chapter will provide a comprehensive overview of the classifications, causes, and risk factors of diabetes. The key principles of patient assessment are established, before exploring best practice to deliver care, prevent acute complications, and minimize long-term complications. Nursing assessments and priorities are highlighted throughout, and the nursing management of the symptoms and common health problems associated with diabetes can be found in **Chapters 19, 22, 24, 25, 26,** and **28,** respectively ⟶.

Understanding diabetes mellitus

Definitions

Diabetes mellitus is a group of metabolic conditions with **hyperglycaemia** occurring as the main feature. It is characterized by chronic increased blood glucose (hyperglycaemia), with disturbance of carbohydrate, protein, and fat metabolism, which results from defects in **insulin secretion**, insulin action, or both (World Health Organization (WHO), 1999). The hormone **insulin**, produced by the **beta cells** in the pancreas, controls blood glucose levels,

keeping them within a narrow range in normal health (4–6 mmol/l before food). When blood glucose levels rise (for example, after a meal containing carbohydrates has been consumed), glucose enters the beta cells, eventually resulting in the release of insulin into the portal circulation.

Classifications of type 1 and 2

The classifications of diabetes mellitus (World Health Organization, 2006) are as follows.

- Type 1 diabetes mellitus, previously known as insulin-dependent diabetes mellitus (IDDM)
- Type 2 diabetes mellitus, previously known as non-insulin-dependent diabetes mellitus (NIDDM)
- Gestational diabetes mellitus
- Others, such as disorders affecting the pancreas, and endocrine conditions

The features of type 1 and type 2 diabetes mellitus are outlined in Table 9.1.

Table 9.1 Features of type 1 and type 2 diabetes mellitus

Type 1 diabetes mellitus	Type 2 diabetes mellitus
Beta cells are destroyed, leading to loss of insulin production; this may be **idiopathic** by nature or resulting from an immune response	Characterized by problems with the secretion and/or action of insulin (insulin resistance)
An infectious or environmental stimulus is the possible trigger to this **autoimmune** response; markers of autoimmunity are usually present	A progressive condition that may eventually lead to beta cell exhaustion; markers of autoimmunity not usually present
Usual absence of **C peptide**	C peptide usually detectable
Onset usually in children and young adults, but may occur in older people; if this is the case, then always consider an organic cause	Onset usually in middle-aged and older people, but occurs earlier in some ethnic groups; with growing levels of obesity, it is now occurring in young people

Gestational diabetes mellitus

Gestational diabetes is carbohydrate intolerance, resulting in hyperglycaemia with onset or recognition during pregnancy (World Health Organization, 2006). However, the condition may have been present prior to pregnancy, but not been diagnosed.

Other forms

Diabetes mellitus may occur for other reasons, including genetic defects and diseases affecting the pancreas. It can be induced by some drugs (e.g. corticosteroids and thiazide diuretics) that may not cause diabetes, but may make individuals more susceptible to developing the condition. Finally, there are endocrine disorders that oppose the action of insulin.

Prevalence and epidemiological profile

There is an epidemic of type 2 diabetes worldwide. The number of people with diabetes in the world was expected to double over the 13-year period from 1997 to 2010 to a total of 221 million people, with prevalence rates expected to rise by 111% in Asia, 93% in Africa, and 51% in Europe. Further increases in the prevalence rate are predicted up to 2030, when the worldwide prevalence of diabetes is expected to be 7.8%, with 438 million people in the world with diabetes (Diabetes Atlas, 2009).

The latest figures suggest that there are currently about 2.8 million people with diabetes in the UK, a prevalence rate of 4.26%. In 2006, the figures were 2.2 million and 3.54%, respectively, highlighting that the epidemic is being seen in the UK as well (Diabetes UK, 2010).

Some key facts and figures about diabetes are as follows.

- Diabetes is the fifth commonest cause of death in the world (Roglic *et al.*, 2005).
- There is increased cardiac mortality after myocardial infarction in people with type 2 diabetes (Capes *et al.*, 2000).
- There are improved patient outcomes when glycaemia is well controlled during a hospital admission (Bruno *et al.*, 2008).
- Life expectancy is reduced for people with diabetes mellitus.
- 'Healthcare systems world-wide are faced with the challenge of responding to the needs of people with chronic medical conditions such as diabetes mellitus.' (World Health Organization, 2002)

THEORY INTO PRACTICE 9.1
Putting theory into practice

What is the prevalence of diabetes mellitus within your client group or where you live?

The pathophysiology of diabetes mellitus

The pancreas is a gland found in the abdominal cavity adjacent to the small intestines (Figure 9.1). The pancreas has several functions (endocrine and exocrine), with the

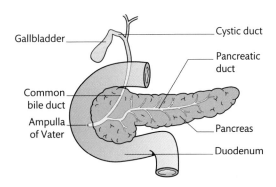

Figure 9.1 The pancreas.

©EMIS 2011 as distributed at **http://www.patient.co.uk/diagram/Pancreas.htm.** Reproduced with permission.

normally functioning pancreas synthesizing and secreting insulin from the beta cells, which are found in the islets of Langerhans.

Insulin is a polypeptide made up of 51 amino acids, which are arranged in two chains and linked by bridges. Insulin acts like a key, allowing the glucose from the bloodstream to enter the cells, where it is utilized to make energy. In normal health, blood glucose levels are maintained within a tight range because there is a balance between glucose entering the bloodstream from the liver and after intestinal absorption (post meals) and glucose uptake into the peripheral tissues (muscles).

Diabetes mellitus occurs when the body fails to control blood glucose levels and levels of blood glucose rise. In type 1 diabetes mellitus, there is a complete destruction of insulin-producing beta cells in the pancreas and hence an absolute deficiency of insulin. Unless insulin is given to a person with type 1 diabetes, he or she will die.

In type 2 diabetes mellitus, there is tissue resistance to the effects of insulin, which is called insulin resistance. The pancreas initially copes with this by producing more insulin. However, there comes a time when the pancreas can no longer produce the amount of insulin needed to overcome this insulin resistance (this is called beta cell dysfunction), and type 2 diabetes ensues.

Causes

The following outlines the risk factors for developing type 2 diabetes mellitus.

- Those with a family history of type 2 diabetes mellitus
- Obesity, particularly central adiposity, which increases the risk of insulin resistance. The waist circumference can be measured by the healthcare professional and used in conjunction with the individual's weight and body mass index to predict those at risk of developing type 2 diabetes mellitus. A waist cirumference over 102 cm for Caucasian men and over 88 cm for Caucasian women is a risk factor for type 2 diabetes (Gautier *et al.*, 2010)—adjustments may need to be made for other ethnic groups; for example, WHO suggests a waist circumference over 90 cm for Asian men.
- Individuals with any degree of impaired glucose regulation
- Increasing incidence with age
- Prevalence in some ethnic groups
- Women who have had gestational diabetes or have given birth to babies weighing 4.5 kg or above

Identifying patients at risk (pre-diabetes mellitus)

Type 1 diabetes mellitus develops suddenly, so there is no prodromal phase (early symptom[s]) in which screening can detect people developing the condition.

Type 2 diabetes mellitus may have a long prodromal phase, in which levels of blood glucose rise above the normal levels seen in healthy people, but do not reach the levels diagnostic of diabetes. If glucose levels are being measured after fasting, this intermediate phase between normal and diabetes is called impaired fasting glucose (IFG). If glucose levels are being measured after a glucose load (in an oral glucose tolerance test), it is called impaired glucose tolerance (IGT). Either of these conditions can progress to type 2 diabetes mellitus. If body weight is lost, blood glucose levels may return to normal.

There is good evidence to suggest that individuals who demonstrate abnormal glucose tolerance can reduce their risk of developing type 2 diabetes mellitus by adopting a healthy lifestyle, for example losing weight if overweight and following a healthy diet (Diabetes Prevention Programme, 2002; Tuomilehto *et al.*, 2002).

Healthcare costs to treat long-term conditions are increasing worldwide, therefore more emphasis needs to be made to prevent or delay individuals developing type 2 diabetes mellitus. A national diabetes screening programme does not currently exist in the UK, but targeting opportunistic screening of individuals at increased risk of developing type 2 diabetes mellitus in primary care is being carried out in some general practices.

Assessing the patient

The signs and symptoms of type 1 and type 2 diabetes mellitus are summarized in Table 9.2, as well as Figures 9.2 and 9.3.

Diagnosis

Diabetes mellitus is definitively diagnosed by measuring blood glucose levels. The blood glucose values for the diagnosis of diabetes mellitus have been determined by the level at which **retinopathy** develops. Table 9.3 gives the World Health Organization guidelines for the diagnosis of diabetes mellitus.

In the presence of symptoms of diabetes mellitus, the following guidelines apply.

- A single random venous plasma glucose equal to or >11.1 mmol/l
- Fasting venous plasma glucose equal to or >7.0 mmol/l
- A 2-hour post glucose load of equal to or >11.1 mmol/l

Table 9.2 The signs and symptoms of type 1 and type 2 diabetes mellitus

Type 1	Type 2
Sudden onset	Slow onset
Severe **polyuria, nocturia,** and thirst; child may start wetting the bed again	May have no or few symptoms; could present with nocturia and possible incontinence in the older person
Recent history of weight loss, which can be very severe	Weight loss not usual
Spontaneous **ketosis** (urinalysis ketones +++)	Ketones not usually present in the urine
Feeling unwell	Blurred vision Problems may be detected on routine examination by the optician
May present with suspected appendicitis owing to abdominal pains, which are caused by the presence of ketones	May present with another condition

In the absence of symptoms of diabetes mellitus, the following applies.

- At least two elevated glucose recordings must be taken on different days before a diagnosis is made.
- The oral glucose tolerance test remains the 'gold standard' test to diagnose diabetes mellitus; this is when the individual is given a glucose load and blood samples are taken 2 hours after its consumption. Different amounts of glucose may be used for this test in different parts of the world. In the UK, a 75 g glucose load is used.
- There is some evidence to suggest that an **HbA1c** level of 5.5–6% (37–42 mmol/mol) increases the risk of developing type 2 diabetes mellitus (Zhang *et al.*, 2010).
- In future, an HbA1c may be used as a test to diagnose diabetes mellitus.

In the UK, there are national targets for the assessment and management of people with diabetes mellitus. These are summarized in Table 9.4, which includes references to source information.

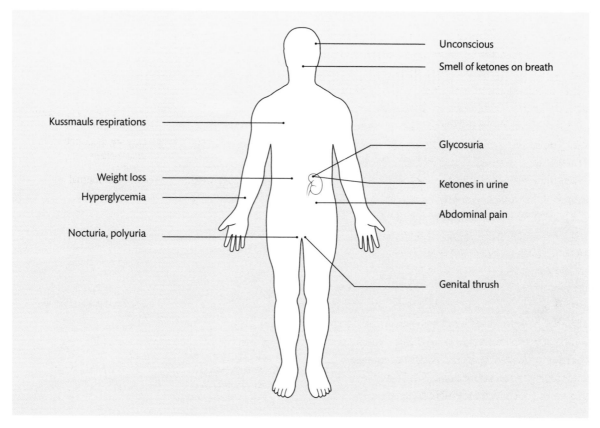

Figure 9.2 Common signs and symptoms of type 1 diabetes.

Table 9.3 Diagnosis of diabetes mellitus

Diabetes	Venous plasma concentrations
Fasting values	≥ 7 mmol/l
2-hour post glucose load	≥11.1 mmol/l
Impaired glucose tolerance 2-hour post glucose load	>7.8 mmol/l
Impaired fasting glucose Fasting	≥6.1 mmol/l, but <7.0 mmol/l

Source: (World Health Organization 2006)

THEORY INTO PRACTICE 9.2
Guidelines

How do guidelines affect the care and treatment received by patients in your clinical area?

Nursing interventions

Type 1 diabetes mellitus

The only treatment option for people with type 1 diabetes mellitus is insulin therapy, with the aim of treatment to achieve normal glycaemia to reduce the risk of the development of acute and long-term complications (DCCT, 1993). Insulin enables glucose to be transported into the cell and lowers blood glucose by suppressing glucose output from the liver. Nurses therefore have a key role to play in monitoring an individual's blood glucose levels and administering appropriate amounts of prescribed insulin. Insulin has to be administered by subcutaneous injections, either by an insulin syringe or an insulin pen device. Continuous subcutaneous insulin infusion (insulin pumps) is also available for some individuals who meet the criteria recommended by the National Institute for Health and Clinical Excellence (NICE) (2008a). Problems with insulin prescribing on hospital wards have been a specific concern. As a result, an Internet-based programme

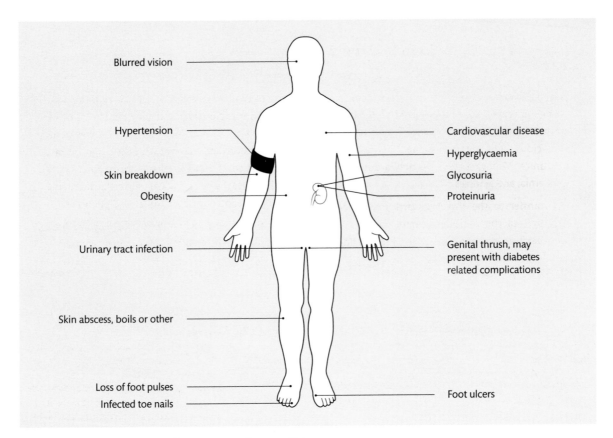

Figure 9.3 **Common signs and symptoms of type 2 diabetes.**

Table 9.4 **National treatment targets for diabetes in the UK**

Measurements	Quality and Outcomes Framework (QOF) (2011), people with diabetes mellitus	National Institute for Health and Clinical Excellence (NICE) (2009), people with type 2 diabetes mellitus
HbA1c	At or below 7.5% (58 mmol/mol)	At or below 6.5% (48 mmol/mol) on lifestyle plus 1 or 2 oral agents At or below 7.5% (58 mmol/mol) on two or more agents
Cholesterol	At or below total cholesterol 5 mmol/l	At or below total cholesterol 4 mmol/l with LDL-C of 2 mmol/l or less in those at high risk (positive microalbuminuria and or strong family history of cerebrovascular disease)
Blood pressure	At or below 140/80	At or below 140/80, but, in those with evidence of end-stage organ damage, 130/80

on the safer administration of insulin has been launched by NHS Diabetes and the National Patient Safety Agency (NHS Diabetes, 2010).

Practising nurses also have a role in encouraging individuals to adopt a healthy lifestyle and to maintain a normal body weight. Individuals with type 1 diabetes will then need to receive appropriate support and education from the multidisciplinary diabetes team to help them to develop the necessary skills to self-manage their condition.

CASE STUDY 9.1 *Joe: 19 years old*

Joe is a university student and is found unconscious by his flatmates. He is transferred to hospital by ambulance and found to be suffering from diabetic ketoacidosis. Emergency treatment in the intensive care unit for 2 days corrects his dehydration, hyperglycaemia, and acidosis.

On transfer to the medical ward, he is seen by members of the multidisciplinary diabetes team who begin the process of helping Joe to adapt to life with type 1 diabetes mellitus. He requires a lot of support at this time, not only coping with the practicalities of managing diabetes on a daily basis, but also in coming to terms with the diagnosis of a long-term condition. Joe will require ongoing social, psychological, and practical support, including monitoring and education from the diabetes team.

What would you include in a care plan for Joe's adaptation to the diagnosis of diabetes mellitus?

Table 9.5 Insulin regimens used in the treatment of type 1 and type 2 diabetes

Insulin regimen	Uses	Advantages	Disadvantages
Once-daily isophane	May be used for individuals with type 2 requiring insulin therapy	Very simple as only one injection daily	Does not control blood glucose levels after meals have been consumed. May not last full 24 hours
Once-daily isophane and oral hypoglycaemic agents	May be used for individuals with type 2 requiring insulin therapy	Very simple as only one injection daily	Useful when oral hypoglycaemic agents not controlling blood glucose levels in individuals with type 2
Twice-daily isophane	May be used for individuals with type 2 requiring insulin therapy Occasionally for individuals with type 1	A simple twice-daily regimen	Does not control blood glucose levels after meals have been consumed
Once-daily long-acting analogue	May be used as basal insulin for people with either type 1 or type 2	Provides background insulin	Does not control blood glucose levels after meals have been consumed
Once-daily long-acting analogue or isophane with short- or rapid-acting insulin before each main meal	Used as basal bolus regimen for people with either type 1 or type 2	Provides background insulin and short- or rapid-acting insulin before or with each main meal Tries to mimic physiological insulin production	At least four injections daily
Short- or rapid-acting insulin with main meals given via subcutaneous injection	May be used for people with type 2 requiring insulin therapy	Offers some flexibility	Poor control of overnight blood glucose levels and between main meals
Short- or rapid-acting insulin in continuous subcutaneous insulin infusion	Usually used for individuals with type 1	Tries to mimic physiological insulin production Offers flexibility	Requires education and support of individual

Dose adjustment for normal eating (DAFNE) is a structured programme that helps individuals to problem-solve and manage their own diabetes on a daily basis (Amiel *et al.*, 2002).

Type 2 diabetes mellitus

Education and lifestyle

Individuals should be encouraged to develop a healthy lifestyle, taking regular physical activity, eating a well-balanced diet, and, if overweight, actively trying to lose weight.

People with type 2 diabetes mellitus are encouraged to receive appropriate group education to help them to manage their condition, and a number of such structured education programmes exist. The two that are most well known are 'DESMOND'—Diabetes education, self management for ongoing and newly diagnosed (Davies *et al.*, 2008)—and the X-pert programme (Deakin *et al.*, 2006). Both programmes are well evaluated and evidence-based.

Glucose-lowering medication for type 2 diabetes mellitus

The aim of treatment is to achieve normal glycaemia whilst minimizing the risk of inducing hypoglycaemia or weight gain. Type 2 diabetes mellitus is a progressive condition and therefore a stepwise approach needs to be taken as treatment options change over time. Details of medications used to treat type 2 diabetes mellitus are given in Table 9.6.

Using oral glucose-lowering therapies

Initial monotherapy

All of the glucose-lowering medications shown in Table 9.6 (apart from acarbose, which is less effective) lower HbA1c by a similar amount (Sherifa *et al.*, 2010). The use of individual therapies is therefore based on parameters of cost and side effects. Nurses have a key role to play in monitoring side effects as part of the assessment process.

All diabetes guidelines recommend that metformin should be the initial therapy of choice in the vast majority of people with type 2 diabetes. This is because it is cheap and weight-neutral, does not cause **hypoglycaemia**, and there is evidence that it protects against cardiovascular ischaemic risk (United Kingdom Prospective Diabetes Study UKPDS 34, 1998). It should not be used in hepatic impairment, renal impairment, ketoacidosis, heart failure, and severe dehydration.

Dual therapy

At the point at which that treatment with lifestyle modification followed by full dose metformin therapy is insufficient to optimize glycaemic control, the National Institute for Health and Clinical Excellence guideline (NICE, 2009) recommends the addition of

Table 9.6 Oral medications for type 2 diabetes mellitus: how they work and common side effects

Drug class	Action of drug	Names of drugs	Common side effects
Biguanides	Decreases hepatic **gluconeogenesis** and also increases peripheral glucose uptake	Metformin Also slow-release formula available	Gastrointestinal side effects
Sulfonylureas	Stimulates beta cells in the pancreas to release insulin	Gliclazide, tolbutamide, glimepiride, glibenclamide	Can cause hypoglycaemia
Alpha glucosidase inhibitors	Delays the absorption of glucose	Acarbose	Gastrointestinal side effects
Glitazones	Helps make the cells more sensitive to insulin	Pioglitazone	Weight gain, use restricted in individuals with heart conditions
DPP-4 inhibitors	Inhibits the breakdown of glucagon-like peptide-1 (GLP-1)	Sitagliptin, vildagliptin, saxagliptin	Gastrointestinal side effects Upper respiratory tract infection and nasopharyngitis

a sulfonylurea agent. The reasons for this include that this group is cheap, and that it acts quickly and effectively to lower blood glucose. The main side effect is hypoglycaemia and, where this is deemed to be a significant risk, NICE (2009) recommends that either pioglitazone or a DPP-4 agent be used instead of the sulfonylurea.

Triple therapy

Once metformin and sulfonylurea dual therapy at maximally tolerated doses is not sufficient for optimal control, other options are available. In the UK, these options include:

1. Add pioglitazone in a 'triple oral therapy' combination
2. Add a DPP-4 inhibitor in a 'triple oral therapy' combination
3. Add insulin, usually by continuing oral agents and adding once-daily long-acting insulin
4. Add an injection of a GLP-1 agonist

Glucagon-like peptide (GLP-1) agonists

Gut hormones known as incretins (GLP-1, glucose-dependent insulinotropic polypeptide; GIP) are produced when food is ingested; they are responsible for increasing insulin secretion as blood glucose levels rise, suppressing glucagon secretion and inducing feelings of satiety in the individual. The hormones are rapidly destroyed by the dipeptidyl peptidase 4 (DPP-4) enzyme found in the gut. The GLP-1 axis is impaired in people with type 2 diabetes mellitus and treatments have now been developed to increase the action of these hormones. This can be done by inhibiting its breakdown using DPP-4 inhibitor agents or by giving a GLP-1-like substance that is not easily broken down by DPP-4.

These agents are called GLP-1 agonists and two are currently available: exenatide, which is given by injection twice a day (or as a once-weekly depot injection); and liraglutide, given by injection once a day. They lower HbA1c by a similar amount to other agents, but are the first glucose-lowering agents to cause weight loss. They are expensive and are therefore recommended for use only as a third line of treatment in people who are significantly obese (NICE, 2009).

Insulin therapy

Insulin therapy may need to be initiated for individuals when blood glucose levels can no longer be controlled

and may be used with some oral hypoglycaemic agents. The National Institute for Health and Clinical Excellence (NICE) 2009 recommends that this can usually be done by adding once-daily long-acting insulin. Table 9.5 gives information on insulin regimens for type 1 and type 2 diabetes mellitus.

Medication for managing cardiovascular risk factors

People with type 2 diabetes mellitus often have several cardiovascular (CVD) risk factors: for example, hyperlipidaemia and hypertension, which increase the likelihood of a heart attack or stroke (see Chapters 6 and 13 ➡). These CVD risk factors require active treatment with statin therapy to lower cholesterol and with agents to lower blood pressure. The National Institute for Health and Clinical Excellence Clinical Guideline 66 (NICE, 2008b) recommends that most people with type 2 diabetes should initially be offered simvastatin (40 mg daily) to manage hyperlipidaemia, and that the initial blood-pressure-lowering therapy should be an angiotensin-converting enzyme (ACE) inhibitor.

Because medication management is such a critical clinical intervention for people with diabetes mellitus, you are encouraged to refer to Chapter 22 ➡ for additional information and advice.

Identifying deterioration and acute complications

There are three potential acute complications in people with diabetes mellitus:

- hypoglycaemia (type 1 and 2);
- diabetic ketoacidosis (type 1);
- hyperosmolar hyperglycaemic state (type 2), previously known as HONK.

Hypoglycaemia

In normal health, as blood glucose levels begin to fall, insulin secretion is suppressed and the counter-regulatory hormones are released, so hypoglycaemia does not occur. In people with diabetes taking insulin and/or sulfonylurea therapy, these medications may lower blood glucose levels too much and precipitate hypoglycaemia symptoms.

In diabetes mellitus, the severity of a hypoglycaemic event is described by the ability of the individual to treat the low blood glucose. The term 'mild' hypoglycaemia is applied when an individual can treat him or herself and 'severe' when he or she requires third-party help to treat the hypoglycaemic episode.

Different blood glucose levels define biochemical hypoglycaemia; however, commonly, a level of at or below 4 mmol/l is often used. The European Medicines Agency defines hypoglycaemia as a blood glucose level of ≤3 mmol/l (Amiel *et al.*, 2002).

Potential causes of hypoglycaemia include:

- an imbalance of carbohydrate foods and insulin intake;
- medication that increases secretion of insulin (sulfonylureas);
- vomiting;
- breastfeeding;
- increased levels of physical activity/exercise;
- alcohol intake.

Factors that increase the risk of hypoglycaemia are renal impairment, hepatic failure, increased intake of alcohol, malabsorption, and anorexia.

If you observe the signs and symptoms detailed in Table 9.7, described as autonomic or neuroglycopenic symptoms in individuals who have diabetes mellitus, acting quickly by monitoring their blood glucose levels and intervening appropriately is critical.

Nursing interventions for hypoglycaemia

Nurses have a role in intervening in the care of people who are experiencing hypoglycaemia. Table 9.8 demonstrates the appropriate evidence-based courses of action.

Diabetic ketoacidosis (DKA)

Diabetic ketoacidosis occurs when diabetes is uncontrolled because of insulin deficiency. It is diagnosed when the following are all present: hyperglycaemia; **ketone bodies**; and metabolic acidosis. It usually occurs in people with type 1 diabetes mellitus; however, it can occasionally occur in people with type 2 diabetes mellitus.

In patients with diabetes mellitus, when there is a deficiency of insulin, glucose is unable to enter the cells to provide energy. The body uses adipose tissue as an alternative source of energy, but fatty acids are

Table 9.7 Autonomic or neuroglycopenic signs of deterioration

Autonomic	Neuroglycopenic
Sweating	Confusion
Palpitations	Drowsiness
Shaking and tremor	Slurred speech
Hunger	May demonstrate unusual behaviour
Feeling hot	Disturbances with vision

Table 9.8 Nursing interventions for hypoglycaemia

Definition of hypoglycaemia	Initial treatment	Further treatment
Mild hypoglycaemia	Take 10–20 g of fast-acting carbohydrate immediately (e.g. sugary drink, glucose tablets)	Follow on with long-acting carbohydrate
Severe hypoglycaemia: conscious and able to swallow	Give 10–20 g of fast-acting carbohydrate immediately (e.g. glucogel, sugary drink) If symptoms persist, then repeat treatment	Follow on with long-acting carbohydrate
Severe hypoglycaemia: unconscious	Place in recovery position, give glucagon 1 mg if available (but ineffective in liver disease) May require emergency services	Once recovered, give long-acting carbohydrate

formed and, as they are taken up by the liver, they are converted to ketone bodies, which are released into the circulation. Low levels of insulin then cause an increase in the levels of **catecholamines, cortisol,** and growth hormone, which causes blood glucose levels to continue to rise.

Hyperosmolar hyperglycaemic state (HHS)

Hyperosmolar hyperglycaemic state affects people with type 2 diabetes mellitus/undiagnosed type 2, usually affecting the middle-aged or elderly. It is not a common condition, affecting approximately 1% of people with type 2 diabetes mellitus, but it has a high mortality rate—11% (Kitabchi *et al.,* 2006)—and is often associated with other comorbidities.

Severe dehydration results from osmotic diuresis as excess glucose and electrolytes are lost via the kidneys.

Ketone bodies are not normally present because some residual insulin is usually present in the body.

Signs and symptoms and interventions for DKA and HHS that would be administered by the multidisciplinary team are summarized in Table 9.9.

Long-term complications of diabetes mellitus

People with type 1 and type 2 diabetes are at risk of developing long-term complications. These risks can be reduced by good glucose control, good control of blood pressure, and control of hyperlipidaemia. The blood test that is used to measure long-term glucose control is called the HbA1c test. It measures glucose that is bound to the haemoglobin of red blood cells, and reflects the average blood glucose level during the previous 3 months.

Table 9.9 Signs and symptoms, and interventions for DKA and HHS

	Diabetic ketoacidosis	Hyperosmolar hyperglycaemic state
Causes	Insulin deficiency Newly diagnosed type 1 Missed doses of insulin Hyperglycaemia Other morbidity No known cause	Newly diagnosed type 2 Infection Large consumption of glucose drinks Drug treatment (steroids, thiazide diuretics) Other morbidity
Signs and symptoms	Hyperglycaemia Severe polyuria, nocturia, thirst Abdominal pains Hypotension Ketonuria Tachycardia Kussmaul respirations Coma pH <7.3	Hyperglycaemia >35 mmol Polyuria, thirst Severe dehydration Gradual loss of consciousness Coma
Interventions	Rehydration with intravenous fluids Replacement of electrolytes Continuous intravenous insulin Treatment of any underlying infection May require admission to intensive care unit Should also consult local protocol for treatment	Rehydration with intravenous fluids Correct electrolyte imbalance Continuous intravenous insulin Treatment of any underlying infection May require admission to intensive care unit Should also consult local protocol for treatment

The Diabetes Control Complications Trial (DCCT, 1993) demonstrated that intensive control with an average HbA1c of 7% reduced the risks of developing microvascular complications in people with type 1 diabetes by over 50% compared with a standard treatment group with an average HbA1c of 9%.

The United Kingdom Prospective Diabetes Study (UKPDS33), a multicentre study with over 5,000 people newly diagnosed with type 2 diabetes mellitus, assessed the benefit of good glycaemic control, with an average HbA1c of 7% compared with standard glycaemic control with a HbA1c of 7.9% on the development of complications. This reduction of HbA1c of 0.9% resulted in a reduction in microvascular complications of around 25%.

Macrovascular complications

People with diabetes mellitus are at increased risk of developing cardiovascular disease, with coronary heart disease being the main cause of death. They are also more likely to experience peripheral vascular disease and a cerebrovascular accident (see **Chapter 13**).

Modifiable risk factors for macrovascular complications are detailed in Table 9.10.

Microvascular complications: retinopathy

Diabetic retinopathy is caused by leakage of blood and fluid from damaged retinal blood vessels. If this occurs in the peripheral retina, eyesight may remain normal, so screening needs to be undertaken to detect it. This is carried out by performing a digital retinal photograph of the retina through a dilated pupil every year. Retinopathy, if present, is classified into: R0—no retinopathy; R1—previously called background; R2—previously called preproliferative retinopathy; and R3—previously called proliferative retinopathy, with M1 being maculopathy, which is graded independently.

In the UK, diabetic retinopathy is the commonest cause of blindness in people of working age (Cheung *et al.*, 2010). Good blood glucose control and good blood pressure control can help to reduce the risk of developing retinopathy. Laser therapy to photocoagulate leaking blood vessels has been demonstrated to preserve sight (Ferris, 1996).

Table 9.10 Macrovascular complications and modifiable risk factors

Macrovascular complications associated with diabetes mellitus	Modifiable risk factors for macrovascular complications
Acute coronary syndrome and myocardial infarction	Hyperglycaemia
Peripheral vascular disease	Hypertension
Cerebrovascular events: strokes and transient ischaemic attacks (TIAs)	Hyperlipidaemia
Death from macrovascular disease	Excess body weight and particularly central adiposity
	Cigarette smoking
	Unhealthy diet, particularly consumption of saturated fats
	Low levels of physical activity

Diabetic nephropathy

Diabetic nephropathy is the commonest cause of end-stage renal failure in the developed world and is also associated with increased risk of cardiovascular disease and other microvascular complications. The aim of diabetes care is to reduce the risk for individuals developing diabetic nephropathy by aiming for good glycaemic control and treating raised blood pressure (see Table 9.4).

Diabetic nephropathy is characterized by the progression from normal albumin excretion to increased urinary albumin excretion, microalbuminuria followed by macroalbuminuria, to reduced glomerular filtration rate, and, finally, leading to end-stage renal failure (see **Chapter 11**). A blood test of serum creatinine is checked yearly to assess and monitor kidney function and, from this, a value of estimated glomerular filtration rate (eGFR) is made. Urine should also be checked yearly to detect protein loss.

Diabetic neuropathy

The commonest manifestation of diabetic neuropathy is sensory neuropathy affecting the feet, leading to numb feet and the loss of protective pain sensation. This can be detected by seeing if the person with diabetes can feel a touch on his or her feet. A 10g nylon monofilament is usually the tool that is used to check for foot sensation every year. Absence of protective pain sensation can lead people to damage their feet without knowing it. Such damage can lead to foot ulceration and potentially amputation. People with neuropathy in their feet need to be referred for support and education, which has been shown to reduce the risk of ulceration (National Institute for Health and Clinical Excellence (NICE), 2004b).

A full range of microvascular complications is detailed in Table 9.11.

Other diabetes-related complications

Erectile dysfunction

Erectile dysfunction is defined as the inability to achieve and maintain an erection that is sufficient for sexual intercourse. Although this is a complication associated with middle-aged to elderly males, it is a common complication of diabetes mellitus. Oral medications, for example sildenafil, can help the condition.

Diabetes and pregnancy

Women with type 1 or type 2 diabetes mellitus should be encouraged to receive pre-pregnancy counselling to ensure that glycaemic control is optimum.

Gestational diabetes mellitus occurs or is first recognized in pregnancy. Women with diabetes should receive 'shared care', with the obstetric and diabetes team working closely together to ensure appropriate treatment is provided. Some women will require oral hypoglycaemic agents, metformin being the only one used in pregnancy, and other women may require insulin therapy. The aim of treatment is to try to maintain blood glucose levels within the normal range (4–6 mmol/l before food).

Women who have experienced gestational diabetes mellitus are at increased risk of developing type 2 diabetes mellitus in later life and should therefore have an annual blood glucose test, and be encouraged to lose weight if overweight and to adopt a healthy lifestyle.

Table 9.11 Microvascular complications and risk factors

Complication	Diagnosis	Related studies	Risk factors
Retinopathy (damage affecting the back of the eye)	Annual retinal screening to detect early changes in the eye and referral to specialist services as required	DCCT (1993) reduction in the development of retinopathy UKPDS33 (1998) reduction in risk of microvascular disease	Duration of diabetes mellitus Hyperglycaemia Hypertension Smoking can accelerate retinopathy High cholesterol
Nephropathy (leading to end-stage renal failure)	Annual microalbuminuria testing Annual blood test for urea and creatinine and eGFR	UKPDS33 (1998) risk of microvascular disease reduced	Duration of diabetes mellitus Hypertension Hyperglycaemia Smoking Ethnicity
Neuropathy (can affect virtually every part of the body)	Annual foot assessment and identification of 'at-risk' feet to identify potential problems	UKPDS33 (1998) risk of microvascular disease reduced	Duration of diabetes mellitus Hyperglycaemia Smoking
Autonomic neuropathy (can present with a range of symptoms)	Annual diabetic review	DCCT (1993) demonstrated risk of autonomic neuropathy reduced if good glycaemic control	Duration of diabetes mellitus Hyperglycaemia

Identifying best practice

Since 2004, GPs have been incentivized through the Quality and Outcomes Framework (http://www.nice.org.uk/aboutnice/qof/qof.jsp) to provide higher quality diabetes care. Since 2004, increased levels of recording of the processes and intermediate outcomes of high-quality diabetes care have been recorded. There are a number of guidelines based on current evidence that provide useful information about best practice in the care of people with diabetes; these are outlined in Box 9.1.

Because research is always ongoing and best practice evolves, it is important that readers stay up to date and know where to find good-quality sources of evidence. Hence we have provided a list of sources that readers should utilize.

Sources of evidence

Organizations

National Institute for Health and Clinical Excellence (NICE) http://guidance.nice.org.uk/

The Scottish Intercollegiate Guidelines Network (SIGN) http://www.sign.ac.uk/guidelines/index.html

NHS Evidence http://www.evidence.nhs.uk/

Agency for Healthcare Quality (AHRQ) http://www.ahrq.gov/

National Institute for Clinical Studies (NICS) http://www.nhmrc.gov.au/nics/index.htm

Registered Nurses Association of Ontario http://www.rnao.org

World Health Organization http://www.who.int/en/

Journals

Diabetes Care
British Medical Journal
The Lancet
New England Journal of Medicine

> **Box 9.1 Useful diabetes guidelines**
>
> - National Institute for Health and Clinical Excellence (NICE) Clinical Guideline (CG) 15 Type 1 Diabetes in Adults and Children (NICE, 2004a)
> - National Institute for Health and Clinical Excellence (NICE) Clinical Guideline (CG) 63 Diabetes & Pregnancy (NICE, 2008a)
> - National Institute for Health and Clinical Excellence (NICE) Clinical Guideline (CG) 66 Type 2 Diabetes (NICE, 2008b)
> - National Institute for Health and Clinical Excellence (NICE) Clinical Guideline (CG) 87 Type 2 Diabetes: rapid update of the glycaemic lowering section for NICE CG 66 (NICE, 2009)
> - International Diabetes Federation (IDF) Global Guideline for type 2 Diabetes (IDF, 2005)
> - Scottish Intercollegiate Guideline Group (SIGN) Guideline 116 Management of Diabetes 2010 (SIGN, 2010)

Conclusion

Nurses have a pivotal role to play in the assessment and monitoring of individuals with diabetes mellitus to ensure that they are receiving appropriate medications and to avoid any potential complications, which can be life-threatening and life-limiting. Nurses also have a crucial role in educating individuals and families to self-manage their condition effectively, including following healthy lifestyle advice.

Online Resource Centre

 In order to help you to develop and apply your knowledge and decision-making skills further, we have provided interactive learning resources online at **www.oxfordtextbooks.co.uk/orc/bullock/**

Whilst these are freely available, you will need to use the access codes at the start of the book.

References

Amiel, S., Beveridge, S., Bradley, C., *et al.* (2002) Training in flexible, intensive insulin management to enable dietary freedom in people with type 1 diabetes: dose adjustment for normal eating (DAFNE) randomised controlled trial. *British Medical Journal* **325**: 746–9.

Bruno, A., Gregori, D., Caropreso, A., *et al.* (2008) Normal glucose values are associated with a lower risk of mortality in hospitalized patients. *Diabetes Care* **31**: 2209–10.

Capes, W., Hunt, D., Malmberg, K., *et al.* (2000) Stress hyperglycaemia and increased risk of death after myocardial infarction in patients with and without diabetes: a systematic overview. *Lancet,* **355**(9206): 1647.

Cheung, N., Mitchell, P., Wong, T.Y. (2010) Diabetic retinopathy. *Lancet* **376**: 124–36.

Davies, M.J., Heller, S., Skinner, T.C., *et al.* (2008) Effects of the diabetes education for ongoing and newly diagnosed (DESMOND) programme for people with newly diagnosed type 2 diabetes: cluster randomised controlled trial. *British Medical Journal* **336**: 491–5.

Deakin, T.A., Cade, J.E., Williams, R., *et al.* G.C. (2006) Structured patient education: the Diabetes X-pert programme makes a difference. *Diabetic Medicine* **223**: 944–54.

Diabetes Control and Complications Trial (DCCT) Research Group (1993) The effect of intensive treatment on the development and progression of long term complications in insulin dependent diabetes mellitus. *New England Journal of Medicine* **329**: 977–86.

Diabetes Prevention Programme Research Group (2002) Reduction in the incidence of type 2 diabetes with lifestyle interventions or metformin. *New England Journal of Medicine* **346**: 393–403.

Diabetes UK (2010) **www.diabetes.org.uk/Professionals/ Publications-reports-and-resources/Reports-statistics-and- case-studies/Reports/Diabetes-prevalence-2010/** (accessed 16 November 2010).

Ferris, F. (1996) Early photocoagulation in patients with either type 1 or type 2 diabetes. *Transactions of the American Ophthalmology Society* **94**: 505–37.

Gautier, A., Roussel, R., Ducluzeau, P.H., *et al.* (2010) Increases in waist circumference and weight as predictors of type 2 diabetes in individuals with impaired fasting glucose: influence of baseline BMI. *Diabetes Care* **33**: 1850–2.

International Diabetes Federation (IDF) (2005) Brussels Global Guideline for Type 2 Diabetes **www.idf.org** (accessed 5 August 2011).

International Diabetes Federation (IDF) (2009) *Diabetes Atlas 2009,* 4th edn. International Diabetes Federation (IDF): Brussels.

Kitabchi, A.E., Umpierrez, G.E., Murphy, M.B., *et al.* (2006) American Diabetes Association consensus statement on hyperglycaemic crises in adults patients with diabetes. *Diabetes Care* **29**: 2739–48.

National Institute for Health and Clinical Excellence (NICE) (2004a) *Type 1 Diabetes in Adults and Children.* NICE Clinical Guideline 15 (CG15). NICE: London.

National Institute for Health and Clinical Excellence (NICE) (2004b) *Type 2 Diabetes: Footcare.* NICE Clinical Guideline 10 (CG10). NICE: London.

National Institute for Health and Clinical Excellence (NICE) (2008) *Diabetes and Pregnancy.* NICE Clinical Guideline 63 (CG63). NICE: London.

National Institute for Health and Clinical Excellence (NICE) (2008a) Continuous subcutaneous insulin infusion for the treatment of diabetes mellitus (review of Technology Appraisal Guidance 57). NICE: London.

National Institute for Health and Clinical Excellence (NICE) (2008b) *Type 2 Diabetes.* NICE Clinical Guideline 66 (CG66). NICE: London.

National Institute for Health and Clinical Excellence (NICE) (2009) *Type 2 Diabetes: Rapid Update of the Glycaemic Lowering Section of NICE CG66.* NICE Clinical Guideline 87 (CG87). NICE: London.

NHS Diabetes (2010) Safe use of insulin. **www.diabetes.nhs.uk/ safe_use_of_insulin** (accessed 5 August 2011).

Roglic, G., Unwin, N., Bennett, P.H., *et al.* (2005) The burden of mortality attributable to diabetes. *Diabetes Care* **28**: 2130–5.

Scottish Intercollegiate Guidelines Network (SIGN) (2010) Guideline 116 Management of Diabetes. Scottish Intercollegiate Guidelines Network: Edinburgh.

Sherifa, D., Nerenberg, K., Pullenayegum, E., *et al.* (2010)The effect of oral antidiabetic agents on A1c levels. *Diabetes Care* **33**: 1859–64.

Tuomilehto, J., Lindstrom, M.S., Eriksson, J.G., *et al.* (2002) Prevention of type 2 diabetes by changes in lifestyle among subjects with impaired glucose tolerance. *New England Journal of Medicine* **344**: 1393–49.

United Kingdom Prospective Diabetes Study UKPDS33 (1998) Intensive blood glucose control with sulfonylureas or insulin compared with conventional treatment and risk of complications in patients with type 2 diabetes. *Lancet* **352**: 837–53.

United Kingdom Prospective Diabetes Study UKPDS34 (1998) Effect of intensive blood glucose control with metformin on complications in overweight patients with type 2 diabetes. *Lancet* **352**: 854–65.

World Health Organization (WHO) (1999) Values for diagnosis of diabetes mellitus and other categories of hyperglycaemia. **http://www.who.int/diabetesactiononline/diabetes/basics/en/index4.html** (accessed 5 August 2011).

World Health Organization (WHO) (2002) *The World Health Report 2002: Reducing Risks Promoting Health Life.* **www.who.int/whr/2002/en/** (accessed 19 October 2011).

World Health Organization (WHO) (2006) World Health Organization/IDF Definition & Diagnosis of Diabetes Mellitus and Intermediate hyperglycaemia. WHO: Brussels.

Year of Care Project (2010) **http://www.diabetes.nhs.uk/year_of_care/** (accessed 5 August 2011).

Zhang, X., Gregg, E.W., Williamson, D.F., *et al.* (2010) A1c level and future risk of diabetes: a systematic review. *Diabetes Care* **33**: 1665–73.

10 *Understanding* Functional Bowel Disorders

Jenny Gordon

Introduction

The aim of this chapter is to provide nurses with the knowledge to be able to assess, manage, and care for people with the group of conditions often described as functional bowel disorders (FBD)—see definitions below—in an evidence-based and person-centred way. The chapter will provide an overview of the causes and impact of FBDs, before exploring best practice to deliver care, as well as to prevent or to minimize further ill-health. Nursing assessments and priorities are highlighted throughout, and the nursing management of the symptoms and common health problems associated with FBDs can be found in Chapters 16, 23, 24, and 25, respectively ➡.

Understanding functional bowel disorders

Defining functional bowel disorders

This chapter discusses the group of conditions often described as functional bowel disorders (FBDs). The term 'functional gastrointestinal disorders' is also used in the literature, but, for the purpose of this book, the term FBDs will be adopted. This refers to a group of disorders that are characterized by chronic gastrointestinal symptoms that currently have an unknown structural or biochemical cause that could explain those symptoms. **Rome III** is an internationally agreed set of diagnostic criteria and related information on functional gastrointestinal disorders (Longstreth *et al.*, 2006). It includes six major domains for adults: oesophageal; gastro/duodenal; bowel; functional abdominal pain syndrome; biliary; and anorectal. This chapter will cover the FBDs that specifically relate to chronic abdominal symptoms. General abdominal symptoms include **functional dyspepsia**, non-cardiac chest pain, which may mimic functional abdominal symptoms, chronic abdominal pain, **functional constipation**, **functional diarrhoea**, functional bloating, and **irritable bowel syndrome (IBS)**. The chapter will concentrate on irritable bowel syndrome. **Coeliac disease** and **Crohn's disease** are included: to give an understanding of these disorders, and to differentiate between inflammatory and non-inflammatory conditions; to highlight the impact of the symptoms on the people who suffer from them; and to give an insight into the contribution that effective nursing makes.

The amount of research and the number of publications concerning FBDs has risen considerably since the mid 1990s, and has contributed to the increasing legitimacy of these conditions as disorders in their own right and not simply by virtue of exclusion of all other possibilities. Scientific advances investigating inflammation, immunology, and alterations in gut flora at a molecular level have helped our understanding of the ways in which FBD symptoms are generated (Drossman, 2006). Technical advances, such as brain imaging with the use of **positron emission tomography (PET)** and **magnetic resonance imaging (MRI)**, offer increased understanding of the brain–gut interactions in FBDs (Drossman *et al.*, 2005).

Integrated view

Psychological tools that measure cognition, emotions, stress, and quality of life have been improved so that researchers are better able to standardize their outcome measures. These have added to our understanding and acceptance of the biopsychosocial model of disease (Jones *et al.*, 2000). In this model, there is a clear link between the body and the mind as part of a complex system, with an understanding that an imbalance in any part of the system can cause illness and disease. The person's experience of his or her condition and the objective pathophysiology found are given equal importance in putting together the full clinical picture (Engel, 1977, 1980). This integrated approach recognizes that symptoms can be determined and modified both by physiological, psychosocial, and cultural influences, and that all of these factors need to be given consideration in the diagnosis and management of any disorder. It also helps to explain how environmental factors, genetic factors, and changes in early life can affect our psychological state, susceptibility to life stress, coping skills, and levels of social support. These factors may also impact on the development of gut dysfunction and explain why different people's experiences of similar symptoms differ (Jones *et al.*, 2006).

Nursing principles

The role of nursing involves understanding the full range of physical, psychosocial, emotional, and spiritual needs of people in your care. All of these aspects are encapsulated in the Principles of Nursing Practice (Royal College of Nursing, 2010). These principles will be used to underpin this chapter because they describe a shared understanding of what all people can expect from nursing in any setting, whether they are colleagues, patients, or families and carers of patients. They were developed in collaboration with nurses, patients, families, professional, and patient organizations. The 'setting' includes any place where care is delivered and received. Nursing is provided by nursing staff, including ward managers in hospitals or team leaders in the community, specialist nurses, community nurses, health visitors, healthcare assistants, or student nurses (see Box 10.1).

However, it is not enough simply to consider the nurses delivering care; consideration must also be given to the care itself. The Principles of Nursing Practice use three domains to identify the different components of care.

- Person-centred care involves: working with people to find out how their individual values, beliefs, and needs relate to their health and social care; providing and discussing relevant information and support; promoting informed choice, shared communication, and decision-making; and enabling participation in the evaluation of care.

- Safe and effective care is care that is evidence-based as far as possible in relation to the treatments provided and the context in which care takes place.

- The context in which care is delivered includes the processes, structures, and patterns of behaviour that allow safe and effective patient-centred care to be sustained.

The principles will be referred to where they contribute to a greater understanding of the nursing role, serving as an overarching guide to best practice.

The anatomy and physiology of functional bowel disorders

To understand the functional gastrointestinal disorders, it is essential to have knowledge and understanding of the structure and functions of the gastrointestinal (GI) tract. This book will cover specific pathophysiology related to the conditions being discussed, but assumes a basic understanding of anatomy and physiology, and readers may wish to consult additional physiology textbooks to supplement their knowledge. A reading list is included at the end of the chapter.

The adult GI tract consists of a fibromuscular tube that starts at the mouth and ends at the anus. The overall

---

Box 10.1 Principles of Nursing Practice (Royal College of Nursing, 2010)

Principle A

Nurses and nursing staff treat everyone in their care with dignity and humanity—they understand their individual needs, show compassion and sensitivity, and provide care in a way that respects all people equally.

Principle B

Nurses and nursing staff take responsibility for the care they provide and answer for their own judgements and actions—they carry out these actions in a way that their patients, and the families and carers of their patients expect, and in a way that meets the requirements of their professional bodies and the law.

Principle C

Nurses and nursing staff manage risk, are vigilant about risk, and help to keep everyone safe in the places they receive healthcare.

Principle D

Nurses and nursing staff provide and promote care that puts people at the centre, involves patients, service users, their families and their carers in decisions, and helps them make informed choices about their treatment and care.

Principle E

Nurses and nursing staff are at the heart of the communication process: they assess, record and report on treatment and care, handle information sensitively and confidentially, deal with complaints effectively, and are conscientious in reporting the things they are concerned about.

Principle F

Nurses and nursing staff have up-to-date knowledge and skills, and use these with intelligence, insight, and understanding in line with the needs of each individual in their care.

Principle G

Nurses and nursing staff work closely with their own team and with other professionals, making sure patients' care and treatment is coordinated, is of a high standard, and has the best possible outcome.

Principle H

Nurses and nursing staff lead by example, develop themselves and other staff, and influence the way care is given in a manner that is open and responds to individual needs.

---

function of the GI tract is ingestion and digestion of nutrients, and the elimination of waste produced during the process. The GI tract is regulated by the autonomic nervous system, together with hormonal control. This chapter concentrates conditions of the small and large bowel, so an overview of the pathophysiology of the intestines follows. Figure 10.1 illustrates the small and large intestines.

The adult small intestine is approximately 3 metres long and is made up of the duodenum (25 cm), the jejunum (1 metre), with the ileum forming the remainder (approximately 2 metres). The inner wall of the small intestine is made up of permanently ridged folds of mucous membrane called plicae circulares that do not flatten when the intestine is distended. They increase the surface area of the small intestine. The surface area is further increased by the lining of the small intestine, which is lined with millions of tiny finger-like projections called villi, which are covered in smaller

microvilli that have a fuzzy coating containing many digestive enzymes. This makes the small intestine a very efficient organ of nutrient digestion and absorption.

The ileocaecal valve is the sphincter between the small and large intestines. It is normally closed, but opens in response to a peristaltic contraction, which allows a one-way flow of intestinal contents from the small intestine to the large.

The large intestine is 1.5 metres long and approximately 6.5 cm wide, and forms a frame around the small intestine. It is divided into the ascending colon (which stretches from the caecum up the right side of the abdomen to the lower edge of the liver), the transverse colon (which extends across the abdomen), and the descending colon (which lies down the left side of the abdomen and leads into an S-shaped sigmoid colon that projects towards the midline and terminates as the rectum). The opening

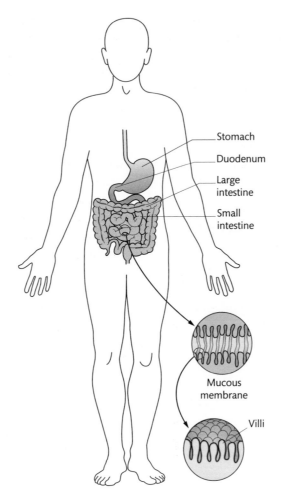

Stomach
Duodenum
Large
intestine
Small
intestine

Mucous
membrane

Villi

Figure 10.1 The small and large intestines.

Reproduced by kind permission of John Heseltine.

from the rectum is called the anus and this allows the elimination of faeces from the colon. The mucosa of the large intestine has neither villi nor digestive enzymes. It is made up of absorptive cells that absorb water and electrolytes. Mucus-producing cells and some endocrine cells are also present, although the hormonal function of the large intestine is not yet understood.

The way in which nutrients work their way through the GI tract (digestion) is controlled by the central nervous system. It relies on a series of autoregulated actions and responses involving the autonomic nervous system. Digestion is also regulated by the specific characteristics of the gut itself, including its own intrinsic nervous system and hormonal interactions. These combined nervous and hormonal systems work together, resulting in an extremely effective gut

motility. Input from the autonomic nervous system can strongly affect the activity of the gut intrinsic nervous system.

The GI tract is well supplied with afferent nerve fibres that transmit important information about the gut, including signals in response to irritation of the gut mucosa or excessive distension. This may result in the increase or decrease of intestinal motility. Other nerve fibres transmit to higher levels of the central nervous system, which, in turn, modulates the signals of the vagus nerve (which controls many GI functions, including peristalsis). **Peristalsis** is the propulsive movement of the GI tract and is the way in which nutrients work their way through the intestines. The movements that keep the intestinal contents thoroughly mixed are also caused by peristaltic movements. Although the process of digestion is described as linear, it is important to remember that each part of the process is separate; although several parts may occur at the same time, the process is synergistic, and if one part of the process is not working properly or is interrupted, this can have a profound effect on the whole of the GI tract. It is also important to consider the fact that people display a wide range of variability in their tolerance of certain nutrients and stooling patterns, and that this may be caused by GI-related differences or learned responses from cultural and environmental experiences.

Defining irritable bowel syndrome

Irritable bowel syndrome (IBS) is a chronic, relapsing, non-inflammatory bowel disease characterized by abdominal pain or discomfort associated with defaecation, bloating, or abdominal distension and altered bowel function (which includes constipation or diarrhoea, or both). It is clearly linked to bowel function and is characterized by symptoms being relieved either by defaecation or with a change in stool form or consistency. Other intestinal symptoms include feelings of incomplete evacuation, **urgency**, and passage of mucus per rectum. Non-colonic symptoms may also present, including back pain, migraine, depression, and urinary and gynaecological problems. It is one of the commonest functional gastrointestinal disorders and may be lifelong. People may present with varying combinations of symptoms, with mainly constipation being predominant, diarrhoea being predominant, or an alternating bowel pattern. These symptoms can cause dehydration, anxiety, lethargy, and sleep disturbance, which in turn may cause considerable disruption to work and social life and result in a significant reduction in quality of life.

IBS commonly affects people between 20 and 40 years of age, although recently there has been an increased prevalence in older people. It is twice as likely to affect women as men (Smith, 2003). Although the prevalence is estimated at somewhere between 10% and 20% of the population, the true prevalence is thought to be much higher because many people rely on self-care rather than seek medical advice.

The cause of IBS is not yet understood because there are currently no objective biochemical markers of the condition. It is thought that altered intestinal motility, intestinal hypersensitivity, bowel dysfunction caused by previous

infections, and/or prolonged use of antibiotics may all contribute. Stress, emotional trauma, and lifestyle are factors that may act as a trigger or aggravate pre-existing symptoms. Food intolerance has also been identified as a contributing factor and many people with IBS use exclusion diets in an attempt to alleviate symptoms. This is often undertaken without the guidance and support of a dietitian, which can lead to dietary imbalance, which, in extreme cases, can lead to malnutrition and exacerbation of symptoms rather than their relief.

The diagnosis and management of IBS can be challenging for patients and clinicians. It is not always easily recognized and a diagnosis has often been made after many inconclusive or negative investigations. A diagnosis of exclusion can leave patients feeling that they have been given a 'wastepaper basket' diagnosis. This may contribute to a lack of confidence in both the diagnosis and the treatments offered. In the recent National Institute for Health and Clinical Excellence (NICE) guideline (2010), positive diagnosis based on identified positive symptoms and targeted (minimal) investigations provides the nurse and other clinicians with a preferred evidence-informed approach. It also includes and incorporates exclusion of any 'red flag' symptoms 🚩 such as unexplained weight loss, rectal bleeding, and abdominal masses (which may suggest suspected carcinoma), and other symptoms that may suggest a differential diagnosis of organic disease such as coeliac and Crohn's disease.

This recent NICE guidance should help to lay a foundation for quicker, more confident diagnosis of the syndrome, and facilitate a much more positive understanding of the chronic nature of this condition. Health professionals and patients need to be equally aware of the current evidence informing decisions about care and management, and actively work together to manage the symptoms that are having the greatest impact for individual patients.

Defining coeliac disease

Coeliac disease is an autoimmune disorder characterized by damage to all or part of the villi lining the mucosa of the small intestine. The damage is caused by an increased immunological response after exposure to gluten and/or related proteins found in wheat, rye, malt, and barley. Gluten is not found in oats, but they are often prepared in the same environment as other cereals, and so cross-contamination can cause a reaction in some people. The exact cause is unknown, but environmental, immunological, and genetic factors are important. For example, it is considered to be more prevalent in people with autoimmune conditions such as type 1 diabetes and in first-degree relatives of people with coeliac disease (Salardi *et al.*, 2008; Biagi *et al.*, 2008). It is a very common condition, occurring all over the world, but is commonest in northern Europe. It is believed to be present in about 1 in every 100 people, with women twice as likely to develop the condition as men. Coeliac disease can be diagnosed at any age after gluten has been introduced into the diet. It is thought that many people have the condition, but are clinically well; however, a significant number may have a range of symptoms, including anaemia, lethargy, abdominal pain, and diarrhoea, which can result in ill-health. This may not be recognized as coeliac disease and so the condition often remains undiagnosed. The delay in diagnosis is a concern because of the possible long-term side effects of untreated coeliac disease. There is evidence that undiagnosed coeliac disease in women can have a negative effect on uterine growth and birth weight, and is associated with increased pre-term birth and increased rates of Caesarean section. There is also evidence to suggest an increase in the risk of fractures and an increased risk of cancers, specifically Hodgkin's and non-Hodgkin's lymphoma, and small bowel cancer, although the risk is small (National Institute for Health and Clinical Excellence (NICE), CG86, 2010).

Defining inflammatory bowel disease (IBD)

Inflammatory bowel disease (IBD) is a general term to describe any disease characterized by inflammation of the bowel. These diseases should not be confused with irritable bowel syndrome (IBS): their aetiology is different and they require different treatment. Examples of IBD include ulcerative colitis and Crohn's disease. Crohn's disease is a chronic inflammatory disease involving any part of the GI tract, but is most commonly found in the terminal ileum or the colon. It can be diagnosed at any age, but is most prevalent in 15–30-year-olds, with a second peak in 55–70-year-olds. It occurs equally in men and women, and in the UK is distributed equally across the social spectrum.

People with Crohn's disease typically have recurring acute episodes of the disease, with varying periods of less active episodes and/or periods of complete remission. The pattern of the disease is highly variable; remission, during which people have no symptoms at all, can last for long periods, but may then be followed by several periods during which they suffer frequent flare-ups. Symptoms include: recurring diarrhoea, with blood and mucus in stools; abdominal pain and cramping, which is usually worse after eating; weight loss; and fatigue. Less common symptoms are skin rashes, inflammation and swelling of joints, fevers, and nausea and vomiting.

The complications of this condition include the development of fistulae, abscesses, intestinal obstruction, and perianal disease. Surgery will be required in a significant number of patients (up to 80%) in addition to medical management. Although surgery is not always completely successful, improvements in surgical techniques have reduced overall mortality from Crohn's disease.

The exact causes of IBD are currently unknown; however, research has identified some factors that may be responsible. Studies have shown that both Crohn's disease and ulcerative colitis occur more commonly in families than would be expected purely by chance; this could be because of predisposing genetic factors within families (Duerr *et al.*, 2006). It is also more common in some ethnic groups than others. There may also be an environmental link; IBD is more common in developed countries and, after family history and ethnic background, smoking is the most important risk factor. Smokers are twice as likely to develop the disease as non-smokers, and people who have Crohn's disease who smoke usually experience more severe symptoms in comparison to non-smokers who have the disease. The immune system is thought to be responsible for the inflammation that occurs. This could be triggered by previous exposure to an infection, which then causes an abnormal immune system response.

Ulcerative colitis is a chronic, inflammatory disease characterized by recurrent ulceration of the colon. It is twice as common as Crohn's disease and similar in its pattern of periods of exacerbation followed by periods of remission. The symptoms are also similar in that the dominant symptom is diarrhoea with blood and mucus in the stools. However, abdominal pain is less significant for most patients with ulcerative colitis, although some may experience mild colic or lower abdominal discomfort that is relieved by defaecation. Guidance is currently in development by NICE in relation to the care and management of individuals experiencing Crohn's disease and ulcerative colitis; these are both due for publication in 2012 at **www.nice.org.uk**. Also see the British Society of Gastroenterology guidelines for the management of inflammatory bowel disease by Mowat *et al.* (2011).

Assessing people who may have functional bowel disorders

We know that functional gastrointestinal disorders (FBDs) are commonly occurring disorders that are characterized by symptoms of abdominal pain and/or discomfort, bloating, and changes in bowel habits. Nurses may be involved in the assessment of people who may have an FBD from the first consultation or at any stage of the process, so it is important to understand all aspects of assessment, diagnosis, and treatment, and the pivotal role that nursing has within the multidisciplinary team. The diagnosis and management of IBS can be frustrating for both patients and health professionals. Everyone needs to recognize the chronic, relapsing nature of the condition and this requires a clear understanding of the current state of knowledge of IBS. The following sections will highlight best practice using national guidance where it exists and will describe particular challenges faced by people with FBDs.

People are often currently diagnosed after a considerable number of tests, which are either inconclusive, negative, or within normal limits. Hence a diagnosis is arrived at by excluding many other differential diagnoses. However, it is much more positive to diagnose a person as having an FBD on the basis of a clinical history of the characteristic symptoms that are described, together with a thorough physical examination and the absence of any of the alarm features or 'red flag' symptoms that would suggest an alternative diagnosis. One of the key symptoms that distinguishes IBS from organic disease is the quality, site, and frequency of the pain and/or discomfort. The site may be described as occurring anywhere in the abdomen and also may vary at different times. Cancer-related pain, for example, usually has a

fixed site. The most important alarm features or 'red flag' symptoms 🚩 include:

- signs of rectal or gastrointestinal bleeding (fresh or altered blood);
- a family history of colorectal or ovarian cancer—if there is significant concern that symptoms may suggest ovarian cancer, a pelvic examination should also be considered;
- a change in bowel habit to looser and/or more frequent stools persisting for more than 6 weeks in a person aged over 60;
- unintentional or unexplained weight loss;
- anaemia;
- abdominal masses;
- rectal masses;
- inflammatory markers for inflammatory bowel disease.

The presence of alarm symptoms obviously does not exclude an FBD, but the symptoms need further investigation before confirmation of any diagnosis.

In the absence of alarm symptoms, establishing a diagnosis of IBS is crucial. The absence of organic changes means that symptom-based diagnostic criteria are often used as the basis for diagnosis (Adeniji *et al.*, 2004). There have been several of these, the first being Manning in 1978 (Manning *et al.*, 1978), followed by the **Rome** series, I, II (Badia *et al.*, 2002), and Rome III (Longstreth *et al.*, 2006) (see Box 10.2).

The primary aim should be to clarify the person's symptom profile, with abdominal pain or discomfort being a key symptom. A diagnosis of IBS should be considered

---

Box 10.2 Rome III diagnostic criteria for irritable bowel syndrome

At least 3 months, with onset at least 6 months previously of recurrent abdominal pain or discomfort* associated with two or more of the following:

- improvement with defaecation; and/or
- onset associated with a change in frequency of stool; and/or
- onset associated with a change in form (appearance) of stool.

*Discomfort means an uncomfortable sensation not described as pain.

only if the person has abdominal pain or discomfort that is either relieved by defaecation or associated with altered bowel frequency or stool consistency. The person should also have had at least two of any combination of the following groups of symptoms for at least 3 days a month in the past 3 months, with the onset of symptoms being at least within the past 6 months:

- altered stool passage (straining, urgency, incomplete evacuation);
- abdominal bloating (more common in women than men), distension, tension, or hardness;
- symptoms made worse by eating;
- passage of mucous.

People with IBS also frequently report symptoms of nausea, lethargy, backache, and urinary/bladder symptoms, and these can be used to help to make a diagnosis of IBS.

The importance of taking a thorough history cannot be overemphasized. The way in which questions are asked is as important as the questions themselves. Asking open questions can help to elicit information that people may not otherwise disclose. Consider asking about how symptoms affect the patient's daily life, leaving the house, travelling, and socializing. Remember that people may be embarrassed or reluctant to talk about bowel habits, so using examples of common problems may help them to feel more comfortable. Using the Bristol Stool Form Scale (Figure 10.2) provides a visual aid to description when determining the consistency and amount of stool passed.

IBS is commonly categorized by the predominant bowel symptom and is described as either constipation-dominant, diarrhoea-dominant, or alternating. Some people experience faecal incontinence, but evidence shows that many are reluctant to talk about it. Only 20% of those experiencing faecal incontinence disclosed the information when asked specifically. Other bowel symptoms include rectal hypersensitivity (pain is experienced when the rectum is distended to a level not normally reported as causing discomfort), incomplete evacuation (a sensation that another bowel movement is necessary soon after a bowel movement, yet there is difficulty passing further stool the second time), and urgency (a sudden urge to have a bowel movement that is so strong that, if a toilet is not immediately available, there will be incontinence). This is more common in people who have diarrhoea-dominant IBS.

Basic laboratory investigations, such as a full blood count (FBC), erythrocyte sedimentation rate (ESR), C-reactive protein (CRP) (which is a general marker for inflammation and infection), and serological tests for coeliac disease (endomysial antibodies, EMA; or tissue transglutaminase, TTG) are useful in the initial evaluation.

Because coeliac disease can be very effectively treated with a gluten-free diet, it is important to identify people with the undiagnosed disease so as to provide satisfactory individual treatment. A gluten-free diet is a lifelong treatment that represents a significant commitment, and the impact of this undertaking should not be underestimated. It is important to remember that it is possible to have coeliac disease and IBS at the same time!

Mucosal intestinal biopsy of the distal duodenum or proximal jejunum, together with a clinical response to dietary withdrawal of gluten, remains the gold standard for the diagnosis of coeliac disease. A diagnostic trial of a gluten-free diet should not be undertaken without first obtaining biopsy evidence consistent with coeliac disease.

Nursing priorities in coeliac disease concern the planning and assessment of care; this will focus on recognition of the disease in undiagnosed patients, management of a gluten-free diet, management of symptoms of diarrhoea, and embarrassment and impact on daily living. People who have been diagnosed with coeliac disease may initially require iron and vitamin B12 and folic acid (Smith and Watson, 2005).

People with predominant and severe diarrhoea who may have inflammatory disease may require further diagnostic investigations, such as colonoscopy with colonic biopsies and a test for bile acid malabsorption. Biopsies will show that the villi may be blunted or the mucosal surface may appear to be flat with a complete absence of villi.

Managing functional bowel disorders

The management of any chronic condition is likely to involve a long-term therapeutic partnership between the person with the condition and a number of healthcare professionals. A key to the success of this relationship is likely to be a shared understanding of what can be expected from the relationship.

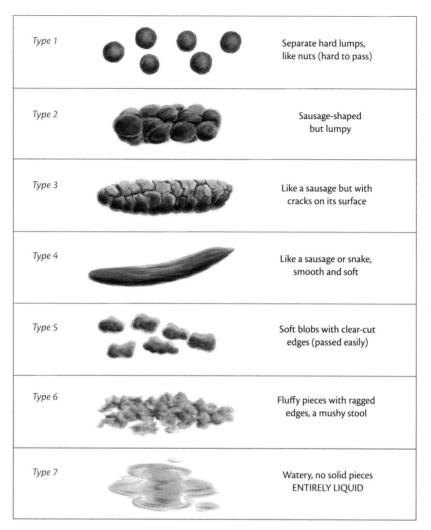

Type 1		Separate hard lumps, like nuts (hard to pass)
Type 2		Sausage-shaped but lumpy
Type 3		Like a sausage but with cracks on its surface
Type 4		Like a sausage or snake, smooth and soft
Type 5		Soft blobs with clear-cut edges (passed easily)
Type 6		Fluffy pieces with ragged edges, a mushy stool
Type 7		Watery, no solid pieces ENTIRELY LIQUID

Figure 10.2 The Bristol Stool Form Scale.

Reproduced by kind permission of Dr K.W. Heaton, Reader in Medicine at the University of Bristol. © Norgine Pharmaceuticals Ltd.

Therapeutic care

The Principles of Nursing Practice discuss providing and promoting 'care that puts people at the centre of care, involving them in decisions and helping them make informed choices about their treatment' (Principle D, Royal College of Nursing, 2010). There are many factors of which healthcare professionals need to be aware to facilitate effective communication. These include being sensitive to the cultural and ethnic needs of all whom they see and recognizing the particular needs of people for whom English is not a first language or who may have cognitive and/or behavioural problems or disabilities. Many people with IBS have been managing their symptoms long before seeking additional support. It may be that a particular symptom has become more severe, so it is helpful to clarify the key issues and challenges; patients may be able to identify triggers. Stress commonly aggravates the disorder, and around half of IBS outpatients attribute the onset of symptoms to a stressful event. Asking people to describe how they have been managing their condition will give insight into coping strategies. They will often have considerable experience and expertise from which healthcare professionals can benefit!

Self-help and activity

Self-help is an integral part of the effective management of IBS, so it is important to build up a picture of a person's general lifestyle, physical activity, diet, and symptom-targeted medication (which may include herbal and over-the-counter medication). For example, work–life balance may be an issue, and it is helpful to encourage people to identify the areas in their daily lives in which they can reduce stress and perhaps identify increased opportunities for relaxation. Physical activity can be a challenge for people with IBS; activity can be assessed using the General Practice Physical Activity Questionnaire (GPPAQ). The General Practice Physical Activity Questionnaire is intended for use in adults (aged 16–74) in routine general practice to provide a simple, 4-level physical activity index (PAI), reflecting an individual's current physical activity. The index can be cross-referenced to 'Read' codes for physical activity and can be used to help to inform the decision as to when interventions to increase physical activity might be appropriate (Department of Health, 2004). People who are sedentary should be supported to increase their activity levels, exploring options for increased activity that improve rather than exacerbate symptoms. Confidence to try a new activity may be an issue, and counselling may be beneficial. Ensuring that people have access to a range of suitable information about activity in general and, specifically, options that are available locally to them is essential, and they may need ongoing encouragement and support.

Diet and nutrition

Diet and nutrition often have a major impact on the quality of life of people with IBS. They have often identified foods that exacerbate their symptoms. It is not uncommon, however, for people to try exclusion diets without seeking dietetic support, and this can lead to insufficient nutritional intake. Nurses serve as a regular point of contact and may be asked about exclusion diets. They should follow the recommendation in the National Institute for Health and Clinical Excellence (NICE) guideline (2010):

> If diet continues to be considered a major factor in a person's symptoms and they are following general lifestyle/dietary advice, they should be referred to a dietitian for advice and treatment, including single food avoidance and exclusion diets. Such advice should only be given by a dietitian. (NICE, 2010: 1.2.1.8, 39)

Giving general dietary advice falls within the remit of all healthcare professionals, and again the NICE guideline gives clear information that can be passed on to people with IBS. This information should be tailored to fit with daily life and it is often helpful to give examples of alternative choices or ideas of foods or meals, particularly when discussing high-fibre foods and resistant starch, which may be less familiar to people.

There has been a long-running and highly effective advertising campaign to encourage the consumption of high-fibre cereal and fruit and vegetables. This is a very positive public health message, and is aimed at reducing the risk of coronary heart disease, colon cancer, and obesity. For many people, particularly those with diarrhoea-dominant or alternating IBS, eating a high-fibre diet may not be the most effective way of managing their symptoms. It may be that a review of the fibre intake of people with IBS means that their intake requires adjustment. Usually, this means reducing the amount of fibre that they eat. Evidence also suggests that the type of fibre that people eat may have an impact on their symptoms and that:

> People with IBS should be discouraged from eating insoluble fibre (for example, bran). If an increase in dietary fibre is advised, it should be soluble fibre such as ispaghula powder or foods high in soluble fibre (for example, oats). (NICE, 2010: 1.2.1.5, 38)

However, it is important that people continue to monitor the effect on their symptoms, and nurses may continue to be the health professionals that provide ongoing support.

Medication and concordance

The range of information required to provide high-quality care for people with IBS highlights another of the Principles of Nursing Practice. Principle F states that 'nurses and nursing staff have up to date knowledge and skills and use these with intelligence, insight, and understanding in line with the needs of each individual in their care' (Royal College of Nursing, 2010). This is further illustrated when we look at the pharmacological therapies that are available to treat the range of symptoms. These include

Box 10.3 **General dietary advice for IBS**

- Have regular meals and take time to eat.
- Avoid missing meals or leaving long gaps between eating.
- Drink at least eight cups of fluid per day, especially water or other non-caffeinated drinks, e.g. herbal teas.
- Restrict tea and coffee to three cups per day.
- Reduce intake of alcohol and fizzy drinks.
- It may be helpful to limit intake of high-fibre food (such as wholemeal or high-fibre flour and breads, cereals high in bran, and whole grains such as brown rice).
- Reduce intake of 'resistant starch' (starch that resists digestion in the small intestine and reaches the colon intact), which is often found in processed or re-cooked foods.
- Limit fresh fruit to three portions per day (a portion should be approximately 80 g).
- People with diarrhoea should avoid sorbitol, an artificial sweetener found in sugar-free sweets (including chewing gum) and drinks, and in some diabetic and slimming products.
- People with wind and bloating may find it helpful to eat oats (such as oat-based breakfast cereal or porridge) and linseeds (up to one tablespoon per day).

(National Institute for Health and Clinical Excellence (NICE), 2010: 1. 2.1.4, 38)

laxatives for constipation, antispasmodics for abdominal discomfort, antimotility agents for diarrhoea, and low-dose tricyclic antidepressants as a second-line analgesic treatment if other treatments have been ineffective. Medicines are prescribed based on the nature and severity of the symptoms, and the doses adjusted according to the response of the person. Medicines may be used singly or in combination. No single drug will alleviate the multiple symptoms often present in those with IBS. As we discover more about the possible underlying causes of IBS and new drugs are developed, the names and actions of the drugs may change, but the role of the nurse remains constant. That role involves maintaining a thorough and up-to-date knowledge of the condition that affects our

patients, in this case IBS, by accessing evidence-based information to support practice and ensuring that we are able not only to communicate the information accurately, but also that we do so in a way that is relevant for each individual, giving consideration to his or her age, lifestyle, culture, and understanding. It is also important that we support patients and their families to find out information for themselves, and that we are willing and able to discuss that information with them. This may present a challenge because there is so much information available, and not all of it is accurate. When people are coping with a long-term chronic condition, they may often feel vulnerable and, if prescribed medication is not having the desired effect on symptoms, they may wish to try alternative treatments. Currently, the evidence for these treatments is scant, although this may change and develop with further research. This means that nurses must help their patients to assess the risk, and they have a responsibility to keep their patients safe. Record-keeping, documentation, and a shared understanding of decision processes, and regular evaluation of treatments are vital components of risk management.

Further specialized treatment options

Many people will respond well to first-line management but for others, whose IBS is described as refractory IBS, there are further specialized treatment options. For these people, referral for cognitive behavioural therapy (CBT) and/or hypnotherapy may be considered. The NICE guideline suggests that these options should be considered for those who have not responded to pharmacological treatments after 12 months and who have developed a continuing symptom profile (NICE, 2010: 1.2.3.1; 40). Figure 10.3 suggests methods for managing IBS.

All patients should have an annual review as part of their follow-up treatment, but more regular follow-up may be agreed on an individual patient basis depending on needs. Patients should be asked about any new or additional symptoms that may prompt further investigation because they may indicate the development of other conditions and comorbidities. Those with chronic conditions may automatically attribute symptoms to their pre-existing condition and may not always disclose additional symptoms.

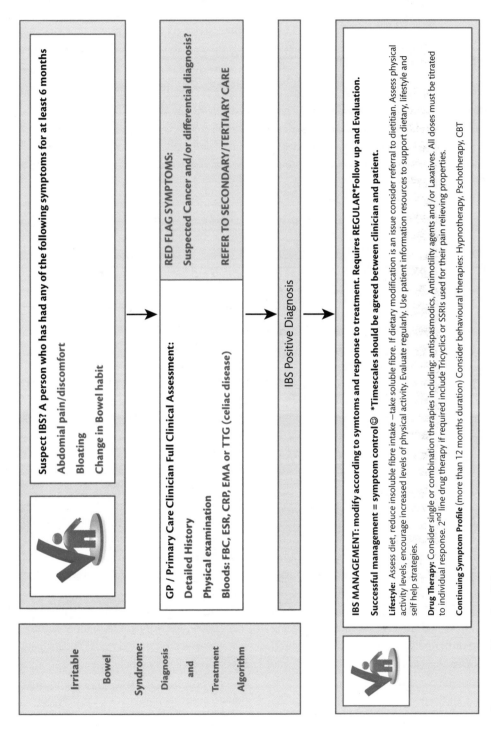

Irritable Bowel Syndrome: Diagnosis and Treatment Algorithm

Suspect IBS? A person who has had any of the following symptoms for at least 6 months

- Abdomial pain/discomfort
- Bloating
- Change in Bowel habit

GP / Primary Care Clinician Full Clinical Assessment:

- Detailed History
- Physical examination
- Bloods: FBC, ESR, CRP, EMA or TTG (celiac disease)

RED FLAG SYMPTOMS:

Suspected Cancer and/or differential diagnosis?

REFER TO SECONDARY/TERTIARY CARE

IBS Positive Diagnosis

IBS MANAGEMENT: modify according to symtoms and response to treatment. Requires REGULAR*Follow up and Evaluation.

Successful management = symptom control☺ *Timescales should be agreed between clinician and patient.

Lifestyle: Assess diet, reduce insoluble fibre intake – take soluble fibre. If dietary modification is an issue consider referral to dietitian. Assess physical activity levels, encourage increased levels of physical activity. Evaluate regularly. Use patient information resources to support dietary, lifestyle and self help strategies.

Drug Therapy: Consider single or combination therapies including: antispasmodics, Antimotility agents and /or Laxatives. All doses must be titrated to individual response. 2nd line drug therapy if required include Tricyclics or SSRIs used for their pain relieving properties.

Continuing Symptom Profile (more than 12 months duration) Consider behavioural therapies: Hypnotherapy, Pschotherapy, CBT

Figure 10.3 Managing IBS.

THEORY INTO PRACTICE 10.1
IBS case studies

Mrs Jones is a 76-year-old woman who is retired and lives on her own in a warden-controlled flat. Anna Lee is a 25-year-old lady who has two young children and works on a part-time basis in a local café. What advice and help could you provide them in relation to lifestyle and diet, and how would this potentially differ for these two individuals experiencing IBS?

Mrs Smith is being discharged home following admission for dehydration secondary to an exacerbation of IBS. What kind of advice would you give her prior to discharge in relation to diet, hydration, and general lifestyle? To what support groups could you point her to help her better manage the syndrome?

Mr Mann has been diagnosed with Crohn's disease, and wants more information about his condition and possibly to meet up with others who also have a diagnosis of Crohn's disease.

Use the 'sources of evidence' signposts at the end of the chapter to shape your responses and find out more about the help available for people with functional gastrointestinal disorders.

Identifying best practice

The National Institute for Health and Clinical Excellence (NICE) continues to update and develop evidence for England and Wales; the Scottish Intercollegiate Guideline Network (SIGN) guidelines in Scotland and Guidelines and Audit Implementation Network (GAIN) in Northern Ireland perform the same function—to guide practice. Nurses have a responsibility to access up-to-date resources; to that end, please see the sources we have highlighted below.

Sources of evidence

Organizations

National Institute for Health and Clinical Excellence (NICE) http://guidance.nice.org.uk/

The British Society for Gastroenterology

The Scottish Intercollegiate Guidelines Network (SIGN) http://www.sign.ac.uk/guidelines/index.html

NHS Evidence http://www.evidence.nhs.uk/

Agency for Healthcare Quality (AHRQ) http://www.ahrq.gov/

National Institute for Clinical Studies (NICS) http://www.nhmrc.gov.au/nics/index.htm

Registered Nurses Association of Ontario http://www.rnao.org

World Health Organization http://www.who.int/en/

Specific resources

General Practice Physical Activity Questionnaire (GPPAQ). http://www.dh.gov.uk/en/Publicationsandstatistics/Publications/PublicationsPolicyAndGuidance/DH_063812

Scottish Nutrition and Diet Resources Initiative (2004) *Irritable Bowel Syndrome (IBS) Your Diet Can Help* http://www.caledonian.ac.uk/sndri/pdf/IrritableBowelSyndrome.pdf

Charitable organizations

The Gut Trust www.theguttrust.org

Core charity funds research into the entire range of gut, liver, intestinal, and bowel illnesses http://www.corecharity.org.uk/

National Association for Colitis and Crohn's Disease (NACC) http://www.nacc.org.uk

Conclusion

This chapter has used IBS to illustrate the principles of nursing that are required to provide care for people with functional gastrointestinal disorders. Although there is still much that we do not know about the causes of these disorders, we can apply what we do know about what constitutes high-quality nursing care. Evidence-based guidance aims to reduce variations in practice, improving patient outcomes related to both the diagnosis and continuous management of IBS.

Online Resource Centre

To help you to develop and apply your knowledge and decision-making skills further, we have provided interactive learning resources online at **www.oxfordtextbooks.co.uk/orc/bullock/**

Whilst these are freely available, you will need to use the access codes at the start of the book.

References

Adeniji, O.A., Barnett, C.B., Di Palma, J.A. (2004) Durability of the diagnosis of irritable bowel syndrome based on clinical criteria. *Digestive Diseases and Sciences* **49**(4): 572–4.

Badia, X., Mearin, F., Balboa, A., *et al.* (2002) Burden of illness in irritable bowel syndrome comparing Rome I and Rome II criteria. *Pharmacoeconomics* **20**(11): 749–58.

Biagi, F., Campanella, J., Bianchi, P.I., *et al.* (2008) The incidence of celiac disease in adult first degree relatives. *Digestive and Liver Disease* **40**: 97–100.

Department of Health (2004) General Practice Physical Activity Questionnaire (GPPAQ). http://www.dh.gov.uk/en/Publicationsandstatistics/Publications/PublicationsPolicyAndGuidance/DH_063812 (accessed 21 March 2012)

Drossman, D.A. (2006) The functional gastrointestinal disorders and the Rome III process. In D. A. Drossman, E. Corazziari, M. Delvaux *et al.* (eds) *Rome III: The Functional Gastrointestinal Disorders*, 3rd edn. Degnon Associates, Inc.: McLean, VA, pp. 1–29.

Drossman, D.A., Morris, C.B., Hu, Y., *et al.* (2005) A prospective assessment of bowel habit in irritable bowel syndrome in women: defining an alternator. *Gastroenterology* **128**(3): 580–9.

Duerr, R.H., Taylor, K.D., Taylor, Brant, S.R., *et al.* (2006). A genone-wide assocation study identifies 1L23R as an inflammatory bowel disease gene. *Science* **314** (5804): 1461–3.

Engel, G.L. (1977) The care of the patient: art or science? *The Johns Hopkins Medical Journal* **40**: 222–32.

Engel, G.L. (1980) The clinical application of the biopsychosocial model. *The American Journal of Psychiatry* **137**: 535–44.

Jones, J., Boorman, J., Cann, P., *et al.* (2000) British Society of Gastroenterology guidelines for the management of the irritable bowel syndrome. *Gut* **47**(Suppl. 2): ii1–19.

Jones, M.P., Dilley, J.B., Drossman, D., *et al.* (2006) Brain–gut connections in functional GI disorders: anatomic and physiologic relationships. *Neurogastroenterology & Motility* **18**: 91–103.

Longstreth, G.F., Thompson, W.G., Chey, W.D., *et al.* (2006) Functional bowel disorders. *Gastroenterology* **130**: 1480–91.

Manning, A.P., Thompson, W.G., Heaton, K.W., *et al.* (1978) Towards positive diagnosis of the irritable bowel. *British Medical Journal* **ii**: 653–4.

Mowat, C., Cole, A., Windsor, A., *et al.* (2011) British Society of Gastroenterology Guidelines for the management of inflammatory bowel disease. **http://www.bsg.org.uk/clinical-guidelines/ibd/guidelines-for-the-management-of-inflammatory.html**

National Institute for Health and Clinical Excellence (NICE) (2009) Recognition and assessment of coeliac disease. NICE Clinical Guideline 86 (CG86). NICE: London.

National Institute for Health and Clinical Excellence (NICE) (2010) Irritable bowel syndrome in adults: diagnosis and management of irritable bowel syndrome in primary care. NICE Clinical Guideline 61 (CG61). NICE: London.

Royal College of Nursing (2010) Principles of Nursing Practice. **www.rcn.org.uk/nursingprinciples**

Salardi, S., Volta, U., Zucchini, S., *et al.* (2008) Prevalence of coeliac disease in children with type 1 diabetes mellitus increased in the mid-1990s: an 18 year longitudinal study based on anti-endomysial antibodies. *Journal of Pediatric Gastroenterology and Nutrition* **46**: 612–14.

Smith, G.D. (2003) measuring quality of life in the healthcare setting. *Gastrointestinal Nursing* **1**(5): 16–19.

Smith, G., Watson, R. (2005) *Gastrointestinal Nursing*. Blackwell: Oxford.

Table 11.1 Stages of chronic kidney disease

Stage	eGFR (ml/min/1.73m²)	Description
1	≥90	Normal or increased GFR, with other evidence of kidney damage
2	60–89	Slight decrease in GFR, with other evidence of kidney damage
3A	45–59	Moderate decrease in GFR, with or without other evidence of kidney damage
3B	30–44	
4	15–29	Severe decrease in GFR, with or without other evidence of kidney damage
5	<15	Established renal failure

If proteinuria is present, the eGFR is followed with the letter 'p'.
Source: National Institute for Health and Clinical Excellence (NICE), 2008a

the risk of later presentation and delayed diagnosis. As eGFR and renal function deteriorates, so the associated symptoms will become progressively worse. Stage 5 CKD will inevitably result in death unless renal replacement therapy (RRT) in one of its forms (e.g. haemodialysis (HD), peritoneal dialysis (PD), or renal transplantation) is instigated. The vast majority of patients with CKD will not develop established renal failure (stage 5 CKD).

Defining acute kidney injury (AKI)

Acute kidney injury (AKI) is a clinical condition characterized by an abrupt (within 48 hours) reduction in renal function associated with an increase in serum creatinine or a reduction in urine output. Prompt recognition and early management of AKI can prove crucial in terms of outcome (Stevens *et al.*, 2001), and nurses can play a pivotal role in identifying the deteriorating patient at risk of AKI and ensuring that he or she is reviewed promptly. AKI is associated with a variety of underlying causes, which can occur across a wide range of clinical settings.

The Acute Kidney Injury Network (AKIN) established an international staging that indicates the severity of AKI, using criteria based on serum creatinine and urine output (**http://www.akinet.org/** Renal Association, 2008). The AKIN staging aims to help to standardize the care of patients with AKI, although any impact of this staging in clinical practice has yet to be fully evaluated (Bradley, 2009). There are limitations in the accuracy of serum creatinine as an absolute measure of GFR (Bellomo *et al.*, 2004), but what is known is that changes in serum

creatinine are associated with increased mortality and increased length of stay in hospital and costs (Chertow *et al.*, 2005).

In AKI, as renal function deteriorates, the patient may become oliguric or anuric. Metabolic waste products rise and the patient is at increased risk from the effects of renal impairment. The early manifestations and management of these problems are discussed later. The patient is likely to require transfer to a critical care or high care environment and may receive specialized RRT treatments such as continuous veno-venous haemofiltration (CVVH) to take over the homeostatic functions of the kidney.

> **Key point!**
>
> CKD and AKI are quite distinct. CKD is characterized by a gradual, but irreversible, decline in renal function. AKI is a sudden loss of renal function, which carries a high mortality rate. If the patient survives and recovers, they will regain normal renal function in the majority of cases.

Prevalence and epidemiological profile of CKD and AKI

The true prevalence of CKD in the earlier stages is difficult to ascertain, given that different criteria and populations have been studied in published research (MacGregor, 2007). However, estimates suggest that between 5% and 11% of the total Western population have moderate to severe CKD (eGFR <60 ml/min/1.73m^2) (Klebe *et al.*, 2007; Stevens *et al.*, 2007). There is an ongoing debate about the true health burden of the older person 'labelled' as having CKD (Khwaja and Throssell, 2009).

Stage 5 CKD (established renal failure) is a relatively rare condition. In the UK in 2008, there were 47,525 adults with established renal failure receiving RRT in the form of dialysis or a renal transplant (Renal Registry, 2009). RRT is expensive, accounting for between 1% and 2% of the NHS budget (Department of Health, 2005a), with a year of dialysis costing between £20,000 and £25,000 for each patient (Department of Health, 2007).

There is an increased risk and incidence of CKD for those of African-Caribbean and South Asian heritage, linked to the increased incidence of hypertension and type 2 diabetes in these populations (Department of Health, 2007; National Institute for Health and Clinical Excellence (NICE), 2008b). Diabetic renal disease is the single commonest cause of established renal failure (Renal Registry, 2009). Given the predicted growth of type 2 diabetes, and diabetes in children (Roberts, 2007), there is an associated predicted increase in the incidence and prevalence of CKD. Further information about diabetes and its complications can be found in Chapter 9 ⟶.

Whilst a screening of the general population for CKD is not yet recommended, there are clear benefits (both in the health of individuals and financial) to be obtained by screening those in the population considered 'at risk' of developing CKD (Heffernan, 2008; National Institute for Health and Clinical Excellence (NICE), 2008a).

The true incidence of AKI is equally difficult to determine, because data are dependent upon the population being studied, the setting in which the patient is managed, and the definition of AKI (Department of Health, 2005a; Renal Association, 2008). Whilst there have been no definitive UK studies of the incidence of AKI (NCEPOD, 2009), some have reported that patients with AKI needing RRT account for 4.9% of all admissions to critical care (Nalker *et al.*, 2007).

Mortality and morbidity in CKD and AKI

In CKD, the absolute risk for death increases exponentially with decreasing renal function (Tonelli *et al.*, 2006). People with CKD are at increased risk of developing cardiovascular

disease, and it is a cause of death in 40–50% of patients with CKD (Go *et al.*, 2004). The Department of Health Vascular Programme (Department of Health, 2008) identifies opportunities and future challenges in key areas of vascular disease, and makes the links between CKD, diabetes, cardiovascular disease, and stroke.

The mortality rate of patients with AKI who are not admitted to critical care environments can be up to 10% (usually when the kidney is the only failed organ). Moreover, AKI in the critical care environment is regularly linked with sepsis and multiorgan failure and has a mortality rate of over 50% (Liano *et al.*, 1998; Stevens *et al.*, 2001). The increased morbidity and mortality associated with both CKD and AKI is the rationale for the focus of care guidelines being directed towards prevention (Department of Health, 2005a; Renal Association, 2008; NCEPOD, 2009). Nurses can play an increasingly important role in the early detection and prevention of both CKD and AKI.

The pathophysiology of renal disorders

To care for the patient with CKD or AKI, it helps to have an understanding of some of the normal and abnormal physiological processes associated with renal function. There are some helpful exercises on the Online Resource Centre to test your knowledge ⓦ. The kidneys have a fundamental role in maintaining homeostasis within the body and are part of the renal and urinary system (Figure 11.1). The microscopic nephron within the kidney produces the urine, and the ureters, bladder, and urethra allow for the passage and storage of urine ready for elimination. It is possible to live healthily with only one kidney; some people are born with just one kidney, while others may lose one through trauma, malignancy, or even donation.

Each kidney has over 1 million nephrons. The flow of blood through the first part of the nephron—the glomerulus—is absolutely crucial to renal function. Alterations in bloodflow will alter GFR. A normal measured GFR is approximately 125 ml/min. While GFR is an indicator of renal function, measuring it accurately can be difficult. The eGFR derived from a specific formula is now a standard measure of renal function in CKD (Levey *et al.*, 2000). However, the correlation between estimated and true GFR can be poor when renal function is relatively well preserved, and so a normal result is taken as >90 ml/min/1.73m^2.

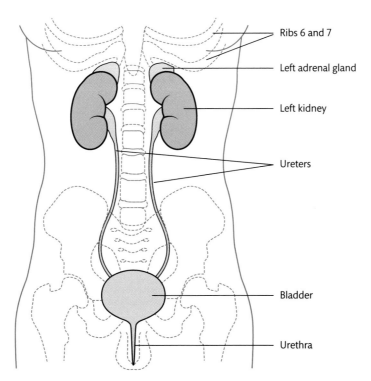

Figure 11.1 The renal and urinary system.

Reproduced with kind permission from *Human Physiology*, 3rd edn, by Pocock and Richards, Oxford University Press.

The physiological mechanisms associated with renal function and the formation of urine are complex and are not within the scope of this chapter. When caring for an individual whose renal function is under threat or who has diminished renal function, it sometimes helps to think about 'what the kidneys do' (Figure 11.3) to recognize why a patient presents in a particular way and to understand the rationale behind the often numerous care interventions.

> **THEORY INTO PRACTICE 11.1**
> **Activity: considering the effects of renal dysfunction**
>
> Think about 'what the kidneys do' and look at Figure 11.3. Review each of the seven individual functions in turn, and consider what you might see or how the patient may feel if there is renal impairment. For example, if there were a problem or imbalance with fluid regulation, how might you recognize this in the patient?

When things start to go wrong with renal function, changes are not immediately evident, because compensatory mechanisms are instigated. The body systems will attempt to address any imbalances, e.g. an increased respiration rate may help to excrete hydrogen ions and reduce blood pH, or the heart rate will increase to circulate increasing fluid volumes. However, should kidney function continue to be impaired, then the individual will become increasingly unwell as toxins and fluid begin to accumulate, and electrolytes and hydrogen ions become deranged. This collection of symptoms is sometimes termed uraemia (see Figure 11.2).

Causes of kidney disorders

The causes of CKD and AKI are numerous, and those more commonly seen are outlined in Boxes 11.1 and 11.2. The multiplicity of causes of CKD and AKI can add to the complexity of nursing care required. When considering treatment and nursing management of CKD and AKI

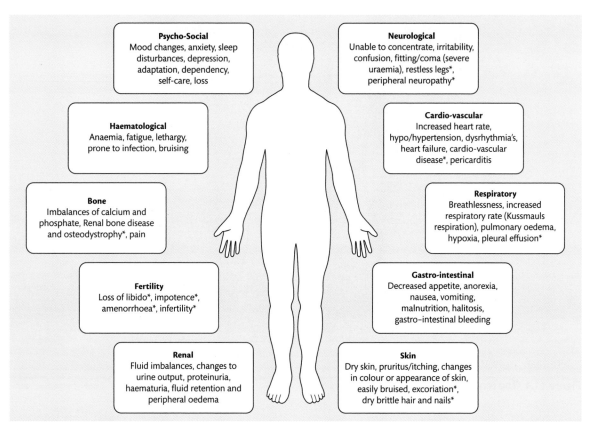

Figure 11.2   The effects of renal impairment.

* more likely associated with CKD.

- Glomerulonephritis (biopsy-proven)
- Diabetes
- Pyelonephritis
- Polycystic kidney
- Hypertension
- Renal vascular disease
- Aetiology uncertain/glomerulonephritis not biopsy-proven

(Renal Registry, 2009)

symptoms, it is essential that any underlying cause(s) is also treated and managed.

The numerous causes of AKI are classically divided into prerenal, renal (intrinsic), and postrenal causes.

Prerenal failure describes a fall in GFR as a result of hypotension or hypovolaemia that can be reversed by correction of the underlying cause (Armitage and Thomson, 2003). This may also be termed 'volume-responsive' AKI (Renal Association, 2008). If there is a prolonged period of hypoperfusion that cannot be corrected, there is a risk of acute tubular necrosis (ATN), and the renal tubules 'shut down' and cease to function (usually temporarily).

Identifying patients at risk of CKD and AKI

The risk factors for CKD are outlined in Box 11.3. In the UK, much of the focus of CKD risk and prevention lies with the primary healthcare team (National Institute

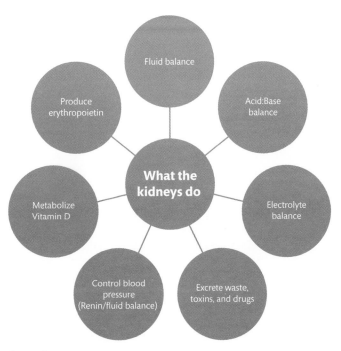

Figure 11.3 What the kidneys do.

Box 11.2 Causes of acute kidney injury

Prerenal (volume-responsive)	**Renal–intrinsic**	**Postrenal**
Hypovolaemia	• Acute tubular necrosis (as a result of volume-responsive cause)	Obstruction
• Vomiting and diarrhoea		• Renal calculi
• Haemorrhage	• Glomerulonephritis	• Prostatic hypertrophy
• Trauma	• Vasculitis, e.g. systemic lupus erythematosus	• Urethral stricture
Decrease in effective circulating volume		• Carcinoma or neoplasm, e.g. bladder, pelvis
	• Haemolytic uraemic syndrome	
• Cardiac failure	• Rhabdomyolysis (crush syndrome)	
• Septic shock		
• Cirrhosis	• Myeloma	
Drugs	• Malignant hypertension	
• ACE inhibitors		

(UK Renal Association, Clinical Practice Guidelines, Module 5—Acute Kidney Injury, 2008)

---

for Health and Clinical Excellence (NICE), 2008a). It is known that patients who present late with CKD do less well, and have increased morbidity and mortality (Kazmi *et al.*, 2004). General practitioners now keep a register of patients with stages 3–5 CKD as part of the Quality and Outcomes Framework, the aim being to monitor progression and ensure timely referral.

One proven nursing intervention that can impact upon the progression of CKD is effective monitoring, management, and control of blood pressure, including the administration

---

Box 11.3   Risk factors for CKD

- Cardiovascular disease
- Proteinuria
- Hypertension
- Diabetes
- Smoking
- Black or Asian ethnicity
- Chronic use of nephrotoxic drugs, e.g. non-steroidal anti-inflammatory drugs (NSAIDs)
- Urinary outflow tract obstruction, e.g. prostatic hypertrophy

(National Institute for Health and Clinical Excellence (NICE), 2008a)

Box 11.4   Top ten risk factors for AKI

1. Age
2. Comorbidity, e.g. cardiovascular disease
3. Medication, e.g. ACE inhibitors
4. Previous CKD
5. Hypovolaemia
6. Sepsis
7. Biochemistry, e.g. changes, monitoring of renal function preoperative and postoperative
8. Abnormal urinalysis
9. Daily weight changes, e.g. if on diuretic therapy
10. Nutritional status, e.g. catabolic patient

(NCEPOD, 2009)

---

of angiotensin-converting enzyme (ACE) inhibitors and angiotensin receptor blockers/antagonists (ARBs) (National Institute for Health and Clinical Excellence (NICE), 2008a; 2008b). (See 'Alert! Blood pressure monitoring in CKD' (page 178 ➡)) Similarly, good glycaemic control for the patient with diabetes can also influence the development of longer term complications such as CKD (DCCT, 1993; National Institute for Health and Clinical Excellence (NICE), 2008b).

The risk factors associated with AKI are also numerous. A 'top ten' of risk factors for AKI have been suggested (NCEPOD, 2009) and are detailed in Box 11.4.

Simple nursing interventions concerned with fluid management (see also Chapter 19 ➡) may help to reduce the risk of AKI. These could include:

- monitoring the length of preoperative 'nil-by-mouth' periods (and the instigation of IV fluids where necessary);
- close attention to medication, fluid balance, and daily weight in patients at risk of dehydration (particularly in older people);
- improving the management of fluid balance in the clinical area through education and audit.

🚩 Alert! Blood pressure (BP) monitoring in CKD

- How often do you need to monitor BP?
- Are you using the right equipment, e.g. cuff size, manual equipment for more accurate 'one-off' readings?

- Do you need to record orthostatic (lying and standing) BP to help with fluid assessment (drop of 20 mmHg systolic = orthostatic hypotension)?
- Which antihypertensive medication is the patient taking? Do you know how it works?
- Is the patient experiencing any difficulties or side effects with his or her medication?
- Is the patient on a low salt diet (DASH, 2001)? Beware: some salt substitutes contain large amounts of potassium.
- What specific lifestyle changes might be necessary to reduce cardiovascular risk?
- In CKD, target: systolic <140 mmHg, diastolic <90 mmHg; in diabetes: systolic <130 mmHg, diastolic <80 mmHg.

🚩 Alert! Monitoring fluid balance

(See also Chapter 19 ➡)

- How is fluid being lost and replaced?
- What measures can you take to ensure an accurate record of fluid intake and output?
- Do you need to increase involvement of the patient/carer? Would daily weight help?
- Review urine output: is it >0.5 ml/kg body weight/hour?
- Is the patient in a positive or negative fluid balance? What needs to be done to correct it?

Think about your clinical environment and the patient population. Compare the patient groups against the risk factors for CKD or AKI.

- Identify one patient whom you think may be at risk. What puts him or her at risk?
- What is his or her current health problem? Has there been any deterioration or change?
- What do you need to do to increase monitoring or what might be the focus of your nursing interventions?

Box 11.5 Investigating renal function

Blood tests
- Urea and electrolytes, serum creatinine
- eGFR (in CKD)
- Full blood count
- HbA1C (in diabetes)
- Bone profile/parathyroid hormone (PTH)
- Lipid profile
- Arterial blood gas (in AKI)

Urine
- Multistix® urinalysis
- Albumin:creatinine ratio (ACR)
- Urine microscopy and culture

Imaging
- Plain abdominal X-ray (KUB = kidneys ureter bladder)
- Intravenous urogram
- Ultrasound

- Does the patient have signs of dehydration or overhydration/fluid overload?
- Review any medication that may affect fluid balance, e.g. diuretics.

Assessing a patient with CKD and AKI

An important stage of patient assessment is to ascertain whether the patient has CKD, AKI, or an acute deterioration of CKD. Also, during any assessment of the patient, any underlying condition or cause of renal impairment needs to be considered.

CKD

In CKD, progression is slower (over years or months) and, as eGFR falls, the patient experiences a worsening of symptoms (Figure 11.2). It should be noted that, in CKD, symptoms do not usually appear until stage 4. If the patient has had previous blood tests, it may be possible to show that renal impairment is long-standing. There may also be evidence of chronic complications such as anaemia and renal bone disease (particularly stages 4–5). The latter is associated with certain biochemical abnormalities, typically high serum phosphate and low serum calcium. A key finding in CKD is bilateral small kidneys on ultrasound.

Full assessment and management of the patient in stages 4 and 5 CKD requires specialist multiprofessional intervention and is beyond the scope of this chapter. Further suggested reading includes: Levy *et al.* (2009) *Oxford Handbook*

of Dialysis; Steddon *et al.* (2006) *Oxford Handbook of Nephrology and Hypertension*; and Thomas (2008) *Renal Nursing*.

AKI

With AKI, the patient is often acutely unwell, becoming ill over hours or days. In addition to the rapid progression of symptoms caused by renal insufficiency, there are also symptoms of the underlying cause. Some of the presenting signs and symptoms are similar to those of CKD, but the speed and severity with which they affect the patient are often much greater. In AKI, anaemia is likely to be caused by blood loss or red blood cell haemolysis and not the reduction in erythropoietin production (or response to erythropoietin) seen in CKD. Typically, an ultrasound of the kidneys will show them to be of normal size.

Monitoring and measurement of renal function

There are many ways in which to measure renal function in clinical practice (Traynor *et al.*, 2006), and some of the blood tests and investigations you may encounter in practice are outlined in Box 11.5.

EVIDENCE BOX 11.1
Measuring eGFR

The estimation of GFR (eGFR) is now commonly calculated by the laboratory using a specific method and formula known as the MDRD (modification of diet in renal disease) formula (Levey *et al.*, 2000). This formula makes adjustments for race, gender, and age. Whilst useful in the ongoing monitoring of CKD, there are some limitations associated with it.

- It is **not** recommended for the monitoring and assessment of AKI.
- It is not validated for use in pregnancy or in children.
- It may not be accurate at low levels of creatinine (such as in early stages of CKD).
- It can also be affected by other factors, such as hydration status, extremes of weight, and the ingestion of meat.

(National Institute for Health and Clinical Excellence (NICE) 2008a; MacGregor, 2007)

For any patient, the frequency of monitoring and the range of investigations required will depend upon the stage of CKD or AKI and the overall clinical picture. In CKD, the frequency and required monitoring for those either at risk or diagnosed with CKD is clearly set out in the Clinical Guidelines for the Management of Adults with Chronic Kidney Disease in Primary and Secondary Care (National Institute for Health and Clinical Excellence (NICE), 2008a). Helpful publications by Crowe *et al.* (2008), Thomas (2009), and de Lusignan *et al.* (2010) summarize these tests and investigations, and provide further guidance.

Key principles of nursing assessment in CKD and AKI

All patients with CKD or AKI require a full and detailed nursing assessment. The nurse needs attuned observational skills, and will often refer to baseline measures and look for trends and patterns of deterioration or improvement (see alerts for fluid balance monitoring and blood pressure monitoring in CKD on page 178 . It is essential to be able to take a good history and gather, review, and compile information from a variety of sources to obtain a clear picture. On a very simple level, we call this 'knowing the patient'.

Alert! 'Know the patient'

- How did the patient get to the point at which he or she is now? What is his or her 'story'?
- Review notes and recent investigations.
- What does the patient understand about his or her condition?
- What is his or her response to information?
- What family and social support does he or she have?
- What does the patient need or want from you?
- What are the priorities for education, self-care management, and preparation for home (as appropriate)?

Psychosocial assessment

Both CKD and AKI have significant effects upon the patient and his or her family. Patients are often in a state of turmoil at the point of diagnosis, and worried about what the future holds for them. Assessing the patient with AKI will require all of your skills and expertise to assess the patient who is deteriorating and critically ill. Those with CKD and established renal failure need time to adapt to living with this long-term condition and the ongoing treatment and potential lifestyle changes (Auer, 2005; McGee and Bradley, 1994). In the earlier stages of CKD (i.e. stages 1–3), individuals may need reassurance that most people do not progress to the point of needing RRT, and that the focus of care is around cardiovascular risk and changing lifestyle behaviours in line with this. Those with stage 4 CKD and evidence of continued deterioration will need to be prepared for life with RRT or, if this is their choice, continued conservative management.

Encouraging self-management

It is now recognized that education for self-management and self-care should begin in the earlier stages of CKD (Thomas, 2008; Hain *et al.*, 2009), and that collaboration between different healthcare teams and healthcare professionals may impact upon patient outcome (Thomas, 2005; Gilbert *et al.*, 2008). Nurses play a central role in caring for and supporting people with long-term conditions, and a case management approach, with personalized care planning, is recommended (Department of Health, 2005b; 2009). Online resources (such as the NHS Choices website) can help individuals to pull together information tailored to their needs.

> **Box 11.6 Key principles of nursing assessment**
>
> - 'Know the patient'—understanding the patient's journey, compiling information—see 'Alert'.
> - Accurate fluid intake and output assessment, and fluid balance monitoring
> - Effective blood pressure monitoring and control—see 'Alert' on page 178 →
> - Recognize deteriorating trends
> - Communication and observation skills
> - Assessing self-care and self-management needs and opportunities

Assessing health status and identifying appropriate nursing interventions

Patients with renal impairment can present with a complex clinical picture (see Figure 11.2) and require assessment that is both systematic and holistic in nature. In AKI and the later stages of CKD, more often than not, the patient feels and looks unwell. Patients and their families and significant others are likely to be very anxious.

Table 11.2 identifies some key elements of assessment with which you will become involved as a nurse. Whilst this table is not exhaustive, it helps to indicate what you might look for, outlines some of the main problems, and then provides links to other chapters within this book, which may supplement and add detail to the information. You may also wish to consult Endacott *et al.* (2009) *Clinical Nursing Skills: Core and Advanced.*

Nursing interventions

Patients with AKI

Nursing interventions for the patient with AKI can be complex. A summary of care interventions for these patients in a ward environment (rather than critical care) is outlined in Table 11.3 (Perkins and Kisiel, 2005; Redmond *et al.*, 2004). Decisive action by the nurse caring for the patient (either referral to local critical care outreach services or requesting prompt medical assessment) may play a role in patient outcome. Even with optimal medical and nursing care, the patient with AKI may continue to deteriorate, and will require transfer and likely RRT. The indications for RRT in AKI are refractory hyperkalaemia, pulmonary oedema, metabolic acidosis, and severe uraemia (Glynne and Lightstone, 2001).

How to detect that a patient with AKI is deteriorating

⚑ As a nurse, you will be key to making a timely and accurate assessment of any deterioration in the patient's condition, as well as escalating prompt review by medical or senior staff. Changes in health status may occur over hours and include these red flag signs:

- a downward trend in BP;
- signs of hypovolaemia/hypervolaemia;
- a failure to respond to correction of fluid depletion;
  - no increase in urine output;
  - no improvement in BP or CVP;
  - no resolution of tachycardia;
- increased respiratory rate or respiratory difficulties (pulmonary oedema or acidosis);
- increasing confusion/disorientation;
- rising blood urea and creatinine levels;
- electrolyte imbalances—particularly hyperkalaemia.

Patients with CKD

In your capacity as a nurse, you can make important decisions in the assessment, monitoring, and management of many of the physical symptoms with which patients with CKD present (Murphy *et al.*, 2008a, b). Referral to the specialist nephrology team is recommended for all patients in stage 4 CKD and in earlier stages, as per National Institute for Health and Clinical Excellence (NICE) Guidelines (2008a).

How to detect that a patient with CKD is deteriorating

⚑ Changes in health status can occur over weeks or months, and are characterized by some or all of the following:

- Decline in eGFR of >5 ml/min/1.73m² within 1 year, or >10 ml/min/1.73m² within 5 years; other indicators include haematuria and proteinuria
- Poor BP control

Table 11.2   **Assessing the patient with renal impairment**

Focus of assessment	What to assess	Potential problems and causes	Links to Part 2 chapters
Respiratory	Respiratory rate and effort; Evidence of peripheral or central cyanosis; O_2 saturations; Arterial blood gases (ABGs) in the acutely ill patient	Acute or chronic breathlessness; Pulmonary oedema; Metabolic acidosis (Kaussmaul respiration); Pneumonia; Anaemia	Chapter 15 Managing Breathlessness
Cardiovascular	Heart rate; Pulse strength and regularity; BP reading and trends; Orthostatic blood pressure; ECG tracing/cardiac monitoring; Serum potassium	Tachycardia; In CKD, clinical picture more commonly long-term hypertension, cardiovascular disease and fluid retention (see below); In AKI, clinical picture more commonly acute hypotension and hypovolaemia (may develop hypervolaemia if high volumes of fluid given in the continued presence of oliguria/anuria); Changes to ECG, e.g. in hyperkalaemia — tented/peaked T wave, widened QRS complex, risk of cardiac arrest	Chapter 19 Managing Hydration Chapter 6 Understanding Coronary Heart Disease
Renal–urinary output	Closely record and review fluid balance; Observe and measure urine output (hourly if AKI suspected); Response to medication, e.g. diuretic; Daily weight; Urinalysis	Imbalances between fluid intake and fluid output; Inadequate urine output <0.5 ml/kg/h (oliguria/anuria); Rising daily weight indicating fluid retention; Peripheral oedema; Presence of abnormalities in the urine, e.g. protein	Chapter 19 Managing Hydration
Skin	Observe colour and feel of skin; Pressure ulcer risk assessment, e.g. Braden Score	Changes to appearance of skin; Clammy to touch (if acutely unwell); Pruritus caused by rising toxins, dry skin; Rashes, bruising; High risk of skin breakdown/pressure ulcer formation	Chapter 27 Managing the Prevention of Skin Breakdown
Nutritional	Changes to appetite; Nutritional history and dietary assessment; Nutritional screening (e.g. MUST; Malnutrition Universal Screening Tool); Weight loss	Loss of appetite; Nausea (vomiting); Increased risk of GI bleeding; In AKI, patient likely to be catabolic	Chapter 24 Managing Nutrition
Neurological	Establish usual neurological state Abbreviated mental test score (AMT) AVPU assessment Glasgow Coma Scale (as indicated)	Rising toxins affect neurological functioning; Impaired cognition. Confused, agitated, disoriented; Disturbed sleep; Limb weakness	Chapter 17 Managing Delirium and Confusion
Psychosocial	Assess patient and family for their understanding of condition; Potential for future behaviour or lifestyle changes depending on the severity or critical nature of current illness	Patient and family may be in acute distress/crisis. Possible shock, denial, grief-type response; Difficulty retaining information; Anxiety	Chapter 14 Managing Anxiety and Agitation Chapter 18 Managing End-of-Life Care

Table 11.3 Key nursing interventions for the patient with AKI in the non-critical care environment

Care need	Key nursing intervention
Acutely unwell and high risk of mortality	Full ABCDE assessment Increased vital signs monitoring—respond to trends and changes Support for patient and family, sharing information
Managing the effects of underlying cause of AKI	Respond to cause of AKI, i.e. appropriate fluid replacement, treat sepsis, identify and stop nephrotoxic medication, e.g. gentamicin
Correcting fluid imbalances	Exact fluid balance monitoring Urinary catheter patent and draining freely Hourly urine output measurements (aim >0.5 ml/kg body weight/h) Increased monitoring, e.g. central venous pressure (CVP) readings Daily (or more frequent) fluid assessment (➡ Chapter 19 Managing Hydration) May require IV fluid challenges (e.g. 250–500 ml bolus) of appropriate replacement fluid crystalloid/colloid/blood Individualized IV regimen, may need to avoid fluids containing potassium May limit fluid intake/input
Assessing the risk/presence of pulmonary oedema	Monitor respiration rate and oxygen saturations Oxygen therapy Fluid/haemodynamic assessment Kidneys may not respond to diuretic therapy used to treat pulmonary oedema Glyceryl trinitrate may be used as an emergency, temporary measure whilst awaiting access to RRT
Managing the effects of rising waste products of metabolism, confusion, and disorientation	AVPU/neurological assessment Patient safety measures Good communication Increased monitoring of blood chemistry Skin care
Managing the effects of hyperkalaemia (normal range 3.5–5.0 mmol/l)	ECG/cardiac monitoring Medication to reduce cardiac instability, e.g. if >6.5 mmol/l—IV calcium gluconate Dextrose and insulin infusion—temporary effect Calcium resonium/Resonium A are best avoided in AKI
Managing the effects of metabolic acidosis	Regular arterial blood gas monitoring (ABG) Sodium bicarbonate IV infusion may be appropriate where there is intravascular depletion RRT will be required if there is continued deterioration (especially if pH<7.2)
Managing the effects of protein catabolism	Dietary/nutritional assessment—referral to dietitian Dietary supplementation, enteral, or parenteral nutrition often instigated early

- Rising blood urea and creatinine levels
- Increasing lethargy/tiredness, possible confusion
- Increasing oedema or evidence of fluid accumulation
- Respiratory difficulties (fluid/anaemia)
- Loss of appetite, nausea, vomiting

Caring for the patient with CKD should focus upon symptom management, and supporting the patient and his or her family with adaptations to living with a long-term condition.

As the patient nears stage 5 CKD and symptoms worsen, a point is reached at which he or she will need to

Table 11.4 Key nursing interventions for the patient with CKD (stages 3b–5)

Care need	Key nursing intervention	Links to other chapters
Adjustment to long-term condition	Sharing information and developing a therapeutic relationship; Identifying self-management opportunities; Education about long-term options; Linking with patient groups and networks	⟶ Chapter 22 Managing Medicines ⟶ Chapter 14 Managing Anxiety
Living with hypertension and increased cardiovascular risk	Accurate and regular BP and eGFR monitoring (see NICE Guidance, 2008a); Antihypertensive medications management and polypharmacy; Lifestyle changes, e.g. low salt diet, smoking cessation, supporting patient to keep active	⟶ Chapter 22 Managing Medicines ⟶ Chapter 24 Managing Nutrition
Managing fluid imbalances (often fluid retention)	Monitoring fluid intake and managing fluid allowances; Daily weight; Skin care; Diuretic medication management	⟶ Chapter 19 Managing Hydration
Decreasing appetite, risk of malnourishment	Referral to dietitian, and usually notable dietary modification; Supporting the patient with changes to diet: high calorie/energy and individual assessment of protein needs—may be 'normal' protein intake (i.e. 0.8–1 g/kg body weight/day), but debate over low protein diet in CKD continues (Fouque and Laville, 2009)	⟶ Chapter 24 Managing Nutrition
Living with the effects of anaemia	Subcutaneous injections of erythropoiesis stimulating agents (ESAs), often known as 'EPO' (NICE, 2006) Self-management is encouraged Aim for target Hb > 11 g/dl in women and > 12 g/dl in men)	
Managing the effects of long-term renal bone disease	Dietary changes (as serum phosphate rises, reduce phosphate intake); Vitamin D analogue supplementation, e.g. alfacalcidol Phosphate-binding medication, e.g. Calcichew®, Phosex®, Renagel® (taken directly with food)	⟶ Chapter 3 Understanding Bone Conditions
Managing skin care	Skin care and use of emollients for pruritus	⟶ Chapter 27 Managing the Prevention of Skin Breakdown ⟶ Chapter 20 Managing Hygiene
Managing acute and life-threatening effects of renal impairment, e.g. hyperkalaemia, increasing uraemia, metabolic acidosis, pulmonary oedema	Full ABCDE nursing assessment; Dietary modification (often to reduce potassium content of food); In acute/severe hyperkalaemia, ECG/cardiac monitoring and medication to reduce potassium, e.g. calcium resonium/Resonium A and/or dextrose and insulin infusion; Oral sodium bicarbonate may be given to treat chronic metabolic acidosis (especially in conservative management); Fluid limitations and diuretic therapy to maintain fluid balance ; Instigation of RRT or continued conservative management as appropriate	⟶ Chapter 24 Managing Nutrition ⟶ Chapter 19 Managing Hydration

commence RRT or continue with conservative management until the need for palliative intervention is reached. This will be determined by the individual clinical picture and by patient choices, and can be a particular challenge.

Dietary manipulation, along with any necessary reduction in fluid intake (to help to control symptoms), also needs targeted and sustained support. Tackling renal diets is about being able to transform a prescription for nutrients into a tasty selection of foods suited to the individual's tastes, finances, cooking ability, and social circumstances (Sutton, 2004). The key nursing interventions for worsening CKD are outlined in Table 11.4.

There are also a number of nursing interventions that can support patients in the self-management of CKD and encourage lifestyle change where appropriate, including the following:

- reducing cardiovascular risk, e.g. smoking cessation and exercise routine;
- medicines management, e.g. antihypertensive medications and often polypharmacy;
- dietary changes and dietary modification (individualized dietary 'prescription');
- erythropoiesis stimulating agent self-administration for treatment of anaemia (EPO);
- education and preparation for longer term—conservative management or RRT options (stage 4).

Medication in CKD

Many drugs and medications are excreted by the kidney; in renal impairment, these may accumulate, become toxic to the patient, and require dose adjustment (e.g. digoxin) or may need to be avoided altogether (e.g. non-steroidal anti-inflammatory drugs, or NSAIDs). The *British National Formulary* (**www.bnf.org**) provides important guidance for dose adjustment in renal impairment. Patients may need advice about the risks associated with over-the-counter medications, herbal, or Chinese medicines. Polypharmacy is common in CKD (see Chapter 22 Managing Medicines ➡).

End-of-life issues for patients with renal disorders

While the majority of patients adapt and live with CKD and RRT, some patients with advanced CKD will have their symptoms managed conservatively (Douglas *et al.*, 2009) rather than commence dialysis, recognizing that the burden of frequent dialysis may outweigh likely survival and quality-of-life benefits (Noble, 2008). Other patients might withdraw from treatment after they have been receiving RRT for a period of time if they experience a progressive deterioration or poor prognosis related to other comorbidities (White and Fitzpatrick, 2006). In a long-term condition such as CKD, end-of-life decisions need to be considered throughout the patient's trajectory (Noble *et al.*, 2007).

EVIDENCE BOX 11.2

Symptom management for adults dying with advanced kidney disease

- Use the Liverpool Care Pathway (LCP) for the Dying Patient (Renal) and Guidelines for LCP Drug Prescribing in Advanced Chronic Kidney Disease.
- Specific symptoms that patients may experience include: pain; terminal restlessness and agitation; respiratory tract secretions; nausea and vomiting; dyspnoea; and pruritus.
- In pain management, fentanyl and alfentanil are less likely to cause problems of toxicity; therefore avoid other strong opioids.
- Other medications for symptom management may require a 50% reduction in dose, e.g. haloperidol, glycopyrronium.
- Pruritus can be managed with emollients, capsaicin cream, antihistamines, and ondansetron.

(Douglas *et al.*, 2009; Marie Curie Palliative Care Institute, 2008; Murtagh *et al.* 2006)

The Liverpool Care Pathway (LCP) for the Dying Patient (Marie Curie Palliative Care Institute) has been adapted and used successfully for people with renal failure (Douglas *et al.*, 2009). As part of the NHS National End-of-Life Care Programme, a new framework has provided much-needed guidance in managing end-of-life care in advanced kidney disease, focusing on patients opting for conservative kidney management and those 'deteriorating despite' dialysis (National Health Service National End-of-Life Care Programme, 2009).

The symptom burden for those dying with advanced kidney disease is similar to that of those dying with other health problems; end-of-life care is discussed in greater detail in Chapter 18 ➡. However, there are some symptoms and care issues that are particular to patients with advanced renal failure (Evidence box 11.2).

The high mortality rate associated with AKI, especially in the critical care environment, will mean a change in focus of care from saving life to preparing for death. Critical care nurses play a central role in managing the process of withdrawal of treatment (Puntillo, 2001; Puntillo and McAdam, 2006) and clearly influence how death may be shaped (Long-Sutehall *et al.*, 2011). The family may need support through feelings of isolation and loss of control, and may be helped by developing a growing partnership with the healthcare team (Ashwanden, 2002).

Identifying best practice

Supporting and caring for patients with renal impairment can be rewarding and challenging work. Individual patients and their families often become well known to you and the healthcare team, and strong bonds and partnerships form. Viewing services from the standpoint of the patient and working in partnership is now an expectation of healthcare professions (NHS Constitution, 2009). The vast range of clinical guidelines and resources can, at times, be overwhelming. You will need to focus on the key aspects or relevant parts of any guidelines before applying them appropriately to individual patients and patient populations.

Throughout the chapter, you will find recent sources of the best evidence to inform the nursing care of patients with renal disorders. Because research is always ongoing and best practice evolves, it is important that readers stay up to date and know where to find good-quality sources of evidence. Hence we have provided a list of resources that readers should utilize.

Sources of evidence

Renal disorders

The Renal Association http://www.renal.org/home.aspx

Department of Health Kidney Care Programme http://www.kidneycare.nhs.uk/

NHS Evidence—Kidney Diseases https://www.evidence.nhs.uk/search?q=Kidney+diseases

Kidney Diseases—Improving Global Outcomes (KDIGO) http://www.kdigo.org/nephrology_guideline_database/compare_guideline_targets.php

NHS Institute for Innovation and Improvement—Toolkit for preparing for end-stage renal disease http://www.institute.nhs.uk/quality_and_value/high_volume_care/focus_on%3a_renal.html

National Service Framework for Renal Services (Parts One and Two) and subsequent supporting documents http://www.dh.gov.uk/en/Healthcare/Longtermconditions/Vascular/Renal/index.htm

CKD and primary healthcare

Chronic Kidney Disease—A Guide for Primary Care http://www.ckdonline.org/home/

Chronic Kidney Disease Frequently Asked Questions (NHS Employers/BMJ Publication) http://www.nhsemployers.org/Aboutus/Publications/Documents/Chronic_kidney_disease_FAQs_2nd_ed.pdf

NICE CKD Guidelines http://guidance.nice.org.uk/CG73

Kidney Research UK, ABLE project: health awareness for minority ethnic communities http://www.kidneyresearchuk.org/special-projects/able.php

AKI

Acute Kidney Injury Network http://www.akinet.org/

End-of-life care

End-of-life care in advanced kidney disease: a framework for implementation (part of the NHS National End of Life Care Programme) http://www.kidneycare.nhs.uk/Library/endoflifecarefinal.pdf

Resources for patients

National Kidney Federation http://www.kidney.org.uk/

Diabetes UK http://www.diabetes.org.uk/

British Kidney Patient Association http://www.britishkidney-pa.co.uk/

NHS Choices http://www.nhs.uk/Pages/HomePage.aspx

NHS guide to long-term conditions and self-care http://www.nhs.uk/tools/pages/longterm.aspx

Journals and organizations

A range of journals is available, some in a highly readable format that makes keeping up-to-date easy.

Journal of Renal Nursing http://www.renalnursing.co.uk/

British Journal of Renal Medicine http://www.bjrm.co.uk/bjrm/default.asp

Royal College of Nursing Nephrology Forum http://www.rcn.org.uk/development/communities/rcn_forum_communities/nephrology

British Renal Society http://www.britishrenal.org/

European Dialysis and Transplant Nurses Association/ European Renal Care Association http://www.edtnaerca.org/

Conclusion

Nurses can play a vital role in the identification and prevention of progression of CKD and AKI. You will also be crucial in helping the patient and family to adapt to his or her health problems, and in his or her education for self-management, particularly in CKD.

The role of the primary healthcare team in the identification, monitoring, and timely referral of patients with CKD is now clearly defined. Interventions that impact upon the progression of CKD focus upon effective monitoring and management of blood pressure, timely referral and liaison with the specialist renal team, and education for patients and their families, preparing them for lifestyle change. The evaluation and impact of the National Institute for Health and Clinical Excellence (NICE) Guidelines (2008a) is currently being assessed.

In patients with AKI, you can play a central role in identifying those who may be at risk of developing AKI, and ensuring that measures are in place to reduce the risk. These may be simple measures such as commencing fluid balance recordings and ensuring a regimen of fluid replacement (oral or IV) for a patient with diarrhoea. In acute and high care environments, nursing care should focus upon effective monitoring, and responding to changes and trends that indicate that a patient is developing AKI. Support for the family is also important.

The effectiveness and appropriateness of the nursing management of these problems will depend on an in-depth knowledge and understanding of renal disorders. We hope that this chapter will help you to develop this expertise. We would like to thank Robert Lewis for his support and valuable comment.

Online Resource Centre

 To help you to develop and apply your knowledge and decision-making skills further, we have provided interactive learning resources online at **www.oxfordtextbooks.co.uk/orc/bullock/**

Whilst these are freely available, you will need to use the access codes at the start of the book.

References

Andrews, P.A. (2008) Early identification and management of chronic kidney disease in adults in primary and secondary care: a commentary on NICE guideline No. 73. *British Journal of Diabetes and Vascular Disease* **8**(6): 257–62.

Armitage, A., Thomson, C. (2003) Acute renal failure. *Medicine* **31**: 43–8.

Ashwanden, C. (2002) The effects of acute renal failure on the family. *EDTNA/ERCA Journal* (Suppl. 2): 56–8.

Atkins, R.C., Briganiti, E.M., Lewis, J.B., *et al.* (2005) Proteinuria reduction and progression to renal failure in patients with type 2 diabetes mellitus and over nephropathy. *American Journal of Kidney Disease* **45**(2): 281–7.

Auer, J. (2005) *Living Well with Kidney Failure: A Guide to Living your Life to the Full.* Class Publishing Ltd: London.

Bollomo, R., Kellum, J.A., Ronco, C. (2004) Defining acute renal failure: physiological principles. *Intensive Care Medicine* **30**: 33–7.

Bradley, J. (2009) Injury time: losing out in acute kidney injury (editorial). *British Journal of Renal Medicine* **14**(3): 3.

Chertow, G.M., Burdick, E., Honour, M., *et al.* (2005) Acute kidney injury, mortality, length of stay, and costs in hospitalized patients. *Journal of the American Society of Nephrology* **16**: 3365–70.

Crowe, E., Forrest, C., McIntyre, N., *et al.* (2008) Early identification and management of chronic kidney disease in primary health care. *Primary Health Care* **18**(10): 29–33.

DASH Trial (2001) Effects on blood pressure of reduced dietary sodium and the dietary approaches to stop hypertension (DASH). *New England Journal of Medicine* **344**(1): 3–10.

DCCT (1993) The effect of intensive treatment of diabetes on the development and progression of long-term complications in insulin-dependent diabetes mellitus: The Diabetes Control and

Complications Trial Research Group. *New England Journal of Medicine* **329**: 977–86.

De Lusignan, S., Gallagher, H., Stevens, P., *et al.* (2010) *Chronic Kidney Disease: Frequently Asked Questions*. NHS Emloyers/BMJ: London. http://www.nhsemployers.org/Aboutus/Publications/Documents/Chronic_kidney_disease_FAQs_2nd_ed.pdf (accessed 17 October 2011).

Department of Health (2004) *National Service Framework for Renal Services Part One: Dialysis and Transplantation*. Department of Health: London. http://www.dh.gov.uk/en/Publicationsandstatistics/Publications/Publications PolicyAndGuidance/DH_4070359 (accessed 17 October 2011).

Department of Health (2005a) *National Service Framework for Renal Services Part Two: Chronic Kidney Disease, Acute Renal Failure and End of Life Care*. Department of Health: London. http://www.dh.gov.uk/en/Publicationsandstatistics/Publications/PublicationsPolicyAndGuidance/DH_4101902 (accessed 17 October 2011).

Department of Health (2005b) *Supporting People with Long Term Conditions: Liberating the Talents of Nurses who Care for People with Long Term Conditions*. Department of Health: London. http://www.dh.gov.uk/en/Publicationsandstatistics/Publications/PublicationsPolicyAndGuidance/DH_4102469 (accessed 17 October 2011).

Department of Health (2007) *The National Service Framework for Renal Services: Second Progress Report*. Department of Health: London. http://www.dh.gov.uk/en/Publicationsandstatistics/Publications/PublicationsPolicyAndGuidance/DH_074811 (accessed 17 October 2011).

Department of Health (2008) *Vascular Programme: Putting Prevention First Vascular Checks/Risk Assessment and Management*. F—VC, RAM Department of Health: London. http://www.dh.gov.uk/en/Publicationsandstatistics/Publications/PublicationsPolicyAndGuidance/DH_083822 (accessed 17 October 2011).

Department of Health (2009) *Achieving Excellence in Kidney Care: Delivering the National Service Framework for Renal Services*. Department of Health: London. http://www.dh.gov.uk/en/Publicationsandstatistics/Publications/PublicationsPolicyAndGuidance/DH_109978.

Douglas, C., Murtagh, F.E., Chambers, E.J., *et al.* (2009) Symptom management for the adult patient dying with advanced chronic kidney disease: a review of the literature and development of evidence-based guidelines by a United Kingdom Expert Consensus Group. *Palliative Medicine* **23**: 103–10.

Endacott, R., Jevon, P., Cooper, S. (2009) *Clinical Nursing Skills: Core and Advanced*. Oxford University Press: Oxford.

Fouque, D., Laville, M. (2009) Low protein diets for chronic kidney disease in non-diabetic adults. *Cochrane Database of Systematic Reviews* Issue 3: Art. No. CD001892. DOI: 10.1002/14651858.CD001892.pub3.

Gilbert, M., Staley, C., Lydall-Smith, S., *et al.* (2008) Use of collaboration to improve outcomes in chronic disease. *Disease Management and Health Outcomes* **16**(6): 381–90.

Glynne, P.A., Lightstone, L. (2001) Acute renal failure. *Clinical Medicine* **1**(4): 266–73.

Go, A.S., Chertow, G.M., Fan, D., *et al.* (2004) Chronic kidney disease and the risks of death, carciovascular events and hospitalization. *New England Journal of Medicine* **351**: 1296–305.

Hain, D., Calvin, D.J., Simmons, D.E. (2009) CKD education: an evolving concept. *Nephrology Nursing Journal* **36**(3): 317–19.

Heffernan, C. (2008) Population Screening for Chronic Kidney Disease. UK National Screening Committee. www.screening.nhs.uk/policydb_download.php?doc=2 (accessed 17 October 2011).

Kazmi, W.H., Obrador, G.T., Khan, S.S., *et al.* (2004) Late nephrology referral and mortality among patients with end-stage renal disease: a propensity score analysis. *Nephrology Dialysis Transplantation* **19**(7): 1808–14.

Khwaja, A., Throssell, D. (2009) A critique of the UK NICE guidance for the detection and management of individuals with chronic kidney disease. *Nephron* **113**(3): c207–14.

Klebe, B., Irving, J., Stevens, P.E., *et al.* (2007) The cost of implementing UK guidelines for the management of chronic kidney disease. *Nephrology Dialysis Transplantation* **22**: 2504–12.

Levey, A.S., Greene, T., Kusek, J.W., *et al.* (2000) A simplified equation to predict glomerular filtration rate from serum creatinine. *Journal of the American Society of Nephrology* **11**: A0828.

Levy, J., Brown, E., Daley, C., *et al.* (2009) *The Oxford Handbook of Dialysis*. Oxford University Press: Oxford.

Liano, F., Junco, E., Pascual, J., *et al.* (1998) The spectrum of acute renal failure in the intensive care unit compared with that seen in other settings: the Madrid Acute Renal Failure Study Group. *Kidney International* **53**: S16–24.

Long-Sutehall, T., Willis, H., Palmer, R., *et al.* (2011) Negotiated dying: a grounded theory of how nurses shape withdrawal of treatment in hospital critical care units. *International Journal of Nursing Studies*, **48**:1466–74.

MacGregor, M.S. (2007) How common is early chronic kidney disease: a backgound paper prepared for the UK consensus conference on early chronic kidney disease. *Nephrology Dialysis Transplantation* **22**(Suppl. 9): ix8–ix18.

Marie Curie Palliative Care Institute Liverpool (2008) The Liverpool Care Pathway for the dying patient. http://www.mcpcil.org.uk/liverpool-care-pathway/ (accessed 17 October 2011).

Marieb, E. (2009) *Essentials of Human Anatomy and Physiology*, 9th edn. Pearson Education Inc: San Francisco CA.

McGee, H., Bradley, C. (1994) *Quality of Life Following Renal Failure*. Harwood Academic Publishers: Chur, Switzerland.

Murphy, F., Jenkins, K., Chamney, M., *et al.* (2008a) Patient management in chronic kidney disease stages 1 and 3. *Journal of Renal Care* **34**(4): 127–35.

Murphy, F., Jenkins, K., McCann, M., *et al.* Sedgewick, J. (2008b) Patient management in chronic kidney disease stages 4 and 5. *Journal of Renal Care* **34**(4): 191–8.

Murtagh, F.E.M., Addington-Hall, J.M., Donohoe, P., *et al.* (2006) Symptom management in patients with established renal failure managed without dialysis. *EDTNA/ERCA Journal* **XXXII/**(2): 93–8.

Nalker, S.S., Liu, K.D., Chertow, G.M. (2009) The incidence and prognostic significance of acute kidney injury. *Current Opinion in Nephrology and Hypertension* **16**: 227–36.

National Confidential Enquiry into Patient Outcome and Death (2009) *Adding Insult to Injury*. National Confidential Enquiry into Patient Outcome and Death: London.

National Health Service Constitution (2009) **http://www.nhs.uk/choiceintheNHS/Rightsandpledges/NHSConstitution/Documents/NHS_Constitution_interactive_9Mar09.pdf** (accessed 28 February 2010).

National Health Service National End of Life Care Programme (2009) End of life care in advanced kidney disease: a framework for implementation. **http://www.endoflifecare.nhs.uk/eolc/kidney.htm** (accessed 17 October 2011).

National Health Service (NHS) Institute for Innovation and Improvement, High Volume Care Kidney Project. **http://www.institute.nhs.uk/quality_and_value/high_volume_care/focus_on%3a_renal.html** (accessed 21 February 2010).

National Institute for Health and Clinical Excellence (NICE) (2003) Pre-operative tests: the use of routine pre-operative tests for elective surgery. NICE Clinical Guideline 3 (CG3). **http://guidance.nice.org.uk/CG3** (accessed 17 October 2011).

National Institute for Clinical Excellence (NICE) (2006) Anaemia management in CKD. NICE Clinical Guideline 39 (CG39). **http://guidance.nice.org.uk/CG39** (accessed 17 October 2011).

National Institute for Health and Clinical Excellence (NICE) (2008a) Chronic kidney disease: early identification and management of chronic kidney disease in adults in primary and secondary care. NICE Clinical Guideline 73 (CG73). **http://guidance.nice.org.uk/CG73** (accessed 17 October 2011).

National Institute for Health and Clinical Excellence (NICE) (2008b) Type 2 Diabetes National clinical guideline for management in primary care and secondary care (update). **http://www.nice.org.uk/nicemedia/pdf/CG66FullGuideline0509.pdf** and partial update 2009 **http://www.nice.org.uk/nicemedia/pdf/CG87ShortGuideline.pdf** (accessed 23 March 2011).

Noble, H. (2008) Supportive and palliative care for the patient with end-stage renal disease. *British Journal of Nursing* **17**(8): 498–504.

Noble, H., Kelly, D., Rawlings-Anderson, K., *et al.* (2007) A concept analysis of renal supportive care: the changing world of nephrology. *Journal of Advanced Nursing* **59**(6): 644–53.

O'Donoghue, D. (2009) Editorial. *British Journal of Primary Care Nursing* (special issue: chronic kidney disease) **6**(4): 3–4.

Perkins, C., Kisiel, M. (2005) Utilising physiological knowledge to care for acute renal failure. *British Journal of Nursing* **14**(14): 768–73.

Puntillo, K.A. (2001) End-of-life issues in intensive care units: a national random survey of nurses' knowledge and beliefs. *American Journal of Critical Care* **10**: 216–29.

Puntillo, K.A., McAdam, J.L. (2006) Communication between physicians and nurses as a target for improving end-of-life care in the intensive care unit: challenges and opportunities for moving forward. *Critical Care Medicine* **34**(11 Suppl.): S332–40.

Redmond, A., McDevitt, M., Barnes, S. (2004) Acute renal failure: recognition and treatment in ward patients. *Nursing Standard* **18**(22): 46–53.

Renal Association UK (2008) *Clinical Practice Guidelines*, 4th edn. Module 5: Acute Kidney Injury. Royal College of Physicians, Renal Association: London. **http://www.renal.org/clinical/Guide lines-Section/Guidelines.aspx** (accessed 17 October 2011).

Renal Registry (2009) *12th Annual Report*. Renal Registry: Bristol. **http://www.renalreg.com/Reports/2009.html** (accessed 4 April 2011).

Roberts, S. (2007) *Improving Diabetes Services: The NSF Four Years On—The Way Ahead: The Local Challenges*. Department of Health: London. **http://www.dh.gov.uk/dr_consum_dh/groups/dh_digitalassets/documents/digitalasset/dh_072779.pdf** (accessed 28 February 2010).

Steddon, S., Ashman, N., Chesser, A., *et al.* (2006) *Oxford Handbook of Nephrology and Hypertension*. Oxford University Press: Oxford.

Stevens L.A., Levey, A. (2009) Measured GFR as a confirmatory test for estimated GFR. *Journal of the American Society of Nephrology* **20**: 2305–13.

Stevens, P.E., O'Donoghue, D.J., de Lusigan, S., *et al.* (2007) Chronic kidney disease management in the United Kingdom: NEOERICA project results. *Kidney International* **72**: 92–9

Stevens, P.E., Tamimi, N.A., Al-Hasani, M.K., *et al.* (2001) Non-specialist management of acute renal failure. *Quarterly Journal of Medicine* **94**: 533–40.

Sutton, D. (2004) Renal nutrition. In N. Thomas, (ed.) *Advanced Renal Care*. Blackwell Publishing: Oxford. pp. 167–83.

Thomas, N. (2005) Can we delay the progression of chronic kidney disease (CKD) by improving collaboration between renal units and primary care teams? *EDTNA/ERCA Journal* **31**(4): 178–81.

Thomas, N. (2008) *Renal Nursing*, 3rd edn. BaillièreTindall Elsevier: Edinburgh.

Thomas, N. (2009) Timetable of tests for chronic kidney disease. *British Journal of Primary Care Nursing* (special issue: chronic kidney disease) **6**(2): 18–19.

Tonelli, M., Weibe, N., Culleton, B., *et al.* (2006) Chronic kidney disease and mortality risk: a systematic review. *Journal of the American Society of Nephrology* **17**(7): 2034–47.

Traynor, J., Mactier, R., Geddes, C.C., *et al.* (2006) How to measure renal function in clinical practice. *British Medical Journal* **333**: 733–7.

White, Y., Fitzpatrick, G. (2006) Dialysis: prolonging life or prolonging dying? Ethical, legal and professional considerations for end-of-life decision-making. *EDTNA/ERCA Journal* **32**(2): 99–103.

12 *Understanding* **Skin Conditions**

Steven J. Ersser

Introduction

The aim of this chapter is to provide nurses with the knowledge to be able to assess, manage, and care for people with skin conditions in an evidence-based and person-centred way. The chapter will provide a comprehensive overview of the commonest skin diseases and their causes before exploring best practice to assess and help patients to manage skin conditions. Nursing priorities are highlighted throughout, and the nursing management of the symptoms and common health problems associated with skin conditions can be found in Chapters 19, 20, 21, 24, 27, and 28 on skin care and the maintenance of skin hygiene, skin barrier integrity, the prevention of skin breakdown, and wound management, respectively ➡.

Skin care is a fundamental area of nursing responsibility. The skin, or integumentary system, is the largest organ of the body and has significant protective and thermoregulatory functions. Skin disease is common, accounting for approximately 24% of GP visits (Schofield *et al.*, 2009). It may have a major psychosocial impact on a person's quality of life through its influence on appearance, body image, and self-esteem. This chapter introduces you to the common skin diseases that you are likely to encounter when caring for adult patients and outlines the nursing problems that you will need to manage.

The causes of skin conditions

The cause or aetiology of common skin conditions lies with the interaction between genetic and environmental factors. For example, a child's eczema is influenced by his or her genotype and his or her exposure to environmental allergens. Within the UK population, 23–25% have a skin problem at some time in their lives that can benefit from medical care (Schofield *et al.*, 2009). Skin problems are the commonest reason for consulting a GP, with 6% referred for specialist advice. As such, all registered nurses should have the knowledge and skills to manage the common conditions. The commonest skin conditions in the Western hemisphere are chronic inflammatory skin diseases (CISDs), such as eczema. In developing countries, the common conditions are infections and infestations. The quality-of-life impact of CISDs can exceed that for life-threatening conditions such as cancer (Rapp *et al.*, 1999; Kingman, 2005).

Skin disease and external factors, such as trauma and the physical environment, disrupt normal skin structure

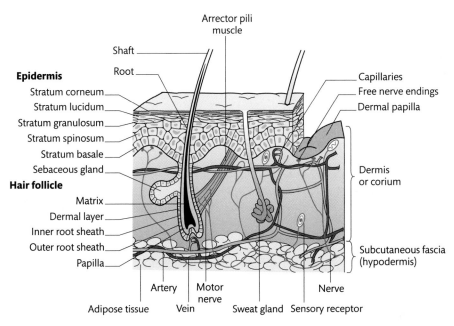

Figure 12.1 The structure of the skin.

Reproduced from Colbert *et al.*, *Anatomy & Physiology for Nurses and Health Professionals* (2009), 1st revision, by permission of Pearson Education.

and affect the skin barrier function. The skin barrier concept is important to your understanding of the integument as a protective system. Figure 12.1 depicts the skin structure (Colbert *et al.*, 2009).

The various skin layers, the outer epidermis and the inner dermis, provide the protective capacity of the skin. The epidermis is comprised of multiple cell layers. The skin is given strength by the organization of its protein fibres, including collagen, which act like the girders of a building, giving it strength; elastin fibres provide elasticity and the reticulin fibres provide a mesh, adding resilience. The skin barrier is comprised of protein and lipids (fat) layers. Other key protective factors include sebum, a natural skin oil or emollient produced by the sebaceous glands, keeping the skin supple. Another key protective system is the acid mantle, in which the pH of the skin inhibits the growth of pathogens (Penzer and Ersser, 2010).

Disease and physicochemical factors, such as pressure and the application of soap and detergents, can disrupt this intricate barrier system (see Chapters 20 and 21 ➡). For example, the inflammatory changes of eczema may lead to behavioural responses such as scratching, which increases infection risk. Immobile patients may have impaired microcirculation to skin and therefore potential poor skin integrity due to pressure from the weight of the body over bony prominences, such as the sacrum. Excessive washing of the skin aggravates these problems by removing sebum and leaving an alkaline residue. An understanding of the skin barrier will help you to appreciate the significance of its disruption by dermatological diseases. The recent advances in understanding the aetiology of atopic eczema may illustrate this (Buxton and Morris-Jones, 2009). Inflammation here results primarily from an inherited skin barrier defect in key proteins, called filaggrins (Elias and Steinhoff, 2008).

Common skin problems

Some of the commonest skin problems are eczema, psoriasis, oedema, infection, infestations, and skin cancers. These are described in the following section, along with detail on their prevalence and causative factors. In each case, nursing intervention can protect the skin barrier through careful skin hygiene, emollient therapy, and supporting patients to understand and use their treatment effectively.

To identify skin conditions accurately, it is important to understand the nature and distinction between a lesion and a rash. A lesion is a localized pathological change in the skin or tissues, whereas a rash is a pattern of skin lesions. Further details on the nature and assessment of lesions and rashes are discussed later to provide the basis for developing your ability to assess abnormalities of the skin.

Eczema

Eczema is the commonest cause of a scaly itchy (pruritic) rash. The main types follow.

Exogenous (contact dermatitis)

This is caused by an external agent—leading to either an irritant or an allergic reaction (Figure 12.2a; Graham-Brown and Burns, 2007).

Endogenous (atopic eczema or dermatitis)

Atopic dermatitis (AD) (Figure 12.2b; Williams *et al.*, 1995) presents as an itchy skin condition, plus three or more of the following:

- past involvement of skin creases;
- personal or immediate family history of asthma or hay fever;
- tendency towards dry skin;
- onset under the age of 2;
- visual flexural dermatitis;

The lesions are typically flat, of varying size, rather diffuse, and red (erythematous) (see Table 12.1). AD has a

(a)

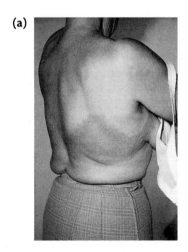

(b)

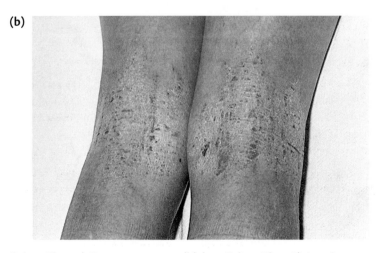

Figure 12.2 **(a) (see Colour Plate 1) Contact eczema. (b) (see Colour Plate 2) Atopic eczema.**

(a) Reproduced from Saxe *et al.* (2007) *Handbook of Dermatology for Primary Care*, with permission from Oxford University Press.

(b) Reproduced from Mackie (2003) *Clinical Dermatology*, with permission from Oxford University Press.

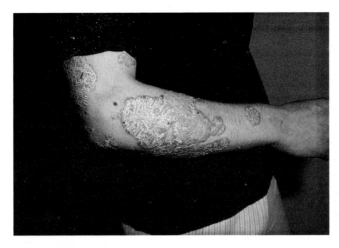

Figure 12.3 **(see Colour Plate 3) Plaque psoriasis.**

Reproduced from Saxe *et al.* (2007) *Handbook of Dermatology for Primary Care*, with permission from Oxford University Press.

prevalence of 15–20% in children aged 7–18 but is higher in the first 5 years (Herd, 2000).

Psoriasis

Psoriasis is an inflammatory disease of skin characterized by an accelerated rate of epidermal turnover owing to genetically based defective maturation of epidermal keratinocytes. It affects 1–3% of the population (Naldi and Chalmers, 2008). It is typically a chronic disease, with chronic plaque psoriasis manifesting as well demarcated, often symmetrically distributed over extensor surfaces, at sites of trauma, Koebner phenomenon and also in the flexures, with thickened, salmon pink, and scaly plaques (Table 12.1 and Figure 12.3). Other forms include guttate psoriasis, which is an acute form, with a droplet-like rash mainly affecting the trunk, but also involving the limbs and scalp, which is triggered by group B haemolytic streptococcus throat infection, affecting younger people (Burge and Wallis, 2011).

Chronic oedema and lymphoedema

Chronic oedema is a broad term used to describe oedema present for more than 3 months and may involve many areas of the body including, for example, the limbs, hands, feet, breast, genitals, and head. It has multiple causes, but common ones include changes in venous pressure related to cardiac or vascular disease, capillary permeability, and factors such as serum protein levels when malnourished.

Lymphoedema is oedema that develops as a result of a failure in the lymphatic system (Figure 12.4), but chronic oedema may have a more complex underlying aetiology (Moffatt *et al.*, 2003). Primary lymphoedema is congenital. Secondary lymphoedema is caused by injury, which may follow surgical removal of the lymph vessels, obstruction by tumours, or obstruction of lymph flow in the vessels, or nodes by parasites, such as worm infestation. Although lymphoedema is not a skin condition, if not managed properly, it can have a significant impact on the condition of the skin.

Skin infections

Skin infections are caused by a range of pathogenic micro-organisms and are a common reason for seeing a GP (Schofield *et al.*, 2009). When washing a patient, you may observe inflamed infected lesions and you can help to prevent these through educating patients on skin hygiene, including adequate drying of the skin. The skin is host to many microorganisms that are harmless to the skin (commensals), but these may invade a damaged epidermis. Bacterial infections are the commonest type of skin infection. They produce signs of acute inflammation: erythema, oedema, heat, and pain. Invasion into the deeper tissues causes cellulitis (Figure 12.5). Common problems include infected eczema, impetigo, boils (furuncles), folliculitis, and erysipelas (Burge and Wallis, 2011).

Viral infections, such as herpes simplex infections, manifest as small vesicles affecting the mouth, face, and

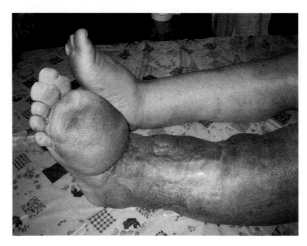

Figure 12.4 **(see Colour Plate 4) Lymphoedema.**

Image courtesy of Professor Christine Moffat.

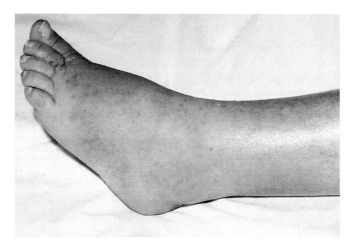

Figure 12.5 **(see Colour Plate 5) Cellulitis.**

Reproduced from Mackie (2003) *Clinical Dermatology*, with permission from Oxford University Press.

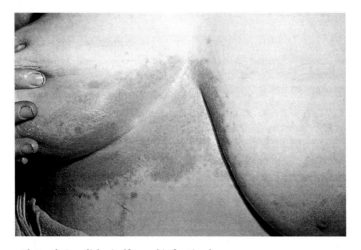

Figure 12.6 **(see Colour Plate 6) Candidosis (fungal infection).**

Reproduced from Mackie (2003) *Clinical Dermatology*, with permission from Oxford University Press.

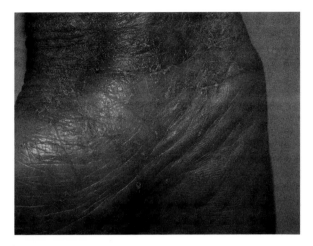

Figure 12.7 (see Colour Plate 7) Scabies.

Reproduced from Saxe *et al.* (2007) *Handbook of Dermatology for Primary Care,* with permission from Oxford University Press.

genitalia. Herpes zoster (shingles) is caused by reactivation of previously acquired varicella zoster virus (chicken pox). Shingles appears as a rash of erythematous papules that usually precede vesicles, which crust as they resolve. Conditions such as infection by HIV (human immunodeficiency virus) commonly manifest as skin conditions (up to 80%), and these become more serious in such a disease: for example, a common skin infection such as a fungal rash and non-infective conditions such as Karposi's sarcoma . You need to be aware of and report repeated or widespread infection, which may reflect immunosuppression.

Fungi can cause infection of the epidermis and mucosa, affecting the skin, hair, nails, and orogenital tract. There are two common types of fungal infection:

- dermatophyte moulds (e.g. tinea infections, such as that affecting the body, groin, and feet—athlete's foot);
- yeasts (e.g. candida infections—which most commonly occur in infants and the elderly, and young to middle aged women in whom it presents as thrush, e.g. Figure 12.6); they are common in hot climates and the immunosuppressed—Seal *et al.*, 2000; Buxton and Morris-Jones, 2009).

Skin infestations

The commonest infestation worldwide is scabies, caused by the *Sarcoptes scabiei* mite. The female burrows into the epidermis, laying eggs that hatch in larvae, spreading readily. They cause intense itching—especially at night.

The finger web spaces and genitals may have mite burrows (Figure 12.7). Another common infestation is of lice, which affect the head, body, and pubic area, accompanied by itching and visible eggs (as nits—the white empty egg cases) (Buxton and Morris-Jones, 2009). The incidence of both scabies and headlice has declined over recent years (Schofield *et al.*, 2001; 2009), but they remain significant health problems. Nurses have a key teaching role to prevent the transfer of infestations and to educate patients on the effective sequencing of anti-scabies treatments such as topical permethrin.

Skin cancer

Skin cancer is the most frequently diagnosed cancer in the UK (Cancer Research UK, 2009). The main types are melanoma (MSC) (Figure 12.8) and non-melanoma skin cancer (NMSC).

The primary cause of skin cancer is ultraviolet (UV) radiation. Melanoma occurs following the malignant transformation of melanocytes (Barnhill *et al.*, 1993). NMSC refers to a number of skin cancers that are not melanomas, and includes basal cell and squamous cell carcinomas, which are common compared to melanoma. Many skin lesions are benign; this includes viral conditions such as warts or molluscum contagiosum with its papules (see Table 12.1), or those caused by solar (ultraviolet) damage, e.g. actinic (solar) keratosis in sun-exposed areas (Poyner, 2000). The All Party Parliamentary Group on Skin (2003) reports that the incidence of skin cancer has doubled over the past

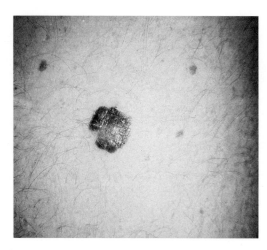

Figure 12.8   (see Colour Plate 8) Melanoma.

Reproduced from Saxe *et al.* (2007) *Handbook of Dermatology for Primary Care*, with permission from Oxford University Press.

20 years. As a nurse, you have a significant role in preventing skin cancer by advising on how to minimize UV exposure. Cancer Research UK is a reliable evidence source (see Table 12.4).

Assessing the patient with a skin condition

Making a physical assessment

You need to be able to undertake a systematic assessment of the skin and be able to recognize common lesions and skin rashes, and to assess the skin barrier.

Understanding lesions and rashes is essential for effective clinical assessment, referral, and planning effective nursing intervention. They are the building blocks, which may be assembled in typical patterns or distributions, which are indicative of specific diseases. The different distributions of rashes can be an important indicator to understanding its causation or nature. Poyner (2000) gives a clear illustration of these. For example, some rashes are localized, such as that owing to contact allergy—affecting, say, a nurse's hand after prolonged washing with harsh detergents or in areas where nickel jewellery is worn. Other localized factors may be caused by the influence of the sun in sun-exposed sites, as in polymorphic light eruption or following herpes simplex infection around the mouth.

In contrast, there are also generalized rashes that have distinctive patterns of distribution, such as atopic eczema, which affects the face, neck, the elbows, and the backs of the knees (the popliteal fossae). Another is illustrated by plaque psoriasis, in which the rash is often symmetrical in distribution, with scaly, well-defined lesions called plaques (Table 12.1) producing silvery scale. By careful description of these lesions, noting their patterns and distribution in clinical notes, you will be able to build up the assessment picture and monitor changes over time.

Given the number and complexity of dermatological symptoms, it is beyond the scope of practice of the non-specialist qualified nurse to diagnose common skin conditions definitively. However, it is vital to pass on clear, useful, and relevant information to the colleagues that will be making the final diagnosis. Understanding lesions is essential for effective clinical assessment and planning intervention, and you should develop the skills needed to identify common rashes (or patterns of lesions) by recognizing their distribution (Lawrence and Cox, 2002). The four main areas of your assessment should be as followes.

- Has the skin's integrity (barrier) been maintained?
- Does the patient have skin lesions and, if so, what type?
- What are their surface features and distribution?
- Are there any red flag skin signs? (See Table 12.2.)

Table 12.1 Common lesion types and their description

Flat: macule	Circumscribed area of altered skin colour <1 cm diameter, e.g. vitiligo, solar lentigo
Flat: patch	Lesion >1 cm in diameter, e.g. port wine stain
Raised: papule	Lesion <1 cm in diameter, e.g. molluscum
Raised: plaque	Slightly raised flat-topped lesion >1 cm in diameter of surface skin, e.g. plaque psoriasis
Raised: nodule	Solid palpable mass >1 cm the greater part of which lies beneath the skin, e.g. basal cell carcinoma
Fluid-filled: vesicle	Small lesion <5 mm diameter, e.g. herpes simplex, eczema herpeticum
Fluid-filled: bullae (blister)	Lesion >5 mm diameter, e.g. bullous pemphigoid
Fluid-filled: pustule	Lesion <1 cm filled with pus, e.g. acne vulgaris
Due to broken surface: ulcer	Loss of at least the epidermis and often the dermis, e.g. decubitus (pressure) ulcer
Due to broken surface: erosion	Loss of epidermis only, e.g. intertrigo (a rash in the body folds)
Colour: due to blood	Petechiae (pinhead size), e.g. meningococcal disease (do not disappear when pressure applied)—purpuric lesions up to 2 mm across
	Purpura (<2.5 mm): red, purple, or brown colour (leaking from blood vessels)
	Haematoma (bruise)
	Telangiectasia: spider-like capillaries (cause, e.g. longer term treatment with topical corticosteroid therapy)
Colour: due to pigment	May be caused by increase in melanin pigment following epidermal inflammation, e.g. lichen planus
Colour: due to lack of blood/ pigment	Depigmentation: complete loss of melanin, e.g. vitiligo

Source: Esser (2010a)

Table 12.1 summarizes commonly observed skin lesions, reflecting their different features, and patterns of variation in size, colour, distribution and elevation. You will also need to determine and describe the skin's surface features using the following descriptors: normal scaly hyperkeratotic or thickened (e.g. psoriasis); warty (e.g. seborrhoeic keratosis); crust (e.g. the skin infection impetigo); exudate (arising from, say, small vesicles in eczema); and excoriation (scraped or scratched skin, as seen in eczema). Your nursing assessment should identify whether the rash is generalized, localized, symmetrical, or asymmetrical and consider whether the rash is confluent (merging into each other) or is interrupted by intervening areas of normal appearing skin.

These observations provide clues to causation and intervention.

Reporting these observations is an important nursing role. Your assessment must consider stage of development (from neonatal to elderly) and ethnic variations (Kelly and Taylor, 2009). People of colour comprise the majority of the world's population, with Asian people making up more than half of the Earth's population, yet the literature on the characteristics of those with skin of colour is limited. Skin assessment therefore requires consideration of the effect of different melanin levels, how this may affect coloration, and the appearance of lesions and rashes among ethnic minorities or non-Caucasian skin. Where possible, use good-quality image sources to aid lesion assessment (see Table 12.4, sections 6 and 7).

Table 12.2 **Some examples of red flag skin signs: requiring urgent referral**

Meningitis 🚩	Rash can start with a few lesions and then may spread quickly, but may also fade and return. The rash that does not fade (blanche) under pressure (glass test) is a sign of meningococcal septicaemic fever, along with headache, photophobia, and stiff neck.
Adverse drug reactions 🚩	Often affect the skin, typically because of an immune reaction, causing generalized or localized rashes, typically maculopapular and erythematous. Note the timing in relation to drug administration. Sometimes purpuric. See Buxton and Morris-Jones, 2009.

Table 12.3 **Topical corticosteroids and their relative potency**

Potency	Generic name (example)	Proprietary name
Mild	Hydrocortisone 1%	Mildison®
Moderate	Clobetasone butyrate 0.05%	Eumovate®
Potent	Mometasone furoate 0.1%	Elocon®
High or superpotent	Clobetasol proprionate 0.05%	Dermovate®

Nurses also need to observe the skin's integrity and examine for breaches or disruption. Assisting patients whilst providing routine skin care provides an excellent opportunity to examine and observe its condition, including dryness (xerosis), loss of elasticity and hydration, or microvasculature status, such as erythema (see Chapters 20 and 27 ➡️).

A key safety issue is the ability to recognize and highlight red flag rashes, which are skin-related signs that require prompt medical referral 🚩. Examples are given in Table 12.2.

Making a psychological assessment

In your capacity as a nurse, you must also be able to identify the person's responses to his or her disease (Royal College of Nursing, 2003). The significance of the quality-of-life impact has been highlighted (and its measurement is discussed below). However, there is a need to identify specific common psychological responses to chronic skin conditions, such as the impact of prolonged anxiety and stress on the immune system and how this may affect disease severity. An example often seen is the deterioration of psoriasis during periods of acute stress. Mental health problems may aggravate some skin conditions or be an adverse consequence of conditions such as depression, owing in part to their impact on body image, social confidence, and on building personal relationships.

Using measurement tools in physical and psychological assessments

There is an array of tools to assist you in the process of examining the skin and people's responses to it, which may help you to make more systematic and informed assessments and evaluations of interventions. Skin samples include skin scrapings for mycology (fungal) assessment, or the use of skin (bacteriology) swabs for, say, an infective wound lesion (Penzer and Ersser, 2010). More advanced technology may include the dermatoscope,

---

CASE STUDY 12.1 *A person living with chronic plaque psoriasis*

David is a 40-year-old single accountant with chronic plaque psoriasis (Table 12.1). His condition emerged in his 30s, but flared following a break-up of a personal relationship. His father had mild psoriasis; the inheritance pattern of psoriasis is complex, but a child with one affected parent has a 16% chance of developing psoriasis. David smokes and consumes excess alcohol; these are known to be precipitating factors (Weller *et al.*, 2008), which may be a trigger and/or a consequence of his condition. The plaque lesions (Table 12.1) on his back, neck, elbows, and scalp are typically scaly and often pruritic. David finds his condition stressful owing to the reaction of others (people wrongly think that it is infectious), the shedding of skin scales, and the itching. At times, he says his sleep is disturbed because his skin is sore, tight, and itchy (Ersser *et al.*, 2002). He feels his situation has led him to lose social confidence in developing new relationships, which, together with the symptoms and the need to apply his greasy treatments daily, has affected his quality of life. This was confirmed by his poor DLQI score (=12, 11–20 indicating very large impact), which he completed while in day care. His condition becomes more unstable and severe at times, when work becomes stressful or he does not keep up with treatment. When this occurs, he arranges through his GP support from the nurse-led dermatology day treatment centre. He sees his GP while his condition is stable. When the psoriasis is unstable, nurses at the day treatment centre reassess his needs, provide support, and teach him effective methods of treatment application.

This case study is typical of the kinds of problems you may encounter as a nurse caring for adults. There is a range of evidence-based treatments and interventions that can be utilized. These are described in the following sections of this chapter and most are relevant to the management of David's care.

---

as used by dermatologists and some specialist nurses to examine suspected cancerous pigmented lesions. Some tools may be in a questionnaire format—to assess key disease factors, such as severity (e.g. the Psoriasis Area Severity Index, or PASI) or disease-related quality of life (e.g. the Dermatology Life Quality Index, or DLQI) (Finlay and Khan, 1994). For a PASI score, a representative area of psoriasis is selected for each body region. The intensity of redness, thickness, and scaling of the psoriasis is assessed as: none (0); mild (1); moderate (2); severe (3); or very severe (4). The percentage area affected by psoriasis is evaluated in the four regions of the body. Clinical improvement in the PASI is measured by the percentage change: the lower the score, the greater the improvement. PASI >12 defines severe; PASI 7–12 is moderate; and PASI <7 is mild chronic plaque-type psoriasis (Schmitt and Wozel, 2005). The DLQI is easy to use. It is calculated by totalling the score of each question, resulting in a maximum of 30 and a minimum of 0. The higher the score, the more quality of life is impaired: a low score (under 5) indicates a small effect on the patient's life; 6–10 a moderate effect; and 11–30 a substantial effect.

Nursing management of an individual with psoriasis

Case study 12.1 illustrates the factors influencing the development of skin conditions, and the psychosocial and physical impact of living with chronic conditions. It provides a basis for assessing the person's nursing needs, planning his or her care, and choosing effective interventions, linked to evidence. This section is intended to be illustrative of treatment options rather than comprehensive. Further detail of the management of the common skin conditions mentioned in this chapter can be found by examining the reference sources in Table 12.4)

Topical treatment and patient education and support

The type of treatment prescribed provides a clue to disease severity. Mild to moderate disease usually requires topical therapy (e.g. coal tar); moderate disease requires photo (light) therapy and topicals; and for those with severe disease, systemic therapy (oral or injected drugs), e.g. methotrexate, may be required. Treatments are often used in combination: for example, calcipotriol and topical steroids may be used initially, because they are easier to apply and not as messy as some coal tar preparations, The focus within this chapter is on topical therapy, which is more likely to be seen in non-specialized clinical environments. Those requiring intensive teaching or support, or with more severe disease requiring phototherapy and systemic therapy, are usually seen in dermatology outpatients or day treatment centres. For key treatment-related evidence, see the tabulated summary of sources (Table 12.4).

Emollient therapy

Emollients are an important therapeutic tool for a nurse to use since they fortify the skin barrier. Invariably, nurses are able to select, in discussion with the patient, those for which the patient has a preference and therefore is likely to use. They are topical medications that reduce the signs and symptoms of dry, scaly skin, making the rough surface soft and smooth (Kligman, 2000). Emollients are prescribed to help to seal the water within the skin, reducing loss through the disrupted barrier (see Ersser *et al.*, 2009; Table 12.4, section 14; and Chapters 17 and 18 ➡). They come in different formulations, with different chemical constituents providing varying therapeutic properties. Creams are a mixture of water in lipid; they are absorbed quickly and are less greasy than ointments. Ointments do not contain any water and are the most greasy emollients (Penzer, 2010a). Creams are often selected when the patient requires a less greasy emollient, which may be more suitable for application when wearing work clothing. They are also used when the skin is wet, as is

sometimes the case with conditions such as eczema, to avoid enhancing the hydration level that results from using ointments. However, where the skin is very dry, it is better to apply a greasier ointment, if this can be tolerated, because this provides better hydration by sealing the skin from transepidermal water loss. Soap substitutes may also be used to avoid soap, which may remove the added oil and sebum; these may come in pots, tubes, or as a shower gel.

To prevent cross-infection due to contamination of the emollient, it is important to keep pots for individual patients. If there are stockpots, then the emollient should be removed using a wooden spatula. Pump dispensers are a useful method of dispensing that avoids contamination. Also for home use, patients need to be taught how to avoid contaminating the emollient, using handwashing and, if pump dispensers are not available, using devices such as a clean spoon.

Other topical treatments and their application

There are wide ranges of topical treatments that contain pharmacologically active ingredients in an emollient base to help to manage the symptoms for dermatological disease. An extensive account is beyond the scope of this chapter, although further details may be obtained from the *British National Formulary* (British Medical Association and Royal Pharmaceutical Society of Great Britain, 2009), or from evidence-based nursing sources such as Penzer and Ersser (2010a). Calcipotriol provides one illustration for a common topical treatment for psoriasis treatment. It is a vitamin D analogue that affects cell division within a formulation product combined with the steroid, betamethasone. It is prescribed as one application per day (up to 15 g or 100 g/week). Some treatments are formulated for specific areas of the body. Again, for scalp psoriasis, a common compound consists of coal tar, salicylic acid, and coconut oil. It is used at night before bed to moisturize, and to reduce inflammation and excessive scale (Table 12.4, sections 2–5).

Typically, topical corticosteroids (steroids) have a limited role in the treatment of psoriasis in countries like the UK; they are typically used for flexural and facial psoriasis. However, as a general topical treatment concept, it is important to be aware that, with some topical treatments such as steroids, there is a need to understand both the different potencies of the steroid—for example, low potency; mild potency, for example hydrocortisone (0.1%–2.5%); and a very potent steroid, for example Clobetasol proprionate (0.05%) —and the strength of the steroid, cited in parentheses here. In the case of hydrocortisone, you will note that there is a range of strengths. Note that the topical steroids of different potency do have similar names (see Table 12.3). The greater the potency, the more effect it has on reducing inflammation, but the greater the risk of side effects with continued use. Lower potency steroids are used on areas of thinner skin, such as the face, with higher potency used on, say, the legs. Typically, treatment commences with low potencies for a period and then builds up, however, sometimes higher potencies are used first in short bursts for a few days to enhance therapeutic impact and convenience. Furthermore, it is important to be aware that continuous daily application of a mild corticosteroid, such as hydrocortisone 1%, is equivalent to a potent such as betamethasone 0.1% that is used intermittently. Table 12.3 highlights the relative potency of different topical steroids.

A key nursing responsibility is to ensure that the appropriate quantity of emollient or active topical is applied. One way of managing this is to use, or to teach the patient to use, the system of fingertip units (FTUs). To dispense 1FTU, the medication is squeezed on the finger top to the first crease, which is equivalent to half a gram (1FTU); this is enough to treat an area of psoriasis equivalent to the size of the flat of an adult's hand (Long and Finlay, 1991). For many topicals, this is applied only once the emollient has penetrated, often after 30 minutes (British Dermatological Nursing Group (BDNG) Nurse Prescribing Sub-group, 2007). However, depending on the chemical formulation of the medication (lipid and water content), sometimes the emollient may be applied after the active topical. Therefore the sequence advised in the manufacturer's guidance must be followed.

Patient education and support

Many patients find their topical treatment regimen a burden because it is often messy and time-consuming, and some treatments, such as coal tar preparations, have a strong odour. To ensure effective use of topical therapy, you will need to teach patients how to apply their treatments effectively around their lifestyle, considering emollient, preference, and timing issues around social roles. For example, messier topicals such as ointments or scalp treatments may be applied at bedtime and washed out in the morning. Another key therapeutic objective is to improve treatment adherence, which is crucial to its effectiveness. Therefore the nurse needs to teach the patient how to apply and use treatments properly, which involves some understanding of how they work and their duration of effect, so that he or she knows what to expect (Ersser *et al.*, 2002). A collaborative approach involving the concordance process can be effective, because this takes account of the patient's beliefs about his or her condition and treatment (e.g. use of steroid medication), and his or her emollient preferences and lifestyle (Taal *et al.*, 1993; Ersser 2010b).

Many people living with chronic skin conditions will cope better if they receive sustained support and teaching from nurses. This includes the use of health education opportunities on managing stress, regulating alcohol intake, and smoking cessation (van Ryn and Heaney, 1997) . All three of these factors may exacerbate psoriasis. Advice on joining a patient support group, such as the Psoriasis Association (UK), may be helpful (The Psoriasis Association, 2010). They provide information sheets, website podcasts, and the opportunity to meet others with psoriasis locally. Joining a virtual social networking group of people living with psoriasis may also be helpful (Idriss *et al.*, 2009) (see Table 12.4).

Identifying best practice

Table 12.4 provides a comprehensive list of the key sources of high-quality evidence for the common skin problems described in this chapter.

Table 12.4 Key sources of quality evidence on skincare problems

Source	Problem type	Nature of evidence and tips for use and review
1. **NHS Evidence (skin disorders)** www.evidence.nhs.uk	Dermatological disease and its evidence-based treatment	Web Portal: The UK NHS 'one-stop' resource bringing together high-quality evidence-based information on all of aspects of skin disorders and their treatment. The new skincare library site is available from May 2011.
2. **Cochrane Library**: internationally recognized source of systematic review www.thecochranelibrary.com/view/0/index.html	Dermatological disease and lymphoedema	The Cochrane collaboration **www.cochrane.org/** is an extensive highly regarded independent source of systemic reviews of healthcare interventions (treatments), synthesizing best evidence from mainly published research sources, e.g. Ersser *et al.*, 2007)
3. **British Association of Dermatologists** www.bad.org.uk	Dermatological disease	Professional association website 1. Clinical Guidelines **www.bad.org.uk//site/495/default. aspx** links to the key sources (primarily journal)—all evidence-based (A–Z, mainly condition-related) 2. Patient information leaflets: written by the British Association of Dermatologists **www.bad.org.uk//site/578/default.aspx**
4. **Health Technology Assessment (HTA)** www.hta.ac.uk/	Dermatological treatments	The HTA programme is part of the National Institute for Health Research (NIHR). It produces independent research information about the effectiveness, costs, and broader impact of healthcare treatments and tests.
5. **NICE (National Institute for Health and Clinical Excellence)** www.nice.org.uk	Dermatological disease	Website (NHS) NICE is an independent organization responsible for providing national guidance on promoting good health and preventing and treating ill-health. NICE issues open access clinical guidance, e.g. Pimecrolimus and tacrolimus for atopic dermatitis **http://guidance.nice.org.uk/TA82**
6. **Dermatology Society of New Zealand (DSNZ)** www.dermnetnz.org/	Dermatological disease	Professional association website: Widely regarded as an authoritative and clear source of information for health professionals and patients/service users
7. **Dermis** www.dermis.net/dermisroot/en/home/index.htm	Dermatological disease	Professional website: extensive image bank. One of the largest dermatology image resources on the Internet. Information is localized on a body map, if diagnosis is unknown.
8. **Centre for Evidence-based Dermatology (CEBD)** www.nottingham.ac.uk/SCS/Divisions/EvidenceBasedDermatology/index.aspx	Dermatological disease	Website and centre: a centre with substantial expertise in evidence-based dermatology. It produces the NHS Evidence-Skin disorders site (above). 1. Cochrane Skin Group Base (see Cochrane Library, above) **www.csg.cochrane.org/en/index.html** 2. Epidemiological expertise (Schofield *et al.*, 2009) 3. UK Dermatology Clinical Trials Network (UKCTN): conduct high-quality trials (randomized controlled trials) answering key clinical questions

Table 12.4 (*continued*)

Source	Problem type	Nature of evidence and tips for use and review
9. **Patient support (and research) charities**	Dermatological disease	1. Skin Care Campaign: an umbrella organization uniting patient, health professionals, pharmaceutical companies, and politicians concerned with skin conditions. Provides information on patient groups and the All Party Parliamentary Group on Skin, which produces key policy documents **http://skincarecampaign.org/** 2. Psoriasis Association (The Psoriasis Association, 2010) **www.psoriasis-association.org.uk/index.html**. Information resources for patients and podcasts 3. National Eczema Society: Fact sheets: **www.eczema.org/factsheets.html** 4. Wessex Cancer Trust: good-quality information sheets on skin cancer **www.eczema.org/factsheets.html** 5. Cancer Research UK: see the SunSmart home page—skin cancer information and prevention **www.sunsmart.org.uk/index.htm**
10. **NHS Quality Improvement Scotland (including SIGN)** http://www.healthcare improvementscotland.org/ home.aspx www.sign.ac.uk	Skincare Dermatological disease	NHS care guideline and evidence synthesis initiative: Best Practice Statement: skin care of patients receiving radiotherapy (NHS Quality Improvement Scotland, 2004) Includes SIGN **www.sign.ac.uk**: Scottish Intercollegiate Guidelines Network produces high-quality user-friendly guidelines based on current evidence, e.g. cutaneous melanoma (Scottish Intercollegiate Guidelines Network (SIGN), 2003)
11. **Established definitive textbooks (reference sources)**	Dermatological disease	Reference books: comprehensive authoritative texts located in specialist health care libraries *Evidence-based Dermatology*, 2nd edn (Williams *et al.*, 2008) and *Rook's Textbook of Dermatology* (Burns *et al.*, 2004)
12. **Lymphoedema guidelines** (international and national)	Lymphoedema	*International Consensus Best Practice for the Management of Lymphoedema* (Lymphoedema Framework, 2006) Care Guideline: Clinical Resource Efficiency Support Team (CREST) (2008) *Guidelines for the diagnosis, assessment and management of lymphoedema* **www.crestni.org.uk**. GAIN (Guidelines and Audit Implementation Network) ((CREST) Clinical Resource Efficiency Support Team, 2008)
13. **Review papers**	For example, on incontinence and skin vulnerability	These collate, distil, and categorize the key sources of evidence and appraise the gaps in evidence (Ersser *et al.*, 2005)
14. **ISNG-BDNG Best practice document**	Emollient therapy	Best Practice in Emollient Therapy is an initiative of the International Skin care Nursing Group and the BDNG (Ersser *et al.*, 2009)

Conclusion

This chapter has highlighted the important role of nurses in the care of those with skin conditions, both in recognizing signs of disease, and in understanding the physical and psychosocial implications for patients and families. Nurses have a responsibility to provide education and support to enable effective self-management by those living with a long-term skin condition. The best practice case illustration of the experience of living with a chronic skin problem reveals how you can help patients to manage the challenges of their disease and treatment.

Because skin problems may arise for patients in every clinical field and setting, they are universal and fundamental nursing problems and not just the concern of those working in the field of dermatology. As a nurse, you are ideally placed to protect the person's skin barrier, identify and manage his or her skin problems, support those living with chronic problems, and prevent some important ones arising. This means being knowledgeable about the scale and causes of skin conditions, and developing competence in making accurate assessments and providing evidence-based interventions.

Online Resource Centre

 To help you to develop and apply your knowledge and decision-making skills further, we have provided interactive learning resources online at **www.oxfordtextbooks.co.uk/orc/bullock/**

Whilst these are freely available, you will need to use the access codes at the start of the book.

References

All Party Parliamentary Group on Skin (2003) *Enquiry into the Treatment, Management and Prevention of Skin Cancer.* All Party Parliamentary Group on Skin, Portcullis: London.

Barnhill, RL., Martin, C., *et al.* (1993) Neoplasms: malignant melanoma. In T. B. Fitzpatrick, A. Z. Sisen, K. Wolff, *et al.* (eds) *Dermatology in General Medicine.* McGraw-Hill: New York, pp. 1078–1115

British Dermatological Nursing Group (BDNG) Nurse Prescribing Sub-group. (2007) Patient information leaflet: How to ... Apply Dovobet Ointment. **www.bdng.org.uk/news/patients/ Dovobet.pdf** (accessed 2 March 2010).

British Medical Association, Royal Pharmaceutical Society of Great Britain (2009) *British National Formulary.* British Medical Journal Publishing Group Ltd, The Royal Pharmaceutical Society of Great Britain: London.

Burge, S., Wallis, D. (2011) *Oxford Handbook of Medical Dermatology.* Oxford University Press: Oxford.

Burns, T., Breathnagh, S., *et al.* (2004) *Rook's Textbook of Dermatology.* Blackwell Publishing Ltd: Oxford.

Buxton, P.K., Morris-Jones, R. (eds) (2009) *ABC of Dermatology.* Wiley-Blackwell & BMJ Books: Chichester.

Cancer Research UK (2009a) Malignant Melanoma: Cancerstats. **http://info.cancerresearchuk.org/cancerstats/types/skin/ incidence/** (accessed 2 March 2010).

Clinical Resource Efficiency Support Team (CREST) (2008) Guidelines for the diagnosis, assessment and management of lymphoedema. CREST & GAIN: Central Medical Advisory Committee, Health Service in Northern Ireland: Belfast.

Colbert, B., Ankney, J., *et al.* (2009) *Anatomy and Physiology for Nursing and Health Professionals.* Pearson Education: Harlow.

Elias, P.M., Steinhoff, M. (2008) Outside-to-inside (and now back to outside) pathogenic mechanisms in atopic dermatitis. *Journal of Investigative Dermatology* **128**: 1067–70.

Ersser, S. (2010a): Assessment and planning care. In R. Penzer, S. Ersser (eds) *Principles of Skin Care: A Guide for Nurses and Health Care Professionals.* Wiley-Blackwell: Oxford, pp. 29–47.

Ersser, S.J. (2010b) : Helping patients make the most of their treatment. In R. Penzer, S. Ersser (eds) *Principles of Skin Care: A Guide for Nurses, Health Care Professionals.* Wiley-Blackwell: Oxford.

Ersser, S.J., Getliffe, K., *et al.* (2005) A critical review of the inter-relationship between skin vulnerability and urinary incontinence and related nursing intervention. *International Journal of Nursing Studies* **42**(7): 823–35.

Ersser, S. J., Latter, S., *et al.* (2007) Psychological and educational interventions for atopic eczema in children. *Cochrane Database of Systematic Reviews*, Issue 3: Art. No. CD004054. DOI: 10.1002/14651858. CD004054. pub2.

Ersser, S., Macguire, S., *et al.* (2009) Best practice in emollient therapy: a statement for health care professionals. *Dermatological Nursing* (suppl.): 1–22.

Ersser, S.J., Surridge, H., *et al.* (2002) What criteria do patients use when judging the effectiveness of psoriasis management? *Journal of Evaluation in Clinical Practice* **8**(4): 367–76.

Finlay, A., Khan, G. (1994) Dermatology Life Quality Index (DLQI): a simple practical measure for routine clinical use. *Clinical and Experimental Dermatology* **19**(3): 201–6.

Graham-Brown, R., Burns, T. (2007) *Lecture Notes Dermatology.* Blackwell Publishing: Oxford.

Herd, R.M. (2000) The morbidity and cost of atopic dermatitis. In H.C. Williams (ed.) *Atopic Dermatitis.* Cambridge University Press: Cambridge. pp. 85–95.

Idriss, S.Z., Kvedar, J.C. *et al.* (2009) The role of online support communities. *Archives of Dermatology* **145**(1): 46–51.

Kelly, A.P., Taylor, S.C. (2009) *Dermatology for Skin of Color.* McGraw-Hill Education: Maidenhead.

Kingman, S. (2005) Growing awareness of skin disease starts flurry of initiatives. *Bulletin of the World Health Organization* **83**(12): 891–2.

Kligman, A.M. (2000). Introduction. In M. Loden, H. Maibach (eds) *Dry Skin and Moisturisers: Chemistry and Function.* CRC Press, Boca Raton, FL, pp. 1–4

Lawrence, C.M., Cox, N.H. (2002) *Physical Signs in Dermatology.* Mosby: London.

Long, C.C., Finlay, A.Y. (1991) The finger-tip unit: a new practical measure. *Clinical and Experimental Dermatology* **16**(6): 444–7.

Lymphoedema: Framework (2006) *International Consensus Best Practice for the Management of Lymphoedema: An International Perspective.* MEP Ltd: London.

Moffatt, C.J., Franks, P. J., *et al.* (2003) Lymphoedema: an underestimated health problem. *The Quarterly Journal of Medicine* **96**(10): 731–8.

Naldi, L., Chalmers, J.G. (2008). Psoriasis. In H.C. Williams, M. Bigby, T. Diepgen *et al.* (eds) *Evidence-Based Dermatology.* Blackwell Publishing: Oxford, pp. 171–88.

NHS Quality Improvement Scotland (2004) *Best Practice Statement: Skin Care of Patients Receiving Radiotherapy.* NHS Quality Improvement Scotland: Edinburgh.

Penzer, R. (2010a) Emollients. In R. Penzer, S. Ersser (eds) *Principles of Skin Care: A Guide for Nurses and Health Care Professionals.* Wiley-Blackwell: Oxford, pp. 7–84

Penzer, R. (2010b) Psychological and social aspects of skin care. In R. Penzer, S. J. Ersser (eds) *Principles of Skin Care: A Guide for Nurses and Health Care Professionals.* Wiley-Blackwell: Oxford, pp. 85–102.

Penzer, R., Ersser, S.J. (2010) *Principles of Skin Care: A Guide for Nurses and Health Care Professionals.* Wiley-Blackwell: Oxford.

Poyner, T.F. (2000) *Common Skin Diseases.* Blackwell Science: Oxford.

Psoriasis Association (2010) The Psoriasis Association. **http://www.psoriasis-association.org.uk/** (accessed 3 March 2010).

Rapp, S.R., Feldman, S.R., *et al.* (1999) Psoriasis causes as much disability as other major medical diseases. *Journal of the American Academy of Dermatology* **41**(3): 401–7.

Royal College of Nursing (RCN) (2003) *Defining Nursing.* Royal College of Nursing: London.

Schmitt, J. Wozel, G. (2005) The Psoriasis Area and Severity Index is the adequate criterion to define severity in chronic plaque-type psoriasis. *Dermatology* **210**(3): 194–9.

Schofield, J., Grindlay, D., *et al.* (2009) *Skin Conditions in the UK: A Health Care Needs Assessment.* University of Nottingham: Nottingham.

Schofield, P.E., Beeney, L.J., *et al.* (2001) Hearing the bad news of a cancer diagnosis: the Australian melanoma patient's perspective. *Annals of Oncology* **12**: 365–71.

Scottish Intercollegiate Guidelines Network (SIGN) (2003) Cutaneous Melanoma: A National Clinical Guideline. **www.sign.ac.uk/guidelines/fulltext/72/section10.html**

Seal, D.V., Hay, R.J., *et al.* (2000) *Skin and Wound Infection. Investigation and Treatment in Practice.* Blackwell Publishing: Oxford.

Sitzia, J., Woods M., *et al.* (1998) Characteristics of new referrals to twenty-seven lymphoedema treatment units. *European Journal of Cancer Care (Engl)* **7**(4): 255–62.

Taal, E., Rasker, E., *et al.* (1993) Health status, adherence with health recommendations, self-efficacy and social support in patients with rheumatoid arthritis. *Patient Education Counseling* **20**: 63–76.

van Ryn, M., Heaney, C.A. (1997) Developing effective helping relationships in health education practice. *Health Education & Behavior* **24**(6): 683–702 .

Weller, R., Hunter, J.A.A., *et al.* (2008) *Clinical Dermatology.* Blackwell Publishing Ltd: Oxford.

Williams, H., Bigby, M., *et al.* (2008) *Evidence-Based Dermatology.* BMJ Books, Blackwell Publishing: Oxford.

Williams, H., Forsdyke, H., *et al.* (1995) A protocol for recording the sign of visible flexural dermatitis. *British Journal of Dermatology* **133**: 941–9.

13 *Understanding* **Stroke**

Christopher R. Burton and Caroline Smith

Introduction

The aim of this chapter is to provide nurses with the knowledge to be able to assess, manage, and care for people with stroke in an evidence-based and person-centred way. The chapter will provide a comprehensive overview of the seven stages of stroke, exploring best practice to deliver care, as well as to prevent or minimize further ill-health. Nursing assessments and priorities are highlighted throughout, and the nursing management of the symptoms and common health problems associated with stroke can be found in Chapters 23, 24, and 27, respectively ➡.

Understanding stroke

Defining stroke

Stroke is defined as the rapid onset of focal neurological deficit lasting more than 24 hours (in which the patient survives the initial event), with no apparent cause other than disruption of blood supply to the brain (World Health Organization, 1978).

Prevalence

As well as being the third commonest cause of death only in middle- and high-income countries (WHO, 1978) (along with cancer and heart disease), stroke is the largest cause of adult physical disability in the world (Bath and Lees, 2000). However, owing to advances in research and evidence synthesis, stroke is now a preventable and treatable disease (National Collaborating Centre for Chronic Conditions (NCCC), 2008).

Pathophysiology

Despite its relative small weight (approximately 2% of body weight), the brain requires 750 ml of bloodflow every minute, and consumes nearly 45% of arterial oxygen (Alexandrov, 2003). Bloodflow to the brain is assured through two circulatory systems (anterior and posterior), which are connected by the circle of Willis, and supplied by the internal carotid and vertebral arteries. Disruption of this bloodflow can be either in the form of a bleed (haemorrhagic stroke) or clot (ischaemic stroke), and the clinical presentation will vary depending on the location of the disruption in the brain. Ischaemic strokes are more common and account for almost 70% of all events (Wolfe *et al.*, 2002). Whilst thorough clinical examination is essential, the only clear tool to identify the type of stroke is to perform a brain scan using either magnetic resonance imaging (MRI) or computed tomography (CT) technology (Figure 13.1a–c).

It is important to note that, often, when a CT brain scan is performed within the first few hours of an event, the scan may not show any significant tissue damage because the changes that occur may take several days to be clearly visible. The rationale for scanning early is to exclude a haemorrhage and to establish an appropriate treatment plan. A normal brain scan within the first day does not necessarily exclude a stroke, and it is essential to obtain a diagnosis through a thorough clinical assessment.

The brain is divided into two hemispheres—left and right—and consists of four lobes—frontal, parietal, temporal, and occipital. Along with the cerebellum and brainstem, each has its own role in body function (Figure 13.2). Damage to different brain structures will precipitate different signs and symptoms relevant to the area that has

been affected. However, Sacco *et al.* (1997) found that, following a stroke, 12–18% of patients were left with speech problems, 25% were unable to walk, and 50% had a residual weakness. Typically, however, after 1 year, 80% of patients are in their own home, 66% have regained the ability to walk, 45–60% are independent, and only 5–9% are totally dependent (Tyson, 1995).

Strokes can also be classified according to which circulatory route is disrupted (Bamford *et al.*, 1991), as follows:

- total anterior circulation (effects include dysphasia, visual disturbance, and loss of consciousness);
- partial anterior circulation (associated with partial motor or sensory defect);
- lacunar (mixed effects, which include weakness or paralysis that typically affects the face, arm, or leg of one side);
- posterior circulation (effects include visual field loss, bilateral motor or sensory defects, and loss of balance).

Despite significant advances in the organization and content of stroke services, nearly 30% of patients will die in the acute phase (11% of all deaths in England and Wales are due

---

Box 13.1 Facts and figures for the UK

Incidence: 150,000 in the UK
Prevalence: 450,000 people in the UK are currently living with the consequences of stroke

(National Audit Office, 2005).

(a)

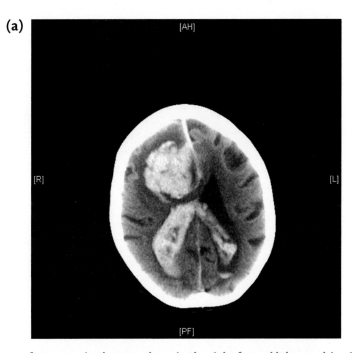

Figure 13.1 (a) A CT scan of an extensive haemorrhage in the right frontal lobe resulting in oedema causing shift of the midline and the bleed extending into the ventricles.

(b)

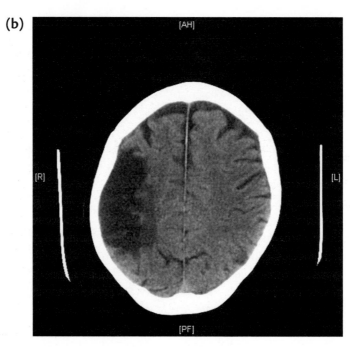

Figure 13.1 (b) An established infarct in the right pariental lobe.

(c)

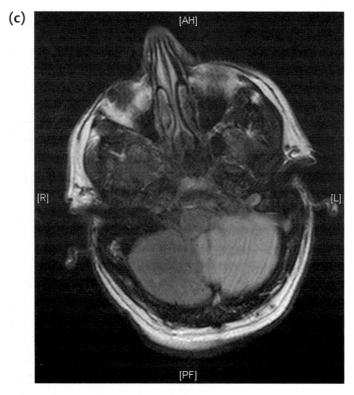

Figure 13.1 (c) An MRI of an infarct involving the cerebellum.

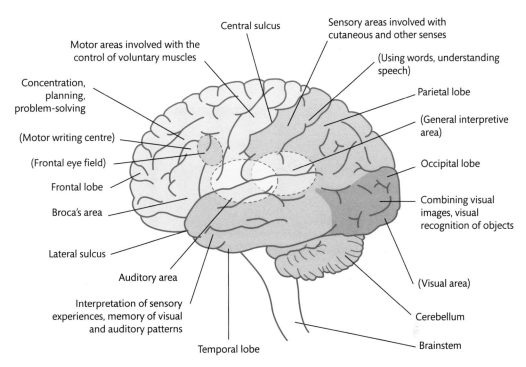

Figure 13.2 Lateral view of the brain, with functional area descriptions in parentheses.

Reproduced from Fitzgerald O'Connor and Urdang (2008) *Oxford Handbook of Surgical Cross-Cover,* by permission of Oxford University Press.

to stroke) (National Audit Office, 2005). Stroke progression, defined as persistent neurological deterioration, can occur in over 25% of patients after admission to hospital (Jorgensen *et al.*, 1996). Other complications following a stroke are numerous and, whilst some are generic, such as pressure sore risk, others are more specific to either stroke, falls risk, or the area in the brain affected, such as cognitive impairment. Early identification of these risks is essential to treat and minimize the risk of harm to the patient.

Impact

Every year in the UK, 130,000 people experience a stroke (National Statistics Health Statistics Quarterly, 2001), which equates to a new event every 5 minutes. The financial burden to statutory healthcare services is extensive, with an estimated £2.8 billion annually in direct costs, an additional £1.8 billion lost from the wider economy owing to lost productivity and disability, and £2.4 billion in informal care costs (National Audit Office, 2005).

Although stroke causes over 60,000 deaths each year in the UK (Allender *et al.*, 2006), most people survive a first

stroke. They can experience significant disability: there are currently estimated to be 900,000 people in England who are living with the effects of a stroke and half of these are dependent on other people for help with everyday activities (National Audit Office, 2005). With stroke patients typically occupying 20% of all acute hospital beds and 25% of long-term beds, it is essential that the management and care of these patients is evidence-based, because any small improvement will result in a significant change to many people.

Stroke management

Stroke provides an excellent example of the potential impacts of the evidence-based practice agenda. In the past 20 years, stroke has emerged from a sense of therapeutic nihilism, under which stroke was viewed as a consequence of ageing, meaning that little could be done for the patient. Systematic reviews of the evidence base for the organization of stroke services, such as stroke units (Langhorne *et al.*, 1993), have underpinned a reinvigorated service model with stroke as an emerging specialism for nursing practice.

Box 13.2 **Best management for stroke**

- General stroke education and awareness campaign
- Early reporting into ED (dialling 999 rather than contacting GP)
- Rapid response by ambulance service
- Early clinical assessment in ED by stroke specialist
- Access to evidence-based treatment such as thrombolysis and rapid admission to a dedicated stroke unit

---

There is now considerable government guidance, such as the UK National Stroke Strategy (Department of Health, 2007), on what are considered to be acceptable standards for stroke services that are relevant to nursing. These emphasize a multifaceted approach to stroke recovery, including early diagnosis, swallow screening and early nutrition, bladder control, and mood assessment (see Box 13.2). Intervention on these improves the outcome for the individual and typically has been found to be financially viable (National Institute for Health and Clinical Excellence (NICE), 2010).

High-profile media campaigns such as the FAST campaign (see Figure 13.4) seam to have been very successful in raising public awareness relating to the speed of reporting early symptoms that will enable potential brain-saving treatment interventions (the principle of 'time lost is brain lost' is very real). Whilst there are some variations across international healthcare contexts, the stages of stroke have been simplified into seven core principles: the seven 'R's (Ford, 2009), as follows.

- Recognize—recognition of the symptoms of stroke
- React—management of stroke as a medical emergency
- Respond—appropriate responses from patients and staff
- Reveal—ensuring timely access to scanning
- Reperfusion—delivery of evidence-based treatments, including thrombolytic therapy if appropriate

- Rehabilitation—to address functional limitations
- Reintegration—enabling the development of meaningful social lives (e.g. work and leisure) after stroke

Increasing knowledge of the risk factors associated with stroke means that stroke prevention should be embedded within the stroke service model.

Stroke prevention

There are numerous modifiable risk factors for stroke, including smoking, high blood pressure, high cholesterol, diabetes, obesity, alcohol, lack of exercise, and atrial fibrillation (AF). In addition to gender and age, ethnicity is a non-modifiable factor, with Afro-Caribbean people being twice as likely to have a stroke compared with Caucasian people; the risk is thought to be related to having a higher incidence of high blood pressure (Cappuccio, 1997).

Ensuring that modifiable risk factors are managed using evidence-based guidance is important in reducing the incidence of stroke. In addition, national guidelines recommend that all patients who have had a stroke should received an individualized stroke risk reduction programme, with special attention paid to anti-platelet, anticoagulant, anti-lipid, and antihypertensive therapy unless contraindicated (Intercollegiate Working Party for Stroke, 2008).

The chapter will look at each of the seven 'R's (Ford, 2009).

Recognition

To minimize the extent of damage caused by stroke, early recognition of signs and symptoms (Figure 13.3) and treatment is crucial. In the UK, the Department of Health has invested £1.2 million in a multimedia campaign to increase public recognition of the symptoms of stroke and the importance of early intervention. This campaign is just one element of the National Stroke Strategy, which was launched in December 2007 with a clear, evidence-based 10-year programme to improve stroke services of all elements—from prevention to long-term life after stroke care.

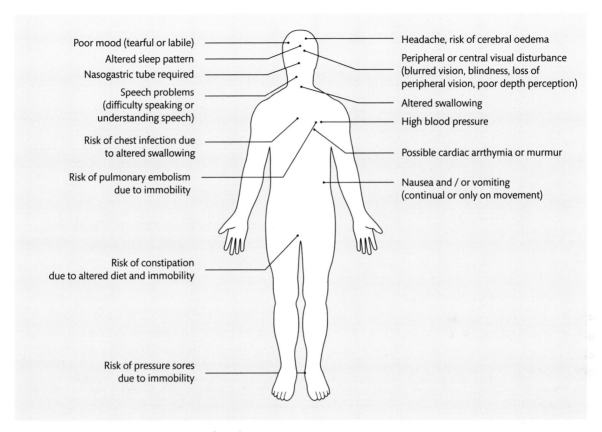

Poor mood (tearful or labile)

Altered sleep pattern

Nasogastric tube required

Speech problems
(difficulty speaking or
understanding speech)

Risk of chest infection due
to altered swallowing

Risk of pulmonary embolism
due to immobility

Risk of constipation
due to altered diet and immobility

Risk of pressure sores
due to immobility

Headache, risk of cerebral oedema

Peripheral or central visual disturbance
(blurred vision, blindness, loss of
peripheral vision, poor depth perception)

Altered swallowing

High blood pressure

Possible cardiac arrthymia or murmur

Nausea and / or vomiting
(continual or only on movement)

Figure 13.3 **Potential complications of stroke.**

In the UK, the public awareness campaign has been built around FAST: the Face, Arms and Speech Test—although the 'T' has been relabelled 'Time' to reinforce the sense of urgency required to any sign of:

- facial weakness (can the person smile? has his or her mouth or eye drooped?);
- arm weakness (can the person raise both arms?);
- speech problems (can the person speak clearly and understand what you say?).

The FAST (NHS Choices, 2011) is one of several structured assessment tools to aid the recognition of stroke (Figure 13.4). When the accuracy of early recognition of stroke by ambulance paramedics and stroke neurologists was compared, it was found that the assessments or diagnoses made by the two groups were very similar. Of the three items, arm weakness was the commonest and was present in 96% of the 217 patients confirmed with stroke (Nor *et al.*, 2004).

React

The FAST campaign was designed to improve public awareness of and attitudes to stroke. In 2005, a MORI poll commissioned by the Stroke Association found that only half of people asked could correctly identify what a stroke is, and only 40% could correctly name three stroke symptoms. When asked what they would do if they had these symptoms, 60% would contact their GP or NHS Direct, only a third would go to hospital or

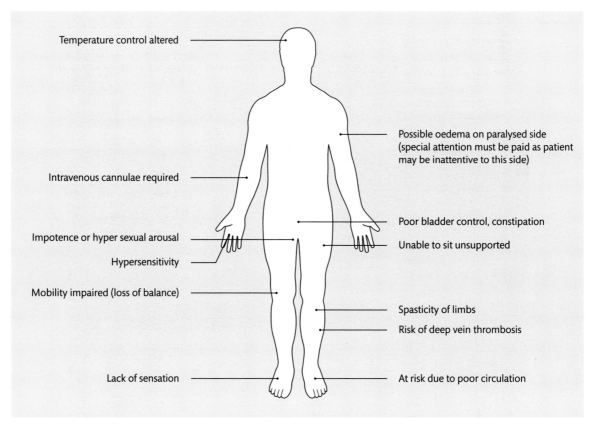

Figure 13.3 (*continued*).

call an ambulance, and a quarter did not believe that specialist treatment or care could make a difference.

Respond

Stroke is a medical emergency, and requires appropriate responses from patients, clinicians, and health services alike. For patients, ensuring that an emergency ambulance is called for rapid transfer to an appropriate stroke facility is crucial, rather than waiting to see if symptoms persist or consulting a primary care physician. For clinical staff, the focus of attention is on ensuring that an accurate diagnosis is made, and that complications from stroke are prevented.

Assessment

There is no such thing as a 'typical stroke patient' because of the potential variability in the location of the stroke in the brain, resulting in different signs and symptoms for each individual. When assessing a patient following a

stroke, it is essential to observe all of the body systems, because any part of the body may be affected and detection is not always easy or apparent on first examination. Clear documentation is essential because deterioration may be an indicator for repeat brain scanning. It is important, for example, that neurological observations are jointly performed at shift change over time to exclude the chance of misinterpretation of the results. (It is worth noting that the pupil size indicator on hospital issue pen torches may, in some organizations, be of a different size from the scale used on the charts.) Assessing the patient can be divided into three key stages, as follows.

1. On admission, for emergency management and diagnosis

2. The acute phase for early identification of deterioration, risk factors, or potential problems

3. In the long term, to identify rehabilitation needs and barriers to developing a meaningful life with stroke

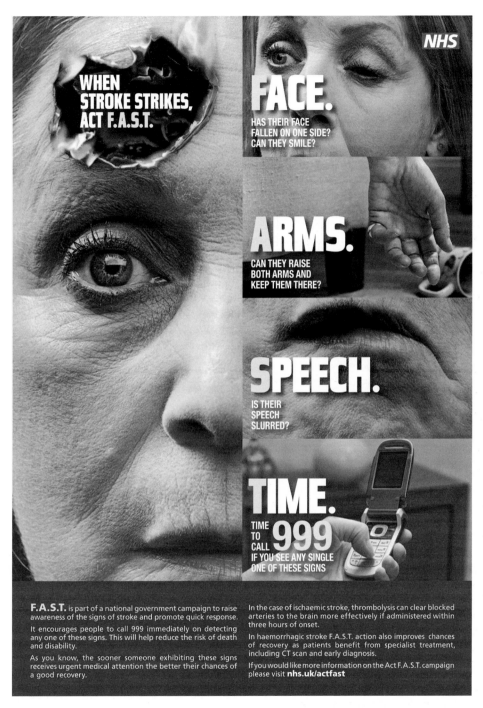

Figure 13.4 FAST.

Crown Copyright.

The hyperacute period refers to the first few hours after admission, and may include treatment with a thrombolytic drug if the patient presents with an ischaemic stroke very quickly after symptom onset. Early diagnosis and treatment is essential in order to maximize the possibility of a good outcome, and the role of the paramedic and emergency department nurse is essential. It is essential that all nurses are able to recognize the key symptoms of stroke and to respond quickly—realizing that 'time is brain'. Cross (2008) highlighted that, for each minute untreated, a person will lose 1.9 million neurons and 14 billion synapses. This is equivalent to an accelerated brain ageing of 3.6 years for each untreated hour. Early presentation to the emergency department and diagnosis can not only provide the option for thrombolysis, but also highlight the need for direct admission to the stroke unit.

There are several acute models of care that provide a dedicated nurse-led stroke service with staff who assess, initiate treatment, and ensure swift transfer to the stroke unit, reducing any delays that may be encountered owing to limited medical personnel. Davis (2005) described one such service in which a 'stroke nurse clinician role' sped up the stroke care process. This 12-hour weekday and 8-hour weekend service included assessing patients, referring to the medical team, arranging brain scan, and obtaining blood tests, ECGs, and X-rays. Following these assessments and investigations, medication is administered, swallow assessment performed, and intravenous fluids are commenced. This has resulted in the patient pathway being improved, increased the number of patients who have received thrombolytic therapy, and increased the number of patients directly admitted to the stroke unit.

Once in hospital, the accuracy of the FAST assessment can be increased further by asking additional questions, and the ROSIER scale is typically used for this higher level information. The Recognition of Stroke in Emergency Room (Nor *et al.*, 2005) involves the need to exclude the commonest stroke mimics of seizure and syncope, and also includes facial and leg weakness, increasing its diagnostic sensitivity of 92% and specificity of 86%. As with any tool, its accuracy is dependent on appropriate training and use, and it is essential that the ROSIER is used routinely for all stroke admissions. It should be noted that neither of these tools is useful for determining the symptoms of posterior stroke, which tend to be visual or balance and coordination problems.

Swallowing difficulties

It is essential that the nurse considers several other potential problems that may occur as a consequence of the stroke. The incidence of dysphagia (swallowing difficulties) varies within the literature, but is commonly quoted as being around 40% (Langdon *et al.*, 2007). Patients with dysphagia are more likely to have a poor outcome from their stroke, having a higher incidence of death, disability, chest infection, and a longer period in hospital (NCCCC, 2008). It is essential that a detailed assessment of a patient's swallowing ability is performed prior to being allowed to eat and drink, and this should be done by a specially trained healthcare professional within 24 hours of admission (Department of Health, 2007). More recent performance targets indicate that this timescale will be reduced further, to assessment within 4 hours of arrival at hospital (National Institute for Health and Clinical Excellence (NICE), 2011). In addition to considering the physical impact of not eating and the need for alternative methods of receiving adequate nutrition such as nasogastric feeding, it is essential to consider associated psychological issues, and consideration should be made of this, especially around the ward mealtimes.

Investigations

The first few hours after admission are also important in obtaining the diagnosis; this will require a brain scan and obtaining blood for tests such as cholesterol, glucose, and ESR. A chest X-ray and ECG are performed; in addition to providing essential information on the status of the patient at that time, these tests are useful in helping to determine the cause of stroke. Cannulation should be performed in the non-affected arm owing to the potential for reduced sensation, preventing early identification of dislocation or a problem with the cannula, and the potential for oedema.

Communication

It is also important during the early stages of admission that there is clear and consistent communication with the patient and his or her family. Family members are particularly helpful if the patient is unable to communicate or is drowsy to provide as much history as possible. This should include current medications, medical history, and previous physical health, such as whether living alone and caring for themselves. This information not only helps to establish a rapport with the family, but also pre-warns the stroke team of additional potential problems such as pain from arthritis if the stroke will result in prolonged immobilization.

Reveal

Brain imaging is essential for stroke care management because it remains the only method available to exclude a haemorrhage or non-vascular conditions that can 'mimic' an acute stroke (e.g. tumours, migraine, or hypoglycaemia); without a scan, treatment cannot be commenced. Initial government guidelines recommended the attainment of a scan within 24 hours; however, the 2010 Sentinel Audit found that this was achieved in only 70% of eligible cases (Royal College of Physicians, 2011). Current recommendations, however, are that a patient should be scanned immediately or at least within 1 hour if he or she meets the criteria set out in Box 13.3.

There is further pressure to improve significantly on scanning performance regardless of the decision to thrombolyse: the Best Practice Tariff (Department of Health, 2010) provides a financial incentive for health provider organizations in the UK to deliver both timely scanning and direct admission to the stroke unit.

Reperfuse

After the publication of the NINDS trial in 1995, which showed that the use of intravenous alteplase (recombinant tissue plasminogen activator, or rt-PA) improves the chances of neurological recovery, its routine use was licensed in the US in 1996 and in the UK in 2003. Thrombolytic therapy works by breaking up, or lysing, the occlusion and reducing the subsequent brain tissue damage. Thrombolysis given within 3 hours of symptoms results in an additional 141 independent stroke survivors and 130 fewer dependent survivors per 1,000 treated (Hacke *et al.*, 2004). Whilst there is already evidence that there is benefit for the use of rt-PA until 4.5 hours (ECASS 3, Hacke *et al.*, 2008), there are further trials in progress increasing the time window to 6 hours (IST-3); the DIAS-4 trial starts soon, and this uses desmoteplase up to 9 hours from stroke onset.

Despite all of the evidence of the benefits of thrombolysis, only 0.8% of patients received this treatment in England in 2008, with a small increase to 3.8% in 2010 (Royal College of Physicians, 2009; 2011). According to the National Audit Office (2005), if thrombolysis level rates in England were to match those of Australia (10%), an additional 1500 patients would make a full recovery, and an additional £16 million a year could be saved by reducing hospital and social services costs. One of the key reasons given for the low number of patients treated is the small proportion who present at hospital within 3 hours of symptom onset; however, recent studies (Batmanian *et al.*, 2007) found that 40% of patients presented within the timescale and audit data for 2010 show that this figure is now 56%. The commonest reasons for exclusion were minor or rapidly resolving symptoms and the presence of haemorrhage on initial CT studies (Batmanian *et al.*, 2007). Unlike thrombolysis for cardiac patients, prior to administration, the stroke patient needs to be assessed to exclude any stroke mimics and, most importantly, to have a brain scan to exclude haemorrhage. In Finland, it is general practice for the ambulance staff to phone ahead with a patient felt to be suitable for thrombolysis and, on arrival at hospital, to go straight into the scanner room and be assessed en route. This practice is currently being trialled in some British hospitals, such as Bournemouth,

---

Box 13.3 **National Institute for Health and Clinical Excellence (2008) Guideline recommendations**

Brain imaging should be performed immediately (ideally the next slot and definitely within 1 hour, whichever is sooner) for people with acute stroke who have any one of the following:

- Indications for thrombolysis or early anticoagulation
- On anticoagulant treatment
- A known bleeding tendency
- A depressed level of consciousness (Glasgow Coma Score (GCS) below 13)
- Unexplained progressive or fluctuating symptoms
- Papilloedema, neck stiffness, or fever
- Severe headache at onset of stroke symptoms

For all people with acute stroke without indications for immediate brain imaging, scanning should be performed as soon as possible (within a maximum of 24 hours after onset of symptoms).

and the initial outcomes are also very positive. In order for any pre-alert system to work, it is essential that the ambulance and hospital staff work closely together with all protocols. Criteria for pre-alert may include:

- patient aged between 18 and 80;
- patient showing signs of stroke;
- witnessed time of onset;
- patient awake at time of onset;
- no history of seizure.

These criteria are changing regularly, with some hospitals now providing thrombolysis with no upper age restriction or witnessed time of onset. The research indicates that thrombolysis in those over the age of 80 remains beneficial, despite a slightly higher rate of intracranial haemorrhage and mortality (Alshekhlee *et al.*, 2010). It is essential, however, that all patients are registered on the SITS-MOST international register to ensure that clinical governance is maintained, and these data will ultimately influence practice in the future.

There is variation in where thrombolysis interventions are provided in the UK, and this includes emergency departments, high-dependency settings, as well as acute stroke units. Patients with a stroke should always be treated in a specialized stroke unit because there is considerable evidence to show that they are less likely to die and more likely to leave hospital independent than if they are cared for on a general ward (Langhorne *et al.*, 1997). Stroke units typically offer access to specialist expertise, earlier feeding, mobilization, and early interventions for infection, as well as significant multidisciplinary working. The number needed to treat for organized stroke units has been calculated to be as low as 15 admissions to avoid one death or disability outcome (Langhorne and Dennis, 1998), and this figure is likely to be even lower since thrombolysis emerged as a treatment option. This is a measure of the clinical significance of evidence-based interventions, and is the inverse of the control event rate minus the experimental event rate, i.e. 1/(CER–EER).

One of the key requirements of an acute stroke unit is that it has continuous physiological monitoring and a higher staff–patient ratio to ensure that regular monitoring of the patient's observations occurs. As part of evidence submitted to the development of the National Stroke Strategy, the UK National Stroke Nursing Forum recommended that two hyperacute patients are cared for by one registered nurse. This recommendation reflects the requirements for intensive monitoring of patients, the potential for thrombolysis, the increased risk of stroke progression, and the profile of interventions required to deliver an appropriate standard of care.

Blood pressure

It is usual for blood pressure to be elevated in acute stroke. In addition, patients may have pre-existing hypertension that may, or may not, have been treated prior to the stroke. In most patients, the blood pressure spontaneously reduces over the first 4–10 days. Lowering of the blood pressure using medication may result in reduction of bloodflow to the brain, reducing oxygen and nutrients to the vulnerable penumbra (the susceptible area immediately around the infarct). This increases its vulnerability and ultimately increases the likelihood of a poor outcome for the patient. Modification is therefore not recommended other than with severe hypertension, such as a systolic blood pressure of greater than 200 mmHg or if the patient has other medical problems. An ECG and telemetry is required to identify AF or other cardiac reason for causing the stroke. For many patients presenting with stroke and AF, the diagnosis of AF is newly identified.

Incontinence

Urinary incontinence is a major problem following a stroke and can affect almost 80% of patients in the initial few days (Kolominsky-Rabas *et al.*, 2003). Whilst it is usual practice to catheterize patients to obtain an accurate fluid balance, this is not usually required for stroke patients and catheterization should be avoided at all costs. Currently, 20% of patients in England and Wales are catheterized within the first week (Royal College of Physicians, 2011). A full continence assessment should be performed on all patients with a loss of bladder control. This should identify the reason for incontinence. The commonest types of incontinence are outlined in Box 13.4.

As with hypertension, it is important to determine wheather incontinence may have preceded the stroke or is a direct consequence. A clinical trial of combined behavioural interventions to improve the management of post-stroke urinary incontinence is currently under way, and will augment the current, patchy evidence base for this clinical problem (Thomas *et al.*, 2011).

(a)

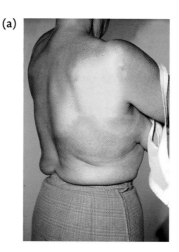

Colour Plate 1 (see Figure 12.2a) Contact eczema.

Reproduced from Saxe *et al.* (2007) *Handbook of Dermatology for Primary Care*, with permission from Oxford University Press.

(b)

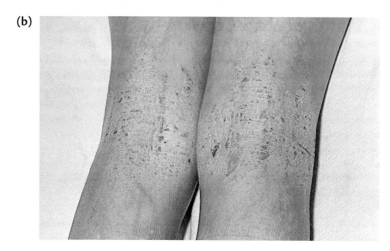

Colour Plate 2 (see Figure 12.2b) Atopic eczema.

Reproduced from Mackie (2003) *Clinical Dermatology*, with permission from Oxford University Press.

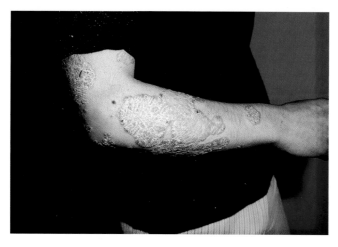

Colour Plate 3 (see Figure 12.3) Plaque psoriasis.

Reproduced from Saxe *et al.* (2007) *Handbook of Dermatology for Primary Care*, with permission from Oxford University Press.

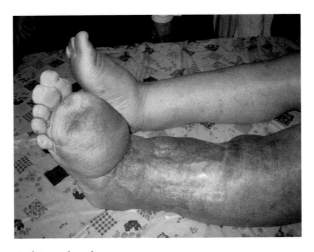

Colour Plate 4 (see Figure 12.4) **Lymphoedema.**

Image courtesy of Professor Christine Moffat.

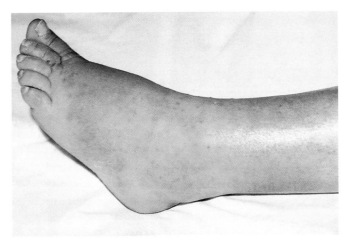

Colour Plate 5 (see Figure 12.5) **Cellulitis.**

Reproduced from Mackie (2003) *Clinical Dermatology*, with permission from Oxford University Press.

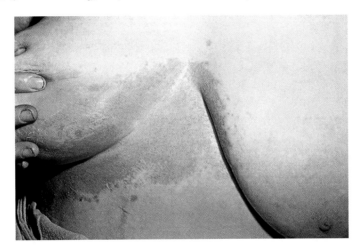

Colour Plate 6 (see Figure 12.6) **Candidosis (fungal infection).**

Reproduced from Mackie (2003) *Clinical Dermatology*, with permission from Oxford University Press.

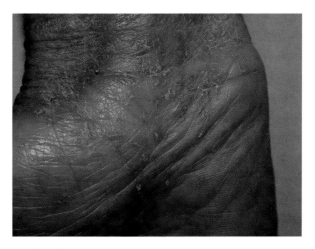

Colour Plate 7 (see Figure 12.7) Scabies.

Reproduced from Saxe *et al.* (2007) *Handbook of Dermatology for Primary Care*, with permission from Oxford University Press.

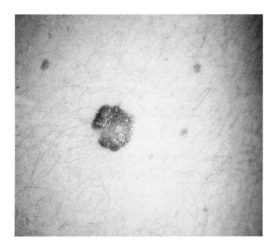

Colour Plate 8 (see Figure 12.8) Melanoma.

Reproduced from Saxe *et al.* (2007) *Handbook of Dermatology for Primary Care*, with permission from Oxford University Press.

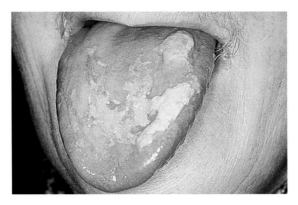

Colour Plate 9 (see Figure 20.3) **Thrush (pseudomembranous candidosis) in an elderly patient.**

Reproduced from Soames and Southam, *Oral Pathology*, with permission from Oxford University Press.

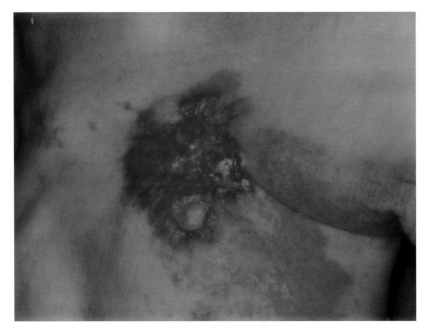

Colour Plate 10 (See Figure 28.1) **Illustration of skin damage from exudate; classified as Code 2 on the TELER indicator.**

Box 13.4 **The commonest types of urinary incontinence (Stroke Association, 2009)**

Frequency—the need to pass urine often

Urge incontinence—an urgent, uncontrollable need to go to the toilet, usually resulting in not giving the person time, and resulting in a wetting or soiling of his or herself

Nocturnal incontinence—wetting the bed whilst asleep

Functional incontinence—resulting from mobility problems, such as difficulty in unfastening clothes

Reflex incontinence or neurogenic incontinence—passing urine without realizing

Overflow incontinence—bladder leakage owing to being too full

Positioning and mobility

Correct patient positioning is essential to minimize damage and to maximize recovery. Pressure areas are vulnerable because it is not uncommon for patients to be found having spent many hours, or occasionally days, lying on the floor. In addition to increasing the risk of chest problems, there is a significant risk of developing pressure sores.

It has been estimated that patients spend only 13% of their working day engaged in activities that contribute to rehabilitation (Bernhardt *et al.*, 2004). Whilst early mobilization is essential, it should be part of an agreed active management plan (Intercollegiate Working Party for Stroke, 2008). All patients should be encouraged to sit up as soon as their condition permits to improve oxygen saturation levels.

Depression

Early detection of post-stroke depression is an important element in the nursing role because it can present a significant obstacle to rehabilitation (Gall, 2005). The causes of mood disturbances may be varied, and may be related to neurotransmitter damage, location of the lesion damage, serotonin levels, or a 'normal' response to adjustment in experiencing a stroke. Research in patients who have experienced aphasia is very limited, and the incidence of depression in this subgroup has not been established. However, it is generally felt that depression has an incidence of 22–55% in hospital and 11–25% in community

studies (Gall, 2005). Whilst specialists such as clinical psychologists are recommended as part of the multidisciplinary team for stroke, this resource may be limited at a local level. There is emerging evidence of the effectiveness of talk-based therapies, including motivational interviewing, in addressing the psychological impacts of stroke (Watkins *et al.*, 2007).

Cognitive deficits and sleep

Cognitive deficits that commonly occur following a stroke include memory problems, language or perception problems, and high-level reasoning and planning difficulties. These patients may lack insight into their condition, which may delay their recovery and increase the risk of harm. It is not unusual for a patient to be quite adamant that he or she does not have a weakness and can walk unaided to the bathroom, and safe management of these patients is essential to reduce the risk of falling. Clear, effective communication between staff, patients, and visitors is essential.

Sleep patterns may also be disrupted, affecting rest and subsequent involvement in rehabilitation. The causes of this are multifactorial, including disturbance from other patients or staff, fear of dying (typically occurring in the night), cognitive disorders, and depression. It is essential to identify any underlying concerns (such as dying fears) and to address them, because medication is not always the best solution.

Rehabilitate

Only a small percentage of patients will receive thrombolysis, and it is essential that all patients have access to the best, evidenced-based rehabilitation as soon as they come into contact with healthcare staff. One of the most comprehensive studies in this area was a retrospective analysis in Calgary, Canada, which found that, after case mix adjustment, the average length of stay was 4 days shorter in the stroke unit than the general ward, and in-hospital mortality was reduced by 4.5% (Zhu *et al.*, 2009). It is essential, however, to ensure that stroke services run effectively 7 days a week. Crowley *et al.* (2009) found that those patients presenting with intracerebral haemorrhage admitted over the weekend had a corresponding increased mortality compared with those admitted during the working week. To ensure standardization of what is expected of a stroke unit, key characteristics have been developed nationally, as follows.

- The rehabilitation unit may be clinically led by a senior non-medical clinician (usually at consultant nurse or consultant therapist grade).
- The rehabilitation unit has regular stroke physician input into the review and medical management of the patient.
- There is a stroke specialist multidisciplinary team.
- There are formal links with patient and carer organizations.
- There are multidisciplinary meetings at least once a week.
- There is provision of information to patients about stroke.
- There is funding for external courses and uptake.

(British Association of Stroke Physicians, 2010; Royal College of Physicians, 2011).

There have been significant improvements in the number of hospitals within England and Wales that have a stroke unit. However, there continues to be room for improvement, with the Sentinel Audit in 2010 finding that fewer than 50% offer an education or vocational programme for patients of working age, a core feature of service provision. In addition, in one-fifth of stroke units patients are mobilized only following an assessment by a physiotherapist. This not only disempowers the stroke nurses, but also risks the patient remaining in bed over the weekend. It is strongly advocated that all nurses working within this specialist area receive the extended skills training in assessing mobility and in screening for swallowing disorders to minimize unnecessary delays for the patient and to enable early commencement of treatment plans.

Early supported discharge

Following a period of acute hospital care, some patients cannot be transferred directly home. However, early supported discharge provides an effective care pathway when less disabled patients can be discharged early to undergo further rehabilitation at home. This results in reducing the hospital length of stay, but can also reduce long-term dependence, admission into institutionalized care, and the risk of further disability after 6 months (Saka *et al.*, 2009). It is anticipated that the stroke pathway will alter significantly over the next decade, with a significantly greater percentage of patients being discharged early and completing their rehabilitation within their own home.

Whilst early supported discharge services should provide specialist stroke care, there is the potential for community nursing to contribute to the stroke pathway. A review of 15 community nursing teams in North Wales (*n* = 15) identified that the average number of stroke patients per team was three (range 1–23). Measures of physical independence suggested that teams were supporting a range of stroke patients in terms of needs and dependency. What was evident was the lack of staff education and training, with only 33% having received stroke education or training. Focus groups highlighted the need for clearer stroke discharge coordination and transfer of care into the community, and leveraging the nursing resources that exist within the district nursing service to enhance the experiences of patients and families (Bampfield and Burton, 2010). District nurses have a role in supporting stroke patients and families in community settings; opportunities to consolidate this role through stroke-specific education and training and clinical leadership should be maximized.

Reintegrate

Life after stroke is a good example of an area in which cross-boundary working is required between primary, secondary, and tertiary services provided by statutory and voluntary organizations. Once care is transferred back into the community, people have little contact with formal services, or access to professional support and advice (Watkins *et al.*, 2002), are unaware of disease consequences, and report an absence of therapy and support. Other challenges include translating rehabilitation to the home and community environment, and renegotiating social and family roles. Longer term challenges include maintaining purposeful leisure activities, returning to work, managing depression and other psychological problems, and limiting social isolation caused by problems with communication and mobility (Stroke Association, 1999).

Implementing best practice

Supporting implementation, there are now a wide variety of sources of evidence for stroke care that, although

---

THEORY INTO PRACTICE 13.1
Learning more

Visit the Stroke Association's website and listen to the available podcasts that describe individual patient journeys following stroke. One example is the story of John Bishop, one of the country's leading fashion photographers, at **http://www. stroke.org.uk/media_centre/podcast/john_ bishop.html;** another is David Festenstein, who underlines the importance of positive thinking and active patient participation in stroke care and rehabilitation. David's story is found at **http://www. stroke.org.uk/media_centre/podcast/david_ festenstein.html**

Think about the key messages from this chapter and apply them to your practice context. Take time to listen to these podcasts or to read more examples of patient stories in The Stroke Association's 'Life After Stroke' publication, available from its website by following this link: **http://www.stroke.org.uk/media_centre/ podcast/life_after_stroke.html**

---

presented within a multidisciplinary context, provide a solid foundation for nursing care.

Examples include the following.

- UK National Clinical Guidelines for Stroke (Intercollegiate Working Party for Stroke, 2008)
- Diagnosis and initial management of acute stroke and transient ischaemic attack (TIA) (National Institute for Health and Clinical Excellence (NICE), 2008)
- Management of patients with stroke or TIA: assessment, investigation, immediate management and secondary prevention (Scottish Intercollegiate Guidelines Network (SIGN), 2008)
- Management of patients with stroke: Identification and management of dysphagia (Scottish Intercollegiate Guidelines Network (SIGN), 2010a)
- Management of patients with stroke: rehabilitation, prevention and management of complications, and discharge planning (Scottish Intercollegiate Guidelines Network (SIGN), 2010b)

- National Sentinel Stroke Audit Organisational Audit, 2010 (Intercollegiate Working Party for Stroke, Royal College of Physicians, 2011)
- Stroke Quality Standard, National Institute for Health and Clinical Excellence (NICE), 2010 **http://www.nice. org.uk/guidance/qualitystandards/stroke/stroke- qualitystandard.jsp**

The National Institute for Health and Clinical Excellence (NICE) is due to publish guidance on stroke rehabilitation in 2012.

Key messages

This chapter has identified several key areas of best practice in which implementation is encouraged by governmental pressure and financial incentives. Strategic direction is provided by the National Stroke Strategy (Department of Health, 2007), which sets out 20 key quality markers for commissioners, stroke networks, and service providers to follow to ensure that they offer the latest, evidence-based care. The strategy concentrates on the four key periods of raising awareness, acute care, life after stroke, and ensuring long-term evidence-based practice. The Stroke Strategy was supported by a significant financial investment from the Department of Health, which provided the media campaigns to help to increase public awareness; their success was so great that they are being repeated in 2011. One key criticism of the strategy was the delay in implementation of the evidence of up to 10 years. However, this has been re-energized by the Best Practice Tariff, which provides additional 'top-up' funding for compliance with the evidence base, including urgent brain scanning, thrombolysis, and direct admission to the stroke unit. It is anticipated that this financial support will aid the decision to invest in stroke care during a time of financial difficulty. Stroke provides a good example of how the latest clinical evidence indicates that investment results in not only a significant improvement to patient outcome, but also a financial saving owing to a reduction in length of hospital stay. Thrombolysis for stroke is the best example of this.

Other implementation strategies include:

- audit and performance feedback of evidence-based clinical standards (the Stroke Sentinel Audit) completed every 2 years by the Royal College of Physicians Clinical Effectiveness and Evaluation Unit;

- the NHS Stroke Improvement Programme;
- a stroke-specific education framework to quality assure all stroke education and training provided in the UK.

The future

Stroke services have altered significantly over the past 10 years and these changes are expected to continue. These changes will not only be in relation to rehabilitation and thrombolysis; the greatest reduction to the disability caused by stroke will be on improving stroke prevention. The second focus of development will be surgical advances. Within the cardiac care setting, patients who have had a myocardial infarction are now routinely receiving primary angioplasty and it is anticipated that more patients who have experienced a stroke will be offered not only intravenous thrombolysis, but also intra-arterial thrombolysis, clot retrieval, or surgical interventions such as decompressive hemicraniectomy.

Sources of evidence

Organizations

National Institute for Health and Clinical Excellence (NICE) **http://guidance.nice.org.uk/**

The Scottish Intercollegiate Guidelines Network (SIGN) **http://www.sign.ac.uk/guidelines/index.html**

NHS Evidence **http://www.evidence.nhs.uk/**

Agency for Healthcare Quality (AHRQ) **http://www.ahrq.gov/**

National Institute for Clinical Studies (NICS) **http://www.nhmrc.gov.au/nics/index.htm**

Registered Nurses Association of Ontario **http://www.rnao.org**

World Health Organization **http://www.who.int/en/**

Journals

Stroke

Journal of Clinical Neuroscience

Neurology

British Medical Journal

The Lancet

Conclusion

A strong government agenda for the improvement of stroke services, financial incentives, and continual national audit has had a profound impact on the organization and delivery of stroke care in the UK. Evidence-based guidance is available to nurses to support a clear pathway for managers and clinicians to plan and deliver effective and appropriate services. The aim is to reduce the incidence of stroke and to improve significantly chances of recovery for the individual patient and his or her family.

Some nurses working within stroke care find it difficult to define their role, perhaps because it is so multifaceted: they are preventionists, identifying early the signs of deterioration; they are coordinators, ensuring the smooth involvement for all of the multidisciplinary staff involved; and most of all they are supporters—for the emotional trauma experienced by the patient and his or her family.

Online Resource Centre

 To help you to develop and apply your knowledge and decision-making skills further, we have provided interactive learning resources online at **www.oxfordtextbooks.co.uk/orc/bullock/**

Whilst these are freely available, you will need to use the access codes at the start of the book.

References

Alexandrov, A. (2003) *Cerebrovascular Ultrasound in Stroke Prevention and Treatment.* Blackwell-Futura: New York.

Allender, S., Peto, V., Scarborough, P., *et al.* (2006) *Coronary Health Disease Statistics.* British Heart Foundation: London.

Alshekhlee, A., Mohammadi, A., Mehta, S., *et al.* (2010) Is thrombolysis safe in the elderly? Analysis of a national database. *Stroke* **41**: 2259–64.

Bamford, J., Sandercock, P., Dennis, M., *et al.* (1991) Classification and natural history of clinically identifiable subtypes of cerebral infarction. *Lancet* **337**(8756):1521–6.

Bampfield, K., Burton, C. (2010) Exploring the role of district nursing in stroke care. *UK Stroke Forum* (1 December 2010): Glasgow.

Bath, P., Lees, K. (2000) ABC of arterial and venous disease: acute stroke. *British Medical Journal* **320**: 920–3.

Batmanian, J., Lam, M., Matthews, C., *et al.* (2007) A protocol-driven model for the rapid initiation of stroke thrombolysis in the emergency department. *The Medical Journal of Australia* **187**(10): 567–70.

Bernhardt, J., Dewey, H., Thrift, A. (2004) Inactive and alone: physical activity within the first 14 days of acute stroke unit. *Stroke* **35**(4): 1005–9.

British Association of Stroke Physicians (2010) *Stroke Service Standards.* http://www.basp.ac.uk/LinkClick.aspx?fileticket=%2FKYTIcgdxg0%3D&tabid=653&mid=1053 (accessed 27 July 2011).

Cappuccio, F. (1997) Ethnicity and cardiovascular risk: variations in people of African ancestry and South Asian origin. *Journal of Human Hypertension* **11**: 571–6.

Cross, S. (2008) Stroke care: a nursing perspective. *Nursing Standard* **22**(23): 47–56.

Crowley, R., Yeoh, H., Stukenborg, G., *et al.* (2009) Influence of weekend hospital admission in short-term mortality after intracerebral haemorrhage. *Stroke* **40**: 2387–92.

Davis C. (2005) Time in mind. *Nursing Standard* **19**(51): 24–6.

Department of Health (2007) *National Stroke Strategy.* Department of Health: London.

Department of Health (2010) *Best Practice Tariffs.* Department of Health: London.

Ford G. (2009) *Joining Forces Networking Together for the Future of Stroke Care.* Stroke Research Network, Peninsula Heart & Stroke Network & National Institute for Health Research Conference, 6 May 2009, Exeter.

Gall A. (2005) Post stroke depression. In R. White (ed.) *Stroke: Therapy and Rehabilitation.* Quay Books: London, pp. 99–112.

Hacke, W., Donnan, G., Fieschi, C., *et al.* (2004) Association of outcome with early stroke treatment: pooled analysis of ATLANTIS, ECASS, and NINDS rt-PA stroke trials. *Lancet* **363**: 768–74.

Hacke, W., Kaste, M., Bluhmki, E., *et al.* for the ECASS Investigators (2008) Thrombolysis with alteplase 3 to 4.5 hours after acute ischemic stroke. *New England Journal of Medicine* **359**: 1317–29.

Intercollegiate Working Party for Stroke (2008) *National Clinical Guidelines for Stroke.* Royal College of Physicians: London.

Jorgensen, H., Nakayama, H., Reith, J., *et al.* (1996) Factors delaying hospital admission in acute stroke: the Copenhagen Stroke Study. *Neurology* **47**: 383–7.

Kolominsky-Rabas, P., Hiltz, M., Neurndoerfer, B., *et al.* (2003) Impact of urinary incontinence after stroke: results from a prospective population-based stroke register. *Neurological Urodynamics* **22**: 322–7.

Langdon, P.C., Lee, A.H., Binns, C.W. (2007) Dysphagia in acute ischaemic stroke: severity, recovery and relationship to stroke subtype. *Journal of Clinical Neuroscience* **14**(7): 630–4.

Langhorne, P., Dennis, M. (1998) *Stroke Units: An Evidence-Based Approach.* BMJ Books: London.

Langhorne, P., Williams, BO., Gilchrist, W., *et al.* (1993) Do stroke units save lives? *Lancet* **342**: 395–8.

National Audit Office (2005) *Brain Damage: Faster Access to Better Stroke Care.* HMSO: London.

National Collaborating Centre for Chronic Conditions (2008) *Stroke: National Clinical Guideline for the Diagnosis and Initial Management of Acute Stroke and Transient Ischaemic Attack (TIA).* Royal College of Physicians: London.

National Institute for Health and Clinical Excellence (NICE) (2008) *Stroke: Diagnosis and Initial Management of Acute Stroke and Transient Ischaemic Attack (TIA).* National Institute for Health and Clinical Excellence: London.

National Institute for Health and Clinical Excellence (NICE) (2010) *Stroke Quality Standards.* http://www.nice.org.uk/guidance/qualitystandards/stroke/strokequalitystandard.jsp (accessed 3 January 2012).

NHS Choices (2011) Stroke Act FAST. www.nhs.uk/actfast/pages/stroke.aspx (accessed 3 January 2012).

Nor, A., Davis, J., Sen, B., *et al.* (2005) The recognition of stroke in the emergency room (ROSIER) scale: development and validation of a stroke recognition instrument. *Lancet* **4**(11): 691–3.

Nor, A., McAllister, C., Louw, S., *et al.* (2004) Agreement between ambulance paramedic and physician recorded neurological signs with fast arm speech test (FAST) in acute stroke patients. *Stroke* **35**: 1355–9.

Royal College of Physicians (2009) *The National Sentinel Stroke Audit 2008.* Royal College of Physicians: London.

Royal College of Physicians (2011) *The National Sentinel Stroke Audit 2010.* Royal College of Physicians: London.

Sacco, R., Benjamin, E., Broderick, J., *et al.* (1997) Risk factors. *Stroke* **28**: 1507–17.

Saka, O., Serra, V., Samyshkin, Y., *et al.* (2009) Cost-effectiveness if stroke unit care followed by early supported discharge. *Stroke* **40**: 24–9.

Scottish Intercollegiate Guidelines Network (SIGN) (2008) *Management of Patients with Stroke or TIA: Assessment, Investigation, Immediate Management and Secondary Prevention.* Scottish Intercollegiate Guidelines Network: Edinburgh.

Scottish Intercollegiate Guidelines Network (SIGN) (2010a) *Management of Patients with Stroke: Identification and Management of Dysphagia.* Scottish Intercollegiate Guidelines Network: Edinburgh.

Scottish Intercollegiate Guidelines Network (SIGN) (2010b) *Management of Patients with Stroke: Rehabilitation, Prevention and Management of Complications, and Discharge Planning.* Scottish Intercollegiate Guidelines Network: Edinburgh.

Stroke Association (1999) *Stroke Care: A Matter of Chance.* Stroke Association: London.

Stroke Association (2009) *Continence Problems after Stroke.* Stroke Association: London.

Thomas, L., Watkins, C., French, B., *et al.* and ICONS Patient Involvement Group (2011) Study protocol: ICONS: identifying continence options after stroke: a randomised trial. *Clinical Trials* **12**: 131.

Tyson, S. (1995) Stroke rehabilitation: what is the point? *Physiotherapy* **81**(8): 430–2.

Watkins, C., Auton, M., Deans, C., *et al.* (2007) Motivational interviewing early after acute stroke: a randomised controlled trial. *Stroke* **38**: 1004–9.

Watkins, C., Leathley, M., Sharma, A. (2002) *Stroke Interface Audit.* University of Central Lancashire: Preston.

Wolfe, C., Rudd, A., Howard, R., *et al.* (2002) Incidence and case fatality rates of stroke subtypes in a multiethnic population: the south London stroke register. *Journal of Neurology, Neurosurgery and Psychiatry* **72**: 211–16.

World Health Organization (1978) *Cerebrovascular Disorders (Offset Publications).* World Health Organization: Geneva.

Zhu, H., Newcommon, N., Cooper, M., *et al.* (2009) Calgary stroke program: impact of a stroke unit on hospital stay and in-hospital case fatality. *Stroke* **40**: 18–23.

PART 2
Managing Health Needs and Symptoms

The key to reframing evidence-based nursing practice

There are 15 chapters in this second part of the book and they are designed to provide you with a definitive guide to your nursing management of a range of the most fundamental problems, symptoms, and health challenges faced by adult patients.

Regardless of what a patient's underlying condition is, you will constantly encounter in your everyday practice these symptoms or challenges. Chapter authors encourage you to recognize that the management of these is the primary responsibility of the nurse, and to shape care interventions on evidence, the basis of expert nursing practice. Expert nursing practice is the ability to identify and deliver contemporary evidence-based nursing interventions that will reduce symptoms and effectively enhance the patient's ability to cope with the challenges that he or she faces. In turn, your nursing expertise has the capacity to improve quality of life and increase health benefits.

To offer the highest quality nursing care to your patients, it is essential that you have the knowledge and confidence both to accurately assess the nature of their symptoms, problems, and challenges, and to identify the most appropriate nursing interventions. Chapter authors guide you through an overview of the symptom recognition, problem identification, or presenting healthcare challenge, developing a comprehensive understanding of both the nature and/or causation. Your nursing responsibility and accountability is emphasized alongside a reliance of evidence-based interventions.

Within this context, where possible, we have indicated how we can 'measure' the impact or effect of these interventions. Within the current healthcare context, the measurement of patient outcomes is increasingly important as the political agenda focuses on quality improvement. This is a developing area of importance, with 'indicators' of measurement being designed alongside service delivery commissioning, so that the quality of patient care can be articulated. The emergence of quality standards has recently focused all areas of health and social care on the importance of measuring the effect of healthcare interventions, and nursing interventions should be treated no differently. Measurement of improvement is something that we actively encourage you to do, ideally over a period of time so that a trend can be determined and improvement demonstrated. Several chapters in Part 2 provide currently used measures or metrics, and the principles explored in these chapters are directly applicable to all chapters in Part 2.

With emphasis on expert clinical assessment, guidance on best practice frameworks for undertaking this is also explored. Good clinical assessment will undoubtedly increase the effectiveness of targeted interventions for your patient. Whilst the body of research evidence is growing in this area, we also address the importance of acknowledging where gaps in the evidence base exist. Consistent with Part 1 chapters, Part 2 chapters provide guidance to definitive sources of trustworthy evidence, often providing the hyperlinks to gold standard sources, thus enabling you to keep up to date.

Studying these chapters will equip you to reframe your understanding of your nursing responsibility for these fundamental areas of care, and will give you the confidence to take a clear leadership role in their management. Patients are reliant on your nursing expertise in these areas of care. We believe that this book will give you the confidence to make sound clinical decisions about the preferred approach, ensuring that the interventions used will lead to healthcare improvement.

Measuring the impact of nursing interventions

The principle of measuring both the effectiveness of nursing intervention and the patient's experience of receiving care is one that you, as a nurse, should, where possible, facilitate. The NHS Information Centre has supported the development of Nursing Quality Metrics (NQMs), which can be used to facilitate quality improvement in patient care and experience: http://signposting.ic.nhs.uk/?k=metrics

This recent move within healthcare to be outcome-focused rather than target-driven is a welcome change in policy direction, initiated by Lord Darzi in his review of the NHS, and sustained by the previous and current UK governments. Metrics have been developed for many aspects of nursing care interventions and cover many inpatient areas, regardless of setting. The collection of these types of data helps healthcare organizations to focus on the delivery of safe and effective care, and can be used for local and national benchmarking, as well as quality improvement.

For further details, visit the NHS Information Centre online at http://www.ic.nhs.uk/, where you will find details relating to nursing audit tools capturing information on documentation for observations, nutrition, medicines administration, pain management, communication, discharge planning, falls, pressure area care, antibiotic prescribing, and infection control.

In determining patient experience of healthcare, The National Institute for Health and Clinical Excellence (NICE) has recently published a Quality Standard online at http://www.nice.org.uk/ that guides service delivery planning to ensure improvements in patient experience. Further commissioned work by the Department of Health has developed a single measure of patient experience. Supplementing these data is the NHS Survey, which captures patient views relating to ward cleanliness, infection control, staff attitudes, pain management, management of privacy, experience of dignity, nutrition, medicines administration, quality of communication, and discharge. Details can be found online at http://www.nhssurveys.org/

14 *Managing* Anxiety

Sarah Kendal and John Baker

Introduction

This chapter explores anxiety, providing a clinical description of its impact on patients with guidance for evidence-based assessment and management. Anxiety has a defined physiological mechanism and merits a planned management approach.

Every nurse should possess the knowledge and skills to identify patients with and/or at risk of anxiety, to select and implement evidence-based strategies to manage anxiety, and to review the effectiveness of these to inform any necessary changes in care.

Understanding the importance of anxiety

It can be useful to think of most mental and emotional phenomena as being a combination of four systems: autonomic, behavioural, cognitive, and environmental (Box 14.1).

Emotions that we experience, such as happiness, sadness, anxiety, and anger, depend on how the systems interact with each other. These four systems combine to form a common model in mental health, known as the ABC-E model of emotion (Briddon *et al.*, 2008) (also see Chapter 8 ➡), which will be used as a framework for the chapter. An ABC-E-based assessment helps to clarify nursing interventions in each one of these four areas. An intervention in one of these systems can often help to alleviate distressing emotions.

Defining anxiety

A commonly used classification system for mental disorders is the International Classification of Diseases version 10 (ICD-10) (World Health Organization (WHO), 2010). An alternative classification system is the Diagnostic and Statistical Manual of Mental Disorders (DSM) (American Psychiatric Association, 1994). The main types of anxiety are listed in Box 14.2.

Many features of anxiety disorder also present in the patient who is agitated. Agitation is a form of anxiety that can raise particular concerns about safety. As illustrated in Table 14.1, the main difference is in the cognitive and behavioural domains, i.e. what the person is thinking and doing. The descriptions in Table 14.1 apply to anxiety as a clinical problem, as in the case of David, whose story is described in Case study 14.1. The difference between non-clinical and clinical anxiety is explained in the 'Making a clinical assessment' section.

Box 14.1   A model of emotion

A The body (Autonomic nervous system)
B The things that people do (Behaviours)
C The thoughts people have (Cognitions)
E The environment (situational and personal circumstances)

(Briddon *et al.*, 2008)

Box 14.2   Defining types of anxiety

Adjustment disorders
Generalized anxiety disorder (GAD)
Mixed anxiety and depressive disorder
Obsessive-compulsive disorder (OCD)
Panic disorder (with or without agoraphobia)
Phobias, including:

- agoraphobia
- social phobias
- specific phobias
- other phobic anxiety disorders

Post-traumatic stress disorder (PTSD)
Reaction to severe stress
Unspecified anxiety disorders

There are other approaches to defining anxiety. For example, the *British Medical Journal* (BMJ) has defined generalized anxiety disorder (GAD) as follows:

> At least 6 months of excessive worry about issues, that causes distress or impairment. The anxiety is not confined to features of another mental disorder or as a result of substance abuse or a general medical condition. At least 3 of the following symptoms are present most of the time: restlessness or nervousness, easy fatigability, poor concentration, irritability, muscle tension, or sleep disturbance. (BMJ, 2010)

These definitions illustrate a focus on clinical symptoms for the purpose of diagnosis.

Alternatively, many user-led or user-focused organizations define anxiety by focusing on how it feels, with less emphasis on listing clinical symptoms. One of the advantages of this approach is that it can encourage clinicians to see the condition from the patient's perspective. Examples of this approach can be found on the following organizations' websites: MIND **www.mind.org.uk**; Anxiety UK **www.anxietyuk.org.uk**; Young Minds **www.youngminds.org.uk**; the Mental Health Foundation **www.mentalhealth.org.uk**; and the Centre for Mental Health **www.centreformentalhealth.org.uk**

Defining agitation

Agitation can be understood as acute anxiety—a form of acute stress reaction (Box 14.3). When people feel anxious or agitated, they can go to extreme measures to reduce the intensity of their feelings. This can extend to behaviours that distract them from their thoughts or emotions, including, for example, self-medicating with drugs or alcohol, risk-taking, acts of harm to self, and violence or aggression. Nurses should not focus on the behaviours without considering the underlying causes. Agitation is therefore a serious condition requiring skilled nursing intervention to relieve the symptoms (thoughts, feeling, and behaviours) before harm occurs.

Prevalence

One in six adults in the UK has a common mental health problem such as anxiety or depression (Office for National Statistics, 2006). This is relatively high compared with much of Europe (King *et al.*, 2008). Figure 14.1 shows UK data collected from general practice that illustrate that women are more likely than men to suffer from common mental health problems. Other data collected from general practice suggest that anxiety is as prevalent as coronary heart disease, and more common than diabetes (Moser and Majeed, 1999).

Research shows the chronic nature of anxiety and reinforces the case for providing effective treatment. For example, a longitudinal study in which 2,406 participants were interviewed about their mental health showed that half with common mental health problems such as anxiety and depression were still unwell after 18 months, although those who received treatment did show improvement (Singleton and Lewis, 2003). These findings demonstrate that depression and anxiety may not resolve spontaneously.

Table 14.1 Typical signs and symptoms of anxiety and agitation

	Anxiety	Agitation
Autonomic	Feeling hot Sweating Muscle tension Tight throat	Feeling hot Sweating Muscle tension
	Sleep disturbance Tiredness	Sleep disturbance
	Raised heart beat Rapid breathing Palpitations Chest pain	Raised heart beat Rapid breathing
	Sensations of not hearing or seeing properly	Hearing or seeing becomes more focused
	Churning stomach	Urgent bowel movements
	Dizziness Feeling unsteady	
Behavioural	Irritability	Irritability
	Pacing Restlessness	Pacing Restlessness
		Clenching fists Shouting
	Avoiding situations that might be stressful	
	Needing constant reassurance Checking	
Cognitive	Pessimistic predictions Sense of impending doom	
	Worry and fear	
	Confusion Disorientation	
	Sense of unreality	
		Perception of not being treated with respect
		Frustration

Causation

Causes of anxiety may be considered to be biological, psychological, and social. These three factors work together in a circular way so that improvement in one aspect of a patient's experience can enhance recovery in other areas (Figure 14.2). The biopsychosocial concept of mental health is endorsed in current UK health policy (Department of Health, 2010) and the application of the ABC-E model and a biopsychosocial approach can enhance holistic assessment and care (Barker, 2009; Gupta, 2010).

Box 14.3 The International Classification of Diseases: acute stress reaction (ICD-10 F43.0)

Acute stress reaction

A transient disorder that develops in an individual without any other apparent mental disorder in response to exceptional physical and mental stress and that usually subsides within hours or days. Individual vulnerability and coping capacity play a role in the occurrence and severity of acute stress reactions.

The symptoms show a typically mixed and changing picture and include an initial state of 'daze' with some constriction of the field of consciousness and narrowing of attention, inability to comprehend stimuli, and disorientation. This state may be followed either by further withdrawal from the surrounding situation (to the extent of a dissociative stupor—F44.2), or by agitation and over-activity (flight reaction or fugue). Autonomic signs of panic anxiety (tachycardia, sweating, flushing) are commonly present.

The symptoms usually appear within minutes of the impact of the stressful stimulus or event, and disappear within two to three days (often within hours). Partial or complete amnesia (F44.0) for the episode may be present. If the symptoms persist, a change in diagnosis should be considered.

(World Health Organization (WHO), 2007)

Biological causes

Physical health difficulties such as illness, pain, debility, or impaired mobility can cause stress, particularly if they are chronic problems (Stark and House, 2000). It is common for people to feel stressed about their physical health: for example, patients with vascular disease may experience headaches, palpitations, feeling hot or unsteady—symptoms that can be attributed to both anxiety and vascular problems. The link between physical and mental health symptoms can also work in the other direction; Stapleton *et al.* (2005) reported that patients with chronic chest disease experienced an improvement in their physical symptoms when they were treated for depression, suggesting that improvement in mental health can have a positive impact on physical health outcomes.

Psychological causes

Low-level, long-term stress, and short, but highly stressful, experiences can lead to anxiety or agitation in some people. Some factors that can contribute to anxiety are excessive responsibility or workload, or chronic feelings of failure, inadequacy, or anger. How a person copes with stress seems to be important: for instance, a study of occupational stress in nurses concluded that stress can be reduced if a person has effective coping mechanisms (Wu *et al.*, 2010).

Anxiety in childhood appears to be linked with anxiety in adulthood. A cohort study of children born in Britain in

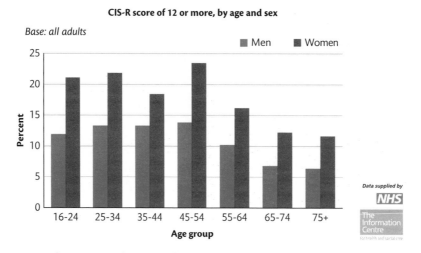

Figure 14.1 CIS-R score of 12 or more, by age and sex.

1970 found that having a mild emotional problem at the age of 5 increased the likelihood of having mild to moderate emotional problems by the time someone reached the age of 30 (Richards *et al.*, 2009).

Traumatic psychological factors may be linked with disruption to the sense of self, owing to relationship break-up, betrayal of trust, estrangement, separation, or bereavement (Tolin and Foa, 2008). All of these can trigger loss of identity, role, and sense of belonging. If an individual is unable to come to terms with the initial shock, he or she may be vulnerable to developing mental health problems.

Social causes

Poor social and economic circumstances are risk factors for developing anxiety and reduced chances of recovery. Problems with employment, debt, housing, long-term illness or disability, family conflict, prolonged court cases, and criminal activity are all identifiable social stressors that, if too much for the individual to cope with, may develop into a clinically diagnosable anxiety disorder.

Childhood adversity is another acknowledged risk factor, having a detrimental effect on a person's chances of a high quality of life, including his or her emotional health. Abuse and personal trauma in childhood can damage self-esteem and the ability to trust, which is likely to make it more difficult to forge helpful, lasting relationships with other people. The political context is relevant, since war or persecution can expose people to violence or displacement. Individuals with many advantages can also develop anxiety, with an extreme fear of failure or disgrace (Lucey and Reay, 2002).

Human and social burden and costs

Unresolved anxiety can reduce quality of life and life chances. Richards *et al.* (2009) reported that anxiety can have a detrimental impact on a person's activities and his or her ability to maintain good physical health, supportive relationships, employment, and social roles. Societal cost is reflected in loss of social capital and cohesion, because people frequently try to cope with anxiety by avoiding social interactions and new situations, leading to isolation and disengagement from their communities.

Societal costs are not factored into calculations of the cost-effectiveness of health interventions. Consequently, they are difficult to measure in health economic modelling, although it is helpful to understand the economic impact of a disorder in addition to the personal burden. A comprehensive review of generalized anxiety disorder (GAD) established that the burden it places on individuals was equivalent to that of other conditions, including peptic ulcers, arthritis, diabetes, and autoimmune disease (Hoffman *et al.*, 2008). It has been suggested that the estimated economic cost of anxiety disorders in adults in the UK in 2006 was 1% of the total national income (London School of Economics, 2006).

The aetiology of anxiety: fight or flight (or fright)

Anxiety is believed to be a survival mechanism that helps a person to fight or flee from danger. The causes of anxiety are likely to be rooted in stressors within a person's

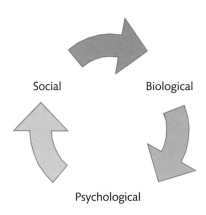

Figure 14.2 **A biopsychosocial model.**
(ONS, 2002).

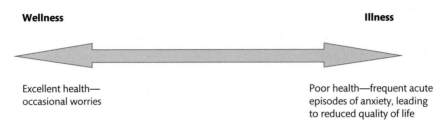

Wellness   **Illness**

Excellent health—   Poor health—frequent acute
occasional worries   episodes of anxiety, leading
                            to reduced quality of life

Figure 14.3 The wellness–illness continuum.

environment. There may be little risk of being chased through the high street by a sabre-toothed tiger, but past difficulties and worries about present or future problems can all cause day-to-day stress.

The wellness–illness continuum

Health professionals understand that health status fluctuates along a continuum, ranging from excellent to poor health (Figure 14.3). Mild or temporary experience of anxiety or agitation does not necessarily indicate a need for a health intervention. Anxiety and/or agitation are normal and healthy human experiences in certain situations and at certain times, but if they become persistent or severe, mental health problems can develop.

An important factor to consider is the impact that anxiety is having on the individual: is it affecting his or her day-to-day functioning, such as their ability to work, or to look after themselves or other people? What about physical health: can the person sleep? Is he or she eating well? Perhaps he or she is trying to manage symptoms with increased use of alcohol, over-the-counter medication, or recreational drugs? What effect is the anxiety having on his or her relationships, work, and finances?

A second important consideration is whether the anxiety seems out of proportion to the problem. This is obviously a subjective judgement, and nurses must take care not to impose their own views and values on a patient. The key is to listen to the patient and try to understand his or her perspective. Sometimes, it is helpful to think about the context. Consider Barney's unfortunate experience, in Box 14.4.

> **Box 14.4 Barney: anxiety, or an anxiety problem?**
>
> A large and inquisitive snake has escaped from a zoo; meanwhile, Barney is standing at a bus stop nearby. If the snake appears and wraps itself around Barney's leg, Barney will probably experience many symptoms of anxiety. However, this does not mean that Barney has an anxiety disorder: the problem is the snake and this can be solved by its safe removal. If we focus on Barney's symptoms without understanding the reality of his situation, we could develop an inappropriate and unhelpful plan of care.
>
> However, what if, 6 months after his experience, Barney has developed such a fear of snakes that he won't go out of his house in case he encounters one, or turn on the television in case he sees an image of one, has abandoned all activities that he can't do at home, and is socially isolated? A clinical assessment may now be called for because it looks as though he may have an anxiety disorder.

Nursing management

Psychological and physical well-being are mutually beneficial, and therefore the responsibility of nurses, regardless of their specialty. With a direct link between physical illness and anxiety established (Mental Health Foundation, 2009), effective nursing management is an important source of support for the patient. Anxiety can coexist with, and worsen, other physical and mental health

> **Box 14.5 Key messages about nursing care of people with agitation (extract from NICE Clinical Guideline 25)**
>
> **Person-centred care**
>
> Service users and their carers should be made aware of the guideline and its recommendations and be referred to the Information For the Public version (IFP). Service users and their carers should be involved in shared decision-making about the preferred choice of intervention for the short-term management of disturbed/violent behaviour through the use of their care plans or advance directives.
>
> **A collaborative interdisciplinary approach to care**
>
> All members of the interdisciplinary team should be aware of the guidelines and all interventions should be documented in the service users' healthcare records.
>
> **Organizational issues**
>
> An integrated approach should be taken to the short-term management of disturbed/violent behaviour in adult psychiatric inpatient settings, with a clear strategy and policy supported by management.
>
> Care should be delivered in a context of continuous quality improvement where improvements to care following guideline implementation are the subject of regular feedback and audit.
>
> Commitment to and availability of education and training are needed to ensure that all staff, regardless of profession, are given the opportunity to update their knowledge base and are able to implement the guideline recommendations.
>
> Service users should be cared for by personnel who have undergone appropriate training and who know how to initiate and maintain correct and suitable preventative measures. Staffing levels and skill mix should reflect the needs of service users and healthcare professionals.
>
> (National Institute for Clinical Excellence (NICE), 2005: 12)

problems, so early recognition and management of the problem is a key responsibility of the nurse.

The amended National Institute for Health and Clinical Excellence (NICE) guidelines for management of anxiety in adults clearly indicate that assessing anxiety is not necessarily a role for mental health specialists. All nurses should be able to identify anxiety characterized by fear, panic attacks, irritability, poor sleeping, avoidance, and poor concentration (NICE, 2007). Nurses who can recognize and manage their own anxieties are more likely to be able to help their patients (refer to websites listed earlier).

The Nursing and Midwifery Council (NMC) Code of Conduct emphasizes the responsibility of all nurses to acquire the skills to meet their patients' psychological needs (NMC, 2008). Further guidance about the nurse's role and accountability is available in the clinical guidelines published by the National Institute for Health and Clinical Excellence (NICE). Relevant guidelines for this chapter include CG22 (Anxiety), and CG25 (Violence), the latter of which concerns the short-term management of violence in emergency departments and inpatient settings.

Clinical assessment of anxiety

What to look for

Assessment of a patient should consider:

- preparation;
- interpersonal skills;
- the interview schedule.

Assessment can be structured around the ABC-E model of emotion, which helps to organize information and see the processes of cause and effect that might be contributing to the problem. The approach below is tried and tested, and is based on key principles of cognitive behaviour therapy (CBT) (Briddon *et al.*, 2008).

Preparation

Many patients dislike having to repeat the same information to several clinicians during the course of assessment (Department of Health, 1999), so, where appropriate, the interviewer should prepare for the assessment in advance by making him or herself familiar with relevant information about the interviewee.

> **Box 14.6   Key features of a therapeutic relationship**
>
> - Warmth
> - Empathy
> - Genuineness
> - Reliability
> - Basic trust
> - Information giving and receiving
> - Attending to immediate needs

Ideally, the assessment should take place in a private interview room. As far as possible, the furniture should be arranged so that both are sitting in similar chairs at the same height, and without a barrier between them. It is often more comfortable for the interviewee if the chairs are at a '10 to 2' angle rather than facing each other, as this enables the patient to break eye contact should he or she so wish.

Interpersonal skills

It is important for the nurse to develop excellent interpersonal skills, to conduct an effective assessment, and to engage the patient in collaborative decisions about treatment. There is emerging evidence to support the idea that a therapeutic relationship between clinician and patient will enhance mental health treatment outcomes (Richardson and Richards, 2006), although this theory has been embedded in nursing models for a long time (Vandemark, 2006). A person-centred approach (Rogers, 1995) can encourage the interviewee to feel that he or she has some control during the interview, which can otherwise be quite disempowering and discourage the interviewee from sharing information. The nurse should be calm, respectful, tactful, and honest. He or she should be skilled in the use of verbal and non-verbal communication techniques, open and closed questioning, pausing, active listening, and showing empathy (Norman and Ryrie, 2009; Barker, 2009). Key features of a successful therapeutic relationship are given in Box 14.6.

Interview schedule

The purpose of a clinical assessment interview is to obtain relevant information from the interviewee, which can be used to form a helpful plan of care. This means that each time we ask for a piece of information, we should understand why we want it and how it will contribute to the patient's care.

When we use a suitable interview schedule, we are more likely to cover the essential topics effectively in the time we have available, with the ABC-E model providing a valuable assessment tool. With practice, the interview can be conducted in a collaborative, conversational style.

The following questions are appropriate for assessment of a patient suffering from either anxiety or agitation (Richards and McDonald, 1990).

1. What is the problem (in your own words)?
2. How long have you had it?
3. How frequently does it occur?
4. How intense is it (e.g. on a scale of 1–10)?
5. How long does it last (e.g. an episode of acute anxiety may last for an hour)?
6. What triggers it (Environment, e.g. anticipation of an unpleasant event)?
7. What physical (Autonomic) reactions do you experience? *Or* How does it make your body feel?
8. What do you do? (Behavioural response)
9. What do you think? (Cognitive response)
10. What is the impact for you (immediate/long term)?
11. What makes it worse/better (e.g. current medication or management strategies)?
12. Who makes it worse/better?
13. When is it worse/better?

Accessing the evidence to support clinical decisions

Guidelines for the management of anxiety (National Institute for Health and Clinical Excellence (NICE), 2006) and for agitation, violence, and aggression (NICE, 2005) report on the best available evidence to support clinical decisions.

Utilizing evidence in the nursing management of anxiety

The National Institute for Health and Clinical Excellence (NICE) recommends a stepped approach to care, in which the aim is to try low-intensity treatments before offering more intense or complex approaches (National Collaborating Centre for Mental Health, 2005). In stepped-care

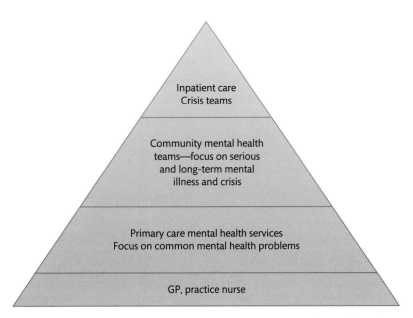

Inpatient care
Crisis teams

Community mental health
teams—focus on serious
and long-term mental
illness and crisis

Primary care mental health services
Focus on common mental health problems

GP, practice nurse

Figure 14.4 Stepped care.

models, first-line treatments may simply involve monitoring the patient. This approach is appropriate for and applicable to the management of anxiety. Specialist practitioners, treatments, and treatment settings are reserved for a very small proportion of mental disorders. The vast majority of mental healthcare takes place in primary care settings, and is delivered by generic practitioners (National Collaborating Centre for Mental Health, 2005). Figure 14.4 illustrates how stepped care can be structured.

Engaging and working with anxious patients

The development of a therapeutic relationship is the basis of all effective nursing interventions. The purpose of a therapeutic relationship is to help the patient. As a practising nurse, you should show empathy (Alligood, 1992) and communicate warmth, genuineness, and unconditional positive regard (Rogers, 1995).

Person-centred care requires that the patient's perspective on his or her situation is acknowledged and respected. Although he or she may be receiving care because of anxiety, this is often a very short interlude in his or her life and so it is inappropriate to assume that he or she sees him or herself as a person with a mental health problem. Indeed, receiving mental healthcare can be extremely demoralizing and can challenge a person's sense of identity, so he or she may resist attempts to be defined by the problem. For

this reason, it is important to recognize what the patient feels as a priority. This could involve, for example, being a member of a church community, having carer responsibilities, or making career plans.

Nurses should strive to appear calm because this has a calming effect on patients. Using a soft tone of voice, a gentle manner, and tactful language is recommended. The use of touch, humour, posture, and eye contact need to be judged carefully to ascertain whether they are appropriate to the particular situation.

The nursing management of anxiety

Psychological approaches: the vicious cycle of anxiety

The best evidence to support non-pharmaceutical interventions for anxiety is derived from cognitive behavioural therapy (CBT), a psychological treatment that targets challenging negative automatic thoughts (such as habitual self-criticism), and encourages behaviour to promote self-confidence and self-esteem (Kaltenthaler *et al.*, 2006). CBT is one of many psychological treatment approaches that may be effective in the treatment of anxiety, but owing to the large, consistent body of evidence to support its effectiveness and acceptability, CBT-based treatments have been particularly strongly promoted in clinical guidelines (Richardson and Richards, 2006; Kaltenthaler *et al.*, 2006; National Institute for Health and Clinical Excellence (NICE), 2006).

The vicious cycle of anxiety is a fundamental theory in CBT. From Figure 14.5, we can see that a triggering event causes us to feel anxious, so we look for a way in which to relieve those feelings. This is likely to involve leaving a stressful situation. The short-term result is that our anxiety symptoms subside and we feel better. However, the next time the trigger occurs, we remember what happened and so we avoid the stressful situation. Over time, we develop a pattern of avoiding behaviours and even thoughts that make us feel anxious, leading to impaired functioning and a potentially devastating impact on our quality of life.

Evidence-based CBT theory argues that we can stop the vicious cycle of anxiety by learning to trust ourselves to cope with unpleasant and frightening anxiety symptoms. This in turn reduces the fear associated with anxiety symptoms and serves to reduce their intensity. Psychological approaches to anxiety management are often based around this theory and are illustrated in Case study 14.1.

Pharmacological approaches

The National Institute for Health and Clinical Excellence (NICE) guidelines recommend that antidepressants should be used only for long-term management

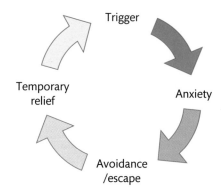

Figure 14.5 The vicious cycle of anxiety.

CASE STUDY 14.1 *David's story*

David was a 32-year-old man who was experiencing intermittent blurred vision and palpitations. This prevented him from functioning effectively at work, where he was a driver for a large car sales business. He visited his GP about his concerns and was referred for tests of his eyes and his heart, but the specialists did not uncover any physical cause of his symptoms. Having clarified this, his GP decided to refer him for an assessment with a mental health nurse. During the assessment, the mental health nurse explained to David that anxiety can cause physical symptoms. This reassured David, who was worried that he had ocular cancer and heart disease.

For 1 week, David kept a diary in which he noted down when his symptoms occurred. He identified that they were worse at work and less severe when he was doing something relaxing. With this information, he and the nurse discussed some of the stressors at work. They then developed a plan to manage his psychological stress, which led to an improvement in his physical symptoms.

of GAD. There is evidence to support the use of a category of antidepressants called **selective serotonin reuptake inhibitors (SSRIs)** to treat GAD, particularly paroxetine, and venlafaxine may also be considered (National Institute for Health and Clinical Excellence (NICE), 2007).

Challenges

Some common challenges to working with anxious patients include:

- managing acute episodes of anxiety while maintaining a therapeutic relationship with the patient;
- supporting carers, who may well have high levels of anxiety of their own;
- working with patients who are intoxicated;
- managing your own feelings in tense situations;
- creating a calm milieu in a busy health setting;
- understanding the threshold for referral to specialist services (e.g. accepting that the mental health team may not accept your referral of an agitated patient).

Strategies for calming situations

The following is a range of strategies useful for calming situations:

- de-trigger;
- distract;
- calm and reassure;
- respond to reasonable needs or demands;
- seek solutions that allow the patient to retain dignity, e.g. provide choices;
- agree to differ/tactical withdrawal;

- challenge without being punitive, putting emphasis on the person's behaviour (e.g. 'I am feeling threatened by what you are saying/doing…');
- as far as possible, avoid changes of staff and maintain a calm and quiet environment.

The importance of communication skills cannot be over-emphasized. Care in selection and use of words, tone, posture, body language, and personal space (give people more space and avoid touching the person: Dix and Page, 2008) is key. Continue to monitor signs and symptoms of agitation, being alert to symptom escalation.

Remember that agitation, like anxiety, requires time; the body is in a state of arousal (the autonomic, or A, response) and adrenaline takes up to an hour to dissipate. It is also useful to think about managing the situation and the environment (E). Often, when individuals are agitated, staff approach in numbers (for protection), but this can be confusing and threatening. It is important to reduce the stimulation, noise, and temperature as far as possible. Other environmental factors to be considered include identifying your exit and knowing how to summon help, if needed (Stevenson, 1991). There may also be times when medication might be useful to help to reduce the physiological arousal that someone is experiencing.

Evaluating impact

Currently, NICE guidance does not recommend the use of specific clinical instruments to measure anxiety, and therefore assessment may rely purely on clinical skills. An instrument that is often used in primary mental health settings in the UK is the **GAD-7**: a seven-item questionnaire specifically focused on GAD (Kroenke *et al.*, 2007).

Summary and key messages

There are a number of key messages from this chapter with which, as a practising nurse, you should be familiar. These include the following.

- Agitation is a form of anxiety.
  Occasionally, people who feel agitated may exhibit aggressive behaviour.

- The ABC-E model can be used to understand, assess, and plan care, and to maintain recovery in people with anxiety.

- Much of the clinical nursing practice associated with anxiety is not based on high-quality evidence, but is supported by theory and expert opinion and NICE guidance.

- Evidence for nursing approaches to the care of people with anxiety and agitation can easily be accessed through electronic databases and websites.

- Interpersonal skills and a good interview schedule are the tools for an effective and therapeutic assessment interview.

- Evidence-based self-help resources can be useful in the prevention and management of anxiety.

Online Resource Centre

 To help you to develop and apply your knowledge and decision-making skills further, we have provided interactive learning resources online at **www.oxfordtextbooks.co.uk/orc/bullock/**

Whilst these are freely available, you will need to use the access codes at the start of the book.

References

Alligood, M. (1992) Empathy: the importance of recognising two types. *Journal of Psychosocial Nursing* **30**(2): 14–17.

American Psychiatric Association (1994) *Diagnostic and Statistical Manual of Mental Disorders, version iv.* American Psychiatric Association: Washington DC.

Barker, P. (ed.) (2009) *Psychiatric and Mental Health Nursing: The Craft of Caring,* 2nd edn. Hodder Arnold: London.

Briddon, J., Baguley, C., Webber M. (2008) The ABC-E Model of Emotion: a bio-psychosocial model for primary mental health care. *Journal of Mental Health Training, Education and Practice* **3**(1): 12–21.

British Medical Journal (2010) *Best Practice: Generalised Anxiety Disorder.* **http://bestpractice.bmj.com/best-practice/monograph/120/basics.html** (accessed April 2010).

Department of Health (1999) *National Service Framework for Mental Health.* HMSO: London.

Department of Health Mental Health Division (2010) *Confident Communities, Brighter Futures: A Framework for Developing Well-being.* Best Practice Guidance Gateway reference 13485. **www.nmhdu.org.uk/silo/files/confident-communities-brighter-futures.pdf** (accessed 20 October 2011).

Dix, R., Page, M. (2008) De-escalation. In: D. Beer, S. Pereira, C. Paton (eds) *Psychiatric Intensive Care.* Cambridge University Press: Cambridge.

Gupta, N. (2010) Don't forget mental illnesses. *British Medical Journal* **340**: c781.

Hoffman, D.L., Dukes, E.M., Wittchen, H.-U. (2008) Human and economic burden of generalized anxiety disorder: research review. *Depression and Anxiety* **25**: 72–90.

Kaltenthaler, E., Brazier, J., Nigris, E.D., *et al.* (2006) Computerised cognitive behaviour therapy for depression and anxiety update: a systematic review and economic evaluation. *Health Technology Assessment* **10**(33): 1–186.

King, M., Nazareth, I., Levy, G., *et al.* (2008) Prevalence of common mental disorders in general practice attendees across Europe. *The British Journal of Psychiatry* **192**(5): 362–7.

Kroenke, K., Spitzer, R.L., Williams, J.B.W., *et al.* (2007) Anxiety disorders in primary care: prevalence, impairment, comorbidity, and detection. *Annals of Internal Medicine* **146**(5): 317–25.

London School of Economics (2006) *The Depression Report: A New Deal for Depression and Anxiety Disorders.* London School of Economics: London.

Lucey, H., Reay, D. (2002). Carrying the beacon of excellence: social class differentiation and anxiety at a time of transition. *Journal of Education Policy* **17**(3): 321–36.

Mental Health Foundation (2009) *In the Face of Fear: How Fear and Anxiety Affect our Health and Society, and What we Can do about It.* Mental Health Foundation: London.

Moser, K., Majeed, A. (ONS) (2009) Prevalence of treated chronic diseases in general practice in England and Wales: trends over time and variations by the ONS area classification. *Health Statistics Quarterly* **2**: 25–32.

National Collaborating Centre for Mental Health (2005) Management of depression in primary and secondary care. National Clinical Practice Guideline 23. National Institute for Health and Clinical Excellence: London.

National Institute for Health and Clinical Excellence (2005) *Violence: The Short-Term Management of Disturbed/Violent Behaviour in In-Patient Psychiatric Settings and Emergency Departments.* Nice Clinical Guideline 25 (CG25) NICE: London.

National Institute for Health and Clinical Excellence (2006) *Computerised Cognitive Behaviour Therapy for Depression and Anxiety.* Review of Technology Appraisal 51. NICE: London.

National Institute for Health and Clinical Excellence (2007). *Anxiety.* Clinical Guideline 22 (CG22). Developed by the National Collaborating Centre for Primary Care. NICE: London.

Norman, I., Ryrie, I. (eds) (2009) *The Art and Science of Mental Health Nursing,* 2nd edn. McGraw Hill, Open University Press: Maidenhead.

Nursing and Midwifery Council (2008) Standards of proficiency for pre-registration nursing education. **www.nmc-uk.org/aDisplayDocument.aspx?documentID=328** (accessed April 2010).

Richards, D., McDonald, B. (1990) *Behavioural Psychotherapy: A Handbook for Nurses.* Heinemann: Oxford.

Richards, M., Abbott, R., Collis, G., *et al.* (2009) *Childhood Mental Health and Life Chances in Post-War Britain: Insights from Three National Birth Cohort Studies.* The Smith Institute, Unison, MRC Unit for Lifelong Health and Ageing, & Sainsbury Centre for Mental Health: London.

Richardson, R., Richards, D.A. (2006) Self-help: towards the next generation. *Behavioural and Cognitive Psychotherapy* **34**: 13–23.

Rogers, C.R. (1995) *On Becoming a Person: A Therapist's View of Psychotherapy.* Houghton Mifflin Company: New York.

Singleton, N., Lewis, G. (eds) (2003) *Better or Worse: A Follow-Up Study of the Mental Health of Adults in Great Britain—Report Based on Surveys Carried out by the Office for National Statistics* in 2000 and 2001 for the Department of Health and the Scottish Executive Health Department. HMSO: London.

Stapleton, R.D., Nielsen, E.L., Engelberg, R.A., *et al.* (2005) Association of depression and life-sustaining treatment preferences in patients with COPD. *Chest* **127**(1): 328–34.

Stark, D.P.H., House, A. (2000) Anxiety in cancer patients. *British Journal of Cancer* **83**(10): 1261–7.

Stevenson, S. (1991) Heading off violence with verbal de-escalation. *Journal of Psychosocial Nursing and Mental Health Services* **29**(9): 6–10.

The Health & Social Care Information Centre (2009) *Adult Psychiatric morbidity in England, 2007 Results of a household Survey.* S. McManus, H. Meltzer, T. Brugha, *et al* (eds). **http://www.ic.nhs.uk/webfiles/publications/mental%20health/other%20mental%20health%20publications/Adult%20psychiatric%20morbidity%2007/APMS%2007%20%28FINAL%29%20Standard.pdf** (accessed 22 March 2012).

Tolin, D.F., Foa, E.B. (2008) Sex differences in trauma and posttraumatic stress disorder: a quantitative review of 25 years of research. *Psychological Trauma: Theory, Research, Practice, and Policy* **S**(1): 37–85.

Vandemark, L.M. (2006) Awareness of self and expanding consciousness: using nursing theories to prepare nurse-therapists. *Issues in Mental Health Nursing* **27**: 605–15.

World Health Organization (2007) ICD version 10: Chapter V: Mental and behavioural disorders (F00-F99); Neurotic, stress-related and somatoform disorders (F40-F48). **http://apps.who.int/classifications/apps/icd/icd10online/index.htm?gf40.htm+** (accessed March 2010).

World Health Organization (2010) *International Classification of Diseases (ICD).* **www.who.int/classifications/icd/en/** (accessed April 2010).

Wu, H., Chi, T.-S., Chen, L., *et al.* (2010) Occupational stress among hospital nurses: cross-sectional survey. *Journal of Advanced Nursing* **66**(3): 627–34.

15 *Managing* Breathlessness

Samantha Prigmore, Vikki Knowles, and Jessica Callaghan

Introduction

This chapter addresses the fundamental nursing in managing breathlessness. Every nurse should possess the knowledge and skills to assess patients holistically, to select and implement evidence-based strategies, to manage breathlessness, and to review the effectiveness of these to inform any necessary changes in care.

Understanding the importance of breathlessness

The nurse has a key role in managing this often frightening symptom, which may be caused by many disorders, including certain heart and respiratory conditions, strenuous exercise, or anxiety.

Definitions

Breathlessness is described as a distressing subjective sensation of uncomfortable breathing (Mosby, 2009) and can be expressed as an unpleasant or uncomfortable awareness of breathing, or of the need to breathe (Gift, 1990). The term dyspnoea, also meaning breathlessness, is derived from the Greek word for difficulty in breathing.

Prevalence

Whilst it is difficult to estimate the prevalence of dyspnoea, it is apparent when we exercise beyond our normal tolerance levels; pathologically, dyspnoea occurs with little or no exertion and is a symptom response to different aetiologies (causes of illness). Breathlessness is a common symptom in patients with both cardiac (McCarthy *et al.*, 1996) and respiratory disease (Dean, 2008), and also in people with neuromuscular diseases approaching the end of life; this can prove difficult and distressing to manage (see Chapter 18 Managing End-of-Life Care ➡). There is a peak incidence of chronic dyspnoea in the 55–69 age group (Karnani, 2005), and the prevalence and severity of dyspnoea increases with age. This is associated with an increase in mortality and reduction in quality of life (Huijnen *et al.*, 2006). It is estimated that 70% of all terminal cancer patients experience breathlessness in their last 6 weeks of life (Davis, 1997). Both physiological and psychological responses (including pain, emotion, and anxiety) can lead to an increase in respiratory rate.

Causes of breathlessness

Breathing is controlled by the respiratory centre in the medulla of the brain. Higher centres in the cerebral hemispheres can voluntarily control respiratory rate so that breathing can be temporarily stopped, slowed,

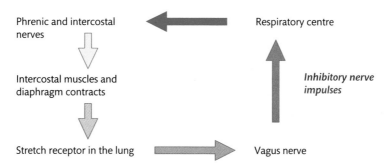

Figure 15.1 Hering–Breuer reflex.

or increased. The respiratory centre generates the basic rhythm of breathing, with the depth and rate being altered in response to the body's requirements, mainly by nervous and chemical control (Ward and Linden, 2008).

Nervous control of breathing is via the phrenic and intercostal nerves, which activate the diaphragm and intercostal muscles, respectively. Stretch receptors in the thoracic wall generate inhibitory nerve impulses once the lungs have inflated (Hering–Breuer reflex), which are then transmitted to the respiratory centre via the vagus nerve (Waugh and Grant, 2006; Figure 15.1).

Chemical control of breathing involves chemoreceptors, which increase ventilation in response to hypercapnia (high levels of carbon dioxide), hypoxaemia (low levels of oxygen), and changes in the pH of the blood. Peripheral chemoreceptors (in the carotid and aortic bodies) mainly respond to hypoxaemia, while central chemoreceptors (on the surface of the medulla oblongata) mainly respond to hypercapnia. In healthy people, hypercapnia is the main respiratory drive. However, some individuals with chronic respiratory disease (e.g. chronic obstructive pulmonary disease, or COPD) depend on hypoxia to drive the stimulation for respiration. In response to the body's demand to increase respiratory effort, the accessory muscles of respiration (sternocleidomastoid muscles), together with the diaphragm and intercostal muscles, are recruited to maximize the capacity of the thoracic cavity (Waugh and Grant, 2006). It is clear that normal respiration depends on a complex interaction between mechanical, neural, and chemotactic pathways, and breathlessness can occur when there is disruption to them.

Breathlessness is a common symptom of disease particularly in those of the cardiorespiratory system. Karnani (2005) reports that approximately two-thirds

Table 15.1 Causes of acute breathlessness

Cardiac	Pulmonary oedema
	Acute myocardial infarction
	Arrhythmias
	Pericarditis
	Pericardial infusion
Respiratory	Pneumonia
	Pneumothorax
	Pulmonary embolism
	Acute asthma
	Exacerbations of chronic obstructive pulmonary disease
	Airway obstruction, e.g. anaphylaxis, foreign body, tumour
	Other respiratory infections, e.g. pulmonary tuberculosis
Endocrine	Diabetic ketoacidosis
	Thyrotoxicosis
Other	Pain
	Anxiety
	Drugs, e.g. aspirin overdose
	Altitude sickness
	Trauma
	Acute blood loss
	Systemic infection

Source: Adapted from **www.patient.co.uk/doctor/breathlessness.htm** (accessed 24 April 2011)

of cases of dyspnoea in adults are caused by a pulmonary or cardiac disorder, and in one-third of cases the diagnosis will be multifactorial. The major causes of dyspnoea, both acute and chronic, are outlined in Tables 15.1 and 15.2.

Table 15.2 Causes of chronic breathlessness

Cardiac	Left ventricular disease
	Valvular disease
	Arrhythmias
	Pericardial disease
Respiratory	Asthma
	Chronic obstructive pulmonary disease
	Bronchiectasis
	Cystic fibrosis
	Interstitial lung disease
	Pleural effusion
	Pulmonary hypertension
	Lung malignancy
	Chronic pulmonary thrombo-embolic disease
Neuromuscular	Motor neurone disease
	Guillain–Barré syndrome
	Myasthenia gravis
Other	Anaemia
	Pulmonary thromboembolic disease
	Thyroid disease
	Obesity
	Malignancy
	Psychogenic, e.g. anxiety
	Lack of conditioning

Source: Adapted from **www.patient.co.uk/doctor/breathlessness.htm** (accessed 24 April 2011)

The choice of treatment will be dependent on the cause of breathlessness. For example, fluid overload secondary to heart failure will be treated with diuretics, whereas bronchoconstriction secondary to acute asthma will be treated with bronchodilators and corticosteroids. Therefore accurate assessment of the patient is key to the reduction on symptom impact and essential for symptom control.

The human and social burden

Breathlessness is a common symptom present in many different conditions (see Tables 15.1 and 15.2); it is a frequent reason to seek nursing and medical assessment. Dyspnoea is almost always associated with fear and anxiety, often because of the unknown cause in acute situations. When chronic, it can lead to significant reduction in the quality of life, resulting in disability (Ries, 2006), which can affect the ability to maintain permanent employment. Chronic breathlessness results in increasing difficulty in undertaking activities of daily living, subsequently resulting in loss of independence, which may impact upon dependent relationships.

Nursing role in the management of breathlessness

Although it can be a normal physiological response, for example during strenuous exercise, in the healthcare setting, tachypnoea (respiratory rate greater than 20 breaths/min) is usually one of the first signs of patient deterioration (Jevon, 2009). Accurate measurement of respiratory rate is a fundamental part of patient assessment and is an important baseline observation. It is a key component of the (UK) Resuscitation Council's systematic approach to the assessment of critically ill patients (Resuscitation Council (UK), 2006). Your role is to measure and interpret an individual's respiratory rate competently (Department of Health, 2009). When breathlessness is acute in origin, the nurse has a crucial role in the identification of a deterioration in health status, in providing prompt first-line intervention, and seeking medical assistance.

With chronic breathlessness, patients will often have varying levels of the condition, which may be increased during exacerbations of their underlying condition or during physical activities. For these patients, support in coming to terms with the chronic nature of the symptom and the need to learn skills to help them to cope with the impact it may have on their quality of life are priorities. The nurse is in an ideal position to provide education relating to the underlying condition and to ensure that adherence to medical treatment is achieved. Advice on adapting to the limitations that breathlessness may cause, with ongoing support, promoting independence and referring on to relevant allied healthcare professionals (e.g. physiotherapists, occupational therapists) for additional treatment or adaptations, are all central to nursing management.

Clinical assessment of breathlessness

Breathlessness in disease is a symptom and not a sign (Cockcroft and Adams, 1989). A sign can be defined as a physical manifestation of an illness, whereas a symptom is a subjective experience. Therefore, accurate, systematic questioning and assessment of the patient will often determine the cause of the breathlessness, enabling appropriate treatment and interventions to be given

Asking the right questions

Taking a thorough history and asking relevant open-ended questions in a systematic manner may help to identify the potential cause of breathlessness, along with assessment of the patient's physical and mental conditions. Example questions are given in Box 15.1.

The key question is whether the breathlessness is acute (sudden in onset) or chronic (long-term).

Exposure to social and occupational irritants can result in conditions that may result in the patient feeling breathless; some of these are displayed in Table 15.3. They can result in allergic responses, as well as irritation of the

airways. It is well documented that smoking increases the risk of respiratory disease, especially obstructive lung disease such as chronic bronchitis and emphysema.

Pharmacological treatments can also result in breathlessness, and common drugs associated with breathlessness are listed in Box 15.2. They may cause deterioration to pre-existing conditions such as asthma.

Nursing role in patient observation and assessment

Temperature

Pyrexia in a breathless patient may suggest infection, either lung in origin or as a consequence of infection elsewhere.

Table 15.3 Social, environmental, and occupational factors that can be associated with breathlessness or breathing disorders

Social	Occupational
Smoking, e.g. tobacco and illicit drugs	Asbestos
Animals, e.g. cats, dogs, birds	Chemicals
Pollution	Moulds
Moulds	

Box 15.1 Taking a history: general questions

- For how long have you been breathless?
- When did it start?
- Are you breathless all of the time?
- Does anything make the breathlessness better/worse?
- How far can walk before you become breathless?
- Can you walk up stairs or inclines without feeling breathless?
- Are you able to sleep flat?
- How many pillows do you need at night?
- Do you get periods of wakefulness due to breathlessness at night?
- Are you breathless on waking?
- Do have any associated symptoms, such as chest pain, cough, sputum production, or blood being coughed up?

Box 15.2 Common drugs associated with breathlessness

- Antibiotics, e.g. nitrofurantoin (potential fibrotic lung changes)
- Anti-arrhythmic agents, e.g. amiodarone (potential fibrotic lung changes)
- Beta-blockers, e.g. atenolol, eye drops (potential bronchoconstriction)
- Cytotoxic chemotherapy (potential fibrotic lung changes)
- Non-steroidal anti-inflammatory drugs (NSAIDs), e.g. ibuprofen or aspirin (potential bronchoconstriction)

Consult the *British National Formulary* (BNF) for other potential pharmacological causes.

Pulse

Pulse rate, rhythm, and regularity should be carefully recorded, because tachycardia and arrhythmias can cause breathlessness.

Respirations

Observation of the respiratory rate (see Figure 15.2), effort, and sound should be included when recording and observing respirations. Inspiration (breathing in) and expiration (breathing out) equals one respiration, and this is recorded as the number of respirations per minute. In particular, you should look at the rate, depth, speed, effort (use of accessory muscles and diaphragmatic support), and pattern of the respirations. The normal respiratory rate of adults is 12–18/min. Healthy spontaneous breathing is quiet with minimal effort, and this should be your baseline for assessment. The recording of respirations has been determined as an important indicator of 'acute illness' (Department of Health, 2009; National Institute for Health and Clinical Excellence (NICE), 2007), and responding to/seeking help in managing an abnormally high or low respiratory rate is a key factor in minimizing complications in acute illness.

Signs of increased work of breathing include an increased respiratory rate and the use of accessory muscles. The following signs suggest respiratory distress:

- the use of accessory muscles (shoulders and neck);
- sternal recession, the sinking in of the sternum during inspiration;
- tracheal tug, the sinking in of the soft tissue above the sternum and between the clavicles during inspiration;
- intercostal recession, the sinking in of the soft tissues between the ribs;
- nasal flaring;
- pursed lip breathing.

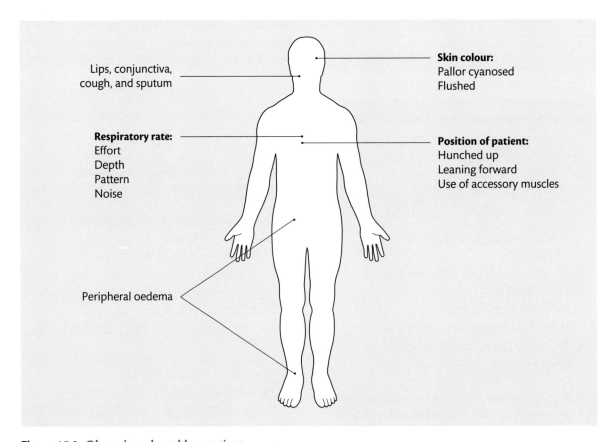

Figure 15.2 Observing a breathless patient.

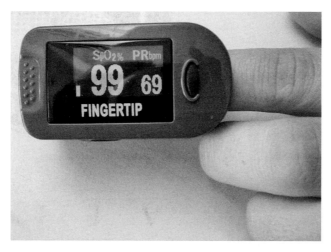

Figure 15.3 **Pulse oximeter probe.**

Reproduced from Endacott, Jevan, and Cooper, *Clinical Nursing Skills (Core and Advanced)*, by permission of Oxford University Press.

Breathless patients may demonstrate different patterns of breathing, as follows.

- Tachypnoea—rapid rate of breathing (>20 breaths/min)
- Orthopnoea—breathlessness when lying flat
- Cheyne–Stokes respiration—periods of absent respiration (apnoea) alternating with rapid respirations (most frequently seen following cerebral events involving the brainstem and severe cardiac failure, but also normal during sleep in the elderly)
- Kussmaul breathing—deep rapid respirations (often referred to as 'air-hungry'), in response to a reduced arterial pH in metabolic acidosis and sometimes present with patients in acute renal failure or diabetic ketoacidosis
- Hyperventilation—irregular, sighing breaths are a common response to anxiety and emotional distress, and can result in respiratory alkalosis, causing light-headedness and pins and needles in the fingers

Stridor (a harsh rasping noise heard on the in-breath) suggests upper airway obstruction.

Blood pressure

Hypotension can be a sign of severe heart failure and life-threatening asthma.

Oxygen saturations

Oxygen saturations should be recorded in the breathless patient. In most individuals, normal oxygen saturations range between 94% and 98% when breathing room air. Some patients may be chronically hypoxic (e.g. COPD patients), with an acceptable oxygen saturation for this group being 88–92% (British Thoracic Society, 2008). Oxygen saturation is measured by a pulse oximeter probe, as shown in Figure 15.3.

Peak expiratory flow rate (PEFR)

PEFR is the maximum flow of air that a patient can expel from his or her lungs following full inspiration. It is a useful tool to measure airway obstruction and is commonly used to determine the severity of an exacerbation of asthma. Figure 15.4 shows an example of a peak flow meter.

Documentation

Observations should be accurately and clearly recorded on the patient's observations chart and in the nursing records, with any abnormalities observed being reported promptly.

Colour

Observe the patient's skin colour, remembering that cyanosis (blue discoloration of the skin and mucous membranes, most noticeable around the lips, earlobes, mouth and fingers) can indicate a severe lack of oxygen. In dark-skinned

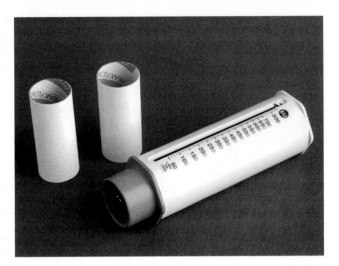

Figure 15.4 Peak flow meter.

Reproduced by permission of Oxford University Press.

patients, signs of poor perfusion or cyanosis may be detected if the area around the lips or nail beds is dusky in colour. Also observe the patient's eyes, looking for conjunctival pallor, a sign of anaemia.

Cough and sputum

Sputum should be examined and may help to identify a cause of breathlessness. Thick sticky purulent (green) sputum is suggestive of infection; sticky casts shaped similarly to the bronchioles could be related to asthma; pink frothy sputum is a classical sign of pulmonary oedema. Blood-streaked sputum or haemoptysis (frank blood in the sputum) is a worrying feature and should be promptly reported.

Peripheral oedema

Amongst hospital patients, peripheral oedema is usually caused by fluid retention, immobility-dependent oedema, and drugs such as steroids or low albumen. In some instances, it is due to cardiac failure. Peripheral oedema, is usually determined by gravity, involving the ankles, legs, backs of the thighs, and the sacral area. It can be detected by pressing firmly on the area with your fingers or thumb for a few seconds, resulting in a marked indentation. This is described as pitting oedema. An elevated jugular venous pressure (JVP) is also associated with cardiac failure.

Listening (auscultation) to the chest

Using a stethoscope, listening (auscultation) to the patient's chest can be very helpful in determining or diagnosing the probable cause of breathlessness. Figure 15.5 demonstrates the ideal positions on the chest for auscultation. The common sounds heard are described in Table 15.4. For more information on how to perform auscultation, see Endacott *et al.* (2009) *Clinical Nursing Skills: Core and Advanced.*

Breathlessness scores

Breathlessness is a subjective experience, and individuals can perceive it differently. Commonly used tools used in daily practice to measure breathlessness include the Medical Research Council (MRC) Dyspnoea Score (Fletcher *et al.*, 1959) (Box 15.3) and the Borg breathlessness scale (1982). In the latter, a visual analogue of 0 equals not breathless; 10 equates to very breathless.

Signs of deterioration

The breathless patient can deteriorate rapidly in acute situations and, equally, the patient with chronic breathlessness may accept an increase in symptoms that may have significant consequences. Examples of 'red flag symptoms' are detailed in Box 15.4.

Summary of clinical assessment

Taking a comprehensive history, observing, and assessing the breathless patient can provide valuable insight to the possible causes of breathlessness. Findings should not be reviewed in isolation, but should inform your decision-making on further investigations and treatment options.

Landmarks for chest auscultation.

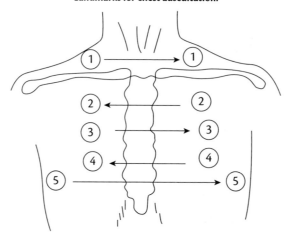

Figure 15.5 **Auscultation positions.**

Reproduced from Crouch *et al., Oxford Handbook of Emergency Nursing* by permission from Oxford University Press.

Table 15.4 **Common sounds heard when listening to the chest**

Observations	Possible causes
Wheeze	Asthma, COPD, pulmonary oedema
Crackles	Pneumonia, bronchiectasis, lung fibrosis, pulmonary oedema
Stridor	Inhaled foreign body, tumour of the upper airway
No additional sounds	Anaemia, pulmonary emboli, neuromuscular disorders, anxiety

Box 15.3 **MRC Dyspnoea Score**

1. Not troubled by breathlessness except on vigorous exercise
2. Short of breath on hurrying or walking up inclines
3. Walks slower than contemporaries because of breathlessness, or has to stop for breath when walking at own pace
4. Stops for breath after walking about 100 metres or stops after a few minutes' walking on the level
5. Too breathless to leave the house or breathless on dressing or undressing

(Fletcher *et al.,* 1959)

Nursing management interventions

Having established that breathlessness impacts both physiologically and psychologically on the individual and his or her carers, traditional models of care have focused on the biomedical model in which the emphasis is on the pathophysiology of breathing. This model isolates the cause of breathlessness and targets the interventions at removing the sensation. This approach, however, fails to take into account the holistic impact of breathlessness, and management tends to be focused on pharmacological interventions. Therapeutic advances in breathlessness management are relatively limited compared to other conditions (Booth *et al.,* 2008). Corner *et al.* (1995) identify the integrative model of management, which considers the mind and body to be inseparable, and suggests that therapy should focus on the meaning behind the breathlessness experience. This approach recognizes the impact or problems that the symptom has on the individual, leading to a partnership approach to management.

Effective nursing management of breathlessness is therefore shaped by a combination of optimal pharmacological management with non-pharmacological interventions and psychosocial support.

Breathlessness management can be approached in a variety of settings across both primary and secondary care although, once the cause has been identified, care of the breathless patient ideally will be closer to home, utilizing all of the services available: for example, community specialist respiratory care services, primary care, and palliative care services for patients with end-stage disease. Coordination of care to ensure continuity is clearly of paramount importance, and clear documentation such as the use of management plans will support successful outcomes.

Pharmacological management of breathlessness

Pharmacological management depends on the underlying cause of breathlessness. Careful assessment of the breathless patient allows the practitioner to identify the underlying health problem and the mechanisms contributing to symptoms, thus highlighting the most appropriate treatment strategy. For example, patients with underlying respiratory disease may require escalation of their respiratory treatments (e.g. bronchodilators), whereas patients with pulmonary oedema should improve with diuretics.

Patients with neuromuscular disease may respond better to non-pharmacological management such as ventilatory support. The aim, however, must be to optimize treatment for the underlying condition and to exclude additional problems such as infection, obstruction (in the case of cancer), anaemia, or pulmonary oedema.

Respiratory diseases

Bronchodilator therapy should be optimized in patients with obstructive lung problems because it can significantly reduce the sensation of breathlessness. This improvement is caused by reduction in air trapping, which reduces the functional reserve capacity of the lungs, thereby improving the work of breathing. Bronchodilatation can be achieved by using β_2-agonists. Anticholinergic treatment should also be considered to dilate the airways, especially in COPD. Either short-acting anticholinergic drugs four times daily or preferably a long-acting anticholinergic, e.g. tiotropium, once daily can be used. These drugs, however, will not be helpful for all respiratory disorders, and patients suffering from interstitial lung disease are not likely to find them helpful.

Infection is a common cause of increased breathlessness for patients with underlying heart and chest disease, and should be treated promptly with the appropriate antibiotics (Scottish Intercollegiate Guidelines Network (SIGN), 2007; National Institute for Health and Clinical Excellence (NICE), 2010). If the infection has failed to respond to first-line antibiotic treatment, sputum should be sent for culture to ensure that additional antibiotic treatment is appropriate. Oral corticosteroids are indicated in acute exacerbations of asthma and may be beneficial during infective exacerbations of COPD or for patients experiencing breathlessness as a consequence of cancer, either to reduce inflammation within the airways or to reduce peritumour oedema (Urie *et al.*, 2000). Thick pulmonary secretions can increase the sensation of breathlessness and, although little research is available on the use of nebulized saline, a trial should be considered. Mucolytics on a short-term basis can also be helpful for patients with obstructive lung disease who have difficulty in epectorating thick secretions (NICE, 2010).

Once treatment is optimized for the underlying condition, a trial of benzodiazepines, opioids, and antidepressants should be considered for palliation of intractable symptoms.

For cardiac-related symptoms, associated pain, and possible associated anaemia, please refer to **Chapters 6 and 25** ➡.

Anxiety and depression

The incidence of mood disorders such as anxiety and depression in patients with chronic lung disease and cancer exceeds that found in the general population (Booth, 2008). Both can exacerbate symptoms of breathlessness if untreated, and there is debate as to which comes first, breathlessness or anxiety (Booth, 2008). There is a developing evidence base that anxiety management utilizing non-pharmacological interventions is effective in relation to clinical outcomes. Cognitive behavioral therapy is likely to be of benefit in self-management and alleviation of symptoms whatever the original cause of breathlessness. This is a recent change in direction to long-term management that fills a gap in which there is typically a limited evidence base (Howard *et al.*, 2010). Twycross and Lack (1990) identified the anxiety–breathlessness cycle, in which the increased need for oxygen triggers breathlessness, leading to the sensation of anxiety. This results in a feeling of lack of control, and the fear of not coping or dying leads to panic, increasing respiratory rate and exacerbating the sensation of breathlessness.

Few studies have been carried out looking at the efficacy of anxiolytics in patients with severe breathlessness; however, current respiratory and cardiac guidelines recommend that anxiolytics such as lorazepam 0.5–2 mg sublingually and diazepam 5 mg should be considered because they can reduce breathlessness by reducing panic and providing sedation. Low doses are recommended to minimize the risk of respiratory depression.

A Cochrane review (Simon *et al.*, 2010) looking at the use of benzodiazepines for the management of end-stage breathlessness concluded that, although evidence was weak, benzodiazepines should still be considered when other first-line therapies have failed to alleviate symptoms. Dean (2008) showed that over 77% of patients with COPD approaching the end of life suffer from low mood; this can aggravate their ability to cope with their symptoms and therefore antidepressant treatment may be helpful.

People with chronic long-term conditions such as heart failure suffer from double the rate of depression when compared to the general population (National Institute for Health and Clinical Excellence (NICE), 2009).

If prescribing antidepressants, remember that tricyclic antidepressants should be avoided for patients with chronic heart failure.

Palliative care

A Cochrane review (2001) looked at the use of oral and parenteral opioids in the management of dyspnoea in advanced disease (of any cause) and found them to be beneficial. Oral opioids such as morphine sulphate solution 2.5 mg four times daily decrease ventilatory demand by altering the processing of central motor signals, which can reduce the central perception of breathlessness and give significant relief (Jennings *et al.*, 2002). Again, low doses will minimize the risk of respiratory complications, but are sufficient to impact on the sensation of breathlessness. The use of nebulized morphine is not recommended because there is little evidence supporting additional benefit from this route over the use of oral preparations. It also carries an increased risk of bronchoconstriction when used at high doses (Cochrane Review, 2001).

There are clear guidelines supporting the use of long-term oxygen therapy in the presence of chronic hypoxaemia (British Thoracic Society, 2006). Evidence is lacking, however, for palliative use of oxygen for relief of breathlessness in respiratory and cardiac disease. Therefore oxygen should be introduced for palliative relief of breathlessness only on a trial basis. Currow *et al.* (2009) suggests that, in palliative care, air is effective and therefore oxygen should be given only if the patient is hypoxic. It should be accompanied by subjective and objective measures of the patient's response by the use of dyspnoea scales and pulse oximetry before being introduced on a long-term basis.

Non-pharmacological management

> It is well recognized that breathlessness is a complex experience and derives from 'interactions among multiple physiological, psychological, social and environmental factors, and may induce secondary physiological and behavioural responses'. (American Thoracic Society statement on dyspnoea, 1999)

Non-pharmacological treatments, which are aimed at these 'interactions' and 'behavioural responses', should be considered by all those involved with the breathless patient and at every stage. Nursing management strategies should be targeted at giving the patient a sense of confidence and control over breathlessness. Non-pharmacological strategies are particularly necessary when breathlessness is severe and has not been sufficiently reduced by pharmacological treatments, and if anxiety, depression, social isolation, or reduced confidence are contributing to a poor quality of life. A multidisciplinary approach to the breathless patient (recommended by chronic heart failure and COPD NICE guidelines) makes available a wide range of non-pharmacological specialist education, advice, and interventions.

An important goal of treatment should be to facilitate the patient's self-awareness and insight into his or her condition, ways of coping, and his or her individual thought–behaviour cycles. Feedback from the nurse as to the patient's natural way of managing breathlessness can be the first step in identifying which strategies the individual patient is likely to find most helpful if he or she has limited awareness.

Education

Education is an important part of any non-pharmacological intervention, because the patient's increased knowledge and understanding can significantly improve his or her confidence in being able to cope with symptoms. Individually tailored education topics may include the mechanisms/mechanics of breathlessness, nutritional advice (e.g. for heart failure patients, salt and fluid restriction advice where necessary), recommendations about vaccinations, medications, smoking cessation, lifestyle balance (e.g. between sleep, rest, exercise, and activity), and support services available (statutory and non-statutory).

Improved knowledge can lead to improved self-efficacy (defined as 'belief in one's capabilities to organize and execute the course of action required to produce given attainments': Bandura, 1977). A part of the health professional's role is to increase a patient's level of self-efficacy either through educating or reinforcing goals and behaviour changes that he or she has successfully achieved. With an improved level of self-efficacy, you can expect to see a patient who finds self-management easier. An individualized self-management plan enables the patient to take responsibility for learning about and improving management of his or her symptoms. The plan may be a standardized pamphlet, such as with the British Lung Foundation's *COPD Self Management Plan*, or it could be a plan created specifically for the individual. It is helpful to

include medications, usual level of function, and coping strategies for managing symptoms such as breathlessness and panic. Any style of self-management plan ought to include an action plan. The action plan is guidance for the patient on what to do if his or her breathlessness (or other symptoms) worsen, for example whether to make changes to medication and when to call the doctor or to contact emergency services. This can obviously be as useful for the carer as for the patient, and can reduce panic by giving basic instruction, set out in a simple format and easy to follow in a crisis.

Rehabilitation

There is a wealth of evidence to support exercise, when used as part of rehabilitation for the patient with chronic disease (Congestive Heart Failure and COPD NICE guidelines). There is strong evidence, mainly for patients with cardiopulmonary disease, that exercise programmes (often combined with self-management education) can be effective in tackling the deconditioning spiral (Figure 15.6).

Figure 15.6 describes the breathlessness–inactivity–reduction in fitness cycle often experienced by the breathless patient, which results in muscles using oxygen less efficiently. Improvement in this spiral through exercise training can reduce healthcare utilization and improve quality of life amongst other benefits (ATS/ERS Guidelines on Pulmonary Rehabilitation, 2004). When engaged in a supported and individualized exercise programme, the patient is desensitized to breathlessness, which reduces fear and provides evidence to challenge negative beliefs about breathlessness being harmful. The patient can begin pushing his or herself to get fitter, experience breathlessness, and try out new coping strategies in a 'safe' environment. In addition to these benefits, the dynamics of groupwork can increase self-efficacy, as the patient observes others with similar symptoms learning to manage breathlessness successfully.

Assessment of the patient's breathing pattern at rest and on exertion can reveal that certain breathing techniques and positioning of the body may assist the patient in improving control of the breathlessness. Knowledge of the patient's underlying condition and physiological reason for breathlessness is vital to know which techniques and positions may be beneficial, and interventions aimed at improving the breathing pattern should be done with careful consideration.

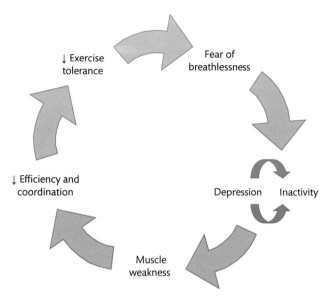

Figure 15.6 The deconditioning spiral of breathlessness.

Physiotherapy

Breathing control (relaxed, gentle breathing) can be very helpful for recovery of breathlessness after exertion and particularly to help to control panic-fuelled breathlessness. Pursed lip breathing has been shown to be beneficial for people with obstructive lung disease (Dechman *et al.*, 2004). Diaphragmatic breathing may be useful for some patients, but is not recommended for use with patients with severe COPD because it can increase the work of breathing (Vitacca *et al.*, 1998). It is useful to remember that, for people with certain conditions (e.g. restrictive lung disease), shallow breaths may be all they can manage. Patients could be more distressed and breathless if they are physically unable to follow instruction, so be cautious about using terms such as 'deep breathing' or 'slow breathing'. A strategy termed 'blow as you go' (to exhale on effort) is advised by many physiotherapists and can be usefully transferred into daily activities, especially those involving reaching, lifting, or bending. For example, a very fatigued, breathless patient may find it useful to blow out on a task as simple as standing from the sitting position. In addition to some of the breathing exercises above, to aid breathlessness on exertion, patients can be encouraged to pace their breathing with steps (e.g. if walking or going up stairs). Forward leaning and fixing of the shoulder girdle while sitting or standing is a commonly used technique and the evidence for these approaches is outlined in the 2009 BTS/ACPRC physiotherapy guideline. A patient at the end of his or her life, and struggling with breathlessness and severe weakness, could be placed in a sitting forward lead position (e.g. onto a table), using a lot of pillows to fix the shoulder girdle. This positioning aims to maximize comfort and to reduce effort, whilst also providing an alternative to the patient being in bed.

Patients with cystic fibrosis, bronchiectasis, or other conditions that result in excessive sputum production and difficulty clearing sputum may benefit from specialist advice on airway clearance techniques. The range of techniques and the evidence to support them can be found in detail in the BTS/ACPRC physiotherapy guidelines, but specific techniques such as the active cycle of breathing technique (ACBT) and positive expiratory pressure devices are commonly used by physiotherapists. The nurse can refer a patient for physiotherapy assessment when appropriate.

Practical support

Many patients living with breathlessness, whatever the underlying cause, also experience fatigue. Energy conservation techniques need to be discussed with the patient alongside breathlessness management strategies. Encourage the patient to consider his or her routines, sleep, balance of personal care, domestic, and leisure tasks, and assist him or her in identifying priorities and goals. Very often, patients are in a process of adjusting to the limitations of their condition, which can involve a lot of frustration, either because they try to do tasks in the way they always have or because they are less independent in tasks. The breathless patient may need permission and encouragement to try new ways of approaching tasks. New approaches can involve doing the task more slowly in stages, sitting rather than standing, or asking for help for some tasks so that he or she has energy to do other activities. Although patients may understand and successfully use strategies to manage breathlessness during exertion (such as walking or stairs), problem-solving how to apply these to daily activities (such as vacuuming or showering) can be more difficult. Turner-Lawler (2004) describes 'activity efficiency' rather than energy conservation techniques, because many strategies useful to patients may focus on comfort doing the task, as well as on reducing the energy required. For the patient identifying specific activities that are problematical and not easily resolved or improved, it is worth considering a referral for occupational therapy.

Practical solutions that form part of the non-pharmacological area of treatment include adaptive equipment. Small items include a long-handled shoehorn or shower stool, while larger adaptations might be a level-access shower or a stair lift. Timing of consideration and discussion with the patient of these large adaptations can be very sensitive and must not be done prematurely, owing to the risk of contributing to reduced fitness. We must also be aware of certain belief systems that the patient or carer may have about accepting something that will change his or her home and be a visual display of disability (e.g. 'it's the beginning of the end'). Certain equipment, such as pillow rests or pillow lifts, may reduce symptoms by addressing positioning problems (e.g. orthopnoea, which patients with heart failure may experience). Mobility aids can provide stability, confidence, and the opportunity to fix the shoulder girdle whilst mobilizing: for example, there is evidence to support the use of a delta frame (Probst *et al.*, 2004).

Ideas such as using a towelling bath robe to minimize the exertion of drying after a bath, or choosing a shallow trolley at the supermarket instead of a deep one to minimize bending and lifting, can be useful. Ensuring that the patient is on the correct benefits and receiving all to which he or she is entitled is also important. Receipt of a benefit could enable the patient to pay for a cleaner so that he or she is able to spend time, energy, and breath on activities that are a higher priority. A disabled parking badge could make the difference between a patient being

dependent or independent for a task such as shopping. Referral to the local social care team can be made if a care package for personal care tasks is required, or if there are other concerns about coping at home.

A further practical solution for managing breathlessness can be the use of cool air or movement of air generally over the face, or specifically onto the side of the face (Schwartzstein *et al.*, 1987). The flow of air affects the trigeminal nerve feedback to the brain, which can result in an altered perception of breathlessness. Patients find a small hand-held fan easy to use.

Psychological input and communication

All of the above non-pharmacological management strategies can increase the patient's feelings of control and confidence in managing breathlessness. This in turn can reduce symptoms of anxiety or depression, which may previously have limited the patient alongside symptoms such as breathlessness and associated fatigue. Because of the links between emotion (especially anxiety and anger) and breathing pattern (with the fight/flight, adrenaline response), most patients recognize that managing stress and emotion is key if they are to improve overall management of breathlessness. Active listening, use of basic counselling skills, and giving the patient time to express emotions, thoughts, and feelings need to be a part of any intervention. Sometimes, it is appropriate to assist the patient in being aware of the links between thoughts, feelings, physical symptoms, and behaviours. When aware of unhelpful thoughts and behaviours, and the impact that these can have on breathlessness, the patient is in a better position to explore coping strategies. It is important to recognize the impact that life events and the patient's social situation will have on his or her overall ability to cope with a complex symptom such as breathlessness.

Sometimes, patients need more specialist psychological work on strategies to manage stress or thoughts and behaviours that contribute to the emotion breathlessness spiral. Psychological interventions can be done by a variety of health professionals with the relevant experience and training.

Low confidence and self-efficacy in managing breathlessness can be experienced by patients at any time, but they are probably most vulnerable to this soon after an acute episode of breathlessness. Recovering from a time when they were more unwell, frightened by breathlessness, and less active/independent can be very distressing and can contribute to an overall sense of hopelessness. A patient would understandably be vulnerable to a more permanent deterioration (as well as to anxiety and depression) on these occasions, and realistic goal-setting can be a useful way in which he or she can measure progress and build motivation. Goal-setting should underpin any rehabilitation intervention. Patients often require assistance in learning how to set SMART (specific, measurable, achievable, realistic, time-limited) goals. When set skilfully and agreed using a collaborative approach, goals can help him or her to work towards making changes that improve quality of

life, restore independence, or simply maintain his or her current level of functioning and coping.

Assessment tools

There are many challenges with which a nurse can be faced when working with a patient to improve breathlessness. The patient's insight and ability to recognize patterns/triggers to his or her breathlessness is vital, and some patients find this difficult. Breathlessness is extremely difficult to measure and, although subjective tools such as those listed in Box 15.5 can be useful in the understanding of a patient's breathlessness experience, improvement or deterioration in breathlessness (and efficacy of interventions) are also hard to measure. The patient's and carer's health beliefs and ability to apply self-management advice will also determine efficacy of treatment, and the nurse may have to try several different approaches to maximize the value of self-management education. A patient's motivation can be variable, and poor motivation or low self-efficacy will impact on how effective an intervention can be. Listening and seeking to understand these sorts of barriers can enable the healthcare professional to offer

---

Box 15.5 Breathlessness assessment tools

- COPD Assessment Test (CAT)
- Visual Analogue Scale
- Modified Borg Scale
- Breathing Problems Questionnaire

CASE STUDY 15.1 *Chronic obstructive pulmonary disease*

M is a 63-year-old woman who has a long history of COPD; she has been independent, with minimal breathlessness. She developed problems with breathlessness and fatigue following a 23-day stay in intensive care being treated for bacterial meningitis. At 3 months post discharge, she remained extremely breathless and was referred to the community respiratory care team.

Initial assessment confirmed the diagnosis of severe COPD and significant loss of function. Her medications (salbutamol, tiotropium, fluticasone/salmeterol combination treatment phenytoin, domperidone, and omeprazole) were reviewed in line with NICE guidelines and minimal changes were made. Inhaler technique was assessed, deemed adequate, and concordance to medication was good. M complained of significant breathlessness and fatigue on minimal exertion. This had

contributed to symptoms of anxiety and depression, which impacted further on her symptoms. M was very motivated to improve and was keen to be referred for pulmonary rehabilitation (PR). She started the next available programme.

At PR, M initially walked 100 metres on the endurance shuttle walking test, rated herself MRC 4, and revealed that she had difficulty managing light household tasks. She required assistance with personal care, but was keen to become more independent. During PR, her fitness increased and she learnt to manage breathlessness on exertion and when anxious. She chose to attend without her husband to increase independence and confidence. Strategies she found helpful included pacing, 'blow as you go', and forward lean positioning (putting hands in her pockets when she walks). Her walking distance at the end of PR was 220 metres.

the appropriate education, support, or advice so that concordance and self-management are maximized.

Prevention of breathlessness

There are three approaches to the prevention of breathlessness:

- primary prevention, which focuses on optimizing lung health and preventing the development of disease;
- secondary prevention, which focuses on early diagnosis to minimize disease progression;
- tertiary prevention, which aims to reduce the negative impact of a disease that is already established and to restore function.

Primary prevention

Health promotion measures such as campaigns to stop maternal smoking are aimed at primary prevention. It is well recognized that optimizing lung function at the age of 25 minimizes the risk for later development of respiratory problems. Lung function declines with age (Fletcher and Peto, 1977), and poor lung health at 25 increases the likelihood of developing chronic respiratory disorders later in life. Interventions to promote optimal lung health include identifying those most at risk and developing strategies to support behavioural change (Department of Healath, 2010a).

Smoking impacts on overall health and well-being, increasing the risk of developing both respiratory and cardiac disease. Over 80% of deaths from lung cancer and COPD are due to smoking; 30% of coronary thrombosis, causing myocardial infarction, is also due to smoking. Prevention of breathlessness must therefore focus on smoking cessation when people continue to smoke and on encouraging young people to remain smoke-free. The National Institute for Health and Clinical Excellence (NICE) (2008) set out recommendations for the provision of smoking cessation services across England and Wales, with specified targets for reduction in smoking rates. Currently, the government has set a target smoking rate of 21% or less by 2010 and 26% in manual workers. Prochaska and DiClemente (1991) described the cycle of change in which people pass through five stages before

successfully changing a pattern of behaviour. All smokers should be asked if they have considered stopping and be offered support if they would like to stop. NICE (2007) looked at the cost-effectiveness of smoking cessation interventions and found that 56% of people who had set a quit date had managed to stop, with an overall quit rate of 17% at 1 year.

Secondary and tertiary prevention

Breathlessness may be a common symptom facing patients with long-term conditions. However, the key to minimizing its impact remains accurate assessment and early intervention. To maintain good health, the patient should pursue an active lifestyle, balanced diet, and avoid unhealthy behaviours such as smoking.

Inactivity can lead to a cycle of deconditioning well recognized in respiratory and cardiac conditions, which exacerbates the sensation of breathlessness, leading to a cycle of activity avoidance and further deconditioning. The benefit of exercise for all ages and abilities is well recognized (**www.nhs.uk**). There are often condition-specific exercise programmes available. For example, there is a strong evidence base for pulmonary rehabilitation, which has been shown to improve exercise capacity, reduce the sensation of dyspnoea, and improve the quality of life in patients with COPD (Griffiths *et al.*, 2001). Although the benefits of rehabilitation have primarily been identified for people with moderate to severe disease, there is evidence that early intervention can help to prevent disease progression, especially when coupled with lifestyle changes such as smoking cessation (Department of Health, 2010b).

Maintaining a healthy weight and following a balanced diet will also minimize the development of breathlessness. Obesity can have an adverse impact on respiratory function and is likely to impact on activity levels, which can lead to deconditioning and breathlessness. Cachexia is a common feature of advanced disease. Low body mass index (BMI), with a history of significant weight loss owing to poor nutritional intake, has a similar adverse effect on respiratory function because of reduced muscle strength with muscle wasting. Age Concern also suggested that 14% of people over 65 in the UK are malnourished, which can be both the cause and result of illness (McWilliams, 2008).

Early intervention and recognition of poor nutritional status will therefore be helpful in preventing the development of breathlessness in patients with chronic illness. One tool available to monitor nutritional status is the Malnutrition Universal Screening Tool (MUST) (Malnutrition Advisory Group, 2003). MUST is five-step screening tool that includes management guidelines that help the nurse to develop a plan of care to improve nutritional status.

Recurrent chest infections have also been shown to impact negatively on lung health, and measures to reduce the frequency of infection will support optimum lung health and help to prevent the development of breathlessness. Strategies to reduce the risk of infection include early diagnosis of lung disease and optimizing treatment in patients with COPD to include the use of combination inhalers containing long-acting β_2 agonist and inhaled cortico-steroid and long-acting anticholinergic inhalers (NICE, 2010). The Department of Health recommends that patients with long-term conditions and younger people who are at risk receive the annual influenza vaccination and single pneumococcal vaccination in an attempt to prevent infection (**http://www.dh.gov.uk/en/Publichealth/Flu/Flugeneralinformation**).

Measuring the impact of nursing interventions

The principle of measuring both the effectiveness of nursing intervention and the patient's experience of receiving care is one that, as a nurse, you should, where possible, facilitate. The NHS Information Centre has supported the development of Nursing Quality Metrics (NQMs), which can be used to facilitate quality improvement in patient care and experience (**http://signposting.ic.nhs.uk/?k=metrics**).

This recent move within healthcare to be outcome-focused rather than target-driven is a welcome change in policy direction, initiated by Lord Darzi in his review of the NHS, and sustained by the previous and current UK governments. Metrics have been developed for many aspects of nursing care interventions and cover many inpatient areas, regardless of setting. The collection of those types of data helps healthcare organizations to focus on the delivery of safe and effective care, and can

be used for local and national benchmarking, as well as for quality improvement.

For further details, visit the NHS Information Centre online at **http://www.ic.nhs.uk/**, where you will find details relating to nursing audit tools, capturing information on documentation for observations, nutrition, medicines administration, pain management, communication, discharge planning, falls, pressure area care, antibiotic prescribing, and infection control.

In determining patient experience of healthcare, NICE has recently published a Quality Standard (**http://www.nice.org.uk/**) that guides service delivery planning to ensure improvements in patient experience. Further commissioned work by the Department of Health has developed a single measure of patient experience. Supplementing these data is the NHS Survey, which captures patient views relating to ward cleanliness, infection control, staff attitudes, pain management, management of privacy, experience of dignity, nutrition, medicines administration, quality of communication, and discharge. Details can be found at **http://www.nhssurveys.org/**

Accessing the evidence to inform nursing decisions

Throughout this chapter, several evidence-based tools have been mentioned. To help you to stay up-to-date with evidence in the field, we have provided a list of reliable sources of evidence.

Sources of evidence

Organizations
National Institute for Health and Clinical Excellence (NICE)
Scottish Intercollegiate Guideline Network (SIGN)
Cochrane Database
British Thoracic Society

Journals
Thorax
Chest
European Respiratory Journal
Primary Care Respiratory Journal
Chronic Respiratory Disease
British Journal of Medicine

Summary and key messages

The nurse plays a key role in managing the individual's experience of breathlessness. Your aim is to minimize the related physiological and psychological impacts and associated symptoms. Breathlessness remains a significant symptom and can be a consequence of many different conditions. Assessment of the patient is key to developing your plan of care, determining targeted interventions designed to improve both functional ability and quality of daily life.

Online Resource Centre

 To help to you to develop and apply your knowledge and decision-making skills further, we have provided interactive learning resources online at **www.oxfordtextbooks.co.uk/orc/bullock/**

Whilst these are freely available, you will need to use the access codes at the start of the book.

References

Aitken, R.C. (1969) Measurement of feelings using visual analogue scales. *Proceedings of the Royal Society of Medicine* **62**: 689–92.

American Thoracic Society Consensus Statement (1999) Dyspnea: mechanisms, assessment and management. *American Journal of Critical Care Medicine* **159**: 321–40.

American Thoracic Society/European Respiratory Society (2006) Statement on pulmonary rehabilitation. *American Journal of Respiratory Critical Care Medicine* **173**: 1390–1413.

Bandura, A. (1977) Self-efficacy: toward a unifying theory of behavioral change. *Psychological Review* **84**: 191–215.

Bausewein, C., Booth, S., Gysels, M., *et al.* (2008) Non-pharmacological interventions for breathlessness in advanced stages of malignant and non-malignant diseases. *Cochrane Database of Systematic Reviews* Issue 2: Art. No. CD005623. DOI: 10.1002/14651858. CD005623.

Booth, P.S., Moosavi, S., Higginson, J. (2008) The aetiology and management of intractable breathlessness in patients with advanced cancer: a systemic review of pharmacological therapy. *National Clinical Practice Oncology* **5**(2): 90–100.

Borg, G.A. (1982) Category scale with ratio properties for intermodal and individual comparisons. In H.G. Geissler, T. Petzoldt (eds) *Psychophysical Judgements and the Process of Perception*. Deutscher Verlag: Berlin.

British Thoracic Society (2006) Clinical component for the home oxygen service in England and Wales: 2-8. **www.brit-thoracic. org.uk** (accessed 3 March 2011).

British Thoracic Society (2008) Emergency oxygen guidelines. *Thorax* **63**(Suppl. VI): vi1–vi68.

British Thoracic Society/Association of Chartered Physiotherapists in Respiratory Care (2009) Guidelines for the physiotherapy management of the adult, medical, spontaneously breathing patient. *Thorax* **64**(Suppl. 1): i1–i51.

Cochrane Reviews (2001) Opioids for the palliation of breathlessness in terminal illness. **http://www.cochrane.org/ reviews/en/ab002066.html**

Cockcroft, A., Adams, L., Guz, A. (1989) Assessment of breathlessness. *Quarterly Journal of Medicine* **77**(268): 669–76.

Corner J., Plant H., Warner, L. (1995) Developing a nursing approach to managing dyspnoea in lung cancer. *International Journal of Palliative Nursing* **1**: 5–10.

Currow, D., Ward, A., Abernathy, A. (2009) Advances in the pharmacological management of breathlessness. *Current Opinion in Supportive and Palliative Care* **3**(2): 103–6.

Davis, C.L. (1997) ABC of palliative care. Breathlessness, cough and other respiratory problems. *British Medical Journal* **315**(7113): 1–4.

Dean, M. (2008) End of life care for COPD patients. *Primary Care Respiratory Journal* **17**(1): 46–50.

Dechman, G., *et al.* (2004) Evidence underlying breathing retraining in people with stable chronic obstructive pulmonary disease. *Physical Therapy* **84**: 1189–97.

Department of Health (2009) Competencies for Recognising and Responding to Acutely Ill Patients in Hospital. Department of Health: London.

Department of Health (2010a) *Consultation on a Strategy for Services: Chronic Obstructive Pulmonary Disease (COPD)*. Department of Health: London.

Department of Heath (2010b) *Coronary Heart Disease and the need for Cardiac Rehabilitation*. **http://www.dh.gov.uk/ prod_consum_dh/groups/dh_digitalassets/@dh/@en/@ps/ documents/digitalasset/dh_118402.pdf** (accessed 1 May 2011).

Endacott, R., Jevon, P., Cooper, S. (2009) (eds) *Clinical Nursing Skills: Core and advanced*. Oxford University Press: Oxford.

Fletcher, C.M., Elme, P., Fairbairn, A., *et al.* (1959) The significance of respiratory symptoms and the diagnosis of chronic bronchitis in the working population. *British Medical Journal* **2**: 257–66.

Fletcher, C.M., Peto, R. (1977) Graph of survival. *British Medical Journal* **1**: 1645–8.

Gift, A.G. (1990) Dyspnoea. *Nursing Clinics of North America* **25**(4): 955–65.

Griffiths, T.L., Philips, C.J., Davies, S., *et al.* (2001) Cost effectiveness of an outpatient multidisciplinary pulmonary rehabilitation program. *Thorax* **56**: 779–84.

Howard, C., Dupont, S., Haselden, B., *et al.* (2010)The effectiveness of a group cognitive-behavioural breathlessness intervention on health status, mood and hospital admissions in elderly patients with chronic obstructive pulmonary disease. *Psychology, Health & Medicine* **15**(4): 371–85.

Huijnen, B., van der Horst, F., van Amelsvoort, L., *et al.* (2006) Dyspnoea in elderly family practice patients: occurrence, severity, quality of life and mortality over an 8-year period. *Family Practice* **23**(1): 34–9.

Jennings, A.L., Davies, A.N., Higgins, J.P.T., *et al.* (2002) A systematic review of the use of opioids in the management of dyspnoea. *Thorax* **57**(11): 939–44.

Jevon, P. (2009) *Clinical Examination Skills.* Wiley-Blackwell: Oxford.

Karnani, N.G., Reisfield, G.M., Wilson, G.R. (2005) Evaluation of chronic dyspnea. *American Family Physician* **71**(8): 1529–37.

Malnutrition Advisory Group (2003) *The 'MUST' Report: Nutritional Screening for Adults—A Multidisciplinary Responsibility.* **http://www.bapen.org.uk/pdfs/must/must_full.pdf** (accessed 1 May 2011).

McCarthy, M., Lay, M., Addington-Hall, J. (1996) Dying from heart disease. *Journal of the Royal College of Physicians* **30**: 325–8.

McWilliams, B. (2008) Assessing the benefits of a malnutrition screening tool. *Nursing Times* **104**(24): 30–1.

Mosby (2009) *Mosbyz's Medical Dictionary,* 8th edn. Elsevier: Oxford.

National Institute for Health and Clinical Excellence (NICE) (2006) NICE RAPID REVIEW The Effectiveness of National Health Service Intensive Treatments for Smoking Cessation in England June 2006. **http://www.nice.org.uk/nicemedia/pdf/SmokingCessationNHSTreatmentFullReview.pdf** (accessed 26 March 2012).

National Insitute for Health and Clinical Excellence (NICE) (2007) Acutely ill patients in hospital: recognition and response to acute illness in adults in hospital. NICE Clinical Guideline 50 (CG50). **www.nice.org.uk/CG50** (accessed 24 April 2011).

National Institute for Health and Clinical Excellence (NICE) (2008) Smoking cessation services in primary care, pharmacies, local authorities and work places, particularly in manual working groups, pregnant women and hard to reach communities. NICE Public Health Guidance 10. NICE: London.

National Institute for Health and Clinical Excellence (NICE) (2009) Depression in adults with a chronic physical health problem: treatment and management. National Clinical Guideline 91 (CG91). NICE: London.

National Institute for Health and Clinical Excellence (NICE) (2010) Chronic obstructive pulmonary disease: management of COPD in primary and secondary care. NICE Clinical Guideline 101 (CG101). **www.nice.org.uk/guidance/CG101.** (accessed 24 April 2011).

Probst, V.S., Troosters, T., Coosemans, I., *et al.* (2004) Mechanisms of improvement in exercise capacity using a rollator in patients with COPD. *Chest* **126**: 1102–7.

Prochaska, J.O., DiClemente, C.C., Norcross, J.C. (1992) In search of how people change: applications to addictive behaviours. *American Psychologist* **47**: 1102.

Resuscitation Council (UK) (2006) *Advanced Life Support.* Resuscitation Council (UK): London.

Ries, A.L. (2006) Impact of chronic obstructive pulmonary disease on quality of life: the role of dyspnea. *American Journal of Medicine* **119**(10 Suppl. (1):12–20.

Schwartzstein, R.M., Lahive, K., Pope, A., *et al.* (1987) Cold facial stimulation reduces breathlessness induced in normal subjects. *American Review of Respiratory Disease* **136**(1): 58–61.

Scottish Intercollegiate Guidelines Network (SIGN) (2007) Management of chronic heart failure: a national clinical guideline. **http://www.cochrane.org/reviews/en/ab002066.html** (accessed 12 February 2011).

Simon, S.T., Higginson, I.J., Booth, S., *et al.* (2010) Benzodiazepines for the relief of breathlessness in advanced malignant and non-malignant diseases in adults. *The Cochrane Database of Systematic Reviews.* Issue 12: Art. No. CD007354. **www2.cochrane.org/reviews/en/ab007354.html**

Turner-Lawler, R. (2004) Occupational therapy in pulmonary rehabilitation. In R. Garrod (ed.) *Pulmonary Rehabilitation: An Interdisciplinary Approach.* Whurr Publications: London, Philidelphia, PA.

Tywcross, R., Lack, S. (1990) *Therapeutics in Terminal Cancer,* 2nd edn. Churchill Livingstone: Edinburgh and New York.

Urie, J., Fielding, H., McArthur, D., *et al.* (2000) Palliative care. *The Pharmaceutical Journal* **265**(7119): 603–14.

Vitacca, M., Clinic, E., Bianchi, L. *et al.* (1998) Acute effects of deep diaphragmatic breathing in COPD patients with chronic respiratory insufficiency. *European Respiratory Journal* **11**: 408–15.

Ward, J., Linden, R. (2008) *Physiology at a Glance.* Wiley Blackwell: Oxford.

Waugh, A., Grant, A. (2006) *Ross and Wilson Anatomy and Physiology in Health and Illness.* Elsevier: Edinburgh.

16 *Managing* Continence

Mandy Fader, Christine De Laine,
Christine Norton, and Jacqui Prieto

Introduction

This chapter addresses the fundamental role of continence management as a core nursing activity. Every nurse should possess the knowledge and skills to carry out an essential, but simple, continence assessment, as well as to select and implement evidence-based strategies to manage continence in all care settings (including hospital and community), and to review the effectiveness of these to inform any necessary changes in care.

Despite being essential for dignity and compassionate care, continence needs are often not prioritized as highly by nurses as they are by patients and their relatives. For adults, the ability to control bladder and bowel emptying is very important to self-esteem and dignity. Continence is a complex specialty involving a number of disciplines, including specialist nurses, specialists in urology, gynaecology, physiotherapy, and elderly care, yet the prevalence of continence problems means that much depends on you as a registered nurse taking responsibility for initiating assessment and management.

Continence issues frequently arise as a result of other healthcare problems, and you should remain constantly aware of this, identifying patients who are at risk of incontinence and helping embarrassed patients to seek help.

Understanding the importance of continence

Bladder and bowel control are taken for granted by most of us. Once continence is achieved during childhood, we expect to remain in charge of these bodily functions for the rest of our life. Temporary loss of continence commonly accompanies acute illness or hospitalization, particularly if mobility and/or cognition become impaired (Resnick *et al.*, 1989), or if the disease or injury impacts directly on bladder or bowel function. If the bladder fails to function normally (such as an overactive bladder), lower urinary tract symptoms may be experienced, and these may include incontinence. If bowel habits are disrupted, this may result in faecal incontinence (FI), constipation, or both. Incontinence is also associated with long-term

> **Box 16.1 Definitions of urinary, faecal, and anal incontinence**
>
> Urinary incontinence (UI) is the complaint of any involuntary leakage of urine (Abrams *et al.*, 2002).
>
> Faecal incontinence (FI) is the loss of stool, which is a social or hygienic problem.
>
> Anal incontinence is the loss of stool or flatus, which is a social or hygienic problem (Norton *et al.*, 2009).

> **Box 16.2 Prevalence of UI in the UK**
>
> For people living at home
> - Between 1 in 20 and 1 in 14 women aged 15–44
> - Between 1 in 13 and 1 in 7 in women aged 45–64
> - Between 1 in 10 and 1 in 5 women aged 65 and over
> - Over 1 in 33 men aged 15–64
> - Between 1 in 14 and 1 in 10 men aged 65 and over
>
> For people (both sexes) living in institutions
> - One in 3 in residential homes
> - Nearly 2 in every 3 in nursing homes
> - Between 1 in 2 and 2 in 3 in wards for the elderly and elderly mentally infirm
>
> (Department of Health, 2000)

conditions, in particular those affecting the neurological system (Fowler *et al.*, 2010).

Dealing with incontinence is a very common activity for nurses, and it is easy to become inured to this, forgetting that, for the patient, the experience can be devastating. It is noteworthy that the International Continence Society defines urinary incontinence (UI) as being *any* involuntary leakage of urine (Abrams *et al.*, 2002), and it is therefore a symptom (however slight) that you should never ignore. See Box 16.1 for definitions of different types of incontinence.

The prevalence of continence problems

Urinary incontinence is very common at all ages, particularly in older people and those in nursing and residential homes, although prevalence has been difficult to determine reliably owing to differences in the definitions of incontinence (e.g. any leakage 'ever' or 'bothersome' leakage in the past month). Box 16.2 summarizes the prevalence of UI in the UK. These data are rather old, but provide the most recent comprehensive account. More up-to-date data have been obtained from a large European survey (Hunskaar *et al.*, 2004). Box 16.3 shows the size of the problem of UI in women. In Figure 16.1, Perry *et al.* (2002) describe the prevalence of FI in the community in the UK, with 2.2% of the overall population reporting regular FI, although prevalence rates of up to 15% have been reported in other studies (Whitehead *et al.*, 2009). In older adults, 4% report FI (AlAmeel *et al.*, 2010).

The human and social burden of incontinence

It is known that incontinence is very damaging to quality of life (Brittain *et al.*, 2000), both for the individual and

> **Box 16.3 Prevalence of UI in women in four European countries**
>
> - Spain 23%
> - France 44%
> - Germany 41%
> - UK 42%
>
> (Hunskaar *et al.*, 2004)

for his or her family and carers (Coyne *et al.*, 2003). Key themes and findings that have emerged from interviews with patients include:

- embarrassment;
- fear of smell;
- fear of visible leakage or a public 'accident';
- low self-esteem;
- anxiety and depression;
- damage to sexual relationships;
- financial costs;
- loss of employment;
- 'toilet mapping'—always needing to know the location of the nearest toilet;
- isolation and reduced socializing;

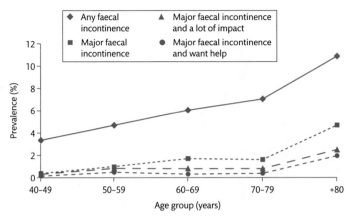

Figure 16.1 Prevalence of faecal incontinence (Perry *et al.*, 2002).

Reproduced from *Gut* 2002; 50: 480–4, with permission from BMJ Publishing Group Ltd.

- concern about the possibility of leakage during intimacy;
- increased need for residential care.

Incontinence is also known to be associated with an increase in falls and fractures (Brown *et al.*, 2000), pressure ulcers, and skin health problems (Gray *et al.*, 2007). Older people with FI are almost twice as likely to be living in a nursing home as those without FI (AlAmeel *et al.*, 2010), and those in institutional care with FI have a higher mortality than those who are continent of faeces (Chassagne *et al.*, 1999), although this does not confirm a causative relationship.

Causes of urinary incontinence

Urinary continence is dependent on normal anatomy and function of the lower urinary tract and the nervous system. Normal bladder function consists of two phases—storage and emptying (voiding)—with the urinary bladder and the urethral sphincter working in a coordinated way, regulated by the central and peripheral nervous systems. During urinary storage, the bladder muscle (**detrusor**) stretches to accommodate increasing amounts of urine at low pressure, while the urinary sphincter mechanisms are activated to maintain high resistance to keep the bladder outlet closed. During voiding, the bladder contracts to expel urine, while the urinary sphincter opens (low resistance) to allow unobstructed urinary flow and bladder emptying.

Continence therefore relies upon competent anatomical and physiological mechanisms, and/or the absence of factors that escalate the risk of incontinence. Figure 16.2 illustrates risk factors for incontinence that have been identified from epidemiological studies (studies that seek to find associations between risks and health problems), as well as known causes of UI.

Types of urinary incontinence

Broadly speaking, UI can be divided into two main categories (which can coexist): storage problems; and voiding problems. Table 16.1 shows the different types of incontinence (and their causes) within each category. Appropriate care planning and treatment depends on accurately identifying the type of incontinence, and a nursing continence assessment is therefore essential to begin this process.

Types of faecal incontinence

There are four main categories of FI, which can coexist in the same individual.

Urge FI means that the patient usually feels an urge to empty the bowel, but cannot hold on and leaks before getting to the toilet. Passive FI denotes loss of stool without feeling or an urge. Reflex FI occurs in people with neurological conditions in which colonic peristalsis results in reflex bowel emptying that the patient does not have the ability to control. Rectal loading with 'overflow' stool leakage may mean that the rectum is full of hard or soft stool. Rectal loading inhibits the anal sphincters and leakage may result.

Causes and Risk Factors associated with Urinary Incontinence

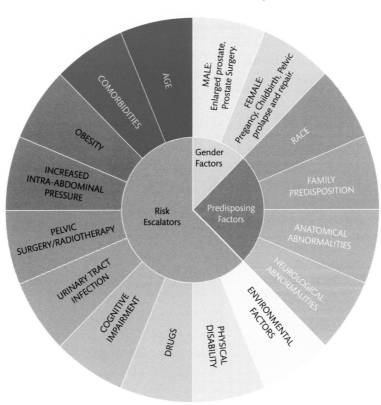

Figure 16.2 **Risk factor wheel.**

(adapted from Abrams *et al.*, 2005). Reproduced with permission from Health Publications Ltd.

Causes of faecal incontinence

Bowel incontinence, as with UI, can result from impaired storage or impaired emptying (evacuation). Table 16.2 shows the commonest underlying causes of FI. As with the UI wheel (see Figure 16.2), cognitive or mobility impairment, an adverse environment, anatomical or neurological abnormalities, obesity, advancing age, medications, and comorbidities each increase the risk of FI.

Nursing responsibilities and accountability for managing continence

While recognizing that many people feel highly embarrassed by their bladder or bowel symptoms, you will need

to enquire about possible problems ('active case finding', NICE FI Guidelines, 2007) and enable the patient to talk about concerns. Many patients in hospital fear incontinence, even if it has not actually happened. They are often uncertain how to raise the subject and some do not have a vocabulary with which they are comfortable. The nurse needs to be sensitive to this and to find ways to enable patients to express their needs.

You have a key role in identifying, assessing, and managing continence in all healthcare settings and for all patients. General surgical and medical nurses will encounter patients with incontinence in all specialties, and will be responsible (as a minimum) for initiating essential assessment and interventions, and for liaising with medical and other professional colleagues. Nurses who work in areas in which specific continence problems commonly occur (e.g. gynaecology, older people, urology, community,

Table 16.1 Types of urinary incontinence

Storage problems	
Stress urinary incontinence (SUI)	**Urge urinary incontinence (UUI)**
• Leaks when coughing/sneezing or with physical activity • Unusual in men except following prostate surgery	• Leaks before getting to the toilet • Affects men and women
Caused by the pressure in the bladder exceeding the closing pressure in the urethra, usually as a result of damage to the pelvic floor from pregnancy and childbirth (Figure 16.3(a)) Contributing factors include: • Female sex • Pregnancy and childbirth • Pelvic organ **prolapse** • Pelvic surgery and radiotherapy • Age • Obesity • Chronic cough • Constipation • Following prostate surgery in males	Caused by involuntary bladder (detrusor) contractions (Figure 16.3(b)). In most cases the reason for this is unknown; however, it may be associated with neurological disease (**neurogenic**) such as multiple sclerosis. A diagnosis of overactive bladder (OAB) can be made when a patient has symptoms of frequency, urgency, and/or urge incontinence provided that there is no infection or other pathology. A diagnosis of **detrusor overactivity** (DO) is only used when these involuntary detrusor contractions have been proven by bladder pressure tests (**urodynamics**). Contributing factors include: • Neurological abnormalities • Functional impairment • Cognitive impairment • Age • Drugs, e.g. diuretics • Fluid intake and type • Anxiety
Voiding problems	
Bladder outlet obstruction (BOO)	**Detrusor underactivity**
• Leaks when finished urinating • Leaks for no obvious reason • Leaks all the time • Leaks when asleep • Leaks before going to the toilet • Recurrent urinary tract infections common • Commonest cause in men is benign prostatic enlargement • Uncommon in women	• Leaks when finished urinating • Leaks for no obvious reason • Leaks all the time • Leaks when asleep • Leaks before going to the toilet • Recurrent urinary tract infections common • Affects men and women
May be caused by: • Enlarged prostate gland (Figure 16.3 (c)) • Urethral stricture (narrowing) • Pelvic prolapse • Severe constipation Contributing variables or risk factors include: • Male sex • Severe constipation • History of urethral trauma • Pelvic organ prolapse in females	May be caused by: • Damage to the peripheral nerves or cauda equina in conditions such as diabetic neuropathy, pelvic injury, or multiple sclerosis. • impaired detrusor contractility in frail older people (Figure 16.3 (d)). Contributing variables or risk factors include: • Anticholinergic medication • Age • Neurological abnormality

(a)

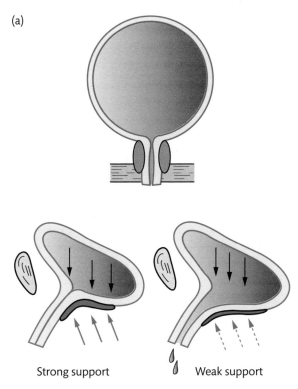

Strong support   Weak support

Figure 16.3 (a) Urethral sphincter supported by pelvic floor muscles and anatomical support.

(b)

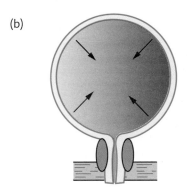

Figure 16.3 (b) Involuntary detrusor contractions.

(c)

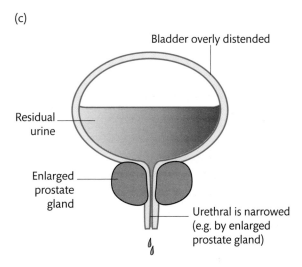

Bladder overly distended

Residual urine

Enlarged prostate gland

Urethral is narrowed (e.g. by enlarged prostate gland)

Figure 16.3 (c) A enlarged prostate.

(d)

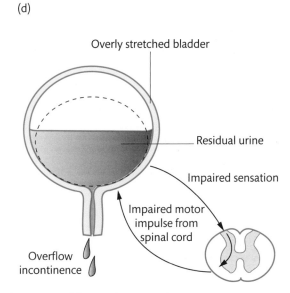

Overly stretched bladder

Residual urine

Impaired sensation

Impaired motor impulse from spinal cord

Overflow incontinence

Figure 16.3 (d) A underactive detrusor.

Table 16.2 **Causes of faecal incontinence**

Pathology	Example causes	Typical symptoms
Damaged external anal sphincter	Childbirth injury, such as third-degree tear	Urgency, urge FI
Damaged internal anal sphincter	Anal surgery, such as haemorrhoidectomy	Passive FI
Diarrhoea or intestinal hurry	Any cause of diarrhoea, e.g. gastrointestinal infection or inflammation; drug-induced; colonic resection; pelvic radiotherapy; irritable bowel syndrome	Urgency, urge FI
Rectal loading	Cognitive impairment leading to ignoring call to stool; immobility; constipating drugs such as opiates; evacuation difficulty or incomplete emptying	Leakage of often liquid offensive-smelling stool
Reflex bowel emptying	Spinal cord injury or other neurological disease or injury	Bowel emptying with no warning: may be day or night

stroke units) will need additional training to provide elements of further assessment and in interventions that require skills and experience, e.g. use of bladder scanner, intermittent catheterization, pelvic floor muscle training, bladder retraining, and digital rectal examination.

Specialist continence nurses are usually responsible for providing continence services in primary (and sometimes secondary) care, including managing caseloads of patients with more complex bladder and bowel problems. Internationally, the UK has been a leader in developing the role of the specialist continence nurse and, uniquely, the NHS funds the provision of continence services in primary care nationwide, which are led by nurses.

All nurses should be able to perform the essential assessments and interventions (listed in Box 16.4) competently. Further assessment and interventions listed in the right-hand column of Box 16.4 require additional training and/or would be undertaken by advanced nurse practitioners or continence specialist nurses.

Making a clinical assessment of continence

Most patients whom you encounter will require nursing support primarily for reasons other than incontinence. However, because so many healthcare conditions are associated with a continence problem, it is important to routinely ask the question: 'Do you have any problems with bladder or bowel control?'

If the answer is 'yes' (or if incontinence is observed), then an 'essential continence assessment' (Figures 16.4 and 16.6) should be completed.

Nursing assessment and management of urinary incontinence

Figure 16.4 outlines essential assessment for urinary continence. When assessing your patient for continence problems, it is important to remember to use words that the patient understands and is comfortable using, and that the following elements are covered:

- recognizing symptoms;
- undertaking urinalysis;
- reviewing medications;
- identifying constipation;
- disimpaction and treating constipation (with appropriate training);
- using a chart;
- toileting interventions;
- observing the patient's skin.

Recognizing symptoms

The symptom questions are those that comprise the ICIQ short form (Avery *et al.*, 2004), which is a standardized brief assessment tool recommended by the most recent International Consultation in Incontinence (Abrams 2009). The symptoms listed under 'context of leakage' indicate the possible type(s) of UI

Box 16.4 Essential and further assessment and interventions

Essential

- Enable patient to report continence symptoms or concerns

- Urinalysis

- Contribute to medications review (in consultation with medical staff)

- Identification of bowel pattern and constipation

- Digital rectal examination to assess contents of the rectum (this clinical skill should only be undertaken after appropriate training)

- Continence chart

- Toileting observation

- Genital, perianal, and skin observation

- Simple interventions such as identification and treatment of urinary tract infection or constipation; lifestyle advice such as: fluid and diet modification, toileting management, establishing a bowel routine, and use of containment products and perineal skin protection

- Provision of written information on pelvic floor exercises and behavioural therapies, e.g. bladder retraining

- Onward referral (if necessary)

Further

- Comprehensive continence-focused history

- Measurement of post-void residual urine

- Monitoring therapeutic effects of medication therapy

- Digital rectal examination to assess contents of rectum, including assessment of anal sphincter tone in FI

- Synthesize all assessment data to identify reversible causes and types of incontinence

- Interpret diagnostic studies such as urodynamic and anorectal physiology tests

- UI: diagnose urge, stress, mixed or functional incontinence, or voiding problem

- Conservative treatments and interventions, including behavioural therapies such as pelvic floor muscle exercise and bladder retraining; prescribing medication; intermittent catheterization; and use of a wide range of containment products

- FI: diagnose urge, passive FI, or impaction with leakage

- Conservative treatments and interventions, including pelvic floor muscle exercise and bowel retraining, rectal irrigation, biofeedback

- Evaluate outcomes of interventions and report to the primary care provider for further specialist referral if necessary

that the patient is experiencing. The symptoms scoring system (questions 1, 2, and 3) provides a quantitative measure of the baseline severity of incontinence and should be repeated once assessment and treatment have been instigated to measure outcome.

Undertaking urinalysis

Incontinence may be a symptom of urinary tract infection or other underlying disease, so routine urinalysis using a reagent strip (indicating pH, protein, nitrites,

leukocytes, glycosuria, ketones, and blood) should be done (Department of Health, 2000). If there is glucose and/or ketones, then report immediately to medical staff. If there are nitrites and/or leukocytes present, then urine should be sent for microscopy, culture, and sensitivity.

Reviewing medications

Many medications are known to contribute to incontinence (e.g. diuretics), and these should be identified and

Name- ______________

DOB- ______________

ESSENTIAL CONTINENCE ASSESSMENT FOR URINARY INCONTINENCE

Date of Assessment ________
Assessor- ____________

1 **How often do you leak urine?**

Never (0), Once a week or less (1)
2-3 times a week (2), Once a day (3)
Several times a day (4), All the time (5)

2 **How much urine do you usually leak ?**

None (0), A small amount (2)
A moderate amount (4),
A large amount (6)

3 **Overall, how much does leaking urine interfere with your everyday life ?**

0-1-2-3-4-5-6-7-8-9-10
(not at all)------------------(a lot)

TOTAL SCORE:

Context : When there is a urine leak
(please tick all that apply)?

- -Urine does not leak ☐
- -Leaks before you get to toilet ☐
- -Leaks when you cough/sneeze ☐
- -Leaks when you are asleep ☐
- -Leak when physically active ☐
- -Leaks when finished urinating ☐
- -Leaks for no obvious reason ☐
- -Leaks all the time ☐

Urinalysis	Medications	Constipation	Chart	Toileting	Observation
Leucocytes Pos ☐ Neg ☐ Nitrites Pos ☐ Neg ☐ Remember incontinence can be a symptom of infection	Look at medication chart, and identify any, Diuretics ☐ Hypnotics ☐ Antidepressants ☐ Drugs for urinary incontinence ☐ Drugs for urinary retention ☐	Ask patient "Are you constipated at the moment?" (or check with carer) Yes ☐ No ☐	Ask patient or carer to complete fluid intake, (amount and type) and urine output (amount voided and incontinent), for three days on a continence chart (Fig. 16.5).	Observe toileting for : Impaired : Mobility ☐ Dexterity ☐ Vision ☐ Cognition ☐ Assistance Required ☐ Carers available ☐	Look at the skin around the genital area for : Erythema ☐ Rashes ☐ Broken skin ☐ Obvious abnrmalities... Describe- ______
Action-	**Action-**	**Action-**	**Action-**	**Action-**	**Action-**
If positive for leucocytes or nitrites obtain MSU and discuss treatment with doctor.	Inform doctor that patient is experiencing continence problems, and request medical review if any of the above are listed.	Do digital rectal examination and bowel clearance (according to local policy). See treating constipation and impaction box (Box 16.7)	Look at chart—see chart box. (Table 16.3)	If reaching the toilet is a problem aim to make this as easy as possible- see toileting action box (Table 16.4)	Treat skin problems- see skin care box, refer any other abnormalities to doctors
Outcome-	**Outcome-**	**Outcome-**	**Outcome-**	**Outcome-**	**Outcome-**
________	________	________	________	________	________
Review Date- ________	**Review Date-** ________	**Review Date-** ________	**Review Date-** ________	**Review Date-** ________	**Review Date-** ________

Figure 16.4 Essential continence assessments.

discussed with medical staff (Rigby, 2007). Routine laxatives may lead to loose stool and FI unless resulting stool form is closely monitored and laxatives adjusted as needed.

Identifying constipation

Constipation is believed to contribute to UI, although there is little clinical research evidence to support this. In addition, it may underlie FI (see below). Constipation needs to be ruled out either by questioning the patient, or (if necessary) by observation of bowel habit or stool, or by digital rectal examination. If constipation is present, then it should be treated as indicated in Box 16.5.

Normal bowel habit should be identified and medication may be required (in consultation with medical staff). Suppositories or an enema may produce a more predictable response. Occasionally, a gentle manual evacuation is needed if the rectum is very loaded. Once the impaction is cleared, then measures must be taken to stop recurrence.

Your nursing actions will include ensuring adequate toileting opportunities linked to the patient's normal habit and with a high level of privacy, provision of fluids, dietary manipulation (such as supplementing an inadequate fibre intake), and optimization of mobility and toilet access.

Disimpaction and treating constipation

If assessment has found a rectum loaded with hard or soft stool, this should be cleared in the first instance because, in many cases, FI will resolve. Oral laxatives can be used, but can lead to FI episodes if the patient is immobile or confused. Suppositories or an enema may produce a more predictable response. Occasionally, a gentle manual evacuation is needed if the rectum is very loaded. Once the impaction is cleared, then measures must be taken to stop recurrence.

Using a chart

A UI chart (Figure 16.5) needs to be completed by the patient with UI or his or her carer for 1–3 days to obtain a baseline of fluid intake, voiding, and incontinence frequency. Chart interpretation and action are shown in Table 16.3. A similar chart for bowels may be useful for the patient with FI, particularly if a relationship between FI and diet or laxatives is suspected. A record for at least 3 days, and preferably for 1 week, may clarify the situation.

Box 16.5 Treating constipation and impaction

- If a patient has impaction, rectal evacuant (suppository or enema) may produce a more predictable effect than oral laxatives.
- Gentle manual evacuation is occasionally required and would be performed by a competent practitioner with additional training.
- Increase fluid intake if patient is dehydrated or drinking less than 1.5 l/day. Be aware of patients with heart failure who may be fluid-restricted: use caution when increasing oral or IV fluids. Excessive fluid intake is not helpful and may cause bloating.
- Increase fibre intake if stool is hard (type 1 or 2). Use a variety of formats. (Note: excessive fibre intake may cause bloating and abdominal discomfort).
- More exercise may help if the patient is sedentary or immobile. Abdominal massage may substitute if mobility is impossible.
- Try to establish an evacuation routine (after breakfast is often the most likely time).
- Sit well supported on the toilet. Feet may need support on a footstool.
- Attempt to maximize privacy and do not rush.
- Educate patient not to hold the breath and strain, but to use the abdominal muscles to expel stool gently.
- If regular laxatives are needed, adjust dose depending on response.

Toileting interventions

Incontinence can be caused by or worsened by difficulties with toileting. If this is suspected (particularly if there are mobility or cognitive problems), a toileting episode should be observed and actions taken to make it easier (Table 16.4).

Observing the patient's skin

Incontinence can cause skin health problems such as dermatitis, especially if faecal incontinence is present and is associated with pressure ulcers. The skin within the 'pant'

Continence Chart									
Patient identification details:									
Time	Date:			Date:			Date:		
	IN-TAKE	OUT-PUT	WET	IN-TAKE	OUT-PUT	WET	IN-TAKE	OUT-PUT	WET
06.00 am									
07.00 am									
08.00 am									
09.00 am									
10.00 am									
11.00 am									
12 noon									
1.00 pm									
2.00 pm									
3.00 pm									
4.00 pm									
5.00 pm									
6.00 pm									
7.00 pm									
8.00 pm									
9.00 pm									
10.00 pm									
11.00 pm									
Midnight									
01.00 am									
02.00 am									
03.00 am									
04.00 am									
05.00 am									
TOTAL									

Figure 16.5 Continence chart.

area should be observed for skin problems and action taken (see **Chapters 20 Managing Hygiene** and **27 Managing the Prevention of Skin Breakdown** ➡).

Obvious genital abnormalities (e.g. prolapse or hydrocele) should be referred to medical staff. Perianal conditions such as haemorrhoids (piles) or an anal fissure may be observed and should be recorded, with medical referral if bleeding is reported.

Nursing assessment and management of faecal incontinence

Figure 16.6 shows the essential continence assessment for anal and faecal incontinence.

Recognizing symptoms

Because there is no evidence-based short assessment for FI, the scoring is based on the UI questions. The symptoms listed may indicate the type of FI (see Figure 16.6).

Digital rectal examination

If the anus is gaping, this may indicate that there is major nerve or muscle damage, or that rectal loading is inhibiting the sphincters. A loaded rectum should be cleared using oral or rectal medications (see Box 16.5). This may resolve FI.

Reviewing medications

Many medications affect the bowel to cause loose stool or constipation. Adjusting medications where possible may resolve bowel symptoms. Frail or immobile people may have FI caused by laxative overuse.

Identifying constipation

Constipation needs to be ruled out by either questioning the patient, or (if necessary) by observation of bowel habit or stool, or by digital rectal examination. If assessment has found a rectum loaded with hard or soft stool, this should be cleared in the first instance because in many cases FI will resolve. If constipation is present, then it should be treated as indicated in Box 16.5. Oral laxatives can be used, but can lead to FI episodes if the patient is immobile or confused.

A chart needs to be interpreted in the light of the individual's normal bowel pattern. Simple interventions are: a gradual increase of fibre (particularly soluble); increase

Table 16.3 Chart actions

Chart shows		Actions
Very abnormal fluid intake	Drinking too much (>3000 ml)	Fluid advice or assistance to achieve normal intake
	Not drinking enough (<1000 ml)	Fluid advice or assistance to achieve normal intake
Night-time symptoms	Nocturia >2 per night	Refer to doctor (may be medical causes)
	FI at night	Refer to doctor (may be medical causes)
	Night-time UI	Establish if patient leaks when he or she is asleep—if so, consider timed waking
		If awake—improve toilet access
Daytime symptoms	High daytime urinary frequency (>7) and 'context' symptom 'leaks before you get to toilet'	Bladder retraining plus pelvic floor muscle training (PFMT) may be appropriate—discuss onward referral with doctor
	Normal urinary frequency (>4<7) and incontinence and 'context' symptom 'leaks when you cough/sneeze' or 'when physically active'	PFMT may be appropriate if patient leaks when coughing/sneezing or physically active—discuss onward referral with doctor
	Low daytime urinary frequency (<4) and incontinence	Ensure adequate toileting opportunities (3–4-hourly) to pre-empt incontinence.
		If cause not known—discuss onward referral with doctor
Bowel symptoms	Frequent (>3 per day) or loose stool for no apparent reason	Refer to doctor (may be medical causes for diarrhoea)
	Loose stool associated with laxatives	Reduce or stop laxatives
	No stool for 3 days or more	Check usual bowel habit
		Treat for constipation

Source: NB. This list is not comprehensive, and is intended as a guide for nurses caring for adult patients in the management and treatment of common continence problems.

fluids where dehydrated; and ensure well-supported feet during attempted defaecation. If the patient has lost all awareness of call to stool, encourage attempted bowel emptying after meals (bowel is most active after eating).

Loose stool will exacerbate urgency and may in some cases be the sole cause of FI. This may be caused by the underlying disease process, but can be the result of overuse of laxatives, or a side effect of other medications such as antibiotics, anxiety, and numerous other causes. Persistent diarrhoea needs medical referral, as does any case of rectal bleeding. Bowel cancer is the second commonest cancer and can be treated if caught early (National Institute for Health and Clinical Excellence (NICE), 2005).

Using a chart and toileting interventions

The principles underpinning these activities mirror those for UI (see Tables 16.3 and 16.4, and Figure 16.5).

Observing the patient's skin

This involves the same observations as in UI, but must include observing the area around the anus (see Chapter 20 Managing Hygiene ⟶ measures for more detailed skin care).

Further treatment and specialist referral

Persistent UI may indicate the presence of a specific storage (SUI or UUI) or voiding (BOO or detrusor underactivity)

Table 16.4 Toileting actions

Patient does not	Action
Recognize the need to use the toilet	Remind patient to go to the toilet every 3 hours during daytime Consider waking patient once at night
Find the toilet	Ensure that location of toilet is known and signs are clear Provide carer help
Get to the toilet	Ensure that mobility aids are available Provide carer help Consider toilet chair/commode, or urinal
Adjust clothes and pants	Simplify clothing Provide carer help
Sit well supported with knees bent for bowel emptying	Consider use of footstool to aid evacuation
Use the toilet/toilet chair/commode/urinal	Optimize privacy (whenever safe, leave patient alone) and dignity (no public exposure, attention to sound, and smell minimization)
Clean adequately after using the toilet;	Provide bidet, wet wipes, washing facilities, or assistance

problem that requires referral onward to a continence specialist. Persistent FI may likewise indicate specialist referral. The completed essential assessment form will provide vital background information on which to start specialist assessment and is designed to accompany the referral. Further treatments and interventions are reviewed below.

Further evidence-based management of urinary incontinence

A summary of treatments for UI is given in Box 16.6.

The role of lifestyle changes

Whilst there are very few randomized controlled trials that assess the impact of lifestyle changes on UI, the interventions involved are generally health-promoting and carry a low risk of adverse effects (Abrams *et al.*, 2005).

Lifestyle changes that may be beneficial to promoting continence include:

- losing weight if obese;
- decreasing caffeine intake;
- smoking cessation, to reduce cough;
- decreasing carbonated fluids;
- avoiding constipation.

The role of pelvic floor muscle training (PFMT)

The aim of PFMT is to strengthen the pelvic floor muscles and therefore the closing pressure of the urethral sphincter. It is the first line treatment for women with stress incontinence (National Institute for Health and Clinical Excellence (NICE), 2006). PFMT may also be used in UUI because contraction of the pelvic floor muscles causes a reflex inhibition of the detrusor (bladder) muscle, aiding urine storage. PFMT is known to be helpful for women with all types of incontinence, but particularly those who have SUI on exercise for more than 3 months (Dumoulin and Hay-Smith, 2010). National Institute for Health and Clinical Excellence (NICE) guidelines recommend that PFMT is taught by experienced practitioners (usually continence specialist nurses or physiotherapists) following digital assessment of the pelvic floor. As a general nurse, you would not normally be expected to offer PFMT unless trained and competent in digital assessment of the pelvic floor. Self-help guidance is available

FAECAL INCONTINENCE- THE ESSENTIALS

Name-
DOB-

Date of Assessment- _____
Assessor- _____

1 How often do you leak stool

Never (0), Once a week or less (1)
2-3 times a week (2), Once a day (3)
Several times a day (4), All the time (5)

2 How much stool do you usually leak?

None (0), A small amount (teaspoonful) (2)
A moderate amount (tablespoonful) (4)
A large amount (whole stool) (6)

3 Overall, how much does leaking stool interfere with your everyday life ?

0-1-2-3-4-5-6-7-8-9-10
(not at all) ——————— (a lot)

TOTAL SCORE: - - - - - - -

When there is a stool leak (please tick all that apply)?

-Stool does not leak ☐
-Leaks before you get to toilet ☐
-Leaks without you realising ☐
-Leaks when you are asleep ☐
-Leak when physically active ☐
-Leaks after bowel action ☐
-Leaks for no obvious reason ☐
-Leaks all the time ☐

Digital rectal	Medications	Constipation	Chart	Toileting	Observation
Anal tone absent (patulous anus) ☐ Anal pain ☐ Rectum empty or small amount stool only ☐ Hard stool loading rectum ☐ Soft stool loading rectum ☐	Look at medication chart, and identify any : Analgesia ☐ Antacids ☐ Antidepressants ☐ Drugs for urinary incontinence ☐ Antibiotics ☐ Laxatives ☐	Ask patient or carer- "Are you constipated at the moment?" Yes ☐ No ☐ If yes ask if - Hard stool ☐ Unable to empty/straining ☐ Loss of urge to empty ☐	Ask patient or carer to record bowel actions (amount and Bristol stool form: type) and any laxatives or evacuants such as suppositories or enemas, (amount and type) for at least three days (preferably 7 days)	Observe toileting for Impaired mobility ☐ Impaired dexterity ☐ Impaired vision ☐ Impaired cognition ☐ Assistance required ☐ Carers available ☐	Look at the skin around the perianal area for : Irritation ☐ Rashes ☐ Broken skin ☐ Bleeding (rectal) ☐ Obvious abnormalities : Describe-_____
Action- If rectum is full clear bowel (according to local policy), see treating constipation and impaction box (Box 16.6) If pain or absent anal tone- refer to specialist	**Action-** Inform doctors or nurse prescriber that patient is experiencing continence problems, prompting a medication review.	**Action-** See treating constipation and impaction box Table 16.5	**Action-** Look at chart-see Table 16.3	**Action-** If reaching the toilet is a problem aim to make this as easy as possible-see toileting action Table 16.4	**Action-** As urinary (9) RED FLAG! Always refer reported or observed rectal bleeding for urgent medical opinion
Outcome-	Outcome-	Outcome-	Outcome-	Outcome-	Outcome-
Review Date-	Review Date-	Review Date-	Review Date-	Review Date-	Review Date-

Figure 16.6 Essential continence assessment for anal and faecal incontinence.

Box 16.6 Summary of further treatments for UI

Treatments for storage problems

Stress urinary incontinence (SUI)
- Lifestyle changes
- Pelvic floor muscle training
- Surgery

Mixed incontinence (SUI + UUI)
- Treat the predominant problem first

Urge urinary incontinence (UUI)
- Lifestyle changes
- Bladder retraining
- Pelvic floor muscle training
- Medication

Treatments for voiding problems

Bladder outlet obstruction (BOO)
- Medication
- Surgery
- Clean intermittent catheterization
- Indwelling catheter

Detrusor underactivity
- Clean intermittent catheterization
- Indwelling catheter

---

through patient organizations such as the Bladder and Bowel Foundation, and patients may find this helpful in addition to or instead of referral to a specialist. Current evidence suggests that the programme needs to build up to at least eight strong contractions three times a day, and that these need to be continued for at least 3 months (NICE, 2006). Because progress can be very gradual, regular follow-up and support by the practitioner may improve compliance.

The role of bladder retraining

Bladder retraining aims to increase the interval between voids by encouraging the patient to 'hold on', resisting the urge to void; this technique is used in the treatment of urge incontinence caused by detrusor overactivity or overactive bladder, although evidence for its efficacy is limited (Wallace *et al.*, 2004).

The patient is asked to keep a bladder diary or chart recording the time at which urine is passed and also the volume passed. He or she is then encouraged to increase the intervals between voiding until he or she is able to hold on to 400–500 ml. Mental distraction, such as writing a shopping list or reciting a times table, may be helpful. Patients can also be helped to reduce their urgency by learning to avoid triggers such as running water (Abrams *et al.*, 2005).

The diary or chart may highlight other contributing factors, such as excessive fluid intake or a large urine production at night.

Box 16.7 Drugs used in the treatment of urinary incontinence

For urge incontinence caused by detrusor overactivity or overactive bladder
- Oxybutynin
- Tolterodine
- Fesoterodine
- Solifenacin
- Trospium
- Darifenacin
- Propiverine

Voiding difficulties caused by benign prostatic hyperplasia

Prostate-relaxing:
- Alfuzosin
- Doxazosin
- Tamsulosin
- Terazosin

Prostate-shrinking:
- Dutasteride
- Finasteride

The role of medication

Medication is rarely used for stress incontinence. Effective medication is available for urge incontinence and targets neurotransmitters in the bladder smooth muscle to reduce unwanted bladder contractions (see Box 16.7). Dry mouth and constipation are common side effects with these drugs. The use of medication in voiding difficulties is limited to the treatment of benign prostatic hyperplasia (enlarged prostate). These drugs work by reducing the tone of the prostatic smooth muscle (thus improving urinary flow) or by shrinking the prostate. Examples are shown in Box 16.7.

The role of surgery

Surgery for SUI has advanced substantially within the past 10 years, with the introduction of low-tension suburethral tapes. The tapes provide a firm supporting layer at the bladder neck and under the urethra, enabling the urethra to be compressed when abdominal pressure rises and urine flow to be 'pinched off' such that no incontinence occurs. This surgery is known to be effective (Ogah *et al.*, 2009) and is commonly used if conservative measures (lifestyle changes and PMFT) have not been successful, although long-term outcomes are not known.

Surgery for benign prostatic hyperplasia usually involves transurethral resection of the prostate (TURP), which is carried out using a resectoscope via the urethra. This surgery is effective in the treatment of BOO (Varkarakis *et al.*, 2004). Prostate cancer or a very large prostate require more invasive surgical techniques. All prostate surgery carries the risk of causing incontinence, although this is usually very short-lived (a few days) following TURP. More radical surgery can result in persistent incontinence, which may be permanent (Miller *et al.*, 2005) There is also a risk of FI after radical prostate surgery.

The role of clean intermittent catheterization

Intermittent catheterization involves the insertion of a urinary catheter (hollow tube) at intervals to drain urine from the bladder. This technique may be used whilst waiting for surgery for BOO or if surgery is not possible, and is usually carried out by the patient (self-catheterization). It is the optimum treatment for detrusor underactivity and when incomplete bladder emptying occurs because the detrusor does not contract in synchrony with relaxation of the sphincter.

Clean intermittent catheterization is preferable to an indwelling catheter (Box 16.8)

Further evidence-based management of faecal incontinence

The role of lifestyle changes

Obesity and smoking are risk factors for FI, but it is not known whether losing weight or stopping smoking helps FI. Exercise stimulates peristalsis in the colon, and may help the constipated immobile person. Eating and drinking stimulate the gastrocolic response, and this can trigger a mass colonic movement, rectal filling, and the urge to defaecate. The bowel is relatively inactive at night and peak peristalsis is usually in the morning. For many patients, eating breakfast and taking a drink will stimulate a predictable bowel action 20–30 minutes later. If eating

---

Box 16.8 Advantages of intermittent catheterization versus an indwelling catheter

- Better for body image and sexuality
- Reduced risk of common catheter-associated problems, including urinary tract infection and urethral trauma
- No risk of catheter blockage due to encrustation (deposits of mineral salts on and inside the catheter)
- Less equipment is needed
- Patient has the potential to be continent between catheterizations

---

Box 16.9 Summary of further treatments for FI

- Lifestyle changes
- Diet and fluids
- Treating constipation
- Pelvic floor muscle training
- Bowel retraining
- Medication
- Surgery
- Irrigation
- Products and devices

stimulates urge FI, taking loperamide before a meal may control this (see 'The role of medication' below).

Patients with hard stool may benefit from additional fibre. Those with soft stool and incontinence may find that additional soluble fibre improves stool consistency (Bliss *et al.*, 2001), but others may find that fibre actually worsens symptoms. Caffeine is a gut stimulant and alcohol can lead to loose stool. It is worth excluding these from the diet to see if continence improves. Other dietary triggers are very individual and it is worth experimenting.

The role of pelvic floor muscle training

Patients with urge and passive incontinence may benefit from exercising the anal sphincter muscle and pelvic floor. These exercises are conducted in exactly the same way as for UI (see above), while concentrating on the posterior portion of the pelvic floor. However, the evidence for benefit is sparse (Norton *et al.*, 2006).

The role of bowel retraining

As with bladder retraining (above), the patient with urge FI may benefit from a progressive programme of delaying defaecation and practising 'holding on'. Instead of running to the toilet at the first urge to empty the bowel, the patient is asked to sit or stand still, and concentrate on contracting the anal sphincter while keeping the abdominal muscles relaxed. Once the immediate urgency has passed, a slow walk to the toilet is advised. If the urgency is so severe that this is impossible, holding on can be started on the toilet and the distance from the toilet gradually increased as control improves. At present, the evidence for this intervention is not well established.

The role of medication

Loose stool can be firmed by using anti-diarrhoeal medication such as loperamide (Cheetham *et al.*, 2002). Care needs to be taken that too much is not used and constipation results. Loperamide works best if taken before eating. A syrup formulation can be given in lower does if tablets constipate the patient. There is a wide variety of different oral laxatives. Stimulant laxatives (e.g. senna) promote gut peristalsis. Osmotic laxatives retain fluid in the stool and thus soften hard stool. Oral laxatives must be used with care in immobile or confused people because FI can result.

The role of surgery

Surgery may be needed to repair a disrupted anal sphincter (for example, after obstetric trauma to the anal sphincter). However, the results do not always last in the long term (Malouf *et al.*, 2000). There are also a number of different operations to reconstruct or stimulate the anal sphincter. Occasionally, a patient with very severe FI that has not responded to treatment will choose to have a stoma formed to achieve social continence. The evidence on long-term surgical outcomes remains sparse (Brown *et al.*, 2010).

The role of irrigation

Some patients with severe FI or constipation can learn to self-irrigate the lower bowel as a means to control bowel emptying. This is being increasingly used in people with neurological conditions such as spinal cord injury (Christensen *et al.*, 2006; Coggrave *et al.*, 2006).

Management with containment products

Some patients, particularly those who are very frail, disabled, and/or cognitively impaired, may not be helped with further specialist referral because the treatment options outlined above are not feasible, and management with containment products is needed. However, it is important to have a positive approach and to aim for continence or a reduction in incontinence. For those for whom continence is not possible, discreet reliable management with continence products and devices is crucial to maintaining quality of life and enabling social continence (i.e. the device is undetectable) (Mitteness and Barker, 1995; Paterson *et al.*, 2003). However, the list of such continence products and devices is long and complicated. Many products have numerous variants and sizes, and it can be difficult for both patients and professionals to make sense of them.

Provision and costs of continence products and devices

In the UK, continence products and devices are provided through the NHS in two main ways: absorbent products are available (and usually delivered to the patient) through the primary care trusts (PCTs), following assessment by a community/district nurse or a continence nurse specialist. There is no statutory obligation to provide absorbent pads, but almost all PCTs do so. However, the range of pads available varies widely across the country, with some PCTs providing all types and designs of absorbent pad, across all absorbency needs (from light to heavy incontinence), including washable as well as disposable products, and others providing perhaps only one type of pad for everyone. The annual cost to the NHS of providing absorbent pads is substantial and is estimated to be around £96 million (Continence Foundation, 2000). To reduce costs, the number of products provided to patients is usually capped and sometimes a waiting list is in use.

Most other products and devices are available on prescription, and this means that, potentially, patients have access to a very wide range of products. However, with relatively few nurse prescribers, the job of selecting the most appropriate product for an individual is often left with GPs, who may have little or no specialist continence knowledge. It is therefore crucially important that you help your patients to gain access to specific direction and advice from specialist continence health professionals to ensure that appropriate products are prescribed. Prescription costs for continence products are estimated to be around £59 million annually, and the combined product costs are much in excess of those of incontinence drug treatment (Continence Foundation, 2000).

Some products and devices (e.g. penile clamps) are not available on prescription; these may be provided through the local continence service or must be purchased by the user. The personal costs of continence products to users is unknown, and many people may purchase products (at relatively high prices) through mail order or in pharmacies, and may struggle financially without being aware that most continence products and devices are available through the NHS.

Selecting products and devices

The flow charts shown in Figures 16.7 and 16.8 (Cottenden *et al.*, 2009) are designed to provide guidance for determining broadly which product(s) is likely to be of benefit to a particular patient.

There are three main questions that you should routinely ask, as follows.

- Is there urinary retention (with or without incontinence)?
- Are there problems with toilet access (e.g. the proximity or design of the toilet, mobility, or urgency problems for the patient)?
- Is there urinary incontinence or faecal incontinence, or both?

Answers to these questions will determine which one (or both) of the flow charts is most appropriate for an individual and will help you to identify the category(ies) of products most likely to help.

Patient assessment

A skilled patient assessment is an important part of the process of product selection, and key features are shown in Table 16.5.

Although needs, priorities, and preferences vary between people with incontinence, it is useful to divide patients into major user groups to help to identify the category(ies) of products most likely to benefit an individual. Broadly speaking, there are seven primary groups:

- people with urinary retention;
- people who need help with toileting/toilet access;
- females with light urinary incontinence;
- males with light urinary incontinence;
- females with moderate/heavy urinary incontinence;
- males with moderate/heavy urinary incontinence;
- people with faecal incontinence.

An individual may belong to more than one group. The products available for children and young people are broadly similar to those for adults.

Skilled assessment is needed not only to help select the most appropriate products for patients, but also to ensure that products are sized and fitted accurately; this can be essential for the good performance of some products. Some companies (particularly those supplying male devices) provide expert assessment to the patient as part of their services.

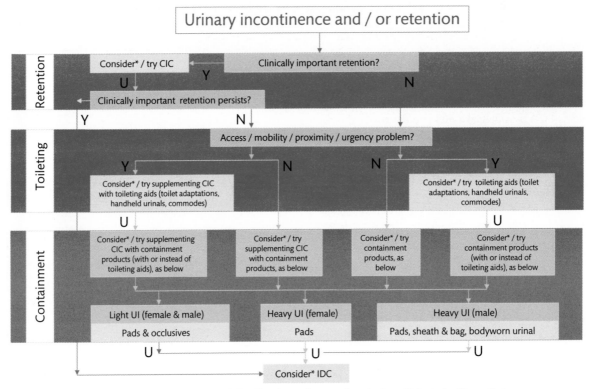

Y = Yes N = No U = Unsatisfactory outcome CIC = Clean intermittent catheterization IDC = Indwelling catheter
* NB physical characteristics; cognitive ability; personal preferences etc

Figure 16.7 **Urinary incontinence and/or retention product flowchart. CIC, Clean intermittent catheterization.**

Reproduced with permission from Health Publications Ltd.

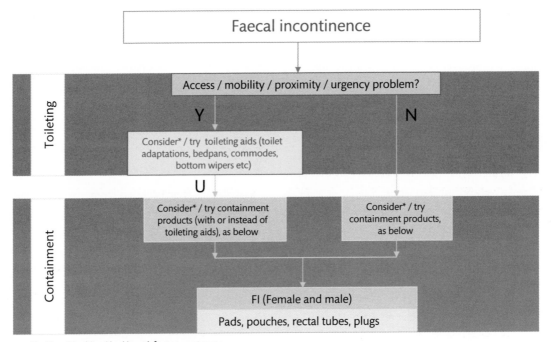

Y = Yes N = No U = Unsatisfactory outcome
* NB physical characteristics; cognitive ability; personal preferences etc

Figure 16.8 **Faecal incontinence product flowchart.**

Reproduced with permission from Health Publications Ltd.

Table 16.5 Patient characteristics and other factors important to assessment for products

Factors	Assessment factors affecting product selection
Incontinence type	The frequency, volume, and flow rate of the urine/faeces
Gender	Some products are gender-specific, e.g. sheaths for men
Physical characteristics	Anthropometrics (e.g. body mass index) will influence the comfort and effectiveness of a product
Mental acuity	Can affect ability to manage product; some products should be avoided if mental impairment is present
Mobility	Impairment can make some product choices impractical or require toilet or clothing modification
Dexterity	Problems with hand or finger movement can make it difficult to use some products, e.g. taps on leg bags, straps with buttons
Eyesight	Impaired eyesight limits effective application and management of some products
Leg abduction problems	Difficulty with abduction can make the use of some products impractical or ineffective
Lifestyle and environments	Daily activities and environments can influence the choice of product and a mixture of products may be optimum
Independence/assistance	If a carer is required to apply or change the product, then his or her involvement in selection is important
Laundry facilities	If washable products are considered, it is important to check that laundry facilities are available
Disposal facilities	Ability to appropriately, safely, and discreetly dispose of the selected products needs to be considered
Storage facilities	Some products can be bulky; adequate space to store supplies between deliveries/purchases needs to be available
Personal preferences	Different people like different products and, where possible, patients should be given a choice of products
Personal priorities	Everyone wants to avoid leakage, but other factors such as discreetness may be more or less important to individuals

Choosing between product categories

Product research has tended to focus on the performance of products in terms of preventing leakage and the extent to which products are problematic to users, including such issues as comfort, skin health, ease of application, odour control, and discreetness. There is no obvious 'control' in that *any* product is likely to be better than no product, and products are therefore usually compared to each other with a view to identifying 'best' performance (with fewest problems) (Fader *et al.*, 2001). Rather than focusing on which product is 'best', it is more useful to think in terms of 'who is this product likely to suit and

under what circumstances' and, conversely, who it will not suit and under what conditions (see Table 16.6).

Managing the use of indwelling catheters

Short-term catheterization

Approaches to managing the care of patients with an indwelling catheter will vary according to whether this is a short-term or long-term issue.

Indwelling urethral catheters are very commonly used in patients in hospital who need fluid monitoring (for

Table 16.6 Products and devices for urinary and faecal incontinence, and indicators for patient selection

People with urinary retention	
Catheters for intermittent use	Optimum management method for urinary retention when surgery is not applicable or possible. Many advantages over an indwelling catheter (Box 16.8). Insufficient evidence to recommend any particular type of catheter (Moore *et al.*, 2007).
Indwelling urethral catheter	Avoid, or remove as soon as possible. High risk of bacteriuria (significant growth of bacteria in the urine without symptoms), which is inevitable after 1 month and increases the risk of symptomatic infection (Saint, 2000).
Indwelling suprapubic catheter	If a long-term catheter is essential, a suprapubic catheter may have some advantages over urethral catheters (comfort, ease of catheterization, sexual activity) (Feifer and Corcos, 2008).
People who need help with toileting/toilet access	
Commodes	Best to wheel patient over normal toilet (without commode pan). Privacy essential. Comfort, safety, trunk support, and pressure areas should be considered, therefore do not use for long periods (Naylor and Mulley, 1993; Nazarko, 1995).
Male urinals	Offer for speedy toileting—no published research.
Female urinals	Offer for speedy toileting, wide range available, different urinals suit different women. Less successful if patient very disabled (i.e. unable to move to edge of chair or bed) (Fader *et al.*, 1999).
Females with light urinary incontinence	
Absorbent products	Most commonly used products for this patient group. Small disposable pads are the most effective (least leaky) type of absorbent product, followed by menstrual pads, washable pants (with integral pad). Washable pads are least effective (Fader *et al.*, 2008). Snug fit important to minimize leakage.
Mechanical devices	Seldom used. Intravaginal and intraurethral devices available to occlude urethra. Little evidence for efficacy and concerns about infection and trauma (Lipp *et al.*, 2011).
Males with light urinary incontinence	
Absorbent products	Most commonly used products for this patient group. Male pad (pouch for penis/scrotum) better than standard absorbent pad and both more effective (less leaky) than washable pants with integral pad (Fader *et al.*, 2006). Snug fit important to minimize leakage.
Male devices	Male body-worn urinals and penile clamps are much less commonly used and require expert fitting (Cottenden *et al.*, 2009; Moore *et al.*, 2004).
Females with moderate/heavy urinary incontinence	
Absorbent products	Preferred option for women. Women prefer 'pull-up' designs or shaped pads worn with close-fitting pants. All-in-one (diaper designs) least preferred (Fader *et al.*, 2008). Snug fit important to minimize leakage.
Urethral or suprapubic catheter	Avoid if possible. The risk of urinary infection is high and there is potential for trauma. Problems of leakage and blockage are common (Cottenden *et al.*, 2009).
Males with moderate/heavy urinary incontinence	
Absorbent products	Men are more likely to find all-in-one (diaper) pads more effective (leak less) than pads worn with pants. Pull-ups are difficult to change with trousers (Fader *et al.*, 2008).
Sheath with leg-bag	May be better/preferred to absorbent pads (Chartier-Kastler *et al.*, 2011). Sizing and skilled fitting are important. Serious skin problems have been reported (Golji, 1981).
Other male devices	Male body-worn urinals used less commonly and require expert fitting.
Urethral or suprapubic catheter	Avoid if possible. Urinary infection is inevitable and there is potential for trauma. Problems of leakage and blockage are common (Cottenden *et al.*, 2009).
People with faecal incontinence	
Absorbent products	Most commonly used, particularly if urinary and faecal incontinence.
Anal plugs	Uncommonly used, reports of discomfort. May be most suitable for people with impaired sensation (Deutekom and Dobben, 2005).
Faecal catheters and collection devices	Used for loose stool, and mainly confined to acute and critical care units.

example, patients with heart failure or acute kidney injury, preoperatively and postoperatively, and in an intensive care unit), or for those patients who are acutely ill and unable to use a toilet, urinal, or commode (comatose, very drowsy, very restricted mobility). They are also used to manage acute urinary retention. However, their use should be minimized because catheter-associated urinary tract infections (CAUTIs) are the major cause of hospital-acquired infection (Plowman *et al.*, 1999). 'Short-term' urinary catheters should usually be used only for 1–2 days, although the term is used for catheters that are in place for up to 14 days.

You should establish the reason for catheter insertion and maintain comprehensive documentation of catheter details to ensure daily monitoring of the need for the catheter and prompt removal or 'trial without catheter'. Aseptic insertions of the catheter, together with prompt removal, are essential to minimize the risk of urinary infection, which increases every day that the catheter remains in place.

Figure 16.9 shows the information required for patients who have a urinary catheter in place in the short term.

Long-term catheterization

Long-term urinary catheterization is to be avoided if possible because it is associated with troublesome and sometimes serious problems that are difficult to prevent and manage. There are few indications for the use of a long-term catheter and these are summarized in Box 16.10.

There are three main problems associated with long-term urinary catheters, and these are summarized in Table 16.7.

Dos and don'ts in the management of patients with long-term catheters

When long-term catheterization cannot be avoided, you will need to be aware of the essential actions to take as well as those that you must *not* take. These are outlined in Table 16.8.

Measuring the impact of nursing interventions

The principle of measuring both the effectiveness of nursing intervention and the patient's experience of receiving care is one that you should, where possible, facilitate. The NHS Information Centre has supported the development of Nursing Quality Metrics (NQMs) that can be used to facilitate quality improvement in patient care and experience **http://signposting.ic.nhs.uk/?k=metrics.**

This recent move within healthcare to be outcome-focused rather than target-driven is a welcome change in policy direction, initiated by Lord Darzi in his review of the NHS, and sustained by the previous and current UK governments. Metrics have been developed for many aspects of nursing care interventions and cover many inpatient areas, regardless of setting. The collection of these types of data helps healthcare organizations to focus on the delivery of safe and effective care, and can be used for local and national benchmarking as well as for quality improvement.

For further details, visit the NHS Information Centre online at **http://www.ic.nhs.uk/**, where you will find details relating to nursing audit tools capturing information on documentation for observations, nutrition, medicines administration, pain management, communication, discharge planning, falls, pressure area care, antibiotic prescribing, and infection control.

In determining patient experience of healthcare, the National Institute for Health and Clinical Excellence (NICE) has recently published a Quality Standard **http://www.nice.org.uk/** that guides service delivery planning to ensure improvements in patient experience. Further commissioned work by the Department of Health has developed a single measure of patient experience. Supplementing these data is the NHS Survey, which captures patient views relating to ward cleanliness, infection control, staff attitudes, pain management, management of privacy, experience of dignity, nutrition, medicines administration, quality of communication, and discharge. Details can be found online at **http://www.nhssurveys.org/**.

Accessing evidence for practice

Below is a list of recent sources of the best evidence to inform the nursing management of continence. Because research is always ongoing and best practice evolves, it is important that readers stay up to date and know where to find good-quality sources of evidence.

Southampton **NHS**
University Hospitals NHS Trust

NHS
Solent Healthcare

Adult Indwelling Urinary Catheter Insertion/Care Record

PATIENT'S NAME AND HOSPITAL NUMBER	Ward:_____
	Date/time catheter inserted: _____
	Signature: _____
	Print name: _____
	Grade: _____

REASON FOR USE *(A urinary catheter should be a last resort when all other options have been considered)*

Short-term indications (1-2 days, up to 14 days)
[Use code for noting overleaf]

☐ [ST1] Surgical procedures and post-op care
☐ [ST2] Hourly urine output monitoring
☐ [ST3] Acute urinary retention (confirmed by bladder scan)
☐ [ST4] Other (please state):

_____

☐ Bladder scan performed (if indicated):

Date:_____ Time:_____ mls:_____

Potential long-term indications (up to 12 weeks)
[Use code for noting overleaf]

☐ [LT1] Bladder outlet obstruction unsuitable for surgery
☐ [LT2] Chronic urinary retention - intermittent catheterisation not possible
☐ [LT3] Open wounds or sores frequently contaminated with urine
☐ [LT4] Severe or terminal illness or disability that prevents toileting
☐ [LT5] Other (please state):

_____

Date next catheter change due: _____
(For long-term indication only)

CONSENT ☐ Informed ☐ Implied	**INSERTION SITE** ☐ Urethral ☐ Suprapubic
ALLERGIES ☐ None known ☐ Latex ☐ Anaesthetic lubricant	**CATHETER STICKER** *(From outer packaging of catheter)*
GAUGE ☐ 10Ch ☐ 12 Ch ☐ 14 Ch ☐ other:____Ch	
BALLOON SIZE ☐ 10mls ☐ other:_____mls	*(Place 2nd sticker in medical notes)*

Sterile water inserted into balloon: _____mls

DRAINAGE SYSTEM USED

Leg Bag   2L Bag   Flip-Flow Valve   Urometer
  ☐   ☐   ☐   ☐

RESIDUAL VOLUME DRAINED _____mls

INSERTION TECHNIQUE ADHERED TO

☐ Hand hygiene before and after procedure
☐ Correct PPE worn
☐ Aseptic technique used
☐ Sterile saline used for meatal cleaning prior to insertion
☐ Sterile lubricant applied
☐ Catheter connected aseptically to drainage system
☐ Foreskin replaced (male patients)

| **URINALYSIS REQUIRED?** | ☐ No | ☐ Yes | Date done: | Results on _____ chart |
| **CSU REQUIRED?** | ☐ No | ☐ Yes | Date sent: | Result: |

Solent Healthcare and Southampton University Hospitals Trust collaborative project to reduce catheter-associated urinary tract infection
Project leads: Jacqui Prieto (Infection Prevention Team, Solent Healthcare) and Julie Brooks (Infection Prevention Team, SUHT)

Figure 16.9 Acute indwelling urinary catheter insertion/care record.

Adult Indwelling Urinary Catheter Insertion/Care Record

Southampton **NHS**
University Hospitals NHS Trust

NHS
Solent Healthcare

Specify any problems, interventions and outcomes in patient's notes / continuation sheet

PATIENT'S NAME:

HOSPITAL NUMBER:

WARD:

Day no.	Date / Time	Catheter still required? If yes, give reason (using codes overleaf) If no, state action taken	Meatal area washed with soap and water?	Catheter secured correctly to ensure it is tension free?	Drainage bag below level of bladder and above floor?	Closed drainage system maintained?	Sign and initial when complete
Day 1							
Day 2							
Day 3							
Day 4							
Day 5							
Day 6							
Day 7							
Day 8							
Day 9							
Day 10							
Day 11							
Day 12							
Day 13							
Day 14							

TRIAL WITHOUT CATHETER (TWOC) ☐ Planned removal ☐ Unplanned removal *(e.g. came out)*

Date TWOC due:	Criterion required for TWOC: *(see medical notes)*

TIME OF DAY OF TWOC:
☐ midnight ☐ early morning ☐ other _____

CONSENT ☐ Informed ☐ Implied

☐ Patient adequately hydrated?
☐ Balloon deflated? _____ mls
☐ Patient advised to monitor urine output?

Date/time removed: _____	Signature: _____ Print Name: _____ Job Title/Grade: _____

TWOC SUCCESSFUL? ☐ Yes ☐ No

If TWOC unsuccessful, document outcome and plan in patient's notes / continuation sheet

Signature: _____ Print Name: _____ Job Title/Grade: _____	Date/time of assessment: _____

Solent Healthcare and Southampton University Hospitals Trust collaborative project to reduce catheter-associated urinary tract infection
Project leads: Jacqui Prieto (Infection Prevention Team, Solent Healthcare) and Julie Brooks (Infection Prevention Team, SUHT)

Figure 16.9 Acute indwelling urinary catheter insertion/care record (*continued*).

Hence we have provided a list of sources that readers should utilize.

- The 4th International Consultation on Incontinence provides a comprehensive review of evidence and recommendations for clinical practice **http://www. icsoffice.org/Publications/ICI_4/book.pdf**

> **Box 16.10 Indications for use of a long-term urinary catheter**
>
> Urinary retention where intermittent catheterization is known not to be possible
>
> Stage 3 or 4 pressure ulcer on hip/buttock/sacrum/ischial tuberosities
>
> Latter stages of terminal illness to avoid burden of toileting
>
> Patient preference (following experience of other options; see Table 16.6)

- There are three NICE guidelines that focus on incontinence:
  - NICE Guideline: CG40 Urinary Incontinence: the management of urinary incontinence in women **http://www.nice.org.uk/CG40**
  - NICE Guideline: CG97 The management of lower urinary tract symptoms in men **http://guidance. nice.org.uk/CG97**
  - NICE Guideline: CG49 Faecal incontinence: the management of faecal incontinence in adults **http://guidance.nice.org.uk/CG49**
- There are more than 90 systematic reviews on incontinence-related interventions: Cochrane Incontinence Group **http://incontinence. cochrane.org**
- The NHS High Impact Action—'Protection from Infection'—focuses on evidence and practice for reducing infections from urinary catheters **http://www.institute.nhs.uk/building_capability/hia_ supporting_info/protection_from_infection.html**

Table 16.7 Problems associated with long-term urinary catheters

Catheter problem	Cause	Prevention and/or management
Infection	Microorganisms from the catheter and peri-urethra migrate into the bladder via the inside of the catheter lumen or external surface of the catheter. Bacteriuria (significant growth of bacteria in the urine without symptoms) is inevitable after 1 month (Saint, 2000). Approximately one in five patients with bacteriuria develop a symptomatic infection (Saint, 2000).	Long-term antibiotics not recommended (Niël-Weise and van den Broek, 2005). Adherence to aseptic technique during catheter insertion and subsequent handling of the system, along with maintenance of a 'closed' drainage system with unobstructed urine flow, is essential to avoid microbial contamination by the healthcare worker/carer (Pratt *et al.*, 2007).
Urethral, bladder, and bladder neck trauma	Trauma to the urethra, bladder, or bladder neck can be caused during insertion, by the catheter tip and balloon damaging the tissues, and by the unsupported tubing and drainage 'pulling' on the urethral meatus and bladder neck.	Catheter insertion is a skilled procedure and should be carried out only by a competent practitioner. Catheter should be 'secured' on the thigh and drainage bags supported with straps or sleeves.
Catheter encrustation and blockage	Microorganisms in the urine (particularly *Proteus mirabilis*) create 'biofilms' in the lumen of the catheter and on the catheter surface, and crystals precipitate under certain conditions and can 'block' the catheter lumen.	There are no known effective ways (including use of special catheters with silver and other coatings) of preventing the formation of biofilms or preventing infection with *Proteus mirabilis* (Jahn *et al.*, 2007).
Leakage around the catheter	May be caused by poor drainage (partial blockage). Also caused by bladder contractions.	Medications to reduce bladder contractions (Box16.7).

Table 16.8 Long-term catheter management: dos and don'ts

Do	Don't
Monitor the catheter 'life' and aim to change the catheter before it blocks (Getliffe and Fader, 2007)	Don't wait until the catheter blocks to change it—blockage may occur inconveniently (e.g. at night) and expensively
Clean the peri-urethral area with usual personal hygiene measures	Don't use any special antibacterial cleaners—they may make things worse (Burke *et al.*, 1981; 1983)
Support the tubing and bag by taping the catheter to the thigh and using well-fitting straps or sleeves to support the bag	Don't use large drainage bags designed for the bedside except at night (attached to the bottom of the leg-bag) or if patient does not leave the bed
Encourage drinking fluids—insufficient evidence for anything special such as cranberry juice (Jepson and Craig, 2008)	Don't do bladder washouts or use catheter management solutions (no evidence of effectiveness) (Hagen *et al.*, 2010)
	Don't break the closed drainage system by disconnecting the catheter from the bag; disconnection may increase the risk of infection (Pratt *et al.*, 2007)

- Chartier-Kastler, E., Ballanger, P., Petit, J., *et al.* (2011) Randomised crossover study evaluating patient preference and the impact on quality of life of unisheaths vs absorbent products in incontinent men. *British Journal of Urology International* **108**(2): 241–7.

Sources of evidence

Journals that specialize in continence nursing

- *Journal of Wound Ostomy and Continence Nursing* http://journals.lww.com/jwocnonline/pages/default.aspx

Useful organizations and associations

Association for Continence Advice: http://www.aca.uk.com/

International Continence Society: http://www.icsoffice.org/

Royal College of Nursing continence forum: http://www.rcn.org.uk/development/communities/rcn_forum_communities/continence_care

Bladder and bowel foundation: http://www.bladderandbowelfoundation.org/

Summary and key messages

- Incontinence is a common problem that all nurses will encounter whatever their specialty.
- It can be difficult for people to admit to bladder and bowel problems, and nurses should therefore help patients to talk about this sensitive subject.

- All nurses should be able to start the process of supporting those with continence problems to achieve continence or to reduce incontinence, and/or effectively to manage leakage.

- The essential elements of nursing assessment and interventions are simple, and may completely resolve continence problems.
- If incontinence persists, expert nursing assessment provides the foundation for further investigation and treatment.

- There is a limited evidence base to inform expert nursing management of continence.
- Further research is needed to inform the most effective intervention to reduce incontinence, to support catheter use, and to determine optimum management with products and product development.

Online Resource Centre

To help you to develop and apply your knowledge and decision-making skills further, we have provided interactive learning resources on the following site: **www.oxfordtextbooks.co.uk/orc/bullock/**
Whilst these are freely available, you will need to use the access codes at the start of the book.

References

Abrams, P., Artibani, W., Cardozo, L., *et al.* (2005) *Clinical Manual of Incontinence in Women*. Health Publications Ltd: Paris.

Abrams, P., Cardozo, L., Fall, M., *et al.* (2002) The standardisation of terminology in lower urinary tract function. *Neurology and Urodynamics* **21**(2): 167–78.

AlAmeel, T., Andrew, M.K., MacKnight, C. (2010) The association of fecal incontinence with institutionalization and mortality in older adults. *American Journal of Gastroenterology* **105**: 1830–4.

Bliss, D.Z., Jung, H., Savik, K., *et al.* (2001) Supplementation with dietary fiber improves fecal incontinence. *Nursing Research* **50**(4): 203–13.

Brittain, K.R., Perry, S.I., Peet, S.M. (2000) Prevalence and impact of urinary symptoms among community dwelling stroke survivors. *Stroke* **32**: 122–7.

Brown, J.S., Vittinghoff, E., Wyman, J.F., *et al.* (2000) Urinary incontinence: does it increase risk for falls and fractures? Study of the Osteoporotic Fractures Research Group. *Journal of American Geriatric Society* **48**(7): 721–5.

Brown, S.R., Wadhawan, H., Nelson, R.L. (2010) Surgery for faecal incontinence in adults. *Cochrane Database of Systematic Reviews* Issue 9: Art. No. CD001757. DOI: 10.1002/14651858. CD001757.pub3.

Burke, J.P., Garibaldi, R.A., Britt, M.R., *et al.* (1981) Prevention of catheter-associated urinary tract infections: efficacy of daily meatal care regiments. *American Journal of Medicine* **70**: 655–8.

Burke, J.P., Jacobson, J.A., Garibaldi, R.A., *et al.* (1983) Evaluation of daily meatal care with poly-antibiotic ointment in prevention of urinary catheter-associated bacteriuria. *Journal of Urology* **129**: 331–4.

Chartier-Kastler, E., Ballanger, P., Petit, J., *et al.* (2011) Randomised crossover study evaluating patient preference and the impact on quality of life of unisheaths vs absorbent products in incontinent men. *British Journal of Urology International* **108**(2): 241–7.

Chassagne, P., Landrin, I., Neveu, C., *et al.* (1999) Fecal incontinence in the institutionalized elderly: incidence, risk factors, and prognosis. *American Journal of Medicine* **106**(2): 185–90.

Cheetham, M., Brazzelli, M., Norton, C., *et al.* (2002) Drug treatment for faecal incontinence in adults (Cochrane review). *Cochrane Database of Systematic Reviews* Issue 3: Art. No. CD002116. DOI: 10.1002/14651858.CD002116.

Christensen, P., Bazzocchi, G., Coggrave, M., *et al.* (2006) A randomized, controlled trial of transanal irrigation versus conservative bowel managment in spinal cord-injured patients. *Gastroenterology* **131**: 738–47.

Coggrave, M., Wiesel, P., Norton, C. (2006) Management of faecal incontinence and constipation in adults with central neurological diseases (Cochrane review). *Cochrane Database of Systematic Reviews*, Issue 2: Art. No. CD002115. DOI: 10.1002/14651858.CD002115.pub3.

Continence Foundation (2000) *Making the Case for Investment in an Integrated Continence Service*. The Continence Foundation: London.

Cottenden, A., Bliss, D., Buckley, B., *et al.* (2009) Management with continence products. In P. Abrams, L. Cardozo, S. Khoury, *et al.* (eds) *Incontinence*, 4th edn. Health Publications Ltd: Paris.

Coyne, K., Zhou, Z., Thompson, C., *et al.* (2003) The impact on health-related quality of life of stress, urge and mixed urinary incontinence. *BJU International* **92**: 731–5.

Department of Health (2000) *Good Practice in Continence Services*. HMSO: London.

Deutekom, M., Dobben, A.C. (2005) Plugs for containing faecal incontinence. *Cochrane Database of Systematic Reviews* Issue 3: Art. No. CD005086. DOI: 10.1002/14651858.CD005086.pub2.

Dumoulin, C., Hay-Smith, J. (2010) Pelvic floor muscle training versus no treatment, or inactive control treatments, for urinary incontinence in women. *Cochrane Database of Systematic Reviews* Issue 1: Art. No. CD005654. DOI: 10.1002/14651858.CD005654.pub2.

Fader, M., Cottenden, R., Brooks, R., (2001) The CPE network: creating an evidence base for continence product selection. *Journal of Wound Ostomy and Continence Nursing* **28**(2): 106–12.

Fader, M., Cottenden, A., Getliffe, K., *et al.* (2008) Absorbent products for urinary/faecal incontinence: a comparative evaluation of key product designs. *Health Technology Assessment* **12**(29): iii–iv, ix–185.

Fader, M., Macaulay, M., Pettersson, L., *et al.* (2006) A multi-centre evaluation of absorbent products for men with light urinary incontinence. *Neurourology and Urodynamics* **25**(7): 689–95.

Fader, M., Pettersson, L., Dean, G., *et al.* (1999) The selection of female urinals: results of a multicentre evaluation. *British Journal of Nursing* **11**(14): 918–20, 922–5.

Feifer, A., Corcos, J. (2008) Contemporary role of suprapubic cystostomy in treatment of neuropathic bladder dysfunction in spinal cord injured patients. *Neurourology and Urodynamics* **27**(6): 475–9.

Fowler, C.J., Dalton, C., Panicker, J.N. (2010) Review of neurological disease for the urologist. *Urologic Clinics of North America* **37**(4): 517–26.

Getliffe, K., Fader, M. (2007) In K. Getliffe, M. Dolman (eds) *Promoting Continence*. Baillière Tindall: London. pp. 239–58.

Golji, H. (1981) Complications of external condom drainage. *Paraplegia* **19**(3): 189–97.

Gray, M., Bliss, D.Z., Doughty, D.B., *et al.* (2007) Incontinence-associated dermatitis. *Journal of Wound and Ostomy Continence Nursing* **34**(1): 45–54.

Hagen, S., Sinclair, L., Cross, S. (2010) Washout policies in long-term indwelling urinary catheterisation in adults. *Cochrane Database of Systematic Reviews* Issue 3: Art. No. CD004012. DOI: 10.1002/14651858.CD00412.pub4.

Hunskaar, S., Lose, G., Sykes, D., *et al.* (2004) The prevalence of urinary incontinence in women in four European countries. *BJU International* **93**(3): 324–30.

Jahn, P., Preuss, M., Kernig, A., *et al.* (2007) Types of indwelling urinary catheters for long-term bladder drainage in adults. *Cochrane Database of Systematic Reviews* Issue 3: Art. No. CD004997. DOI: 10.1002/14651858.CD004997.pub2.

Jepson, R.G., Craig, J.C. (2008) Cranberries for preventing urinary tract infections. *Cochrane Database of Systematic Reviews* Issue 1: Art. No. CD001321. DOI: 10.1002/14651858.CD001321.pub4.

Lipp, A., Shaw, C., Glavind, K. (2011) Mechanical devices for incontinence in women. *Cochrane Database of Systematic Reviews* Issue 7: Art. No. CD001756. DOI: 10.1002/14651858.CD001756.pub5.

Malouf, A.J., Norton, C., Nicholls, R.J., *et al.* (2000) Long term results of overlapping anal sphincter repair for obstetric trauma. *Lancet* **355**: 260–5.

Miller, D.C., Sanda, M.G., Dunn, R.L., *et al.* (2005) Long-term outcomes among localised prostate cancer survivors: health-related quality of life changes afer radical prostatectomy, external radiation and brachytherapy. *Journal of Clinical Oncology* **23**(12): 2772–80.

Mitteness, L. S., Barker, J.C. (1995) Stigmatizing a 'normal' condition: urinary incontinence in late life. *Medical Anthropology Quarterly* **9**(2): 188–210.

Moore, K.N., Fader, M., Getliffe, K. (2007) Long-term bladder management by intermittent catheterisation in adults and children. *Cochrane Database of Systematic Reviews* Issue 4: Art. No. CD006008. DOI: 10.1002/14651858.CD006008.pub2.

Moore, K.N., Schieman, S., Ackerman, T., *et al.* (2004) Assessing comfort, safety and patient satisfaction with three commonly used penile compression devices. *Urology* **63**(1):150–4.

National Institute for Health and Clinical Excellence (2005) *Referral for Suspected Cancer*. NICE Clinical Guideline 27 (CG27). **www.nice.org.uk/CG027** (accessed 8 May 2007).

National Institute for Health and Clinical Excellence (2006) *Urinary Incontinence: The Management of Urinary Incontinence in Women*. NICE Clinical Guideline 40 (CG40). **www.nice.org.uk/CG40** (accessed 5 July 2011).

National Institute for Health and Clinical Excellence (2007). *Faecal Incontinence: The Management of Faecal Incontinence in Adults*. NICE Clinical Guideline 49 (CG49). **www.nice.org.uk/CG49** (accessed 5 July 2011).

Naylor, J.R., Mulley, G.P. (1993) Commodes: inconvenient conveniences. *British Medical Journal* **307**: 1258–60.

Nazarko, L. (1995) Commode design for frail and disabled people. *Professional Nurse* **11**(2): 95–7.

Niël-Weise, B.S., van den Broek, P.J. (2005) Urinary catheter policies for long-term bladder drainage. *Cochrane Database of Systematic Reviews* Issue 3: Art. No. CD004203. DOI: 10.1002/14651858.CD004203.pub2.

Norton, C., Cody, J.D., Hosker, G. (2006) Biofeedback and/or sphincter exercises for the treatment of faecal incontinence in adults. *Cochrane Database of Systematic Reviews* Issue 3: Art. No. CD002111. DOI: 10.1002/14651858.CD002111.pub2.

Norton, C., Whitehead, W. E., Bliss, D. Z., *et al.* (2009) Conservative and pharmacological management of faecal incontinence in adults. In P. Abrams, L. Cardozo, S. Khoury (eds) *Incontinence*. Health Publications: Paris.

Ogah, J., Cody, J.D., Rogerson, L. (2009) Minimally invasive synthetic suburethral sling operations for stress urinary incontinence in women. *Cochrane Database of Systematic Reviews* Issue 4: Art. No. CD006375. DOI: 10.1002/14651858.CD006375.pub2.

Paterson, J., Dunn, S., Kowanko, I., *et al.* (2003) Selection of continence products: perspectives of people who have incontinence and their carers. *Disability Rehabilitation* **25**(17): 955–63.

Perry, S., Shaw, C., McGrother, C., *et al.* (2002) The prevalence of faecal incontinence in adults aged 40 years or more living in the community. *Gut* **50**: 480–4.

Plowman, R., Graves, N., Griffin, M., *et al.* (1999) The socio-economic burden of hospital acquired infection. *Journal of Urology* **164**(4): 1254–8.

Pratt, R.J., Pellawe, C.M., Wilson, J.A., *et al.* (2007) National evidence-based guidelines for preventing healthcare-associated infections in NHS hospitals in England. *Journal of Hospital Infection* **65** (Suppl. 1): 1–64.

Resnick, N.M., Yalla, S.V., Laurino, E. (1989) The pathophysiology of urinary incontinence among institutionalized elderly persons. *New England Journal of Medicine* **320**(1): 1–7.

Rigby, D. (2007) Medication for continence. In K. Getliffe, M. Dolman (eds) *Promoting Continence*. Baillière Tindall: London. pp. 239–58.

Saint, S. (2000) Clinical and economic consequences of nosocomial catheter-related baceriuna. *American Journal of Infection Control* **28**(1): 68–75.

Varkarakis, J., Bartsch, G., Horninger, W. (2004) Long-term morbidity and mortality of transurethral prostatectomy: a 10-year follow-up. *The Prostate* **58**: 248–251.

Wallace, S.A., Roe, B., Williams, K., *et al.* (2004) Bladder training for urinary incontinence in adults. *Cochrane Database of Systematic Reviews*, Issue 1: Art. No. CD001308. DOI: 10.1002/14651858. CD001308.pub2.

Whitehead, W.E., Borrud, L., Goode, P.S., *et al.* (2009) Fecal incontinence in US adults: epidemiology and risk factors. *Gastroenterology* **137**: 512–17.

17 *Managing* Delirium and Confusion

Emma Ouldred and Catherine Bryant

Introduction

This chapter focuses on the assessment, management, and diagnosis of delirium, one form of confusion that commonly presents in healthcare settings. It will equip you with the skills required to differentiate between dementia, delirium, and depression through comprehensive assessment, and will improve the confidence of practising nurses in the management of this debilitating condition. This chapter will help you to select and implement evidence-based strategies to manage patients presenting with confusion regardless of the cause of confusion, such as dementia (see Chapter 7 Understanding Dementia ➡).

- acute disorders usually associated with acute illness, drugs, and environmental factors;
- more slowly progressive impairment of cognitive function, such as that seen in dementia syndromes;
- impaired cognitive function associated with affective disorders and psychoses such as depression.

Regardless of aetiology, confusion can be very distressing for the person exhibiting these symptoms (Figure 17.1), his or her relatives and carers, and for health and social care practitioners. It is important to differentiate between different causes of confusion for appropriate treatment plans to be developed.

Understanding confusion

Confusion is derived from the Latin verb *confundere*, meaning 'to mingle'. It is a descriptive term that has a variety of different definitions. It has been defined as a disturbance of consciousness characterized by impaired capacity to think clearly and with customary rapidity, and to perceive, respond, to, and remember current stimuli, and some degree of disorientation (Faber and Faber, 1953).

Types of confusion

Disorders causing confusion can be categorized into three groups:

Understanding delirium

The word *delirium* is derived from Latin, meaning 'off the track', and is often referred to as acute confusional state. Delirium is a common and distressing disorder associated with increases in physical morbidity, length of hospital stay, and entry to long-term care, and therefore increases in cost to health services. However, it can be prevented and treated if dealt with urgently (National Institute for Health and Clinical Excellence (NICE), 2010a).

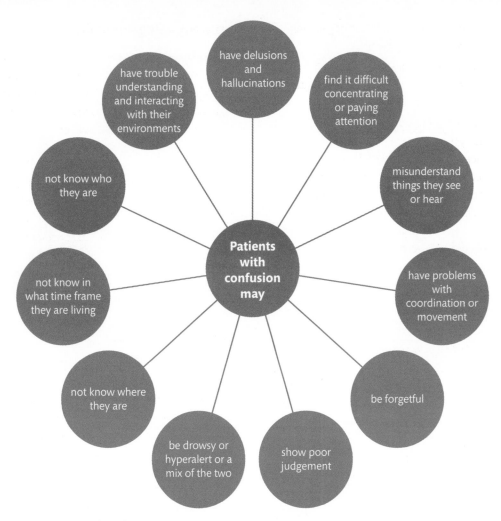

Figure 17.1 Symptoms of confusion.

Classification of delirium

The *Diagnostic and Statistical Manual of Mental Disorders*, 4th edition text revision (DSM-IV TR), is used by clinicians and psychiatrists to diagnose psychiatric illnesses. Delirium is defined by DSM-IV TR as:

a disturbance of consciousness and a change in cognition that develops over a short period of time. The disorder has a tendency to fluctuate during the course of the day, and there is evidence from the history, examination or investigations that the delirium is a direct consequence of a general medical condition, drug withdrawal or intoxication.

The DSM-IV TR specifies delirium further by type based on aetiology, i.e.:

- delirium caused by a general medical condition (including physiological effects of a medication, or delirium owing to

multiple aetiologies, including multiple medical conditions, multiple medications, or a combination of both);

- substance withdrawal delirium (substances of abuse);

- delirium not otherwise specified (cause[s] not confidently identified/classified).

DSM-IV TR also has additional codes for the co-occurrence of dementia and delirium.

For a patient to satisfy the DSM-IV TR classification of delirium, he or she must show all of the four features as follows.

1. Disturbance of consciousness (i.e. reduced clarity of awareness of the environment), with reduced ability to focus, sustain, or shift attention

2. Change in cognition (e.g. memory deficit, disorientation, language disturbance, perceptual disturbance)

that is not better accounted for by a pre-existing, established, or evolving dementia

3. Disturbance developing over a short period (usually hours to days) and tending to fluctuate during the course of the day

4. Evidence from the history, physical examination, or laboratory findings that indicates the disturbance is caused by a direct physiological consequence of a general medical condition, an intoxicating substance, medication use, or more than one cause

Subtypes of delirium

Four different psychomotor behavioural subtypes of delirium have been described (Breitbart *et al.*, 1997): normal, hypoactive, hyperactive, and mixed.

- **Normal:** no psychomotor disturbance
- **Hyperactive delirium:** symptoms range from simple restlessness to agitation and aggression
- **Hypoactive delirium:** characterized by a slowing or lack of movement, paucity of speech, with or without prompting and unresponsiveness
- **Mixed delirium:** elements of both hyperactive and hypoactive forms of delirium are exhibited

Hypoactive delirium is least likely to be detected by practitioners (Inouye *et al.*, 2001), and patients may be misdiagnosed as being depressed. In addition, hypoactive delirium in patients with dementia may have a higher mortality (Yang *et al.*, 2009)

Prevalence of delirium

The prevalence of delirium among medical inpatients varies between 11% and 42% (Siddiqi *et al.*, 2006). In post-fracture neck of femur patients, the prevalence of delirium varies from 10% to 50% (Lindesay *et al.*, 2002). Delirium in critically ill ventilated patients ranges from 60% to 80% (Ely *et al.*, 2001), whilst prevalence is up to 85% in patients who are approaching the last few weeks of their lives (Breitbart and Alici, 2008). Delirium is also common in long-term care, with an estimated median point prevalence of 14% (Siddiqi *et al.*, 2009). The prevalence of delirium in the community is between 1% and 2%, but the prevalence of delirium in the community setting increases with age, rising to 14% in individuals aged over 85 (Inouye, 2006).

Pathophysiology of delirium

The pathophysiology of delirium is not well understood. There is evidence to suggest that there is disruption to higher cortical function affecting several structures in the brain. Multiple pathogenic mechanisms may contribute to the development of delirium, and more research is needed to understand why some people (e.g. those with dementia) are more at risk of developing delirium than others. There is evidence for neurotransmitter dysfunction, especially acetylcholine deficiency and dopamine excess, in delirium. Systemic inflammation mediated by cytokines, high cortisol levels, direct neuronal injury, and reduced cerebral bloodflow and metabolism have also been implicated to some degree in the pathophysiology, but more research is needed (Fong *et al.*, 2009).

Causes of delirium

The cause of delirium is often multifactorial. The development of delirium involves the complex interaction between a patient with predisposing risk factors for delirium and exposure to precipitating factors or noxious insults (Inouye, 2006). Therefore, in vulnerable or high-risk patients such as those with dementia, a simple physical illness such as a urinary tract infection or exposure to a single dose of sleeping tablets may induce delirium. Conversely, a patient with no identified risk factors may develop delirium only when exposed to several noxious insults such as anaesthesia and severe illness. Common causes of delirium are listed in Box 17.1.

Alcohol withdrawal: delirium tremens

Alcohol withdrawal is a set of symptoms that may occur when a person suddenly stops drinking after using alcohol for a long time. If left untreated, alcohol withdrawal can lead to serious symptoms known as delirium tremens (DTs). These symptoms usually appear about 2–10 days after the drinking stops. A person with DTs may exhibit the following symptoms:

- confusion;
- difficulty sleeping, including nightmares;
- disorientation with visual hallucinations;
- excessive sweating;
- fever;

Box 17.1   The CONFFUSED mnemonic

Mnemonics can be helpful to remember key common causes of delirium.

C   **CNS,** such as stroke, subdural haematoma, and meningitis

O   **Organ dysfunction,** such as heart, lung, kidney, and liver disease

N   **Nutritional lack,** such as thiamine deficiency

F   **Fever or infection**

F   **Fluids, electrolyte, or metabolic abnormalities,** such as hyponatraemia

U   **Urinary problems,** which might include infection and urinary retention

S   **Sensory and sleep deprivation**

E   **Endocrine problems** (either overproduction or underproduction of any gland, such as hypothyroidism or hyperglycaemia)

D   **Drugs,** including drug withdrawal or intoxication

- hallucinations and delusions that arouse fears and restlessness;
- severe depression.

Pharmacological management of acute alcohol withdrawal will not be discussed in detail, but practitioners are directed to NICE guidance (2010b) 'Alcohol-use disorders. Diagnosis and clinical management of alcohol-related physical complications'. Pharmacological management of symptoms is usually with benzodiazepines such as lorazepam or chlordiazepoxide. In addition, all patients with acute alcohol withdrawal should be treated with thiamine (vitamin B_1) to help to prevent development of Wernicke's encephalopathy (a serious condition comprising of ophthalmoplegia, confusion, and ataxia), which can lead to permanent memory loss. However, generic non-pharmacological strategies might also be useful when a patient is experiencing DTs. Such strategies are illustrated further on in the chapter.

Clinical assessment of delirium

Nurses are in an ideal position to recognize behavioural and physical changes in patients. The following signs and symptoms are suggestive of delirium. They may fluctuate over hours and days, and this is a key feature of delirium. Such symptoms should be reported immediately to the nurse in charge and/or medical staff. Likewise, nurses should encourage family members and caregivers to report these symptoms to a member of staff.

- Cognitive function: for example, worsened concentration, slow responses, disorientation, rambling speech, inability to follow simple instructions, memory loss
- Perception: for example, visual or auditory hallucinations
- Physical function: for example, reduced mobility, reduced movement, restlessness, agitation, changes in appetite, sleep disturbance
- Social behaviour: for example, lack of cooperation with reasonable requests, withdrawal, or alterations in communication, mood, and/or attitude (Emotional lability is exhibited by intermittent symptoms of fear, paranoia, anxiety, depression, and euphoria.)

Delirium assessment tools

Delirium assessment tools can help to make a diagnosis, although no single diagnostic test for delirium exists. If any of the above changes are present, a healthcare professional who is trained and competent in diagnosing delirium should carry out a clinical assessment based on DSM-IV criteria or short CAM to confirm the diagnosis (NICE, 2010a). In critical care or in the recovery room after surgery, CAM-ICU should be used. A diagnosis of delirium should be accurately recorded in patient records.

Confusion Assessment Method (CAM)

The Confusion Assessment Method (CAM; Inouye *et al.*, 1990) is a useful validated screening instrument based on the DSM-IV diagnostic criteria for delirium that enables a diagnosis of delirium to be made quickly and accurately by non-psychiatrically trained clinicians (although training in the use of the CAM is required). The CAM is a structured assessment approach that can achieve up to 95% sensitivity and specificity. The CAM-ICU can be used in critical care or the recovery room after surgery. CAM can be used on admission to hospital and long-term care, and for serial measurements in patients at risk to help to detect a development of new delirium or its resolution.

Box 17.2 **Confusion Assessment Method**

To have a positive CAM result, the patient must display the following.

1. **Presence of acute onset and fluctuating course** (It might be useful to talk to a family member, carer, or GP.) Do the symptoms come and go or increase and decrease in severity over a 24-hour period? Are there moments of lucidity? Is behaviour/confusion worse in the evening? **AND**

2. **Inattention (e.g. 20-1 test with reduced ability to maintain attention or shift attention** Can the patient maintain conversation or follow commands? Is the patient distractible? **AND EITHER**

3. **Disorganized thinking (disorganized or incoherent speech)** Does the patient show signs of illogical flow of ideas, rambling conversation? **OR**

4. **Altered level of consciousness** Is the patient fully alert, hypervigilant, comatose, lethargic, stuporous?

Long and short versions of the CAM are available. The short version, known as the short CAM (diagnostic algorithm), includes the only four features found to be best able to distinguish between delirium and other types of cognitive impairment. The long version is more comprehensive and is used to screen for clinical features of delirium. It also further defines the four features of delirium outlined in the short CAM. The short CAM is given in Box 17.2.

Administration of the CAM

Go to **http://icam.geriu.org/** to view a video of how to use the CAM.

Assessment with the CAM is made in two parts. Part one is an assessment instrument that screens for overall cognitive impairment, such as the mini mental state examination (MMSE; Folstein *et al.*, 1975) or the abbreviated mental test (AMT; Hodkinson, 1972). Part two covers the four features identified in the short CAM in Box 17.2. Many cognitive tests are patented and protected

by copyright, so practitioners should first check whether their workplace has a licence to use these.

Risk factor assessment

Patients should be assessed for the following risk factors when they first present to hospital or long-term care. If any of these risk factors are present, the patient is considered at risk of delirium (National Institute for Health and Clinical Excellence (NICE), 2010a). It is also important to monitor people for any changes in the risk factors for delirium (such as deterioration in clinical condition).

1. Aged 65 years or older
2. Cognitive impairment: a previous history of cognitive impairment or, if cognitive impairment is suspected, confirm it using a standardized and validated cognitive impairment measure such as the MMSE (Folstein *et al.*, 1975) or the AMT (Hodkinson, 1972)
3. Severe illness
4. Current hip fracture

History-taking

It is important to establish previous functional status and how it compares with a patient's current level of function. Patients should be assessed for deficiencies in activities of daily living, hearing impairment, or vision impairment. Many patients with delirium might be unable to provide an accurate history, and it is therefore important to obtain a detailed corroborative history from a reliable caregiver, relative, and/or GP. Communication between staff from different disciplines is essential to avoid unnecessary repetition of information gathering. There is often difficulty distinguishing between the symptoms of dementia, delirium, and depression. If in doubt, treat as delirium (NICE, 2010a). Delirium assessment is multifactorial and should include the following.

History of confusion

To differentiate between causes of confusion, it is important to establish timelines regarding the onset and course of confusion: for example, did the symptoms come on suddenly (such as hours or days) or progressively over time? Does the patient have a known diagnosis of dementia? Is there a history of delirium? It is useful to ascertain a patient's previous intellectual function, e.g. his or her ability to manage finances, adherence with medication, or ability to use the telephone.

Social history

A person's social history is important because it helps to build up a picture of a patient's background and ability to live independently. Key questions include whether the person is already known to social services, whether there is a history of self-neglect, or if he or she is known to the local memory services or to the local community mental health team.

Drug history

Drugs are an important risk factor and precipitant for delirium in older people, with medication being the sole precipitant for 12–39% of cases of delirium (Alagiakrishnan and Wiens, 2004). A full drug history, including non-prescribed drugs such as illegal drugs and alcohol, should be obtained. Recent changes in drugs, such as the cessation of benzodiazepines, should also be documented. The commonest drugs associated with delirium are psychoactive agents, such as benzodiazepines, narcotic analgesics, and drugs with anticholinergic action (Ancelin and Artero, 2006).

Medical history

It is important to explore symptoms suggestive of comorbid conditions. A review of comorbidities should be conducted, with an emphasis on neurological diseases (e.g. stroke, Parkinson's disease, dementia), cardiovascular diseases (e.g. myocardial infarction, angina), and renal/metabolic diseases (e.g. hyponatraemia, hypernatraemia, chronic renal failure). Information gathering should also include a person's diet and fluid intake, including recent weight loss, self-neglect, bladder and bowel voiding problems such as constipation, and tendency to develop urinary tract infections. History gathering may include formal assessments such as the mental state examination and these should be undertaken by staff formally trained to do so.

Mental state examination

This should consider the following.

- State of consciousness
- General appearance and behaviour: simple unobtrusive observation of a patient's behaviour during assessment can aid diagnosis. Is the patient dressed appropriately? Alert? Focused on the conversation?
- Orientation (to time/place/person)

- Memory (short- and long-term)
- Language: is speech clear? Can the patient read and write or understand?
- Visuospatial functions: for example, can the patient copy intersecting pentagons or draw a clock face?
- Executive control functions (e.g. planning and sequencing of tasks)
- Other cognitive functions (e.g. calculations)
- Insight and judgement
- Thought content
- Mood and affect

Cognitive function should be assessed using a standardized screening tool (such as the AMT or MMSE), including tests for attention: for example, counting backwards from 20 to 1, or spelling 'world' backwards, or serial 7s, which involves counting down from 100 in 7s.

Physical examination

Physical examination should focus on looking for underlying physical causes of confusion, but it should also cover the following areas.

- Rectal examination—if impaction is suspected
- Search for infection, including lungs, urine, abdomen, skin
- Evidence of alcohol abuse or withdrawal (e.g. signs of delirium tremens)
- Neurological examination (including assessment of speech)
- Evidence of sensory impairment, such as visual or hearing deficits
- Pain: severe pain is associated with delirium, and certain analgesics (such as morphine) can be precipitants for delirium, as outlined above

Investigations

The following investigations are almost always indicated in patients with delirium to identify the underlying cause (British Geriatrics Society (BGS), 2006).

- Full blood count, including C-reactive protein
- Urea and electrolytes, calcium
- Liver function tests
- Glucose
- Chest X-ray

- Electrocardiogram
- Blood cultures
- Pulse oximetry
- Urinalysis

Other investigations may be indicated according to the findings from the history and examination rather than performed routinely (BGS, 2006), including:

- a CT head scan if intracranial haemorrhage is suspected and when patients show focal neurological signs, confusion following a head injury or fall, or evidence of raised intracranial pressure;
- an EEG to differentiate delirium from other neurological conditions, such as encephalitis or epilepsy, and also when there is concern that a patient might have an intracranial lesion;
- a chest X-ray to exclude pneumonia, congestive cardiac failure, or other possible causes of hypoxia;
- thyroid function tests;
- blood test for levels of B_{12} and folate;
- arterial blood gases to evaluate for hypoxia and lactate;
- specific cultures, e.g. urine, sputum;
- lumbar puncture might be indicated if a diagnosis of meningitis is suspected. A patient might show signs of meningism, such as stiff neck, photophobia, and headaches. It might also be indicated where encephalitis is suspected.

Differential diagnosis

Dementia, delirium and depression: the 3Ds

Dementia, delirium, and depression are the three most prevalent mental disorders in the elderly (Johnson *et al.*, 1994) (see also Chapter 7 Understanding Dementia and Chapter 8 Understanding Depression ➡). It must also be remembered that depression and delirium are potentially treatable. However, a recent systematic review of research pertaining to frequency and prognosis of persistent delirium in older hospital patients at discharge, and at 1, 3, and 6 months, showed the prevalence of persistent delirium to be 44.7%, 32.8%, 25.6%, and 21%, respectively (Cole *et al.*, 2009). Certain symptoms of the three disorders may overlap, but they also have significant differences. Often, practitioners mistake one disorder for the

other, but it is important to remember that these three conditions can coexist, and therefore accurate assessment and diagnosis is crucial. Table 17.1 outlines the main distinguishing features of dementia, delirium, and depression. It must also be noted that other diagnoses, including schizophrenia, dysphasia, hysteria/mania, and non-convulsive epilepsy, can also be mistaken for delirium. However, if the diagnosis is uncertain, treat for delirium first (NICE, 2010a).

Accessing the evidence to inform clinical decisions

Guidelines for the management, prevention, and diagnosis of delirium were published by the National Institute for Health and Clinical Excellence (NICE) in 2010. NICE issues guidelines that are based on a systematic review of the evidence and consults extensively with expert clinicians, patients, and industry within the specialized field. Many of the recommendations in the NICE guidelines on delirium are based on consensus opinion because (in some areas) there is lack of good-quality research evidence about the management of delirium.

Management of delirium: prevention and treatment

Management of delirium should always be person-centred, giving patients the opportunity to make informed decisions about their healthcare and taking into account their needs and preferences (NICE, 2010). Patients with delirium often lack capacity to make complex decisions, and practitioners are guided towards the summary information provided on the Office of the Public Guardian website (**www.publicguardian.gov.uk**) regarding the Mental Capacity Act 2005. Family and caregivers should all be given the opportunity to be involved in decisions about treatment and care (with patient consent). They should also be encouraged to be actively involved in the provision of care and be reassured that such involvement is a positive addition to care already provided by formal staff.

The NICE clinical guideline on diagnosis, prevention, and management of delirium (2010a) covers adult

Table 17.1 The distinguishing features of dementia, delirium, and depression

History	Dementia	Delirium	Depression
Onset	Vague, insidious, gradual with slow progression of symptoms over months or years	Sudden onset over hours or days	Onset and decline gradual over weeks or months. Often an identifiable trigger such as bereavement
Presentation of symptoms	May go unnoticed for years	Obvious if hyperactive delirium, but more difficult if hypoactive delirium	Evident at an early stage
Cognition and orientation	Lack of insight. Attempts to hide problems or may be unaware. Often disorientated in time, place, and person. Processing of internal and external information is impaired—multiple cognitive problems including memory impairment.	Disorientated in time, place, and person. Short-term memory impaired. Processing of internal and external information is impaired	Subjective complaints of memory loss
Thinking	Problems with memory and thinking	Disorganized, jumping from one topic to another	Slower—preoccupied by negative thoughts
Symptoms	Worse in evening (sundowning)	Worse at night	Early morning wakening
Consciousness	Normal. Difficulty concentrating	Impaired. Can fluctuate between alertness and drowsiness. Poor attention	Normal, but some difficulty concentrating
Sleep pattern	Often disturbed. Night-time wandering	Sudden change in sleep pattern, new/unusual confusion at night	Early morning waking
Mental state	Possible labile mood	Emotional lability. Anxiety, fear, depression, aggression	Distressed/unhappy
Speech	Word-finding difficulty	Changed rate	Normal
Delusions/ hallucinations	Delusions common. Hallucinations rare in early dementia	Illusions, delusions, and hallucinations common	Rare except in severe depression
Psychomotor disturbance	More evident in later stages	Very evident. Purposeless movement. Apathetic/ hypoactive. Hyperactive	May get psychomotor retardation in severe depression

patients over the age of 18 in a hospital setting and adults over the age of 18 in long-term care residential care. It does not cover children and young people (younger than 18), people receiving end-of-life care, or people with intoxication and/or withdrawing from drugs or alcohol, and people with delirium associated with these states.

The clinical guideline is focused on the prevention of delirium. Practitioners are encouraged to 'Think delirium'—that is, to identify high-risk patients on admission to hospital and long-term care settings (within 24 hours of admission to these care settings), to assess high-risk

patients for clinical features that might precipitate delirium, and to implement person-centred delirium prevention strategies if clinical indicators of delirium are not currently present. Such patients should then be assessed daily for any change in clinical indicators.

Patients at risk of delirium should be cared for in an environment that avoids unnecessary room changes and maintains a team of healthcare professionals who are familiar to the patient (continuity of care). Table 17.2 outlines indicators that can contribute to delirium, and preventative interventions and strategies (NICE, 2010a).

Table 17.2 Clinical indicators that can contribute to delirium

Clinical indicators	Preventative interventions and actions
Disorientation	Provide clear signage, soft lighting, a 24-hour clock and calendar, which are clearly visible to the patient and set appropriately.
	Avoid moving patient within the ward environment and between wards. Is it more appropriate for another patient to be moved instead?
Dehydration and/or constipation	Ensure adequate fluid intake to prevent dehydration by encouraging the person to drink. Establish preferences. Consider subcutaneous or intravenous fluids if necessary.
	Take advice where necessary when managing fluid balance in people with comorbidities such as heart failure or chronic kidney disease.
Infection	Look for and treat infection.
	Avoid unnecessary catheterization.
	Implement good infection control procedures.
Pain	Find out whether the patient is in pain. Look out for non-verbal signs of pain such as agitation, especially in patients with limited communication such as those on a ventilator or patients with dementia.
	Consider using a validated pain assessment tool such as the Abbey Pain Scale.
	Administer analgesia as prescribed and review regularly.
Polypharmacy effects	Carry out a drugs review for people on multiple medications.
Poor nutrition and/or constipation	Ensure that the patient has adequate diet and has appropriate assistance at mealtimes. Establish usual bowel pattern and aperient usage.
Restricted or limited mobility or immobility	Encourage patients to walk around.
	Carry out active range-of-motion exercises and early mobilization after surgery.
Sensory impairment	Assess visual or hearing impairment.
	Ensure hearing and visual aids are available to and used by patients who need them and that they are in good working order.
Sleep disturbance	Promote good sleep patterns and sleep hygiene by:
	• establishing usual sleep pattern;
	• provision of appropriate lighting;
	• appropriate stimulation during the day;
	• reducing noise to a minimum during sleep periods;
	• scheduling medication/vital signs rounds to avoid disturbing sleep.

Source: Adapted from NICE (2010a)

Delirium prevention

There is some evidence that delirium can be prevented in up to one-third of cases (Inouye *et al.*, 1999; Royal College of Psychiatrists, 2005). Prevention of delirium is the most effective strategy for reducing its frequency and complications (Inouye, 2006). The identification of high-risk patients, early attention to possible precipitants, and adoption of specific tailored strategies may prevent the development of delirium and significantly improve clinical outcomes

(Marcantonio *et al.*, 2001; Milisen *et al.*, 2001; NICE, 2010a). A Cochrane review (Siddiqi *et al.*, 2007) to determine the effectiveness of interventions designed to prevent delirium in hospitalized patients concluded that robust research evidence on the effectiveness of such interventions is sparse.

Evidence from one study included in the review suggested that proactive consultation by a consultant geriatrician before, or within 24 hours of, operation may reduce the incidence and severity of delirium in patients undergoing surgery for hip fracture. The Yale Delirium Prevention Trial was the first clinical controlled trial to show that delirium can be prevented in older hospitalized people (Inouye *et al.*, 1999). This study showed that a unit-based proactive multifactorial intervention (termed HELP, The Hospital Elder Life Program) actually reduced the incidence of delirium among hospitalized patients ≥70 years old by 40%. In this study, six intervention components were used selectively on the basis of (individualized) patient risk factors determined at an admission assessment: cognitive impairment; sleep deprivation; immobility; visual impairment; hearing impairment; and dehydration. These included the formulation of a non-pharmacological sleep protocol that involved trained volunteers offering patients warm milk and soothing music at bedtime. This intervention reduced the use of night-time sedative-hypnotic medication. This approach has been adopted widely, and practitioners can obtain further information and training resources online (**www.hospitalelderlifeprogram.org**). However, further robust research is required into delirium prevention strategies. Table 17.2 illustrates useful strategies to prevent delirium.

Pharmacological prevention of delirium

Evidence from pharmacological prevention reviews is limited and of low quality. One hypothesis for the pathogenesis of delirium is related to neurotransmitter dysfunction, especially acetylcholine. However, evidence from studies investigating the effects of cholinesterase inhibitors (such as donepezil) versus placebo on prevention of delirium is inconclusive (NICE, 2010a). Other drugs, such as haloperidol and risperidone, have also been investigated, but the evidence is inconclusive because of the paucity of reliable data.

Management of symptoms of delirium

Delirium should be treated as a medical emergency whereby the underlying cause or causes of delirium are identified and managed as soon as possible (Maher and Almeida, 2002). Practising nurses are reminded that delirium is often multifactorial and that while one reason (such as urinary tract infection) has been identified, there might be other causes still present (such as constipation and dehydration) that also need to be addressed. Consideration

> **Box 17. 3 Seven steps to the management of delirium**
>
> 1. Identify the cause/s of delirium where possible.
> 2. Address the cause and any precipitating factors for delirium.
> 3. Manage the symptoms of delirium—non-pharmacological and pharmacological interventions.
> 4. Provide a supportive care environment—psychological, physical, and sensory support.
> 5. Prevent complications—such as falls.
> 6. Educate the patient/client and his or her carers/family.
> 7. Ensure appropriate follow-up.

should also be made regarding appropriate symptomatic relief of delirium.

Many of the strategies to manage delirium symptoms are the same as those recommended to prevent delirium (as outlined in Table 17.2). Figure 17.3 illustrates the key components of delirium management, while Box 17.3 gives the key steps for delirium management.

Non-pharmacological management of delirium

There is limited research evidence about non-pharmacological interventions for the management of delirium. However, because delirium is often multifactorial with varied outcomes, there have been suggestions that multicomponent interventions might be appropriate. Such interventions could include environmental modifications, comprehensive geriatric review pain assessment, and nurse-led interventions and monitoring. Current evidence suggests that enhanced treatment strategies for people with delirium are more successful than usual care, but the evidence is of low quality. However, NICE (2010a) identifies key areas from the multicomponent studies to incorporate in its recommendations, as outlined in a treatment algorithm (Figure 17.4). The current advice is to explore non-pharmacological ways of managing a patient with delirium first, using verbal and non-verbal de-escalation techniques (see Box 17.4).

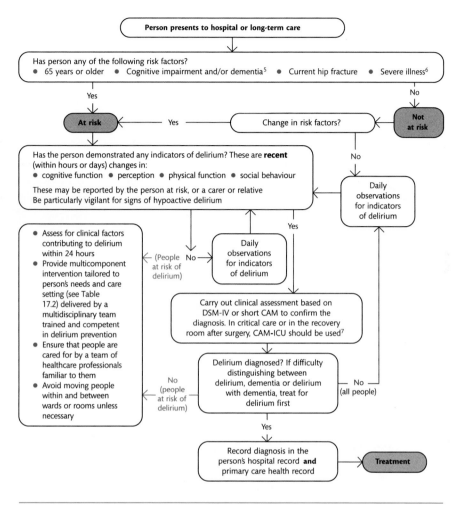

Figure 17.2 Preventing and diagnosing delirium.

National Institute for Health and Clinical Excellence (2010a) *Delirium Diagnosis, Prevention and Management*, NICE Clinical Guideline 103. NICE: London. Reproduced with permission.

Involvement of family members and caregivers

It is important that effective communication, reorientation, and reassurance is given to the patient and family members/caregivers (Box 17.4). Delirium can be a very frightening experience. Written information provided should clearly explain what delirium is, and that delirium is common and usually temporary, and should encourage family members and caregivers to report changes to healthcare practitioners (NICE, 2010a). Families should be encouraged to bring in familiar mementos (such as photographs) to aid orientation. Caregivers should also be encouraged to be as actively involved in care as appropriate (such as accompanying the patient to CT scan or being present during physiotherapy or phlebotomy).

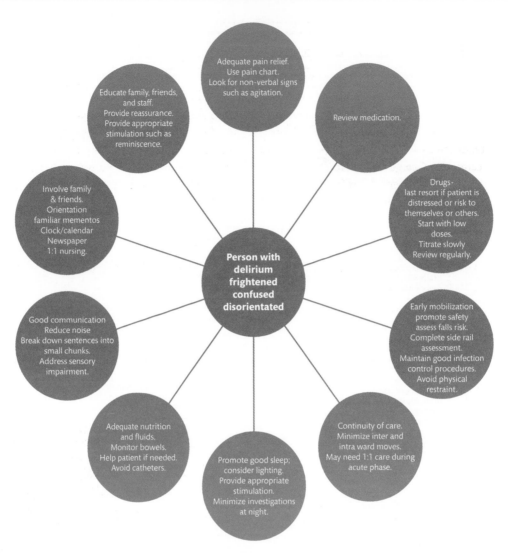

Figure 17.3 The key components of delirium management.

Pharmacological interventions

Good-quality evidence for the use of specific drugs to treat the symptoms of delirium is limited. It must be remembered that certain drugs (for example, anticholinergics and narcotics) can *cause* delirium.

However, drug treatment may be required in certain situations, including:

• in order to carry out essential investigations and treatment;

• to prevent a patient endangering him or herself or other people;

CASE STUDY 17.1 *Mr George*

Mr George is a 78-year-old gentleman who has moderate Alzheimer's disease. He has some visual impairment and wears glasses. He is also diabetic. He attends the local memory clinic. His wife is his main carer. Mrs George reports to the dementia nurse specialist that, over the past few days, her husband's behaviour and function have deteriorated significantly. He has lost his appetite and developed worrying symptoms of urinary incontinence. He does not recognize his own home, and he reports to his wife that he can see people stealing objects from his home. He was recently started on amitriptyline for depression and he is on several other drugs.

Questions

➤ What might have caused the dramatic loss of function/deterioration in behaviour/increased confusion?

➤ Identify two possible risk factors.

➤ What advice would you give Mrs George?

Answers are at the end of the chapter.

- to alleviate distress in patients exhibiting symptoms such as agitation or hallucinations.

Sedating drugs should always be started at the lowest dose, titrated accordingly, and under regular review. NICE (2010a) recommends pharmacological treatment only as short-term treatment (stated as a maximum of 7 days). There is some evidence to suggest that haloperidol (first-generation antipsychotics) and olanzapine (second-generation antipsychotics) are effective in treating delirium (Hu, 2006) and are cost-effective (NICE, 2010a). However, antipsychotics should be used cautiously or not at all in patients with conditions such as dementia with Lewy bodies or Parkinson's disease (NICE, 2010a) (see Chapter 7 Understanding Dementia ➡). Antipsychotic drugs have potential adverse effects, including extrapyramidal side effects, ECG abnormalities, sedation, and increased mortality. Patients need close monitoring and regular review.

Follow-up

Discharge planning for people who have experienced delirium should include follow-up, professional monitoring, and treatment. Post-delirium counselling should be considered for people who have experienced delirium. Good communication with primary care is vital, especially because delirium can persist beyond discharge. People who have had delirium may experience unsettling flashbacks. Depression and post-traumatic stress disorder have been described post delirium (Breitbart *et al.*, 2002). Patients and caregivers need to be aware that the symptoms of delirium may not fully resolve even after treatment of the underlying cause(s), and the consequences of delirium include:

- increased risk of dementia following an episode of delirium;

- increased mortality for patients with delirium;

- increased risk of delirium in the future.

Measuring the impact of nursing interventions

The principle of measuring both the effectiveness of nursing intervention and the patient's experience of receiving care is one that you should, where possible, facilitate. The NHS Information Centre has supported the development of Nursing Quality Metrics (NQMs), which can be used to

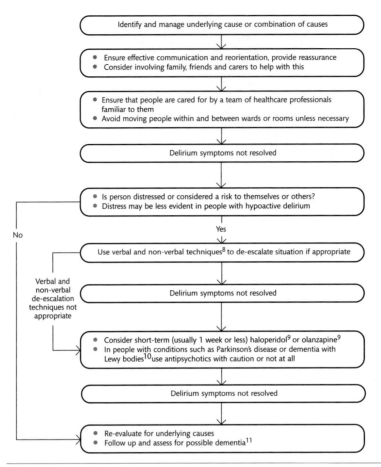

Figure 17.4 Treating delirium.

National Institute for Health and Clinical Excellence (2010a) *Delirium Diagnosis, Prevention and Management*, NICE Clinical Guideline 103. NICE: London.
Reproduced with permission.

facilitate quality improvement in patient care and experience http://signposting.ic.nhs.uk/?k=metrics.

This recent move within healthcare to be outcome-focused rather than target-driven is a welcome change in policy direction, initiated by Lord Darzi in his review of the NHS, and sustained by the previous and current UK governments. Metrics have been developed for many aspects of nursing care interventions and cover many inpatient areas, regardless of setting. The collection of these types of data helps healthcare organizations to focus on the delivery of safe and effective care, and can be used for local and national benchmarking, as well as for quality improvement.

For further details, visit the NHS Information Centre online at http://www.ic.nhs.uk/, where you will find details relating to nursing audit tools capturing information on documentation for observations, nutrition, medicines administration, pain management, communication, discharge planning, falls, pressure area care, antibiotic prescribing, and infection control.

In determining patient experience of healthcare, NICE has recently published a Quality Standard http://www.nice.org.uk/ that guides service delivery planning to ensure improvements in patient experience. Further commissioned work by the Department of Health

Box 17.4 **Advice about communication**

- Introduce yourself.
- Try to catch and hold the attention of your patient before starting to communicate.
- Give your patient time to answer.
- Break down tasks into manageable chunks.
- Keep environmental noise to a minimum, e.g. turn TV down.
- Avoid hostile body language.
- Remain pleasant, calm, and supportive.
- Maintain eye contact with your patient.
- Use short sentences.
- Speak slowly and wait for response.
- Ask only one question at a time.
- Keep the pitch of your voice low, but ensure that the patient can hear you.
- Point, touch, show, initiate a movement for the patient.
- Allow time for unhurried interaction.
- Position yourself so that you can see the patient.
- Avoid challenging the patient or do it in a non-threatening way.
- Double check instructions to ensure understanding.
- Answer repetitive questions consistently.
- Use written instructions as appropriate.

has developed a single measure of patient experience. Supplementing these data is the NHS Survey, which captures patient views relating to ward cleanliness, infection control, staff attitudes, pain management, management of privacy, experience of dignity, nutrition, medicines administration, quality of communication, and discharge. Details can be found online at http://www.nhssurveys.org/.

Resources

- NICE **www.nice.org.uk** provides additional resources to be used to complement the delirium guidelines.
- The European Delirium Association **http://www.europeandeliriumassociation.com/** contains useful information regarding delirium and resource materials.
- The Office of the Public Guardian provides guidance on mental capacity and an overview of the Mental Capacity Act 2005 **www.publicguardian.gov.uk**
- The Alzheimer's Society **www.alzheimers.org.uk** provides information on all forms of dementia and useful coping strategies.

CASE STUDY 17.2 *Mrs Lions*

Mrs Lions is a 60-year-old lady. She was transferred to your ward from the high dependency unit following surgery for coronary artery bypass grafts. She also has Parkinson's disease. On arrival on the ward, she is highly agitated, confused, and paranoid. She keeps trying to remove her Venflon and catheter. She is accompanied by her husband, who is distressed and anxious.

Questions

➤ What is your first consideration?

➤ Where would you place Mrs Lions?

➤ How would you assess her? Would you consider pharmacological management? What would you consider in light of her medical problems?

➤ What would you say to Mr Lions?

Answers are at the end of the chapter.

Summary and key messages

In this chapter, you have been encouraged to consider and implement in your practice the evidence from key national guidance for the management, treatment, and prevention of delirium. The key messages for management of delirium include the following:

- Identification of high-risk patients and frequent monitoring for changes in clinical indicators will help to prevent delirium.

- Assessment is multifactorial and involves input by all members of the multidisciplinary team.

- Non-pharmacological management of delirium is the preferred option. However, where pharmacological treatment is necessary, drugs should be started at low doses, titrated slowly, and reviewed at regular intervals.

- Delirium is distressing, and patients may have recall of this that needs follow-up and monitoring.

- Relatives and caregivers should be encouraged to be fully involved in patient care, and should be provided with written information about delirium.

Answers to Case studies

Case study 17.1 Mr George

➤ Possible causes include urinary tract infection, erratic blood sugars secondary to physical illness, dehydration, amitriptyline. Consider what other drugs Mr George is taking. Consider also constipation and urinary retention. Remember there are likely to be a combination of causes for his delirium.

➤ Risk factors: age, dementia.

➤ Provide written information on delirium for Mrs George and family. This should explain how carers/relatives can help with care by bringing in familiar possessions and orientating Mr George. Be present when investigations are being carried out. This information should give reassurance that delirium is usually temporary and common, but takes time to settle.

Case study 17.2 Mrs Lions

➤ Consider the safety of Mrs Lions, staff members, and other patients. What is causing the delirium? Provide ongoing reassurance to Mr Lions, who may be extremely distressed by the changes he is seeing in his wife.

➤ Mrs Lions should be placed somewhere quiet, but easily visible.

➤ Obtain a detailed history from staff on HDU and Mr Lions. Consider undertaking a cognitive assessment and CAM at the earliest opportunity when Mrs Lions can participate. Consider non-pharmacological management first. If this is not effective and pharmacological management is required, extra care is needed when considering medication because of her Parkinson's disease.

➤ Explain what delirium is. Provide reassurance. Encourage Mr Lions to be involved in his wife's care and show him how he can support his wife through orientation, reassurance, and feeding back any concerns to staff.

Online Resource Centre

 To help you to develop and apply your knowledge and decision-making skills further, we have provided interactive learning online at **www.oxfordtextbooks.co.uk/orc/bullock/**

Whilst these are freely available, you will need to use the access codes at the start of the book.

References

Alagiakrishnan, K., Wiens, C. (2004) An approach to drug induced delirium in the elderly. *Postgraduate Medical Journal* **80**: 388–93.

American Psychiatric Association (1994) *Diagnostic and Statistical Manual of Mental Health Disorders*, 4th edn. APA: Washington DC.

Ancelin, M.L., Artero, S. (2006) Non-degenerative mild cognitive impairment in elderly people and use of anticholinergic drugs: longitudinal cohort study. *British Medical Journal* **332**: 455–9.

Breitbart, W., Alici, Y. (2008) Agitation and delirium at the end of life: 'We couldn't manage him.' *Journal of the American Medical Association* **300**(24): 2898–910.

Breitbart, W., Gibson, C., Tremblay, A. (2002) The delirium experience: delirium recall and delirium-related distress in hospitalized patients with cancer, their spouses/caregivers, and their nurses. *Psychosomatics* **43**(3): 183–94.

Breitbart, W., Rosenfeld, B., Roth, A., *et al.* (1997) The Memorial Delirium Assessment Scale. *Journal of Pain and Symptom Management* **13**: 128–37.

British Geriatrics Society (2006) *Guidelines for the Prevention, Diagnosis and Management of Delirium in Older People in Hospital*. BGS: London.

Cole, M.G., Ciampi, A., Belzile, E., *et al.* (2009) Persistent delirium in older hospital patients: a systematic review of frequency and prognosis. *Age and Ageing* **38**(1): 19–26.

Ely, E.W., Inouye, S.K., Bernard, G.R., *et al.* (2001) Delirium in mechanically ventilated patients: validity and reliability of the confusion assessment method for the intensive care unit (CAM-ICU). *Journal of the American Medical Association* **286**: 2703–10.

Faber and Faber (1953) *The Faber Medical Dictionary*. Faber and Faber Ltd: London.

Folstein, M.F., Folstein, S.E., McHugh, P.R. (1975) 'Mini-Mental State': a practical method for grading the cognitive state of patients for the clinician. *Journal of Psychiatric Research* **12**: 196–8.

Fong, T.G., Tulebaev, S.R., Inouye, S.K., *et al.* (2009) Delirium in elderly adults: diagnosis, prevention and treatment. *Nature Reviews Neurology* **5**: 210–20.

Hodkinson, H.M. (1972) Evaluation of a mental test score for assessment of mental impairment in the elderly. *Age and Ageing* **1**(4): 233–8.

Hu, H. (2006) Olanzapine and haloperidol for senile delirium. A randomised controlled observation. *Chinese Journal of Clinical Rehabilitation* **10**(42): 188–90.

Inouye, S.K. (2006) Delirium in older persons. *New England Journal of Medicine* **354**: 1157–65.

Inouye, S.K. Bogardus, S., Jr, Charpentier, P., *et al.* (1999) A multicomponent intervention to prevent delirium in hospitalized older patients. *New England Journal of Medicine* **340**(9): 669–76.

Inouye, S.K., Foreman, M.D., Mion, L.C., *et al.* (2001) Nurses' recognition of delirium and its symptoms. Comparison of nurse and researcher ratings. *Archives of Internal Medicine* **161**(20): 2467–73.

Inouye, S.K., van Dyck, C.H., Alessi, C.A., *et al.* (1990) CAM confusion assessment test for diagnosis of delirium. *Annals of Internal Medicine* **113**: 941–80.

Johnson, J., Sims, R., Gottlieb, G. (1994) Differential diagnosis of dementia, delirium and depression. Implications for drug therapy. *Drugs Aging* **5**(6): 431–45.

Lindesay, J., Rockwood, K., Rolfson, D. (2002) The epidemiology of delirium. In J. Lindesay, K. Rockwood, A. Macdonald (eds) *Delirium in Old Age*. Oxford University Press: Oxford, pp. 27–50.

Maher, S., Almeida, O. (2002) Delirium in the elderly: another emergency. *Current Therapeutics* **43**: 39–45.

Marcantonio, E.R., Flacker, J.M., Wright, R.J., *et al.* (2001) Reducing delirium after hip fracture: a randomised trial. *Journal of the American Geriatric Society* **49**: 516–22.

Milisen, K., Foreman, M.D., Abraham, I.L. *et al.* (2001) A nurse-led interdisciplinary intervention program for delirium in elderly hip fracture patients. *Journal of the American Geriatric Society* **49**(5): 523–32.

National Institute for Health and Clinical Excellence (NICE) (2010a) *Delirium Diagnosis, Prevention and Management*. NICE Clinical Guideline 103 (CG103). NICE: London.

National Institute for Health and Clinical Excellence (NICE) (2010b) *Alcohol-Use Disorders: Diagnosis and Clinical Management of Alcohol-Related Physical Complications*. NICE Clinical Guideline 100 (CG100). NICE: London.

Royal College of Psychiatrists (2005) *Who Cares Wins: Guidelines for the Development of Liaison Mental Health Services for Older People*. Royal College of Psychiatrists: London.

Siddiqi, N., Clegg, A., Young, J. (2009) Delirium in care homes. *Reviews in Clinical Gerontology* **19**: 309–16.

Siddiqi, N., Holt, R., Britton, A.M., *et al.* (2007) Interventions for preventing delirium in hospitalised patients. *Cochrane Database of Systematic Reviews* Issue 2: Art. No. CD005563. DOI: 10.1002/14651858.CD005563.pub2.

Siddiqi, N., House, A.O., Holmes J. F., *et al.* (2006) Occurrence and outcome of delirium in medical inpatients: a systematic literature review. *Age and Ageing* **35**(4): 350–64.

US Department of Health and Human Services (2004) *CMS Statistics 34*. CMS Publication No. 03445. Centers for Medicare & Medicaid Services: Washington, DC.

Yang, F.M., Marcantonio, E., Inouye, S.K., *et al.* (2009) Phenomenological subtypes of delirium in older persons: patterns, prevalence and prognosis. *Psychosomatics* **50**: 248–54.

18 *Managing* End-of-Life Care

John W. Albarran and Marika Hills

Introduction

This chapter addresses the fundamental nursing role of managing end-of-life care. Death is as fundamental a part of life as living, and while caring for a dying patient and their family is demanding, complex, and emotionally exhausting, it can also be a gratifying and privileged experience for nurses. Specifically, nurses have a centre-stage role in leading and informing care delivery at the end of life. Care will typically embrace assessing the needs of the patient and family, providing symptom relief and comfort care, and providing cultural and spiritual support. Additionally, caring functions should also extend following death to caring for the deceased in a dignified manner and supporting the newly bereaved, demonstrating genuine concern, compassion, and effective communication skills (Hills and Albarran, 2010a; Maben *et al.*, 2010). To examine the key themes and challenges of practice, it is important to understand the political, professional and societal influences, and contextual nature of death and dying in the UK.

Understanding the importance of end-of-life care

Defining end-of-life care

At present, there is neither a clear nor universally accepted definition of end-of-life care, but it is generally understood to be the care of a person who is identified as having failing health and who is in a progressive state of decline (Shipman *et al.*, 2008). Establishing the last phase of a patient's life can be a difficult and complex process, and this might occur:

- after the diagnosis of a life-limiting condition;
- during the transition or deterioration of a chronic disease illness;
- when there is an increasing frailty combined with greater dependence on care provision, particularly in the older adult;
- following a sudden infective episode, cardiac event, or a life-threatening accident.

The last phase of end-of-life care is referred to as the dying phase. Consideration of the end-of-life care needs of people with chronic terminal conditions should begin at diagnosis, and must embrace after-death care and family support.

Mortality rates

Over the past century, progress and advancement in disease management, together with improvements in living standards, have resulted in changes to the national death profile, with currently two-thirds of the 0.5 million annual deaths in the UK occurring in people over 75 years of age. Demographic trends indicate that there are 1.5 million people over the age of 65 (Office for National Statistics, 2009). The fastest growing age group is among the over-85s, with figures for 2008 revealing that this group makes up 1.3 million (5%) of the total population. It is expected that this number will double in the next decade (Office for National Statistics, 2009). The consequence of an ageing population is that the number of people with specific long-term care needs will also grow; dementia care is a good example. Currently, 820,000 are diagnosed with this condition; this represents 1.3% of the population (Luengo-Fernandez *et al.*, 2010). With people living longer, the prevalence of illnesses will increase, as will the complexity of care of older adults suffering from multiple chronic medical conditions (comorbidities) which are likely to impact on their care needs at the end of life. Currently, most people die from illnesses that follow a progressive chronic disease trajectory. This determines whether the death trajectory entails a rapid decline in health, whether it is in the long term with sporadic serious episodes, or prolonged, involving gradual disability, declining physical, and cognitive functioning (Murray *et al.*, 2005). With over half a million people dying annually, it is important that nurses are equipped and prepared to manage the complex physical, emotional, and spiritual needs of patients nearing the end of life, regardless of setting, or whether young or older adult. Caring and supporting the families through these difficult times is a core component of your activity.

Location of deaths

Changes in death demographics have, to a degree, coincided with a change in societal attitudes and outlooks towards death and dying, with people becoming much less familiar with the issues of dying (Department of Health, 2008a). Approaches to the management of dying patients away from the medicalized model of care, which is largely cure- and disease-orientated, towards a holistic approach that considers the whole person have been influential in trying to address challenges in the delivery of care. Currently, 58% of all deaths occur in acute hospitals; however, it is widely accepted that these environments do not provide a good quality of dying (Department of Health, 2008a). While care in a hospice is considered the model of excellence, only 4% of all deaths occur in these settings (Department of Health, 2008a). Whilst most relatives report satisfaction with the care that their loved one received in a hospice (Rhodes *et al.*, 2008), the reverse is often true in acute care hospitals. Indeed, a report by the Health Care Commission (2007) suggests that over 8,500 complaints from acute hospitals centred on end-of-life (EoL) care, after-death care, and care of the newly bereaved.

Policy

The document *Building on the Best* (Department of Health, 2003) led the Department of Health (2005) to recognize the importance of developments in end-of-life care across the country and also initiated a national end-of-life care programme to improve levels of end-of-life care. The impetus for a national strategy, however, was advocated in the Darzi NHS review (Department of Health, 2008b), which promoted improvements in the patient's experience in healthcare services, beginning with maternity all the way through to end of life. The End-of-Life Care Strategy (2008a) was introduced, offering a working framework for improving the delivery of end-of-life care for the patient and family from the point of diagnosis of life-limiting illness, through the dying process, after death, and into bereavement. Recommended tools are discussed later.

The Department of Health (2008a) has developed a national end-of-life care core competency framework (Skills for Care, 2009), as well as programmes to enhance training for pre-registration nurses. This is augmented by the national e-learning package for end-of-life care.

Prevalence

Patients approaching the end of life in a community or hospital setting, whether this involves weeks or days, may experience a combination of physical and emotional health-related problems caused by the presence of distressing and debilitating symptoms. Differences in manifestation and in the degree of severity will vary between individuals according to the underlying medical condition. Clarity in your plan of care should be focused on retaining the dignity of terminally ill patients, managing their symptoms by the application of your skills and knowledge, and by accessing specialist services as appropriate to their needs. Use of evidence-based assessment tools is necessary to identify actual/potential symptoms and problems, to plan individualized care, to control and reduce the burden of distress, while preserving the dignity and comfort of patients (Douglas *et al.*, 2009; Von Gunten, 2005). This is challenging when patients are either semi-comatose or too ill to report their symptoms, so your essential nursing skills (interpersonal, monitoring, analysis, problem-solving, proactivity, and clinical expertise) are all employed in caring for patients at the end of life.

According to Von Gunten (2005), the prevalence of moderate to severe symptoms in the weeks and months before death is high, with an estimated 1.4 million being affected by **dyspnoea** and 1 million suffering pain (see **Chapters 15 Managing Breathlessness** and **25 Managing Pain** ⟶). A high prevalence of five symptoms, including pain, fatigue, dyspnoea, confusion (restlessness or agitation), and death rattle, has been reported for a range of terminal conditions such as cancer, heart failure, human immunodeficiency virus, chronic obstructive pulmonary disease, and renal disease (Chang *et al.*, 2007; Douglas *et al.*, 2009; Von Gunten, 2005). End-of-life symptoms can typically include:

- dyspnoea;
- pain;
- gastrointestinal disturbances (e.g. nausea and vomiting, constipation, loss of appetite, swallowing difficulties, and constipation);
- altered mental state (e.g. agitation, seizures, delirium, and confusion);
- fatigue;
- anxiety and depression;
- increased respiratory tract secretions leading to 'death rattle'.

Research using the Memorial Symptom Assessment scale among patients with cancer and end-stage diseases identified some key differences (Table 18.1) in symptom reports (Trammer *et al.*, 2003).

Another study examining heart failure medical records reported that, on average, patients suffered from 6.7 symptoms in the last 6 months of life, with 88% and 75%

Table 18.1 Differences in key symptoms among patients with cancer and end-stage diseases

Symptom	Patients with cancer (%)	Patients with end-stage diseases (%)
Pain	78	49
Nausea	61	43
Vomiting	41	10
Constipation	48	30
Shortness of breath	24	86
Coughing	52	72

reporting breathlessness and pain, respectively (Nordgren and Sörensen, 2003). However, some of the treatments aimed at ameliorating symptoms associated with end of life produce undesirable side effects, which in many instances can be anticipated and treated accordingly (Douglas *et al.*, 2009; Von Gunten, 2005).

There is increasing evidence among cancer patients that individuals experience 'symptom clusters' that influence functional status, prognosis, and quality of life. Clusters are defined as two or more coexisting symptoms that are interrelated and may possibly have a shared cause (Fan *et al.*, 2007). Cheung *et al.*'s (2009) research identified the major cluster of anxiety and depression, and a grouping that embraced the symptoms of fatigue, drowsiness, nausea, dyspnoea, and loss of appetite among patients with advanced cancer. Targeting symptom clusters in cancer patients may lead to improved therapeutic outcomes rather than treating individual symptoms; however, owing to the complex nature of comorbidity presentations, many symptoms may be either unrecognized, unanticipated, underinvestigated, and/or untreated (Ingham and Foley, 1998; Nordgren and Sörensen, 2003; Von Gunten, 2005).

Causation

The causes of symptoms at the end of life are complex and multifactorial, but often are the result of illness progression, treatments, and complications (Figure 18.1). Within hospice and nursing home settings, environmental features such as noise levels, a lack of privacy, restful surroundings, facilities for prayer, and staffing levels have been found to be influential in how patients respond to and cope with their symptoms (Kayser-Jones *et al.*, 2002; Rigby *et al.*, 2010).

The assessment of a patient's health status can be considered to be the cornerstone of your nursing practice. The aim of identifying patient symptoms or health problems is not only to provide relief and prevent recurrence, but also primarily to implement evidence-based interventions. Using validated assessment tools and standardized criteria for symptom presentation will inform decisions when planning and implementing individualized treatments. Since end-of-life symptoms are burdensome and can be agonizing, guidelines prioritize undertaking regular assessment of needs as important to the delivery of high-quality patient care (Qaseem *et al.*, 2008). Continued evaluation and monitoring are nursing responsibilities, and are vital for confirming the effectiveness of clinical interventions and whether these need discontinuing or modifying (Figure 18.1).

Principles of good assessment include:

- conveying unconditional positive regard (non-judgemental);
- forming a close and trusting relationship to communicate commitment to addressing patient problems/ symptoms;
- active listening and demonstrating empathy;

- communicating and explaining nursing activities using simple, clear, and lay terms;
- demonstrating respect and sensitivity of individuals regardless of age, gender, or culture;
- competence with appropriate use of assessment tools for end-of-life symptoms;
- documenting and sharing findings and patient preferences with the health team.

Tools for delivery of end-of-life care

The End-of-life Care Strategy (DH, 2008a) acknowledges that, whilst differences of individual disease trajectories exist, a stepped end-of-life care pathway (Figure 18.2) with core components should be addressed at each phase. You should embrace themes across the pathway as part of your practice. High-quality care provision for those who are diagnosed with a life-limiting illness should encompass:

- being treated with dignity and respect;
- having appropriate information to allow for personal choice and control;
- having personal needs assessed and reviewed;
- receiving optimal comfort care and symptom control;
- receiving care from professionals with specialist training;
- having psychological, social, and spiritual needs met;
- having the needs of family/carers adhered to and met.

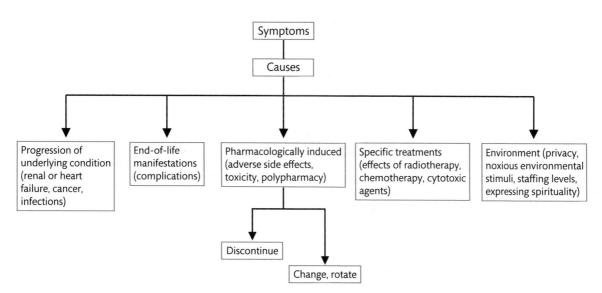

Figure 18.1 Causes for symptoms at end of life.

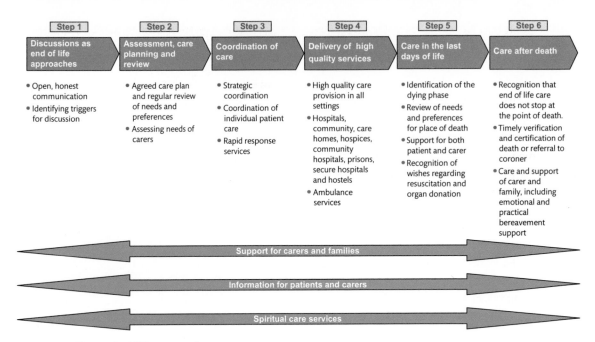

Figure 18.2 The end-of-life care pathway.

(Department of Health, 2008a © Crown Copyright)

Within the strategy (DH, 2008a), three tools are endorsed for supporting hospital- and community-based clinical teams in delivering excellence in end-of-life care and which are integral to the pathway.

- The Gold Standards Framework http://www.gold-standardsframework.nhs.uk/
- The Preferred Priorities of Care http://www.endoflifecareforadults.nhs.uk/tools/core-tools/preferredprioritiesforcare
- The Liverpool Care Pathway http://www.liv.ac.uk/mcpcil/liverpool-care-pathway/

The Gold Standards Framework (GSF) aims to support patient and family choice, and to promote professional communication and collaboration in coordination of care needs, with the aim of supporting people to die where they choose using a three-step approach. Evidence suggests that using the GSF can reduce crisis admissions to hospital, support people to die at home if they wish, and provide a structure to the management of care (Badger *et al.*, 2007; 2009).

Trigger points for using the GSF include increasing frailty, repeated hospital admissions with progressive symptoms that may be associated with the disease, and difficulties in the care setting, such as carer coping. To address some of these concerns, the GSF promotes open and honest communication with the patient and family in making important decisions regarding his or her care. A national prognostic indicator has been developed to help health professionals to identify the dying phase.

Once the prognosis has been determined, a plan of care will be devised in accordance with the level of need. The patient details will be kept in a GP-based register and regular meetings will involve case discussions with those engaged in care delivery. The framework promotes teamwork by adhering to seven elements. (See the Gold Standards Framework website for more information.)

The Preferred Priorities of Care (PPC) embraces a holistic approach to assessment and is mindful that patient preference is not just about the place of care. Open discussion between the patient and care providers is necessary about what key processes might be implemented once the onset of a life-limiting condition has been diagnosed. A record of what is important to the patient, his or her personal values and goals, and which family members and friends are to be involved in discussions is made that informs the care plan. Once detail is confirmed and documented, the care plan will support the patient's wishes regardless of home, hospital, or hospice setting. Application of the PPC facilitates patients and their families being well informed, supported, empowered, and confident in their healthcare. Additionally, this can increase the confidence among professionals involved in delivering quality end-of-life care (Dale *et al.*, 2009; Shaw *et al.*, 2010).

In the community setting, the district nurse's role is pivotal in assuring that all aspects of care are coordinated, including medication and equipment, and that a trusting relationship with patients and carers is developed that includes providing information and practical advice (Eyre, 2010).

The Liverpool Care Pathway (LCP) aims to provide a hospice/specialist palliative care approach, providing a multidisciplinary tool to aid decision-making, documentation, communication, and care planning for the end of life for all patients, particularly those being cared for in a generalist setting (Ellershaw and Wilkinson, 2003). The pathway has been adopted as a national framework for delivering best practice for the last days of life (DH, 2008a). It is recommended for all patients in the final days of life regardless of diagnosis or care setting; however, adaptations have been developed in accordance to clinical environments like community settings, intensive care (ICU), and subsequently for paediatric settings.

Key components of the LCP support the clinical team in the following four key areas.

1. Identifying patients who are in the last days of their life

2. Making an initial assessment of needs that includes:
   - assessing patient and family insight
   - reviewing comfort needs such as the discontinuation of unnecessary interventions and medications
   - anticipatory prescribing as required medication for comfort care
   - assessing religious spiritual needs
   - documentation of communication needs of family

It is important for the nurse to check patient and family understanding, and to follow up with written information regarding the LCP approach and issues related to visiting, parking, where the family can stay, and facilities for their use such as canteen and washing facilities.

1. Ongoing care of the dying person and family involves regular assessment of comfort, including emotional and spiritual needs. Any identified variances are documented with appropriate interventions recorded. For example, an assessment might reveal a change in patient and family coping abilities owing to emotional distress. A practical intervention might be to provide them with an opportunity to express their fears and worries, or to involve the chaplain or religious leader for spiritual support (Pattison, 2008).

2. After-death care involves providing supportive care to the newly bereaved, including facilitating family members to view and say their goodbyes and providing information on what the next steps are (Pattison, 2008; Hills and Albarran, 2010a; 2010b). Care of the deceased is important to communicating dignity and respect for the person who has died, and also to facilitate preparation of the body for onward safe journey to the mortuary. Cultural practices need to be addressed sensitively at this stage. Nurses should assess for spiritual needs and document the patient's wishes, so that his or her religious/spiritual needs can be addressed and so that, after death, the body and the newly bereaved are managed in a dignified manner (Searight and Gafford, 2005; Hills and Albarran, 2010a).

This pathway aims to facilitate prompt communication with primary care staff by ensuring that the GP is informed as soon as the patient is diagnosed as being in the dying phase and as soon as death occurs. During this period, GPs and district nurses are important sources of family support.

Making the clinical assessment

This section will explore the nursing assessment of individual end-of-life symptoms and tools that can support nurses in gathering relevant patient data to inform decisions.

Making the clinical assessment of problems: pain

Pain is highly prevalent at the end of life, with rates varying between 40% and 70% for a range of terminal conditions; controlling and relieving this symptom is therefore a hallmark of effective palliative care (Chang *et al.*, 2007). For patients with malignant or other terminal conditions, the frequency of pain increases markedly over time, escalating in the final days of life. Some patients may have

CASE STUDY 18.1   *Applying the Gold Standards Framework*

Mr Smith is a 72-year-old man with progressive heart failure, which limits his activities. He has been admitted to hospital twice over a 2-month period with increasing breathlessness. You are a district nurse who is asked by the GP to visit him and make an assessment, because he has now decided to register Mr Smith on the Gold Standards Framework. Mr Smith lives with his wife, who has early symptoms of dementia; he has a caring daughter who lives close by. During your interaction, Mr Smith tells you that he wishes to stay at home with his wife of 50 years.

Questions

➤ Look at the Gold Standards Framework website and prognostic indicator guidance. How has this supported the GP's decision-making process?

➤ In what stage of end of life do you think Mr Smith may be?

➤ what sort of symptoms might Mr Smith be experiencing?

➤ How can you assess for the effects that breathlessness might be having on this patient?

➤ As a professional involved with making the assessment and communicating with the Smith family, what skills might you use when you first go to see them?

➤ How would you explain advanced care planning to Mr Smith?

➤ Look at the preferred priorities for the care document to support Mr Smith to stay at home. What sort of care and equipment might he need?

➤ What other professionals do you think may be important in Mr Smith's care?

➤ In consideration of Mrs Smith's needs, is there any care that needs to be put in place to support her?

 See the Online Resource Centre for the answers to these questions.

CASE STUDY 18.2   *Applying the Liverpool Care Pathway (LCP)*

Mrs Jones is an 82-year-old lady admitted via the emergency department following a collapse at home. A scan reveals that she has had a catastrophic cerebral vascular event and has difficulty communicating. The medical team have made a decision that she is probably in the last days of her life, because her condition is deemed unrecoverable. You have been asked to commence the Liverpool Care Pathway (LCP) approach to care.

Questions

➤ Look at the LCP document. How is it structured? Does it incorporate the elements of care needed for this lady?

➤ How would you communicate the information to the family?

➤ What considerations do the family need at this time?

➤ What sorts of symptoms are commonly experienced at the end of life?

➤ What drugs could be prescribed in anticipation of potential health problems and symptoms?

➤ What drugs could be prescribed in anticipation of potential health problems and symptoms?

 See the Online Resource Centre for the answers to these questions.

experienced pain for a number of years; for others, this may be a recent event. Being free from pain, shortness of breath, and anxiety have been ranked as highly important, and as quality end-of-life care measures from both the patient and recently bereaved relatives (Steinhauser *et al.*, 2000).

Causation

Patient distress and discomfort at the end of life may be aggravated by the presence of other chronic illnesses (e.g. back pain), disabilities, limited mobility, emotional concerns, and the side effects of specific (e.g. oncology) treatments (Chang *et al.*, 2007). Performing regular assessment, responding to physical or emotional changes, and adjusting treatments and care accordingly are therefore vital elements of the nursing care plan.

Criteria used to assess severity of pain symptoms/problems

A strategy that involves physical examination, pain history, and the use of validated assessment tools can enable nurses to capture the many aspects of this symptom. Assessment should enable nurses to differentiate whether the presenting pain is disease-related, caused by disability, a side effect, has a psychological component, or is due to other causes (Glare *et al.*, 2003; Sherman *et al.*, 2004; Miller *et al.*, 2001).

Pain assessment tools also direct nurses to consider features of quality, intensity, location, radiation, frequency, precipitating factors, and measures that bring relief. (For more information on assessment tools, see Chapter 25 Managing Pain ⬄.) Open-ended questions, sensory and affective verbal descriptors, body maps, and numerical rating scales all enable the nurse to consider/understand the nature and severity of pain symptoms on the physical and emotional well-being of patients with terminal illnesses (Miller *et al.*, 2001). In developing an understanding of the possible source and origin of the pain, you can be more specific with your questions and discriminate differential causes. Pain observation scales are useful for patients who lack capacity or have cognitive impairment; this includes the Abbey pain scale (Abbey *et al.*, 2004), which is suitable for individuals suffering with dementia. Using descriptors that patients use when reporting the quality of their discomfort is essential. A burning sensation can be applied in cases of bladder discomfort, to neuropathic pain caused by shingles, or linked with oesophageal reflux. Careful assessment, alertness to the terms used, and locating the affected region will assist in identifying whether the patient's symptoms can be relieved by antibiotics, antiviral medications, or antacids.

Making the clinical assessment of problems: dyspnoea

Dyspnoea is one of the most distressing symptoms experienced by the terminally ill. The prevalence of dyspnoea in the advanced stages of oncological and non-oncological conditions is high, and it afflicts a sizeable number of individuals with life-limiting illnesses (Abernethy *et al.*, 2010; Trammer *et al.*, 2003). The symptom is subjectively experienced as difficult or distressed breathing and is reported to affect 50–70% of cancer patients (Abernethy and Wheeler, 2008), but it is more common in those with end-stage lung disease (Ross and Alexander, 2001a). The severity of breathing distress escalates as patients near death. In those with advanced stages of lung cancer, for example, it can increase from 15–30% at the time of diagnosis to 65–90% during the later stages of illness (Kvale, 2007). It is also noted that prevalence of breathing difficulties will be higher if pain and anxiety are high. The significance of this symptom is becoming clinically important because increasingly, based on evidence involving a spectrum of conditions, it is being viewed as a predictor of poor quality of life and mortality (Abernethy *et al.*, 2010).

Causation

The presence of dyspnoea suggests that pathophysiological mechanisms mediate a series of responses to regulate either breathing, the mechanics of breathing, and/or the pattern of breathing (Abernethy and Wheeler, 2008; Ross and Alexander, 2001a). Patients experiencing breathlessness are rarely hypoxaemic when assessed against standard criteria of arterial blood gas findings and saturation readings from pulse oximetry (Ferris *et al.*, 2010), but the results are useful in eliminating other causes. Although the reasons for dyspnoea are multifactorial, they may be classified as pulmonary and non-pulmonary (Table 18.2), but most causes are due to involvement of cancer in the respiratory system, an indirect complication resulting from lung cancer, the effects of standard therapies, respiratory complications, and other comorbidities (Kvale *et al.*, 2007). This is most likely to result from a complex

Table 18.2 Causes of the symptom of dyspnoea

Pulmonary causes	Non-pulmonary causes
Bronchospasm	Hypoxia
Pleural effusion	Anaemia
Chronic obstructive pulmonary disease	Heart failure
Chest infections (e.g. pneumonia)	Superior vena cava compression
Pulmonary embolism	Anxiety
Lung cancer	Lymphangitic tumour spread
Pulmonary oedema	Pulmonary oedema
Lung toxicity induced by radiation and chemotherapy	Pericardial effusion

interface between physiological, social, psychological, and environmental factors (Abernethy *et al.*, 2010; Kvale *et al.*, 2007). Your aim is to identify the underlying cause and to apply targeted evidence-based interventions that will resolve and control dyspnoea (Abernethy *et al.*, 2010).

Criteria used to assess severity of dyspnoea problems

While the use of assessment tools can illuminate the dyspnoea experience and subjectively score its effects on individuals, the lack of a globally valid, reliable, and responsive measure hinders the management of patients and research that aims to determine the value of specific clinical interventions (Dorman *et al.*, 2007). Available assessment tools, of which 29 have been reviewed, can be divided into three subgroups according to their purpose (Dorman *et al.*, 2007); examples of each group are described below.

- Scales that measure severity of dyspnoea
  - Visual analogue scales (horizontally or vertically) (Figure 18.3)
  - Numeric rating scales (Modified Borg Scale)
  - Faces scale
- Descriptions of breathlessness scales
  - Cancer dyspnoea scale (CDS; Tanaka *et al.*, 2000)
- Scales that measure functional abilities or limitations linked with breathlessness

- Medical Research Council Dyspnoea Scale (Mahler and Wells, 1988)
- Chronic Respiratory Disease Questionnaire (CRD-Q; Guyatt *et al.*, 1987)

In terms of scales that measure severity, one validated tool used to quantify the effects of exercise on dyspnoea is the Modified Borg Scale (Borg, 1982; Kvale *et al.*, 2007). Scoring difficulty with breathing relies on a 0–10-point visual analogue scale (Figure 18.4). This instrument was developed as a ratio scale, so that a score of 8 represents twice as much dyspnoea as a score of 4. Additionally, the use of anchoring descriptors along the scale is valuable for assessing trends and response to treatments. Since its inception, the tool has undergone various modifications; however, it cannot be used to discern rapid changes either in terms of health status or based on treatments because measures are linked to specific activities and a time frame (Meek, 2004). For scores to be of use, the tool must be applied consistently, and clear instructions need to be given to patients (Ries, 2006). This measure also provides an indication of functional (exertion) ability/limitation associated with physical activities (Dorman *et al.*, 2007; see **Chapter 15 Managing Breathlessness** (→)).

A systematic review of measurement scales to determine breathlessness identified that many are ideal for palliative care (including numerical rating scales, the Modified Borg Scale, the CDS, and CRD-Q), but that further research is required prior to their wide adoption into clinical practice (Dorman *et al.*, 2007). When dealing with patients from multicultural backgrounds, it is important that nurses explain what purpose the tool serves and that the patient also understands the results of the assessment.

The following clinical tests should augment findings from application of assessment tools:

- full blood count and haemoglobin;
- chest X-ray;
- peak flow;
- electrocardiogram;
- pulse oximetry;
- arterial blood gases;
- measuring respiratory rate.

The collection of data sources will help either to include or to exclude possible organic diagnoses such as congestive heart failure and evidence of acute/chronic

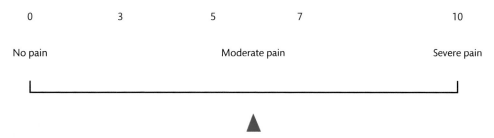

Figure 18.3 Example of a visual analogue scale.

0	Nothing at all (no breathing difficulty)
0.5	Very, very slight
1	Very slight
2	Slight
3	Moderate
4	Somewhat severe (moderately severe)
5	Severe
6	
7	Very severe
8	
9	Very, very severe/difficult
10	Maximal (breathing difficulty)

Figure 18.4 Modified Borg Scale.

Reproduced with permission from Borg, G.V. (1982) Psychological basis of perceived exertion. *Medicine and Science in Sports and Exercise* 14: 377–81.

respiratory disease. Feelings of anxiety, the presence of pain, and apprehension over impending death may precipitate breathlessness, and therefore it behoves nurses during their assessment to consider both disease-related and external factors that may provoke dyspnoea. Limiting the assessment to the scoring breathing difficulties will not address the underlying causes, therefore it is necessary to use a combination of validated instruments. Once assessment baseline is completed, the data will provide the basis for managing breathlessness and

guide decisions that focus on effective symptom relief and control.

Making the clinical assessment of problems: nausea and vomiting

Nausea and vomiting are unpleasant and emotionally distressing symptoms, which are common in around 60% of terminally ill cancer patients, with a prevalence of around 40% in the last 6 weeks of life (Trammer *et al.*, 2003; Von

Gunten, 2005; Wood *et al.*, 2007a). These symptoms occur regularly in patients with other terminal illnesses, but not all of those with cancer will experience nausea, vomiting, or both symptoms. There is a higher incidence for the symptom of nausea than vomiting, but both are important in determining quality of life and are easily corrected and controlled.

Causation

The causes of nausea and vomiting in the terminally ill are diverse (Table 18.3). Wood *et al.* (2007a) discuss the most cited aetiological factors as being the following.

- Biochemical derangements: 33% (metabolic and electrolyte disorders, drug side effects, infections)
- Impaired gastric function: 44%
- Visceral and serosal-related: 31% (bowel obstruction, gastric bleed, enteritis and constipation)

However, the interaction of neural pathways located in brain structures (chemoreceptor trigger zone, cerebral cortex, vestibular apparatus, and vomiting centre) and the lining of the gastrointestinal tract are significant contributors of these symptoms (Figure 18.5; Wood *et al.*, 2007a). Key neurotransmitters within the brain and gastrointestinal

tract have an important function in mediating nausea and vomiting. These include:

- dopamine;
- serotonin;
- acetylcholine;
- histamine.

While all are located across the brain, some are more predominant at specific sites, although cerebral cortex mediation of nausea and vomiting is likely to be more complex and will not involve neurotransmitter activity (Ferris *et al.*, 2002). Understanding the pathophysiological basis and cause for these symptoms is necessary in deciding what pharmacological interventions would be most effective in relieving and controlling nausea and vomiting in individuals (Ross and Alexander, 2001a).

Criteria used to assess nausea and vomiting problems

Determining the underlying cause for these symptoms, including whether they are of primary origin or secondary to an illness, is a clear objective in planning future treatments. The nurse plays a vital role in the assessment of the patient with nausea and vomiting and coexisting medical

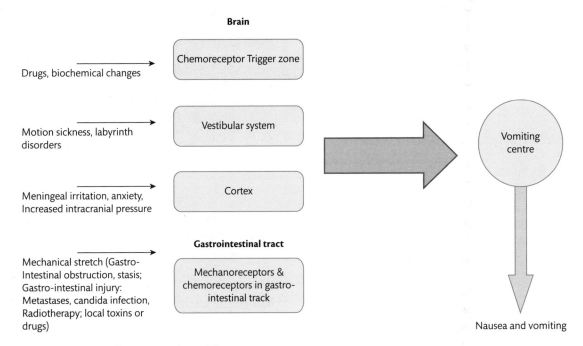

Figure 18.5   Causes of nausea and vomiting.

Modified from Wood *et al.* © (2007a). Management of intractable nausea and vomiting in patients at the end-of-life: 'I was feeling nauseous all of the time … nothing was working'. *Journal of the American Medical Association* **298**(10): 1196–207.

conditions, with physical examination and history-taking crucial (Wood *et al.*, 2007a).

- Physical examination
  - Oral cavity assessment determining whether there are signs of viral/fungal infections or lesions
  - Abdominal examination for the presence of distension, a mass, or malnourishment (also pain and rigidity)
  - Auscultation and percussion: high-pitched or overactive sounds may suggest partial or complete bowel obstruction; a lack of bowel sounds is indicative of an **ileus**
  - Decreased skin elasticity may be a sign of dehydration
  - Evidence of postural hypotension (lying and standing blood pressure)
  - Evidence of bowel impaction

    (Miller and Miller, 2002; Wood *et al.*, 2007a)

- Symptom history
  - Precipitating factors (for example, does this occur before/after meals?)
  - Other factors that provoke nausea and vomiting (e.g. movement, medications such as opioids, NSAIDs, cytotoxic drugs)
  - Associated symptoms (dizziness, epigastric pain, bloating, changes in bowel habits)
  - What relieves/prevents nausea and vomiting?
  - Is there any accompanying of heartburn or reflux?
  - Have bowel habits changed?
  - Has altering/reducing diet and fluid intake helped with nausea and vomiting?
  - Frequency of episodes over a 24-hour period
  - Volume and content of vomit during a 24-hour period

    (Miller and Miller, 2002; Wood *et al.*, 2007a)

Laboratory investigations may determine specific causes, including renal or hepatic failure, electrolyte disorders, and pancreatitis. Similarly, elevated serum levels of some medications (e.g. digoxin) may also result in episodes of nausea and vomiting. Abdominal X-rays are sometimes useful with regard to mechanical problems such as constipation and squashed stomach syndrome resulting from an enlarged liver (Wood *et al.*, 2007a). The aim is to identify the cause of nausea and vomiting (Table 18.3) and to select medications or non-pharmacological interventions that are most effective for relieving the distress for individuals nearing death.

Making the clinical assessment of problems: delirium

Terminal delirium is another common symptom experienced by patients in the later stages of life and presents a sudden deterioration in mental state that is often accompanied by confusion, restlessness, and agitation. Reports suggest that between 28% and 85% of terminally ill patients become delirious as their disease progresses, and just under half will experience agitation (Casarettt and Inouye, 2001; Clary and Lawson, 2009). Symptom manifestation varies according to the population being studied and the criteria used to define delirium. Delirium may be evident as hyperactivity, hypoactivity, or a combination of both behaviours (see **Chapter 17 Managing Delirium and Confusion** ⮕). Managing this syndrome can be difficult, challenging, and distressing: families may feel anxious and concerned because the patient may be confused, incoherent, in apparent pain, and behaving out of character. This can affect the quality of personal interactions between patients and family members. Explanations about the possible trajectory of symptoms and causes for delirium will help to develop understanding, and you should encourage family members to communicate with the patient about familiar aspects that can be helpful.

Causation

Factors responsible for the onset of delirium can be linked to step-up increases in opioids to manage pain. Other causes precipitating a change in mental state include: opioid toxicity; polypharmacy; underlying conditions; **hyponatraemia**; **hypocalcaemia**; **hypoxaemia**; infection; constipation; urinary retention; dehydration; sleep deprivation; pain; and stress. Some of these may be reversible and therefore careful assessment to exclude contributing factors is important (Clary and Lawson, 2009; Ferris *et al.*, 2002). Generally, signs of delirium or confusion tend to herald that the end of life is near (Ross and Alexander, 2001b).

Table 18.3 Eleven Ms of causes and pathophysiology for nausea and vomiting

Cause	Pathophysiology
Metastasis	
• Cerebral	Increased intracerebral pressure causing effect on chemoreceptor trigger zone or meningeal mechanoreceptors
• Liver	Toxin build-up activating chemoreceptor trigger zone
Meningeal irritation	Raised intracranial pressure probably activating meningeal mechanoreceptors
Movement	Vestibular irritation, which may be provoked by morphine or affecting tumour bulk and thus activating stretch receptors
Mental state (anxiety)	Multiple receptors within the cerebral cortex
Medications	
• Opioids	Chemoreceptor trigger zone, vestibular irritation, reduced bowel motility
• Chemotherapy	Chemoreceptor trigger zone, gastrointestinal tract disturbance
• Others, e.g. NSAIDs	Gastrointestinal disturbance, e.g. gastritis
Mucosal irritation	
• NSAIDs	Gastrointestinal tract, gastritis
• Gastro-oesophageal reflux	Gastrointestinal tract, gastritis, oesophagitis
Mechanical obstruction	
• Within intestinal system	Constipation, tumours
• Outside intestinal system	Tumour exerting external pressure on bowel, fibrotic structure (all of the above thus activating gastric mechanoreceptors in the bowel, causing nausea and vomiting)
Motility (decreased)	Gastrointestinal tract, central nervous system
• Opioids	
• Ileus	
• Other medications	
Metabolic derangements	Chemoreceptor trigger zone
• Hypercalcaemia	
• Hyponatraemia	
• Renal/hepatic failure (uraemia, ascites)	
Microbial-related	Chemoreceptor trigger zone
• Local irritation (oral infections, oesophagitis, gastritis due to infections)	
• Systemic sepsis	
Myocardial dysfunction	Vagal stimulation, cerebral cortex, chemoreceptor trigger zone

Source: Adapted from Ross and Alexander, (2001a)

Criteria used to assess delirium

Chapter 17 Managing Delirium and Confusion ⮕ highlights the importance of clinical examination, and natural and clinical history (Glare *et al.*, 2003). Assessment tools such as the mini-mental state examination are extremely useful and these are discussed later in the chapter.

Making the clinical assessment of problems: anxiety and depression

A diagnosis of a terminal condition can be devastating for individuals and their families, and such patients are more predisposed to psychiatric disorders than the general population. Patients will inevitably experience grief and be anxious about many things, but two particular fears will relate to reduced life expectancy and unpredictability about the future. The possibility of death, disfigurement, disability, and dependence on others are typical areas of worry and concern. Additionally, where medical interventions can offer only palliation rather than a cure or when response to therapeutic measures produces limited health gain, this will increase the severity of distress and anxiety for the patient and family (Roth and Massie, 2007).

The prevalence of anxiety levels among individuals with a terminal condition is being reported to be higher than that among healthy individuals. Specifically, patients with advanced cancer are more likely to exhibit a combination of anxiety and depressive symptoms rather than only anxiety (Roth and Massie, 2007). It is also suggested that anxiety levels fluctuate, with increases apparent during disease progression, but falls as physical condition deteriorates. Anxiety can manifest in different ways, including depressive disorder, generalized anxiety disorder, panic, and post-traumatic stress disorder (Roth and Massie, 2007). Nurses must therefore convey a compassionate, dignified, sensitive, and non-judgemental approach when supporting patients and their families.

Depression is a psychological manifestation for which patients with advanced life-threatening conditions remain at high risk. The prevalence rates are estimated to range from 3% to 53% (Block, 2005; Rayner *et al.*, 2009). Individuals can experience periodic and intense moments of tearfulness, social isolation, worthlessness, sadness, guilt, and low withdrawn moods, which, if they persist, may lead to serious and grave consequences, including suicidal ideation (Block, 2005; Noorani and Montagnini, 2007). For example, the presence of depression can adversely influence compliance with treatment, self-perceptions of disability, and prognostic and mortality outcomes (Rayner *et al.*, 2009). Depression increases the risk of suicide and of requests to accelerate death (Block, 2005; Noorani and Montagnini, 2007). One of the main obstacles to treatment of this symptom is poor recognition in terminal ill and palliative groups (Block, 2005; Lorenz *et al.*, 2008; Rayner *et al.*, 2009). Symptom underreporting and concealment from clinicians and family members also explains some of the difficulties in establishing a diagnosis of depression, and, as a consequence, reliable and accurate data on the prevalence in palliative populations are unknown (Noorani and Montagnini, 2007).

Causation

The causes of anxiety among patients at the end of life can be varied and complex (Ferris *et al.*, 2002). In many cases, there are intense feelings of dread, terror, helplessness, and uneasiness, which may become magnified if death is perceived as impending. Terminally ill patients may also experience anxiety symptoms that can be divided into somatic and psychological (Roth and Massie, 2007). Somatic symptoms may be linked to panic attacks, resulting in tachycardic episodes, clamminess, shortness of breath, feelings of nausea, and vomiting. Anxiety symptoms can also cover problems with sleeping, restlessness, concentration difficulties, loss of appetite, and libido. Poor pain control, metabolic derangements, substance withdrawal, and the effects of some medications (i.e. corticosteroids) may precipitate anxiety symptoms, including restlessness and agitation (Ferris *et al.*, 2002; Roth and Massie, 2007). The symptoms of depression are similarly characterized by prolonged low mood states, disinterest in the world, disrupted sleep pattern with early waking, lethargy, poor concentration span, low self-esteem, pathological crying, and thoughts of death (Block, 2005; Rayner *et al.*, 2009).

Criteria used to assess anxiety and depression

Anxiety can be assessed by considering possible underlying causes such as suboptimal pain relief, metabolic derangements, and whether the patient's mood may be drug-induced. The assessment should also determine whether there is a known history of phobias, pre-existing panic disorders, generalized anxiety disorders, or drug misuse, because all of these can intensify feelings of anxiety and influence patient mood and behaviour. A series of specific questions can help to assess and diagnose anxiety within the palliative care context (Roth and Massie, 2007: 52). Examples include the following.

- Do you feel nervous or jittery?
- Do you avoid certain activities or people because of fear?
- Have you felt a lump in your throat or a knot in the pit of your stomach when getting upset?

Other more established and validated instruments for screening and monitoring patients include the Hospital Anxiety Depression Scale (HADS), which has been validated for the palliative care population (Noorani and

Montagnini, 2007). This widely used self-reported assessment tool comprises two subscales of 14 items (anxiety and depression), and focuses specifically on cognitive symptoms.

Assessment of depression requires excluding and differentiating between other possible diagnoses such as grief, delirium, anxiety, and the side effects of some drugs (Block, 2005). The assessment should include determining cognitive functioning, and eliminating organic causes and a previous history of emotional problems (Noorani and Montagnini, 2007). Asking patients directly whether they are 'depressed' provides a sensitive and specific measure of depression among those with advanced cancer nearing the end of life (Block, 2005; Noorani and Montagnini, 2007). Other questions that may be asked have a future orientation and can help to gauge depressive states. However, the *Diagnostic and Statistical Manual of Mental Disorder IV* (DSM-IV) is recognized as reliable in diagnosing major depression when used by trained clinicians (Noorani and Montagnini, 2007). The tool comprises a number of criteria, and evidence of five symptoms for a period of 2 weeks or more, such as depression or an inability to experience pleasure (**anhedonia**), confirms the diagnosis. Simpler and validated depression screening tools for use in palliative care populations have been proposed, including HADS and a 100-mm visual analogue scale.

Accessing the evidence

There are a number of evidence-based sources to guide the management of patients prior to end of life and after-death care. These may include systematic reviews, original research, meta-analyses of studies, and evidence-based guidelines. In particular, systematic reviews of the literature appraise research studies according to specific criteria to determine the strength of evidence in support of a specific intervention. Quality information, in the form of guidelines, research, and systematic reviews that will inform the delivery of patient care, may be obtained from websites (general and specialist interest) and journals. However, for ethical reasons, it may not always be possible to undertake clinical trials on patients who are vulnerable and dying.

- Websites provided by organizations committed to developing evidence to inform decision-making and specialist interest groups can offer a range of learning materials and resources to support the development of practice, but caution is required in evaluating sources of evidence.
- Evidence-based websites include:
  — Cochrane Library **www.cochrane.org.docs/ descrip.htm**
  — National Library of Medicine (National Institutes of Health) **http://www.nlm.nih.gov/cancer**
  — TRIP Clinical Search Engine **http://www.tripdatabase.com/**
  — National Guideline Clearinghouse **http://www. guideline.gov**
  — Nursing, Midwifery and Allied Health professionals gateway **http://www.intute.ac.uk/nmah/**
  — Joanna Briggs Institute **http://www.joannabriggs. edu.au/**
  — Centre for Evidence Based Nursing **http://www. york.ac.uk/healthsciences**
  — National Institute for Health and Clinical Excellence **http://www.nice.org.uk** (re the 'End-of-Life Quality Standard')

Evaluating sources of evidence

Evaluation of evidence in the public domain requires application of specific tools. For example, in judging the quality of content on a website, the following criteria need to be assessed to ensure confidence in the quality of materials.

- Authority (institution, publishers, domains with gov ac, edu, and org are controlled and reputable)
- Currency (Is the material credible, up to date, and produced by respected authorities? Is there any evidence of editorial supervision, professional affiliations, and regular maintenance? Is it regulated by an international code of practice? For example, Health on the Net (HoN) is an award given for ethical standards and quality of content of websites that is reviewed on a regular basis.)
- Coverage (consider depth, breadth, and scope—is this extensive and relevant?)
- Accuracy (is the content factual, comprehensive, directed at a targeted audience, and are purposeful, listed resources available?)
- Objectivity (fair/balanced, depth, wide scope, no conflicts of interest)

Consensus guidelines may be developed by expert opinions in the absence of strong evidence from research and these can offer guidance on pharmacological interventions, approaches to communication, breaking news, processes for withdrawing treatment, after-death care, and providing supportive information for the bereaved (Douglas *et al.*, 2009; Truog *et al.*, 2008).

Some journals, such as those listed below, will produce short reviews of recently published research that are presented in a short, concise, and accessible format:

Bandolier: **http://www.jr2.ac.uk/bandolier**
Evidence-based Nursing **http://ebn.bmjjournals.com/**

Utilizing the evidence base in managing end-of-life care

Defining or diagnosing the dying phase during the transition into the final days of life can prove very difficult owing to the differences in disease trajectories (Murray *et al.*, 2005). For those with a cancer diagnosis or terminal illness, the last days of life can usually be identified by a number of clinical indicators. The evidence base to prevent, control, or effectively manage these is not always available or robust.

Pain symptoms

Controlling, managing, and preventing pain has been guided by the World Health Organization analgesic ladder (2011), with morphine being the drug of choice in those with moderate to severe pain with advanced and terminal conditions. The ladder comprises three steps.

- Step I (mild pain): initiating pain relief with a non-opioid (paracetamol, aspirin, or non-steroidal anti-inflammatory drugs, e.g. ibuprofen)
- Step II (moderate pain): if measures in step I are ineffective, progress to a weak opioid (codeine, dihydrocodeine, tramadol, co-codamol) with or without non-opioid/adjuvant
- Step III: transition to strong opioid (morphine, diamorphine, fentanyl), with or without opioid/adjuvant

Lorenz *et al.* (2008) conducted a systematic review to address the validity of standard interventions in end-of-life care. To assess what treatments work well for treating pain in palliative care, they reviewed 17 studies that explored a variety of pain-relieving strategies in cancer. Data synthesis identified that the use of NSAIDs, opioids, biphosphonates, radiotherapy, or radiopharmaceuticals were strongly supported by evidence from well-conducted studies. There was a weaker evidence base to support the routine use of biphosphonates for bone-related pain. The systematic review identified that some methodological limitations, in particular the heterogeneity of study design, forbade comparison of specific opioids or opioid delivery systems. From this work, Qaseem *et al.* (2008) have developed a practice guideline for pain, dyspnoea, and depression. Inconclusive evidence supported the routine prescription of morphine or diamorphine for patients at end-stage renal failure (Douglas *et al.*, 2009). Based on available evidence, use of alfentanil by continuous infusion is recommended as a substitute for this group of patients.

Non-opioids with NSAIDS are effective in mild pain, which is defined as less than 3 on a 0–10-point visual analogue scale; however, because pain is subjective, a score of 3 for some may require stronger analgesia. Should pain increase to a moderate level range of 4–6, then a weak opioid such as codeine can be added. If this measure proves to be ineffective and pain exceeds 7, initiation of a stronger opioid should not be delayed (Sherman *et al.*, 2004). Equally, for patients initially presenting with severe pain, there should be no delay in the administration of intravenous opioids, which are titrated until symptom relief is achieved (Ferris *et al.*, 2002; Welsh Medicine Resource Centre, 2006).

Practical principles

There are practical principles that inform the management, prevention of pain, and use of opioids in end-of-life situations.

- When pain is constant and rated as moderate to severe, patients should begin with immediate-release formulations (such as oral morphine or subcutaneous morphine) because they are ideal for rapid pain relief due to their quick onset, reduced time to peak effect, and rapid attainment in titrating optimum dose (Glare *et al.*, 2003; Welsh Medicine Resource Centre, 2006). Morphine is a strong oral opioid and

---

Box 18.1   Online sources of guidelines and learning materials for end-of-life care provision

End-of-Life/Palliative Education Resource Centre: **http://www.eperc.mcw.edu**

National Cancer Institute: **http://www.cancer.gov/cancertopics/pdg/supportive care**

Palliative drugs: **http://www.palliativedrugs.com**

Palliative care matters: **http://www.pallcare.info**

Cancer improvement: **http://www.improvement.nhs.uk/cancer**

New Hampshire Hospice and Palliative Care Organization (opioid guidelines): **http://www.nhhpco.org/opioid2010.htm**

Department of Health End-of-Life Care Programme—Examples of Good Practice Guidance: **http://www.endoflifecare.nhs.uk/eolc**

Gold Standards Framework: **http://www.goldstandardsframework.nhs.uk**

Liverpool Care Pathway—Marie Curie Palliative Care Institute Liverpool: **http://mcpcil.org.uk**

International Institute for End-of-Life Care Lancaster: **http://www.eolc-observatory.net**

Sue Ryder Care Centre for Palliative and End-of-Life Studies: **http://www.nottingham.ac.uk/NMP/Research/SPC/index.aspx**

Department of Health End-of-Life Care Strategy: **http://www.dh.gov.uk/en/publicationsandstatistics/publications/publicationspolicyandguidance/dh_086277**

National Council for Hospice and Specialist Palliative Care: **http://www.ncpc.org.uk**

Map of Medicine—Palliative/End-of-Life Care: **http://healthguides.mapofmedicine.com/map/palliative_and_end_of_life_care1.html**

---

should be given 4-hourly or as necessary, starting with:

— 2.5 mg if the patient is an older adult (in the advanced stages of chronic kidney disease, subcutaneous infusion of fentanyl is recommended: Douglas *et al.*, 2009);

— 5 mg if there are no contraindications;

— 5–10 mg if step II of analgesic ladder was omitted.

- Once pain levels are stable and controlled, a sustained-release opioid preparation can be introduced as twice-daily maintenance therapy (Welsh Medicine Resource Centre, 2006). To swap from immediate release to sustained release involves totalling the dose (e.g. morphine) given in the previous 24 hours and dividing this by 2 (e.g. 200 mg ÷ 2 = 100 mg). The result will give the dose that should be administered 12-hourly and must begin when the next immediate release medication was due.

- Immediate-release opioid preparations for episodes of 'breakthrough pain' or 'rescue' pain (e.g. caused by sudden position change or retching) must be prescribed to be administered 'as necessary' or PRN (Glare *et al.*, 2003). Calculation of the dose involves totalling the amount of sustained-release morphine/subcutaneous morphine given in a 24-hour period and dividing this by 6 (e.g. 300 mg ÷ 6 = 50 mg doses for breakthrough pain to be administered as PRN).

- If there are problems with oral ingestion, inconsistencies in drug absorption, or the parenteral route is considered high risk, continuous subcutaneous opioids via syringe driver should be commenced or transdermal patches can be used (Glare *et al.*, 2003). For morphine conversion to the subcutaneous route, the dosage of the previous 24 hours (e.g. 300 mg of sustained-release morphine) is divided by 2 and delivered over 24 hours. In the case of conversion to diamorphine, because this is three times more powerful than morphine, the equivalent dose is one-third of the total oral dose, this being equivalent to 100 mg subcutaneously over a 24-hour period (Glare *et al.*, 2003; Welsh Medicine Resource Centre, 2006).

- Because of the risk of toxic effects among patients with chronic renal disease at the end of life, morphine and diamorphine are not recommended (Douglas *et al.*, 2009). Fentanyl through the subcutaneous route is recommended instead.

Managing the use of opioids

When caring for patients receiving opioids, the responsibilities of nurses are many and involve the following:

- Ensuring that the dose of prescribed opioids is titrated, against pain scale, until the patient's pain is satisfactorily controlled

- Pain relief strategy should comprise opioids and non-opioid medications

- Increasing the prescribed dose of analgesia prior to clinical procedures and, where appropriate, encouraging individuals to verbalize any symptoms can help to manage and control pain levels

- Continuously monitoring trends in pain levels because opioids can become ineffective or tolerance may develop in some patients; it may be necessary to rotate to a new agent, to change the route of administration, or both, to attain symptom control (Miller *et al.*, 2001; Sherman *et al.*, 2004)

- Being proactive and not waiting for patients to report any discomfort or distress

- When breakthrough doses are ineffective, contacting the specialist palliative care team/hospice team is advisable

- Anticipating the side effects of nausea and constipation associated with opioids by administering prescribed antiemetic therapy and laxatives (Clary and Lawson, 2009; Sherman *et al.*, 2004). If a patient is suffering with diarrhoea, laxatives should be omitted. (Maintaining bowel activity is essential, because risks of constipation are high owing to reduced fluid/food intake/physical activity and use of opioids. Seventy per cent of a dry weight stool comprises bacteria, therefore promoting bowel functioning can enhance patient comfort.)

- Being alert and responding appropriately to the warning indices of opioid toxicity, which include a decrease in respiratory rate, unresponsiveness, hallucinations, pinpoint pupils, and involuntary twitching

- Educating/correcting misconceptions among patients and their families about the low risks of addiction, tolerance, and dependence, because, for many, the stigma associated with opioids can lead to them refusing pain relief (Clary and Lawson, 2009; Ferris *et al.*, 2002; Sherman *et al.*, 2004)

Not all pain experienced by patients is opioid-sensitive, and other medications are usually incorporated into the overall treatment plan, but nurses should be mindful of polypharmacy issues, intolerance problems, drug interactions, and adverse effects. Consideration of other routes to achieve pain relief will overcome difficulties of a failing gastrointestinal system, but alternatives may depend on the type of pain, the availability of analgesic formulations, and the risks to the patient. Options include subcutaneous and parenteral routes, rectal suppositories, and dermal patches. Non-pharmacological options are discussed in Chapter 25 Managing Pain and Chapter 22 Managing Medicines ➡.

Dyspnoea symptoms

The evidence to support the treatment and management of dyspnoea at the end of life is dominated by pharmacological therapies, although non-pharmacological treatments (see below) have been reported in a series of experimental studies to be highly beneficial and valuable to patients (Corner *et al.*, 1996; Bredin *et al.*, 1999; Moore *et al.*, 2002). A core component of supportive patient care involves addressing the perceptions of breathlessness and associated anxiety triggers (Glare *et al.*, 2003). Patients may experience either rapid respiratory rates (greater than 24 breaths 1 min), shallow respirations, or prolonged gaps in between breaths lasting up to 60 seconds. These can be distressing for patients and families, so regular reassurance is important. Nurses also have a valuable role through promoting comfort, regulating patient activities, and creating a relaxed environment.

Pharmacological interventions

Established pharmacological measures include the routine use of either oral or parenteral opioids, which should be titrated until the desired effect is achieved, while avoiding the side effects of toxicity. A three-pronged approach to treating breathlessness for patients with advanced terminal illnesses involves:

- opioids;
- benzodiazepines;
- oxygen therapy.

Opioids

Because of the strength of the evidence base, opioids remain the mainstay of treatment for decreasing subjective reports of breathlessness, with oral route the preferred method for administration (Abernethy *et al.*, 2003; 2010). When the patient is semi-comatose or becomes progressively fragile, subcutaneous or rectal methods should be considered as alternatives.

Systematic reviews of published studies into the effects of opioid preparations in treating dyspnoea for advanced lung diseases and terminal cancer demonstrate moderate quality of evidence (Qaseem *et al.*, 2008). Findings from a systematic appraisal of guidelines, and a number of randomized and non-randomized controlled trials, further support the systematic use of opioids to treat dyspnoea among cancer patients (Viola *et al.*, 2008). Another analysis concluded that opioids can reliably and safely decrease breathlessness for individuals with different life-limiting illnesses (Currow *et al.*, 2009). Use of nebulized opiates is not supported by the current evidence base.

Benzodiazepines

Traditionally, benzodiazepines have been given in combination with opioids and titrated to help to relieve anxiety-induced breathlessness (Glare *et al.*, 2003). According to Abernethy *et al.* (2010) and Viola *et al.* (2008), however, at present there is a lack of conclusive evidence to recommend the routine use of these agents in treating dyspnoea at the end of life.

Oxygen

One recent systematic review (Lorenz *et al.*, 2008) reported that the use of oxygen in cancer was weak and that there was an absence of robust studies exploring its role. Abernethy *et al.* (2010) report data from an international double-blind controlled trial that compared oxygen and room air to assess whether oxygen benefited patients with **refractory breathlessness**. The study identified that both air and oxygen had a positive effect on dyspnoea and quality of life. The role of palliative oxygen is therefore one of perceived benefit, but it is not an intervention endorsed by research except for patients presenting with hypoxaemia (Ben-Aharon *et al.*, 2008). The administration of oxygen may have a placebo effect, and the movement of cool air across the face (delivered via face mask or fan) may induce a sense of relaxation in patients. As Abernethy *et al.* (2010) advise, health professionals must continuously examine the rationale for their practice and develop research questions that enhance the quality of care.

Non-pharmacological interventions

The role for nurses is strongest in this area, and responsibilities are linked with promoting comfort, relieving anxiety, and educating patients and their families. Studies have shown that nurse-led interventions for patients with chronic obstructive pulmonary disease, including psychological support, breathing control, and coping strategies, led to significantly improved outcomes against standard treatments (Bredin *et al.*, 1999; Corner *et al.*, 1996; Moore *et al.*, 2002). Additionally, there is strong evidence, from a Cochrane review, for use for neuroelectrical muscle stimulation and chest wall vibration to relieve breathlessness for malignant and non-malignant diseases (Bausewein *et al.*, 2009).

Other practical suggestions for supporting patients include:

- positioning, sitting upright, using pillows to support;
- breathing training;
- involving physiotherapist to advise on breathing exercises;
- encouraging patients to discuss anxieties;
- monitoring pain and anxiety levels;
- monitoring effects of opioid therapy on breathing.

In some cases, a combination of factors (e.g. opioids) may mean that the respiratory system may become depressed, resulting in the accumulation of secretions, which in turn cause noisy respirations or 'death rattle' (Glare *et al.*, 2003). In these situations, keeping the mouth moist is essential to maintain mucosal comfort. Suction of secretions is generally not recommended; however, drug treatments may provide relief.

Nausea and vomiting symptoms

Pharmacological medications used to control nausea and vomiting are many, and tend to exert their effects at various different sites, including the chemoreceptor trigger zone, vomiting centre in the medulla, serotonin receptors, or gastrointestinal smooth muscle (Miller and Miller, 2002). Where an underlying cause cannot be readily established, a broad-spectrum antiemetic may be initially prescribed.

In the UK, cyclizine (an antihistamine) is broadly prescribed because it acts on the vomiting centre medulla to exert its antiemetic function; it also has antimuscarinic properties (Glare *et al.*, 2003). It may also be combined with glycopyrronium in cases of severe vomiting due to bowel obstruction. Sedation is a side effect of antihistamine-based medications and this may limit their use (Miller and Miller, 2002).

The group of phenothiazines, although widely used for managing nausea and vomiting among patients, are not generally used in palliative care. Their function is aimed at the chemoreceptor trigger zone and they may be administered orally, rectally, or topically. They tend to have a short life and sedative effects (Miller and Miller, 2002; Ross and Alexander, 2001a).

Metoclopramide and haloperidol (dopamine antagonists) may also be prescribed to control nausea and when vomiting is precipitated by a variety of causes (Miller and Miller, 2002). Metoclopramide is a **prokinetic**; this means that it is also suitable if the cause of nausea and vomiting is the result of gastric stasis. However, it can precipitate drowsiness, nervousness, and extrapyramidal effects, and consequently it needs to be selectively prescribed (Glare *et al.*, 2003; Ferris *et al.*, 2002).

Levomepromazine, another antiemetic, has a wide effect on pathway sites that induce vomiting, and it is therefore ideal in palliative care (Glare *et al.*, 2003). However, one drawback is its sedative effects, which may be helpful when patients become restless and agitated.

Specific agents such as ondansetron (this blocks serotonin receptors in the central nervous system and is linked with the chemoreceptor trigger zone and vomiting centre) have been identified to have superior effects for patients with chemotherapy-induced nausea and in cases in which initial antiemetic medications have failed. However, it is expensive and should be discontinued if the symptoms remain uncontrolled after a trial period (Ferris *et al.*, 2002).

Because many patients may be anxious and frightened by persistent vomiting, it is important for nurses to:

- create a calm relaxing atmosphere;
- minimize anxiety by encouraging patients to verbalize any worries;
- if appropriate, administer anxiolytics as prescribed;
- prevent smells (e.g. food) that may precipitate nausea, ensureing, that the room is well ventilated;
- ensure that patients have access to vomit bowls and tissues, and replace these regularly;
- provide mouthwash to freshen the oral cavity;
- maintain nutritional intake with small, but regular, meals;
- ensure hydration is maintained with high-calorie drinks;
- record losses from vomiting;

- keep a diary of episodes and triggers of nausea and vomiting.

With disease progression, a decreased need for food and fluids may follow. Extravascular fluid may be retained in the body, causing oedema, and may compromise skin integrity. The decision to administer artificial nutrients and fluids has to be considered against expected benefits. For example, such measures may be implemented if symptoms are being caused by dehydration. A key role of nurses is to ensure that good oral hygiene and care of skin is always maintained (see **Chapters 20 Managing Hygiene** and **27 Managing the Prevention of Skin Breakdown** ➡). Additionally, a combination of reduced nutritional intake and the effects of terminal illness and medications mean that muscle tone changes or becomes relaxed, so the ability to control bladder/bowel function is decreased (see **Chapter 16 Managing Continence** ➡). To minimize embarrassment, appropriate hygiene needs to be maintained, and urethral catheterization may be necessary in some instances (Glare *et al.*, 2003). Finally, as a result of inadequate oral intake, limited mobility, the presence of oedema, and reduced circulation, skin integrity becomes more vulnerable, and therefore regular assessment and appropriate intervention is mandatory.

Delirium symptoms

Interventions are currently divided into pharmacologically and non-pharmacologically based approaches. Pharmacological measures used in managing delirium aim to enhance the patient's mental state in the last days of life (Casarett and Inouye, 2001). If the patient is severely distressed and agitated, a subcutaneous infusion of midazolam can be started; however, because of cumulative effects, caution is required for patients with chronic renal failure—titration is therefore recommended (Douglas *et al.*, 2009). Midazolam has a role in minimizing anxiety and emotional distress, and is commonly prescribed for intermittent (subcutaneous) injections (Bruce *et al.*, 2006; Glare *et al.*, 2003). Most practitioners aim to relieve symptom distress and to minimize the burden of side effects. It is therefore vital for nurses to keep the patient and family informed about effects of sedative agents while the patient is simultaneously receiving opioids. The role of the nurse is central monitoring of the patient's physical and emotional response to palliative sedation, and to be alert to signs of oversedation (Bruce *et al.*, 2006). For patients who are mildly to moderately delirious, haloperidol, an antipsychotic tranquillizer, can be prescribed as first-line medication (Clary and Lawson, 2009). Haloperidol has been reportedly identified as the drug of choice rather than benzodiazepines for HIV patients with delirium, and is also very effective for opiate-induced confusional states (Casarett and Inouye, 2001; Ross and Alexander, 2001b).

Non-pharmacological protocols seek to encourage and promote cognitive functioning through orientation to routines, time, place, and environment. The role of the nurse involves discussing the aims of care with the patient and family, and is vital in maintaining patient safety and minimizing emotional problems (Bruce *et al.*, 2006). Practical interventions to improve quality of sleep involve using relaxation techniques, breathing exercises, and soothing music. Creating a restful atmosphere that minimizes environmental noise, light, and other factors can enable patients to enjoy uninterrupted sleep. Maintaining staff continuity, promoting hydration and nutritional intake, and building day and night routines have also been reported as being effective in decreasing the potential for delirium. In combination, these interventions can also translate to reduced need for sedative medication, which can be contributory to delirium (Casarett and Inouye, 2001; Ross and Alexander, 2001b). Because patients suffering with delirium are at risk of unintentional harm, it is important that nurses provide a presence while patients are agitated because this can be reassuring and comforting to individuals and families. Nurses can also provide family members with emotional support during anticipatory grief that the delirious state will highlight. Should patients become drowsy and sleepy due to sedation, talking to them, particularly when undertaking procedures, is important, and families should be encouraged to do so as well and to communicate with their loved one by comforting touch (see Chapter 17 Managing Delirium and Confusion ➡).

Anxiety and depression symptoms

The approach to managing anxiety involves providing counselling, behavioural therapy, and pharmacological measures (Roth and Massie, 2007). It is important to identify the source of anxiety: for instance, patients may have concerns over finances, future dependency on others, disability, spiritual worries, being in pain and discomfort in the last days of life, and fear of death. Referral to counselling services, appropriate agencies, or spiritual leaders can help to resolve some of the underlying patient worries. Providing a supportive and relaxing environment, facilitating close family relationships, offering regular information updates, effective nurse–patient communication, and outlining anticipatory strategies to prevent symptom distress are also helpful. Allowing patients to discuss their worries and fears about dying is also helpful, and requires nurses to demonstrate listening, communication, and empathic skills.

Decisions about which anxiolytic agent to use may be governed by the severity of the anxiety and the effects that this is having in optimizing the patient's well-being. Whether the patient has renal or hepatic impairment needs to be taken into consideration prior to the initiation of drugs. Benzodiazepines, particularly those with an intermediate half-life (including lorazepam, temazepam, and clonazepam), are commonly prescribed, usually starting with low doses. Monitoring for side effects is important because worsening confusion, poor memory recall, and reduced concentration may develop (Ferris *et al.*, 2002; Roth and Massie, 2007). Drowsiness and sleepiness may also be observed once patients commence benzodiazepines. There are other medications that can be used to manage anxiety, which are long-acting and may be more suitable at different stages following diagnosis and health status.

Research into the effectiveness of treatment for patients with depression and who are terminally ill has received attention, with modern approaches identifying three main strategies:

- psychotherapy and counselling;
- pharmacological measures;
- interdisciplinary team involvement.

(Block, 2005)

A review of clinical trials, for example, reported moderate to consistently strong evidence to support psychological interventions, tricyclic antidepressants, and selective serotonin reuptake inhibitors (SSRIs) in managing cancer patients whose depression has been diagnosed and whose treatment lasts 6 weeks or more (Lorenz *et al.*, 2008). One systematic review of 15 behavioural interventions conducted on behalf of the National Institute of Clinical Effectiveness (Gysels and Higginson, 2004) identified that there was good evidence of effectiveness for using psychological interventions in managing patient depression among cancer patients in enabling adjustment and enhancing control.

The provision of comforting, emotionally supportive, flexible, and individualized counselling that facilitates patients with advanced terminal conditions with acceptance of the dying process, imminent death, and closure is beneficial for some (Block, 2005). However, for those with profound depression, engaging with psychotherapy or counselling may be difficult, so initial intervention with medications may be more appropriate.

Tricyclic antidepressants (for example, amitriptyline and imipramine) have played a major role in managing depression; however, because of problems associated with tolerance, sedative, and autonomic effects, they have become less popular. In contrast, SSRIs (including fluoxetine and paroxetine) are often prescribed as the first-line choice for patients who are terminally ill, when reaching maximal therapeutic levels is not an immediate priority and because of less toxic effects (Block, 2005).

Patients suspected of being depressed need to be assessed by specialists. This may include a psychiatrist or others trained to assess and provide counselling or psychotherapeutic services. All those providing health and social care, as well as carers and religious staff, need to be consulted to obtain a comprehensive appraisal of the patient's cognitive state, mood, and capacity to manage his or her own affairs and to make decisions. The contributions of the team can offer a more detailed insight of the patient's concerns (see **Chapter 14 Managing Anxiety** ➡️).

Ethical issues

Caring for patients at the end of life presents practitioners with a number of ethical and moral issues that typically revolve around a number of areas, including:

- decisions relating to cardiopulmonary resuscitation (CPR);
- withdrawing and withholding treatment;
- exercising autonomy and making decisions.

Decisions relating to cardiopulmonary resuscitation (CPR)

Situations can arise in which a failure to either care plan in advance and/or to communicate CPR decisions can result in the patient being inappropriately resuscitated. The use of tools such those endorsed by the End-of-Life Strategy (Department of Health, 2008a) aim to ensure that the patient and family's wishes, as part of the end-of-life care plan, are recorded, documented, and communicated with all members of the team, so that interventions are appropriate to the individual. These discussions need to be managed with sensitivity, compassion, and respect. Please see **www.resus.org.uk/pages/dnar.pdf.**

Withdrawing and withholding treatment

Another challenge for nurses relates to withdrawing and withholding treatments for patients at the end of life. 'Withholding' refers to not initiating an intervention; the reason might be because this might lead to more adverse side effects or it may be futile, for example prescribing antibiotics. 'Withdrawing' encompasses discontinuing any treatment or intervention that has been provided, but is considered inappropriate. Certain oral medications might be stopped, e.g. when a patient may have difficulty swallowing multivitamins or statins. Other oral medication may need to be converted and delivered by alternative routes.

Contention exists regarding the withdrawing and withholding of fluids and nutrition. This can cause anxiety to family members and clinical staff because they are regarded as essential requirements of patient care. One recent study about practices of ICU nurses across Europe reported that there was a division among participants regarding the continuation of nutritional support for patients at the end of life (Latour *et al.*, 2009). Another area that may precipitate some debate among health professionals and relatives is the extent to which terminally agitated patients should be sedated (Latour *et al.*, 2009).

Exercising autonomy and making decisions

Decisions about managing such circumstances will be more complex if the patient lacks mental capacity. The Mental Capacity Act 2005, however, provides a legal framework for those who are unable to make decisions for themselves. It is important to be aware that patients may be deemed incapable of making decisions only for specific issues and at particular times. Moreover, if an individual's capacity is compromised owing to cognitive impairment, the duty for making decisions will rest with the medical team. There are four aspects that determine ability to make decisions:

1. Understand information about the decision to be made
2. Retain the information
3. Use or weigh the information as part of a decision-making process OR
4. Communicate decisions with others (orally, written, using sign language, or through other means)
    (Department of Constitutional Affairs, 2007: 45)

The dilemma here is that, in some cases, the treatments given to relieve pain or other distressing symptoms may have an adverse effect on the patient's ability to reason, respond appropriately, and exercise autonomy.

Measuring the impact of nursing interventions

The principle of measuring both the effectiveness of nursing intervention and the patient's experience of receiving care is one that you should, where possible, facilitate. The NHS Information Centre has supported the development of Nursing Quality Metrics (NQMs), which can be used to facilitate quality improvement in patient care and experience **http://signposting.ic.nhs.uk/?k=metrics.**

This recent move within healthcare to be outcome-focused rather than target-driven is a welcome change in policy direction, initiated by Lord Darzi in his review of the NHS, and sustained by the previous and current UK governments. Metrics have been developed for many aspects of nursing care interventions and cover many inpatient areas, regardless of setting. The collection of these types of data helps healthcare organizations to focus on the delivery of safe and effective care, and can be used for local and national benchmarking, as well as for quality improvement.

For further details, visit the NHS Information Centre online at **http://www.ic.nhs.uk/**, where you will find details relating to nursing audit tools capturing information on documentation for observations, nutrition, medicines administration, pain management, communication, discharge planning, falls, pressure area care, antibiotic prescribing, and infection control.

In determining patient experience of healthcare, the National Institute for Health and Clinical Excellence (NICE) has recently published a Quality Standard **http://www.nice.org.uk/** that guides service delivery planning to ensure improvements in patient experience. Further commissioned work by the Department of Health has developed a single measure of patient experience. Supplementing these data is the NHS Survey, which captures patient views relating to ward cleanliness, infection control, staff attitudes, pain management, management of privacy, experience of dignity, nutrition, medicines administration, quality of communication, and discharge. Details can be found online at **http://www.nhssurveys.org/**.

Summary and key messages

Caring for patients at the end of life can be emotionally draining, particularly when confronted with ethical dilemmas. The key aspect to end-of-life care is for you to focus on timely care planning that identifies the symptoms/problems that present and, with the multidisciplinary team, to address these through evidence-based interventions. The reality of facing someone's anticipated death is never easy, and caring for a dying patient and family will be demanding, complex, and emotionally exhausting. In applying the principles laid out in this chapter, you will also find it is both a gratifying and privileged experience. Your centre-stage role in leading and informing care delivery at the end of life will have an enormous impact on both the patient and his or her relatives/friends. Care will typically embrace assessing the needs of the patient and family, providing symptom relief and comfort care, and providing cultural and spiritual support, extending to promoting patient dignity and supporting the newly bereaved.

Critical reflection on care situations is essential to maximize expertise in practice and to consider alternative approaches in future situations. A structured approach to your reflection will enable you to describe the experience and reflect on aims, feelings, decision-making, actions and outcomes, whilst considering alternative strategies and new knowledge gained. You may wish to complete the reflective exercise that is offered on the Online Resource Centre .

Online Resource Centre

To help you to develop and apply your knowledge and decision-making skills further, we have provided interactive learning resources online at **www.oxfordtextbooks.co.uk/orc/bullock/**

Whilst these are freely available, you will need to use the access codes at the start of the book.

References

Abbey, J., Piller, N., De Bellis, A., *et al*. (2004) The Abbey pain scale: a 1-minute numerical indicator for people with end-stage dementia. *International Journal of Palliative Nursing* **10**(1): 6–13.

Abernethy, A., Currow, D., Frith, P., *et al*. (2003) Randomised, double blind, placebo controlled crossover trial of sustained release morphine for management of refractory dyspnoea. *British Medical Journal* **327**: 323–30.

Abernethy, A., Wheeler, J.L. (2008) Total dyspnoea. *Current Opinion in Supportive and Palliative Care* **2**: 110–13.

Abernethy, A., Wheeler, J.L., Currow, D. (2010) Common approaches to dyspnoea management in advanced life-limiting illness. *Current Opinion in Supportive and Palliative Care* **4**: 53–5.

Badger, F., Clifford, C., Hewison, A., *et al*. (2009) An evaluation of the implementation of a programme to improve end-of-life care in nursing homes. *Palliative Medicine* **23**: 502–11.

Badger, F., Thomas, K., Clifford, C. (2007) Raising standards for elderly people dying in care homes. *European Journal of Palliative Care* **14**(6): 238–41.

Bailey, F.P., Burgio, K.I., Woodby, C.C., *et al*. (2005) Improving the processes of hospital care during the last hours of life. *Archives of Internal Medicine* **165**(15): 1722–7.

Bausewein, C., Booth, S., Gysels, M., *et al*. (2009) Non-pharmacological interventions for breathlessness in advanced stages of malignant and non-malignant disease. *Cochrane Database of Systematic Reviews* Issue 2: Art. No. CD005623. DOI: 10.1002/14651858.CD005623.pub2.

Ben-Aharon, I., Gafter-Gvili, A., Mical, P., *et al*. (2008) Interventions for alleviating cancer-related dyspnoea: a systematic review. *Journal of Clinical Oncology* **26**: 2396–404.

Block, S.D. (2005) Assessing and managing depression in the terminally ill patient. *Focus: The Journal of Lifelong Learning in Psychiatry* **3**(2): 310–19.

Bredin, M., Corner, J., Krishnasamy, M., *et al*. (1999) Multicentre randomised controlled trial of nursing intervention for breathlessness with lung cancer. *British Medical Journal* **318**: 1–5.

Bruce, S., Hendrix, C., Gentry, J. (2006) Palliative sedation in end-of-life care. *Journal of Hospice and Palliative Nursing* **8**(6): 320–7.

Casarett, D.J., Inouye, S. (2001) Diagnosis and management of delirium at the end of life. *Annals of Internal Medicine* **135**: 32–40.

Chang, V.T., Brooke, S., Rosenfeld, K. *et al*. (2007) Pain and palliative medicine. *Journal of Rehabilitation, Research and Development* **44**(2): 279–94.

Cheung, W., Lu, L.W., Zimmerman, C. (2009) Symptom clusters in patients with advanced cancers. *Support Care Cancer* **17**: 1223–30.

Clary, P., Lawson, P. (2009) Pharmacologic pearls for end-of-life care. *American Family Physician* **79**(12): 1059–65.

Corner, J., Plant, H., A'Hem, R., *et al*. (1996) Non-pharmacological intervention for breathlessness in lung cancer. *Palliative Medicine*, **10**(4): 299–305.

Currow, D.C., Ward, C., Abernethy, A.P. (2009) Advances in pharmacological management of breathlessness. *Current Opinions in Supportive and Palliative Care* **3**: 103–6.

Dale, J., Petrova, M., Munday, D., *et al*. (2009) A national facilitation project to improve primary care: impact of the Gold Standards Framework on process and self ratings scale of quality. *Quality Safe Heath Care* **18**: 174–80.

Department of Constitutional Affairs (2007) Mental Capacity Act Code of Practice. HMSO: London. Available at **http://www. justice.gov.uk/guidance/protecting-the-vulnerable/mental-capacity-act/index.htm** (accessed January 2011).

Department of Health (2003) *Building on the Best: Choice responsiveness and equity in the NHS*. HMSO: London.

Department of Health (2008a) *End-of-Life Care Strategy: Promoting Quality of Care for all Adults at the End of Life*. HMSO: London.

Department of Health (2008b) *High Quality Care for All: NHS Next Stage Review*. HMSO: London.

Dorman, S., Byrne, A., Edwards, A. (2007) Which measurement scales should we use to measure breathlessness in palliative care? A systematic review. *Palliative Medicine* **21**(3): 177–91.

Douglas, C., Murtagh, F.E., Chambers, E.J., *et al.* (2009) Symptom management for the adult patient dying with advanced chronic kidney disease: a review of the literature and development of evidence based guidelines by a United Kingdom Expert Consensus Group. *Palliative Medicine* **23**: 103–10.

Ellershaw, J., Wilkinson, S. (eds) (2003) *Care of the Dying: A Pathway to Excellence* Oxford University Press: Oxford.

Endacott, R., Benbenishty, J., Seha, M. (2010) Preparing research instruments for use with different cultures. *Intensive and Critical Care Nursing* **26**: 64–8.

Eyre, S. (2010) Supporting informal carers of dying patients: the district nurse's role. *Nursing Standard* **24**(22): 43–8.

Fan, G., Filipczak, L., Chow, E. (2007) Symptom clusters in cancer patients: a review of the literature. *Current Oncology* **14**(5): 173–9.

Ferris, F.D., von Gunten, C.F., Emanuel, L. (2002) Ensuring competency in end-of-life care: controlling symptoms. *BMC Palliative Care* **1**: 5.

Glare, P., Dickman, A., Goodman, M. (2003) Symptom control in care of the dying. In J. Ellershaw, S. Wilkinson (eds) *Care of the Dying: A Pathway to Excellence*. Oxford University Press: Oxford, pp. 42–61.

Guyatt, G.H., Townsend, M., Keller, J., *et al.* (1987) Measuring functional status in chronic lung disease: conclusions from a randomised control trial. *Respiratory Medicine* **42**: 773–8.

Gysels, M., Higginson, I.J. (2004) *Improving Supportive and Palliative Care for Adults with Cancer: Research Evidence*. National Institute for Clinical Effectiveness: London.

Health Care Commission (2007) *Spotlight on Complaints: A Report on Second Stage Complaints about the NHS in England*. **www. chi.gov.uk/_db/_documents/spotlight_on_complaints.pdf** (accessed July 2010).

Hills, M., Albarran, J.W. (2010a) After death I: Caring for bereaved relatives and being aware of cultural differences. *Nursing Times* **106**(27): 19–20.

Hills, M., Albarran, J.W. (2010b) After death II: Exploring procedures laying out and preparing the body for viewing. *Nursing Times* **106**(28): 22–4.

Ingham, J.M., Fotey, K.M. (1988) Pain and the barriers to its relief at the end of life: lessons for improving end-of-life health care. *Hospice Journal*, **13** (1–2): 89–100.

Johnson, S., Sherwin, E. (2010) *Preferred Priorities for Care: West Essex Evaluation*. **www.endoflifecare.nhs.uk/eolc/files/NHS-WE-PPC_Evaluation-Feb2010** (accessed July 2010).

Kayser-Jones, J., Schell, E., Lyons, W., *et al.* (2002) Factors that influence end-of-life care in nursing homes: the physical environment, inadequate staffing and lack of supervision. *Gerontologist* **43**(Suppl. 2): 76–84.

Kvale, P.A., Selecky, P.A., Prakash, U. (2007) Palliative care in lung cancer: ACCP Evidence-Based Clinical Practice Guidelines, 2nd edn. *Chest* **132**: S368–S403.

Latour, J., Fulbrook, P., Albarran, J.W. (2009) EfCCNa survey: European intensive care nurses' attitudes and beliefs towards end-of-life care. *Nursing in Critical Care* **14**(3): 110–21.

Lorenz, K., Lynn, J., Dy, S., *et al.* (2008) Evidence for improving palliative care at the end of life: a systematic review. *Annals of Internal Medicine* **148**(2): 147–59.

Luengo-Fernandez, R., Leal, J., Gray, A. (2010) *The Relevance, Economic Cost and Research Funding of Dementia Compared with Other Major Diseases*. Alzheimer's Research Trust: Cambridge.

Maben, J., Cornwell, J., Sweeney, K. (2010) In praise of compassion. *Journal of Research in Nursing* **15**(1): 9–13.

Mahler, D.A., Wells, C.K. (1988) Evaluation of clinical methods for rating dyspnoea. *Chest* **93**: 580–6.

Meek, P.M. (2004) Measurement of dyspnoea in chronic obstructive pulmonary disease: what is the tool telling you? *Chronic Respiratory Diseases* **1**: 29–37.

Miller, K.E., Miller, M. (2002) Managing common gastrointestinal symptoms at the end of life. *Journal of Hospice and Palliative Nursing* **4**(1): 34–48.

Miller, K.E., Miller, M., Jolley, M. (2001) Challenges in pain management at the end of life. *American Family Physician* **64**(7): 1227–34.

Moore, S., Corner, J., Haviland, J., *et al.* (2002) Nurse-led follow up and conventional medical follow up for patients with lung: a randomized trial. *British Medical Journal* **325**: 1145–52.

Murray, S.A., Kendall, M., Boyd, K., *et al.* (2005) Illness trajectories in palliative care. *British Medical Journal* **330**: 1007–11.

Noorani, N.H., Montagnini, M. (2007) Recognizing depression in palliative care patients. *Journal of Palliative Medicine* **10**(2): 458–64.

Nordgren, L., Sörensen, S. (2003) Symptoms experienced in the last six months of life in patients with end-stage heart failure. *European Journal of Cardiovascular Nursing* **2**: 213–17.

Office for National Statistics (2009) *Death Registrations by Case England and Wales*. Statistical Bulletin. HMSO: London.

Pattison, N. (2008) Caring for patients after death. *Nursing Standard* **22**(51): 48–56.

Qaseem, A., Snow, V., Shekelle, P., *et al.* for the Clinical Efficacy Assessment Subcommittee of the American College of Physicians (2008) Evidence-based interventions to improve the palliative care of pain, dyspnea, and depression at the end of life: a clinical practice guideline from the American College of Physicians. *Annals of Internal Medicine* **148**(2): 141–6.

Rayner, L., Loge, J., Wastesib, E., *et al.* on behalf of the European Palliative Care Research Collaborative (2009) The detection of depression in palliative care. *Current Opinion in Supportive and Palliative Care* **3**: 55–60.

Rhodes, R.L., Mitchell, S.L., Miller, S.C., *et al.* (2008) Bereaved family members evaluation of hospice care: what factors influence overall satisfaction with services? *Journal of Pain and Symptom Management* **35**(4): 365–71.

Ries, A.L. (2006) Impact of chronic obstructive pulmonary disease on quality of life: the role of dyspnoea. *American Journal of Medicine* **119**(10a): S12–S20.

Rigby, J., Payne, S., Frogatt, K. (2010) What evidence is there about the specific environmental needs of older people who are near the end of life and cared for in a hospice or similar institution? A literature review. *Palliative Medicine* **24**(3): 268–85.

Ross, D.D., Alexander, C.A. (2001a) Management of common symptoms in terminally ill patients: part I—Fatigue, anorexia, cachexia, nausea and vomiting. *American Family Physician* **64**(5): 807–14.

Ross, D.D., Alexander, C.A. (2001b) Management of common symptoms in terminally ill patients: part II—Constipation, delirium and dyspnoea. *American Family Physician* **64**(6): 1019–26.

Roth, A.J., Massie, M.J. (2007) Anxiety and its management in advanced cancer. *Current Opinion in Supportive and Palliative Care* **1**: 50–6.

Searight, H.R., Gafford, J. (2005) Cultural diversity and the end of life: issues and guidelines for family physicians. *American Family Physician* **71**: 515–22.

Shaw, K., Clifford, C., Thomas, K., *et al.* (2010) Improving end-of-life care: a critical review of the Gold Standards Framework. *Palliative Medicine* **24**(2): 317–29.

Sherman, D.W., Matzo, M.L., Paice, J., *et al.* (2004) Learning pain assessment and management: a goal of the end-of-life nurse education consortium. *Journal of Continuing Education in Nursing* **35**(3): 107–19.

Shipman, C., Gysels, M., White, P., *et al.* (2008) Improving generalist end-of-life care: national consultation with practitioners, commissioners, academics, and service user groups. *British Medical Journal* **337**(7674): 848–51.

Skills for Care (2009) *Core Competencies for End-of-Life Care: Training for Health and Social Care Staff.* http://www.skillsforcare. org.uk/developing_skills/endoflifecare/endoflifecare.aspx (accessed September 2010).

Steinhauser, K., Christakis, N., Clipp, C., *et al.* (2000) Factors considered important at the end of life by patients, family physicians and other care providers. *Journal of the American Medical Association* **284**(19): 2476–82.

Tanaka, K., Akechi, T., Okuyama, T., *et al.* (2000) Development and validation of the cancer dyspnoea scale: a multidimensional, brief, self-rating scale. *British Journal of Cancer* **82**(4): 800–5.

Trammer, J., Heyland, D., Dudgeon, D., *et al.* (2003) Measuring the symptom experience of seriously ill cancer and noncancer hospitalised patients near the end of life with the Memorial Symptom Assessment Scale. *Journal of Pain and Symptom Management* **25**(5): 420–9.

Truog, R.D., Campbell, M.L., Curtis, J.R., *et al.* and American Academy of Critical Care Medicine (2008) Recommendations for end-of-life care in the intensive care unit: a consensus statement by the American College [corrected] of Critical Care Medicine. *Critical Care Medicine* **36**(3): 953–63.

Veerbeek, L., van Zuylen, L., Swart, S.J., *et al.* (2008) The effect of the Liverpool Care Pathway for the dying: a multi-centre study. *Palliative Medicine* **22**(2): 145–51.

Viola, R., Kitely, C., Lloyd, N., *et al.* for the Supportive Care Guidelines Group of Cancer Ontario Programme in Evidence-Based Care (2008) The management of dyspnoea in cancer patients: a systematic review. *Support Care in Cancer* **16**: 329–37.

Von Gunten, C.F. (2005) Interventions to manage symptoms at the end-of-life. *Journal of Palliative Medicine* **8**(Suppl. 1): S88–S94.

Welsh Medicine Resource Centre Bulletin (2006) *Palliative Care 1– Pain Control.* Academic Centre, Llandough Hospital: Penarth.

Wood, G., Shega, J.W., Lynch, B., *et al.* (2007a) Management of intractable nausea and vomiting in patients at the end-of-life: 'I was feeling nauseous all of the time…nothing was working'. *Journal of the American Medical Association* **298**(10): 1196–207.

Wood, J., Storey, L., Clark, D. (2007b) Preferred place of care: an analysis of the first 100 patient assessments. *Palliative Medicine* **21**: 449–50.

World Health Organization (2011) WHO's Pain Ladder. Available at www.who.int/cancer/palliative/painladder/en/ (accessed January 2011).

19 *Managing* Hydration

Debra Ugboma and Michelle Cowen

Introduction

This chapter addresses the fundamental nursing role of managing hydration. Water is a basic nutrient and is essential to sustaining human life. In the developed world, we often take for granted the basic commodity of clean and plentiful water, but in other parts of the world water can have a profound effect on human health, in both the reduction and the transmission of disease (World Health Organization, 2011). For health, body water and electrolytes must be maintained within a limited range of tolerances. For nurses working in acute or primary care settings anywhere in the world, it is important to have a clear understanding of fluid and electrolyte homeostasis to assess haemodynamic status, to anticipate and recognize deterioration in status, and to implement appropriate corrective interventions.

Understanding the importance of hydration

Developing knowledge and associated skills around this topic will be facilitated by reflecting upon your clinical experiences as a student or as a qualified nurse, and your ability to link theory and practice. Your basic foundation of knowledge should include an understanding of how fluid is gained and lost from the body, the distribution of water between different compartments within the body, the processes by which fluid and electrolytes move between the intracellular and extracellular environments (Pocock and Richards, 2009; Cowen and Ugboma, 2011), and knowledge of the different types of intravenous replacement fluid (Endacott *et al.*, 2009: 249–73). Equally important is an insight into the use of criteria such as clinical/outcome indicators and benchmarking, what to use on what occasions, and how to use such tools to your best advantage. Armed with this knowledge, you will be well equipped to assess each patient's needs and to make clinical decisions about the most appropriate evidence-based nursing interventions to be used.

The state of water balance within the body is principally maintained by the osmoreceptors in the hypothalamus. These are best described as 'sensors' that detect the osmolarity (concentration) of the blood to stimulate or suppress the thirst mechanism, as well as regulate the amount of antidiuretic hormone (ADH) released by the posterior pituitary gland. When a person is becoming dehydrated, the thirst centre will be stimulated and usually he or she will seek fluid to rehydrate him or herself. If this is not possible, and the dehydrated state is not improved, more ADH will be released. ADH acts directly on the renal tubules, increasing the amount of water being reabsorbed, and reducing the amount of urine produced. The reverse will occur in a state of overhydration, i.e. less ADH will be released and urine output will increase.

Other quite complex physiological mechanisms, such as the renin—angiotensin—aldosterone mechanism, also play an important role in maintaining fluid balance within the body. This particular mechanism becomes problematic for patients with cardiac failure, who have poor cardiac output and low blood pressure. The kidney responds to the low blood pressure by releasing **renin**, setting off a chain of events that results in increased sodium and water retention by the kidney tubules. This fluid retention exacerbates the patient's condition and, because of this, many patients with cardiac failure are treated with ACE (angiotensin-converting enzyme) inhibitors. These drugs act upon this particular physiological mechanism, preventing the conversion of angiotensin I to angiotensin II. For further detail of associated physiology, we suggest you refer to physiology texts such as Pocock and Richards (2009).

Problems arise when people have difficulties maintaining their own hydration; the underlying problem may be physical, pathophysiological, or psychosocial in origin (Box 19.1). Some people may be affected by a number of different problems across the spectrum.

Patients with fluid imbalances that are fluid deficits or fluid overload can experience a variety of signs and symptoms; these will be covered in more detail in the section on assessment. Nurses are in a position to be the first to recognize and respond to signs of fluid imbalances. However, there is evidence emerging that there are inadequacies in the skills and ability of nurses and junior medical staff to do this well (National Confidential Enquiry into Patient Outcome and Death (NCEPOD), 2001; National Institute for Health and Clinical Excellence (NICE), 2007; National Patient Safety Agency (NPSA), 2007).

The relationship between fluid imbalance and patient outcomes

More and more evidence is emerging about the impact of dehydration upon well-being and patient outcomes. In 2009, one of the key findings of the National Confidential Enquiry into Patient Outcome and Death (NCEPOD)

> **Box 19.1 Risk factors for fluid imbalance**
>
> - Impaired mobility or ability for self-care
> - Confusion or loss of cognitive ability
> - Advanced age
> - Loss of motor function due to injury or a neurological condition
> - Cardiac and/or renal impairment
> - Artificially imposed state of fluid restriction (e.g. nil by mouth pre- or post-surgery)
> - Gastrointestinal disturbances (e.g. diarrhoea and/or vomiting)
> - Mental health issues
> - Trauma and/or severe blood loss
> - Burns
> - Difficulty managing medications
> - Dysphagia
> - Multiple comorbidity
> - Specific treatment regimens (e.g. chemotherapy)
> - Incontinence
> - Infection
> - Acute illness

---

report into deaths in hospital within 4 days of admission was that some basic aspects of clinical care continue to be neglected. Particularly implicated was the monitoring, recording, and management of fluid balance in the elderly and those with multiple comorbidities (NCEPOD, 2009). Previous NCEPOD reports (NCEPOD, 2001, 2002) also identified that fluid charts were poorly maintained and completed, and were a contributory factor in the failure to recognize that a patient was dehydrated and deteriorating.

Dehydration in acutely unwell patients is significantly associated with increased morbidity and mortality (NCEPOD, 2002; NPSA, 2007). Further evidence highlighted in the Royal College of Nursing and National Patient Safety Agency Hospital Hydration Best Practice Toolkit (2007) has also shown that dehydration can double the risk of death in patients admitted to hospital with a stroke, and increase length of stay for patients with community-acquired pneumonia. Moreover, Mentes and Culp (2003) found that an increased risk of urinary tract infection, confusion, delirium, renal failure, and prolonged wound healing were associated with dehydration in older adults.

Table 19.1 Evidence surrounding the potential consequences of underhydration or overhydration

Topic area	Reference	Summary of methods	Principal findings
Postoperative mortality in older adults	National Confidential Enquiry into Perioperative Deaths (NCEPOD, 1999b). Available at www.ncepod.org.uk/1999ea.htm	NCEPOD collects audit data related to all deaths occurring in hospital within 30 days of a surgical procedure. Its aim is to review clinical practice and identify potentially remediable factors in the practice of anaesthesia, surgery, and other invasive medical procedures.	Fluid management in the elderly is often poor and should be afforded the same status as drug prescriptions. **Hypovolaemia** should be corrected before surgery whenever possible. Particular care is required when general anaesthesia is combined with epidural analgesia. Documentation on fluid charts was often poor. Medical and nursing staff need to recognize the clinical importance of fluid charts, and ensure that accurate recording of fluid intake and output are carried out.
Failure to recognize signs of deterioration in acutely ill patients	National Patient Safety Agency (2007) Safer Care for the acutely ill patient: learning from untoward incidents. Available at http://www.nrls.npsa.nhs.uk/resources/?entryid45=59828	NPSA completed a detailed analysis of 576 deaths that could be interpreted as potentially avoidable and related to patient safety issues.	It found 64 deaths related to patient deterioration, which was not recognized or was not acted upon. By identifying patients who are deteriorating and by acting early, staff and their organizations can make a real difference. Patients whose deterioration is not picked up will have increased avoidable morbidity, increased length of stay, and associated avoidable healthcare costs.
Outcomes of post-admission dehydration in older people	Wakefield *et al.* (2009)	Case control design. Medical case notes review of older people admitted to hospital over a 4-year period. Inclusion into the case relied upon one of three 'coding' parameters. Controls were matched on age, ward location, and admission month. There were 335 patients included in the study and 334 controls.	Mortality rates were significantly higher among patients who developed dehydration during their hospital stay.

Table 19.1 highlights some of the key evidence surrounding poor fluid management.

For patients undergoing surgery, avoiding postoperative dehydration and optimizing preoperative hydration can enhance recovery and improve outcome (Powell-Tuck *et al.*, 2006). More recently, excessive fluid infusion, which can lead to sodium and water overload, has been recognized as a significant cause of postoperative morbidity, delayed recovery, and even mortality (Lobo *et al.*, 2006). Correct and individualized IV fluid regimens are important to help to avoid such problems, and you have an impor-

tant role in *ensuring that standard maintenance regimens are followed* for patients without complications. The British Consensus Guidelines on Intravenous Fluid Therapy for Adult Surgical Patients (Powell-Tuck *et al.*, 2006) provide clear guidance for managing surgical patients. The Map of Medicine (**http://app.mapofmedicine.com**;) also provides up-to-date guidance for postoperative fluid management.

Dehydration is not the only problem that people with ill-health may experience; imbalances in extracellular fluid and salt, which can manifest as a state of overhydration, are recognized complications of heart failure (National Institute for Health and Clinical Excellence (NICE), 2003) and renal insufficiency (Renal Association, 2007). Persistent or low-level fluid retention (fluid overload) will impact upon health and functioning. In both primary and acute care, you will have a key role in helping to support patients with fluid management as part of their individual self-management plan. This may include daily/regular weighing, managing diuretic therapy and fluid allowances, dietary manipulation (e.g. sodium intake), and recognizing of clinical signs of increasing fluid retention.

Clinical assessment of hydration status

As discussed and outlined in Table 19.1, there is a wide body of evidence highlighting that assessment of hydration is not always adequate (NCEPOD, 2001; Mentes and Culp, 2003; NPSA, 2007). To carry out a comprehensive and reliable assessment, it is therefore essential that a nurse knows 'what to look for'. Clinical assessment is a bit like doing a jigsaw puzzle: the more pieces you connect, the better idea you have of the whole 'picture'. You can sometimes get a quick overview and, in an emergency, this may be all that you have time for. If the situation allows, you should gather as much data as you can to strengthen your initial suspicions and assessment. A comprehensive assessment is based on an in-depth understanding of relevant physiology, including how the body compensates for disturbances to its normal state of equilibrium. This understanding will enable you to recognize and differentiate between early or later clinical signs (Figure 19.1), and also your ability to assess the effectiveness of any interventions that are made to plan further care for your patient. Finally, fundamental to this assessment is the ability to judge the severity of a given situation and thereby determine how closely you need to assess/monitor your patient at that point in time.

Detecting dehydration

Dehydration occurs when fluid intake is insufficient to balance fluid loss, and may occur as a result of an excessive loss of fluid or a low fluid intake. Dehydration may be accompanied by disturbances in osmolarity, acid–base balance, and electrolyte balance, and, if severe, can lead to haemodynamic instability. In the majority of cases, dehydration occurs over a period of time and, if the warning signs are detected, it can be easily rectified.

Figure 19.1 is an algorithm that details a three-stage assessment process to help to assess the patient's hydration.

- Stage 1 assessment—routine observations that can be carried out in any setting and which may highlight potential or developing dehydration
- Stage 2 assessment—a more detailed holistic assessment, performed to build up a more comprehensive picture
- Stage 3 assessment—the final pieces of the 'jigsaw' that may help to confirm if the patient is dehydrated (It will take time to obtain these results and so, whilst they are classified as stage 3, they may be initiated at any stage of the assessment process.)

Detecting fluid overload

Fluid overload can commonly occur when there has been excessive or inappropriate IV fluid administration, or where there is abnormal renal or cardiac function. In susceptible patients, it may lead to pulmonary oedema and cardiac failure. Detection of fluid overload is usually based on the history to determine whether the patient has received excessive fluid or has associated pathology. Clinical signs to seek include presence of oedema (peripheral or pulmonary), bounding pulse, hypertension, and neck vein distension. Blood tests may reveal a reduced haematocrit due to haemodilution, hyponatraemia owing to excessive water retention and reduced serum osmolarity. Blood urea is decreased because the blood is diluted with excessive water. Finally, specific gravity of the urine is decreased as the kidneys attempt to excrete the excess fluid (Pocock and Richards, 2009). Box 19.2 outlines some clinical signs of fluid overload.

Table 19.2 identifies some commonly encountered signs of dehydration, which are categorized as 'early' or 'later' changes to provide an indication of when you might notice them. However, it must be stressed that these are not absolute indicators and that other factors may influence their presence. For example, thirst cannot be relied upon as an indicator of dehydration in older adults because

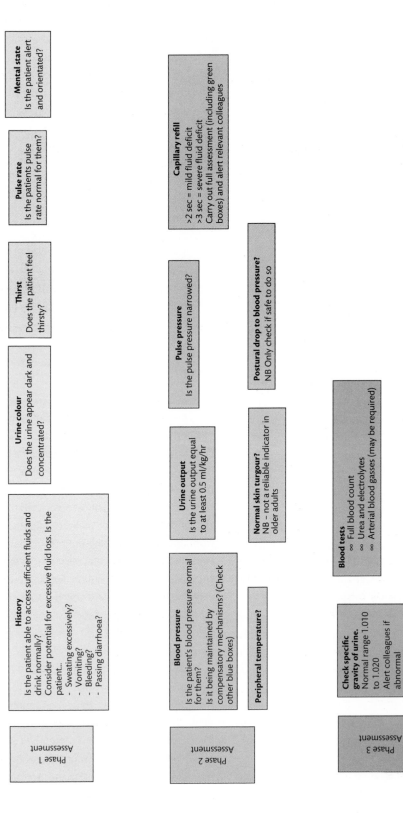

Figure 19.1 Assessment of hydration.

Box 19.2 Recognizing fluid retention/overload

- Breathlessness, dyspnoea, bounding pulse
- Peripheral/pitting oedema
- Raised jugular venous pressure (or central venous pressure, if monitored)
- Rising blood pressure (BP)—in heart failure, shock, or the critically ill patient, the blood pressure may/will remain low
- Rising weight
- Fatigue
- Pulmonary oedema

the sensation of thirst is diminished in this age group. It is therefore imperative that your assessment is holistic and takes full account of the patient's 'normal' state of health, including any pre-existing illnesses or medication that may alter these signs. You should also remember that some of these signs may be quite subtle and that not all of them will be present. If you suspect that your patient may be dehydrated, carry out an in-depth assessment such as the one detailed in Figure 19.1 (a more detailed version of which is available on the Online Resource Centre).

Nursing role in the management of hydration

Ensuring that a patient receives adequate hydration is a fundamental aspect of nursing care. Whilst those who require complex fluid management to address their specific needs may require a multidisciplinary approach, for most patients it is the nurse who has sole responsibility for ensuring that this aspect of care is met in a holistic, caring, and dignified manner, utilizing the best available evidence to inform his or her practice. Nursing interventions in relation to optimizing hydration may range from encouraging the patient to drink an afternoon cup of tea to managing a complicated intravenous fluid regimen. In some areas of nursing, it has been found that the nurse's role in fluid and electrolyte management can be ill-defined (Cook, 2005). However, in many nursing environments, nursing responsibility for managing hydration

often centres upon the accurate recording of fluid intake and output, or the 'fluid balance chart'. Despite their frequent use, research has identified that, although fluid balance charts are rated highly by nurses (Daffurn *et al.*, 1994), they can be inaccurate, inconsistent, and poorly completed (Reid *et al.*, 2004; Eastwood, 2006). It has also been highlighted that fluid balance charts can be commenced or continued unnecessarily and that doctors may not hold them in good regard (Daffurn *et al.*, 1994; Chung *et al.*, 2002).

Physiological 'track and trigger' tools (e.g. the Early Warning Score, EWS) recommended by the National Institute for Health and Clinical Excellence (NICE) (2007) for acutely ill patients in hospital can incorporate a measured urine output as part of the assessment. If this is based upon the information gained from fluid balance charts, and these charts are as poorly completed as the literature suggests, this has the potential to result in inaccuracies in data collection and in the assessment of individual patients.

More recent studies and reviews have identified the benefits of supplementary methods of assessing hydration, either as an alternative to or to support fluid balance charting. These methods include urine-specific gravity testing in older people (Hodgkinson *et al.*, 2003), and daily weight for people with heart failure to help to pre-empt hospital admission (Chaudhry *et al.*, 2007), or to trigger patient contact with healthcare professionals (White *et al.*, 2010). It is important that you support and educate your patients and their carers about the importance of adequate hydration and how this can be achieved. Good communication skills that take into account the individual's cultural needs and personal choices will help to encourage patients to participate in their own fluid management. In 2007, the Royal College of Nursing (RCN), along with the National Patient Safety Agency (NPSA), launched the Water for Health initiative after evidence from the NPSA identified that dehydration is a real patient safety issue. It is now becoming evident that there is considerable human and financial cost as a result of poorly managed fluid balance and hydration in patients or clients in our care. Boxes 19.3 and 19.4 outline some principles of managing the patient who is dehydrated or has fluid retention. However, it is important to remember that best practice nursing management should focus upon prevention of dehydration.

Table 19.2 Recognizing dehydration

Sign/symptom	Cause	Cautions in interpretation	Early/later
Dry mouth	Reduced saliva production		Early
Thirst	Reduced saliva production Osmoreceptors trigger thirst sensation in response to reduced circulating volume	Older adults	Early
Capillary refill in excess of 2 seconds	Mild fluid deficit	Low ambient temperature	Early
Darker urine colour	More concentrated urine in response to release of ADH to preserve circulating volume	**Haematuria**, prescribed medication, e.g. rifampicin may make the urine appear orange	Early
Increased pulse rate (see tachycardia)	Compensatory mechanism to maintain cardiac output	Check patient's normal prescribed drugs, e.g. beta-blockers, which slow the heart rate	Early
Cool peripheries (see cool limbs)	**Baroreceptors** trigger release of renin in response to falling BP, which leads to peripheral vasoconstriction	Peripheral vascular disease. Prescribed drugs, e.g. ACE inhibitors	Early
Normal systolic BP/ slight rise in diastolic (narrowing pulse pressure)	Other compensatory mechanisms maintain systolic BP within normal limits Vasoconstriction owing to renin release increases diastolic BP; gap between systolic and diastolic narrows	Prescribed drugs, e.g. ACE inhibitors	Early
Falling central venous pressure	Reduction in **preload**	Prescribed drugs, e.g. anti-hypertensive medication	Early
Orthostatic hypotension, leading to more marked hypotension	Fall in systolic BP of >20 mmHg Hypovolaemia exceeding compensatory mechanisms	Prescribed drugs, e.g. antihypertensive medication Other underlying pathology	Early/later
Urine output less than 0.5 ml/kg/h	Decreased glomerular filtration in kidney. Release of ADH to preserve circulating volume Effect of **aldosterone** on kidney tubules (increasing sodium and water retention)	Prescribed drugs, e.g. diuretics Renal impairment	Early/later
Tachycardia	Further increase in heart rate to maintain cardiac output	Prescribed drugs, e.g. beta-blockers	Later
Reduced skin **turgor**	Reduction in interstitial fluid	Older adults owing to reduced skin elasticity	Later
Cool limbs	Further release of renin leads to more powerful vasoconstriction	Prescribed drugs, e.g. ACE inhibitors	Later
Confusion	Reduced cerebral perfusion Build-up of toxins from anaerobic metabolism	Diabetes/hypoglycaemia	Later

(continued)

Table 19.2 *(continued)*

Sign/symptom	Cause	Cautions in interpretation	Early/later
Capillary refill in excess of 3 seconds	Major fluid deficit		Later (may be early if sudden loss)
Sunken eyes	Reduced intraocular pressure		Later
Shrunken tongue	Severe fluid loss		Later

Box 19.3 Managing dehydration

- Appropriate fluid replacement—consider route (IV, oral, subcutaneous) and type of fluid (IV regimen, water, rehydration solution)
- Identify cause(s) and treat underlying cause when possible
- Review medication if required, e.g. give antiemetic, stop diuretics
- Increase intake–output monitoring, e.g. fluid balance chart, hourly urine output measurements, daily weight
- More intensive assessment/monitoring of signs and symptoms for improvement or deterioration (may include more invasive monitoring, such as CVP)
- Preventative measures/self-care to reduce risk of dehydration in the future

Box 19.4 Managing fluid overload/ fluid retention

- Identify and treat possible cause
- Manage respiratory symptoms
- Review medication, e.g. give diuretic, ACE inhibitor in cardiac failure
- No salt diet
- Daily weight
- Fluid restriction as advised
- Education in managing fluid intake/ self-care

Utilizing the evidence base in the nursing management of hydration and prevention of fluid disturbances

The most effective nursing interventions in the management of hydration will be based upon up-to-date evidence. Some of the key literature and guidance related to hydration management has already been highlighted and further examples are given at the end of the chapter.

Because eating and drinking are fundamental aspects of nursing care, the management of hydration (along with nutrition) is the focus of a number of national initiatives. The Essence of Care (Department of Health, 2010a) provides benchmarks or 'statements of good practice' in relation to food and drink, and these can help you to take a structured approach to comparing your practice to that of others. This allows you to identify elements of good practice and to develop action plans to remedy poor practice. The High Impact Actions for Nursing and Midwifery (Institute for Innovation and Improvement, 2009) initiative emphasizes how care can be transformed across a range of core nursing themes. One of these themes is 'keeping nourished–getting better', and there are accessible examples of high-quality and cost-effective care that may be shared amongst clinical nurses. There are also proposals for the development of 'nurse sensitive outcome indicators' linked to these High Impact Actions (**http://www.ic.nhs. uk/services/measuring-for-quality-improvement**).

The RCN/NPSA Hydration Best Practice Toolkit (RCN/ NPSA, 2007) (see the Online Resource Centre) is particularly important because this relates to all aspects of nursing, and is helpful in that it provides strategies that you can use to support and educate patients and their families in hydration management. However, the evidence for the basis of these strategies is in line with 'good practice' and is therefore lower in the hierarchy of evidence than vigorous research. Box 19.5 outlines some of the strategies that you can employ to encourage fluid intake. The Toolkit itself provides much more information, and it is strongly recommended that you access it and embrace it as appropriate to your clinical environment.

Care and quality improvement initiatives, such as some of those mentioned above, should always be used with an element of prudence, realism, and with reference to your own clinical environment or patient caseload. Given the increasing plethora of quality measurement tools, the Nursing Roadmap for Quality (Department of Health, 2010b) is a guide that has been developed to clarify the tools and measures for improving the quality of care. This Roadmap can help you to make sense of the quality agenda, and support (or signpost) you and your team to choose appropriate tools that will help you to demonstrate how you are making a difference in the quality of care.

Managing hydration for patients undergoing surgery

Key evidence-based documents related to caring for patients undergoing surgery are the British Consensus Guidelines on Intravenous Fluid Therapy for Adult Surgical Patients (Powell-Tuck *et al.*, 2006) and the RCN Clinical Practice Guidelines for Perioperative Fasting in Adults and Children (Royal College of Nursing, 2005) (see the Online Resource Centre ⓦ). Evidence box 19.1 outlines some important aspects in relation to preparation for surgery, whilst Table 19.3 identifies opportunities to improve hydration management.

Much of the available evidence indicates that aspects of nursing care, such as fluid balance recording, have significant scope to improve. Alongside this, it has been noted that failure to recognize that a patient is dehydrated can impact upon patient outcome (NCEPOD, 2001; 2002; 2009). Table 19.3 outlines some key opportunities for examining and improving how hydration is managed within your clinical environment, linking to the supporting evidence where possible. Figure 19.2 summarizes the key principles of preventing fluid imbalances.

> **Box 19.5 Strategies to encourage fluid intake in adults (adapted from RCN/NPSA Hydration Best Practice Toolkit, 2007)**
>
> - Set an easy-to-remember specific target for fluid intake, e.g. 6 glasses of water per day.
> - Serve water fresh and chilled.
> - Encourage water consumption in the morning for those patients worried about increased use of the toilet at night.
> - Serve small quantities of water alongside tea and coffee—explaining the benefits of increasing water intake.
> - Inform families and visitors about promoting hydration so that they can help achieve any intake target.
> - Hot water, with a piece of lemon, lime, or orange, can appeal to those who wish for a hot drink.
> - Offer water and fluid at all mealtimes.
> - Support individuals to increase fluid intake during periods of hot weather.
> - Hang a picture of a drop of water near patients' beds to remind staff to encourage more fluid intake.
> - Use a positive approach to offering fluids, e.g. 'here's a nice cool drink of water for you'. If you do this when giving medications, offer a fuller glass (and offer to top it up) because many people will finish a glass when taking their tablets.

Measuring the impact of nursing interventions

There is little vigorous research that examines the process and outcomes of different types of nursing intervention. There is therefore a need to undertake such research to provide an evidence base that can inform best practice in the nursing management of preventing dehydration and safe rehydration.

Recognizing the potential for, and acting to prevent, fluid imbalance is a key nursing role, but intervention must be linked to measurable patient outcomes.

The study by Daffurn *et al.* (1994), whilst much quoted in nursing texts, is now over 16 years old and it is timely for further research in this area. Locally, you can choose to audit fluid balance charts in your clinical environment to establish

Table 19.3 Utilizing the evidence: identifying opportunities to improve hydration management

Opportunities	Possible actions	Source of evidence
Identify specific strategies to encourage patients in your care to drink more Consider outcome measures	Use RCN/NPSA Toolkit to assess your clinical environment with regard to your water facilities. Lead or facilitate discussions with the ward team about how you manage hydration in your clinical area. What (and how) do you need to measure to reflect that you are providing the right level of care to achieve your standards?	Water for Health: Hydration Best Practice Toolkit for Hospitals and Healthcare (RCN/NPSA, 2007) High Impact Intervention: Keeping nourished, getting better (Institute for Innovation and Improvement, 2009) Nursing Roadmap for Quality (Department of Health, 2010b)
Improve the accuracy of your fluid balance charts/recording	Raise awareness of accurate fluid balance recording at handover. Consider which patients have priority for fluid balance chart recording and target these. Avoid a 'custom and practice' approach to fluid balance charts. Develop an education resource related to fluid balance recording, e.g. quiz, worksheet, teaching board display. During a shift, give responsibility for a patient's fluid balance monitoring to a specific individual. In some environments, you might consider whether the patient can take responsibility for recording his or her own fluid intake and output (although there is no evidence to say that this is more accurate). Consider how, as a ward team, you will measure or estimate unspecified fluid output, e.g. 'wet bed' or 'incontinent'.	Daffurn *et al.* (1994) Chung *et al.* (2002) Nursing and Midwifery Council (NMC) (2010)
Be proactive in monitoring and improving hydration in those patients at increased risk	Make an assessment, and have a team discussion, to consider which patients in your environment are at particular risk of fluid imbalances. Develop (as a suggested minimum) a three-point strategy/plan to minimize the risk for each individual (try using strategies outlined in the RCN/NPSA Toolkit).	NCEPOD (2009) NICE (2007) Department of Health (2010a) Essence of Care
Take action for surgical patients	Audit your preoperative nil by mouth (NBM) periods—do they reflect the current guidelines? If not, what can you do to improve the situation? Is the prescription for, and delivery of, postoperative fluid replacement regimens individualized? Develop a teaching resource to increase understanding of postoperative physiological oliguria and assessment of hydration status.	Powell-Tuck *et al.* (2006) Johnson and Monkhouse (2009) Royal College of Nursing (2005)
Increase the use of daily weight for patient assessment, e.g. in cardiac failure, older person, diuretic medication	Identify which patients may benefit from daily weight monitoring. How, and by whom, is the daily weight recorded and reviewed? How may self-management be developed for the patient recording daily weight?	NICE (2003) Hodgkinson *et al.* (2003) Chaudhry *et al.* (2007)
Develop skills in assessment of hydration	Utilize the algorithm (Figure 19.1) in your assessment of patients' hydration status. Organize teaching and learning activities related to assessment of hydration. Undertake formal 'physical assessment' modules of study to improve skills such as auscultation, and a holistic approach to assessment.	NCEPOD (2009) NICE (2007)

EVIDENCE BOX 19.1
Preparation for surgery

1. Patients should be adequately hydrated prior to surgery.

2. In patients without disorders of gastric emptying undergoing elective surgery, clear, non-particulate fluids should not be withheld for more than 2 hours prior to the induction of anaesthesia.

3. A minimum preoperative fasting time of 6 hours for food (solids, milk, and milk-containing drinks).

4. In the absence of disorders of gastric emptying or diabetes, preoperative administration of special carbohydrate-rich beverages 6 hours before induction of anaesthesia may improve patient well-being and facilitate recovery.

5. Routine use of preoperative mechanical bowel preparation may complicate intraoperative and postoperative fluid and electrolyte balance, and its use should be avoided whenever possible. If used, any fluid and electrolyte disturbances should be corrected simultaneously with appropriate intravenous fluid replacement.

(from Powell-Tuck *et al.*, 2006 RCN Peri-Operative Fasting Clinical Guideline, 2005)

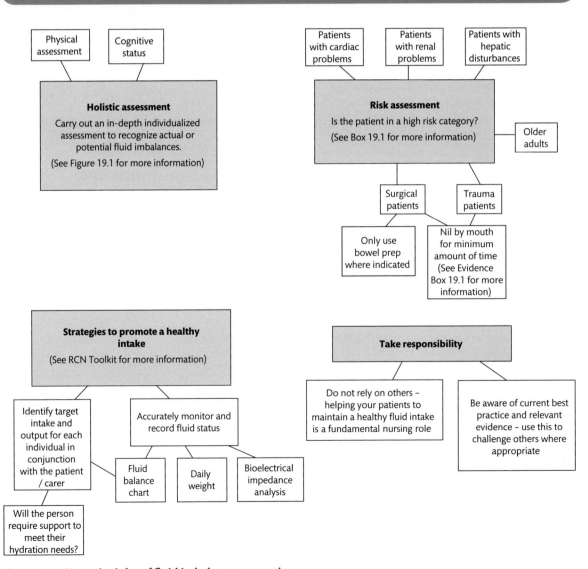

Figure 19.2 Key principles of fluid imbalance prevention.

CASE STUDY 19.1 *Assessing and managing fluid needs for an older adult with dehydration*

Mrs Gwen Jones is a 73-year-old lady admitted to hospital. She was admitted from home, having been found on her bedroom floor. When she arrives on the ward, she is sitting up in bed and is answering questions, although she has some obvious confusion, and is disorientated in time and place. You discover from her family that she has recently had a 'stomach bug'. Until this admission, she was independent, doing her own cooking and cleaning with a little support from her family. She has recently been prescribed bendroflumethiazide by her GP to control her blood pressure.

Her vital signs are as follows:

- Blood pressure 100/55
- Pulse 98
- Resps 18
- Temperature 36.8°C
- Her urine appears concentrated and she is passing small volumes—150 ml since admission 4 hours ago

Her blood results include:

- Urea 14 mmol/l
- Creatinine 120 µmol/l
- Sodium 125 mmol/l
- Potassium 3.5 mmol/l
- Hb 12.6 g/dl

Questions

➤ How will you assess Mrs Jones and what additional information might you require to make a full assessment?

➤ What is your initial management/care plan?

➤ Analyse some of the physical, physiological, and environmental factors that may have contributed to her current problems.

➤ What advice could you give Mrs Jones and her family to help prevent similar episodes in the future?

 See the Online Resource Centre for the answers to these questions.

their accuracy and to identify any potential need for staff education. Similarly, you can examine the scope to develop your own or other nurses' skills in the methods of assessment of fluid balance or haemodynamic status. This may be particularly pertinent in the community, where evidence suggests that fluid gains in patients with heart failure may pre-empt admission to hospital (Chaudhry *et al.*, 2007). You can also audit or undertake clinical studies related to some of the RCN Clinical Guidelines for Perioperative Fasting (Royal College of Nursing, 2005) or the strategies proposed in the RCN/NPSA Hydration Best Practice Toolkit (RCN/NPSA, 2007).

There is significant capacity to increase and develop the evidence base pertaining to the nursing role in managing hydration and assessing fluid status. Exciting develop-ments include an RCN-supported study being undertaken in the West Country (Cornwall Hydration Project for Vulnerable Infirm Patients), which is developing and piloting a new drinking aid specifically suited to the frail vulnerable patient. There is also emerging evidence surrounding the use of a novel drinking mechanism (**http://www.hydrateforhealth.co.uk/**) that may reduce length of stay and inpatient infection rates for hospitalized patients. Similarly, valuable data may emerge from the East of England 'Intelligent Fluid Management Bundle', which is expected to publish soon (see the Online Resource Centre for details).

Table 19.4 identifies groups of patients with specific hydration needs, and signposts where you can access the

Table 19.4 **Further information about groups of patients with specific hydration needs**

Patient group	Further information can be found in:
Patients with mental health problems	➡ Chapter 17 Managing Delirium and Confusion ➡ Chapter 14 Managing Anxiety ➡ Chapter 7 Understanding Dementia ➡ Chapter 8 Understanding Depression
Patients with cardiac disease	➡ Chapter 6 Understanding Coronary Heart Disease
Patients with cognitive impairment	➡ Chapter 7 Understanding Dementia ➡ Chapter 17 Managing Delirium and Confusion
Patients with renal disease	➡ Chapter 11 Understanding Renal Disorders
Patients with swallowing difficulties	➡ Chapter 13 Understanding Stroke
Patients requiring end-of-life care	➡ Chapter 18 Managing End-of-Life Care
Patients receiving nutrition via a PEG	➡ Chapter 24 Managing Nutrition

additional information about their care management in other chapters in this book.

Identifying evidence for best practice

- High Impact Actions: Keeping nourished, getting better http://www.institute.nhs.uk/building_capability/hia_supporting_info/keeping_nourished_getting_better.html
- Essence of Care: Benchmarks for food and drink http://www.dh.gov.uk/prod_consum_dh/groups/dh_digitalassets/@dh/@en/@ps/documents/digitalasset/dh_125313.pdf
- Hospital Hydration Best Practice Toolkit http://www.rcn.org.uk/newsevents/campaigns/nutritionnow/tools_and_resources/hydration#Download
- Nursing Roadmap for Quality http://www.dh.gov.uk/en/Publicationsandstatistics/Publications/PublicationsPolicyAndGuidance/DH_113450
- National Patient Safety Executive http://www.nrls.npsa.nhs.uk
- Patient Safety First: A how to guide for reducing harm from deterioration (2008) http://www.patientsafetyfirst.nhs.uk/ashx/Asset.ashx?path=/How-to-guides-2008-09-19/Deterioration%201.1_17Sept08.pdf

- Scales, K., Pilsworth, J. (2008) The importance of fluid balance in clinical practice. *Nursing Standard* 22(47): 50–7
- Scott, W.N. (2010) *Fluid and Electrolytes Made Incredibly Easy*. London: Wolters Kluwer-Lippincott Williams and Wilkins
- **www.waterforhealth.org.uk**
- NHS Evidence in Health and Social Care **http://www.evidence.nhs.uk/default.aspx**

Systematic reviews

Good, P., Cavenagh, J., Mather, M., Ravenscroft, P. (2008) Medically assisted hydration for adult palliative care patients. *Cochrane Database of Systematic Reviews*, Issue 2. Art. No.: CD006273. DOI: 10.1002/14651858.CD006273.pub2

Hodgkinson, B., Evans, D., Wood, J. (2001) Maintaining oral hydration in older people: a systematic review. Adelaide, SA: Joanna Briggs Institute for Evidence Based Nursing and Midwifery. Systematic Review, 12

Zacharias, M., Conlon, N.P., Herbison, G.P., *et al.* (2008) Interventions for protecting renal function in the perioperative period. *Cochrane Database of Systematic Reviews*, Issue 4. Art. No.: CD003590. DOI: 10.1002/14651858.CD003590.pub3

Summary and key messages

In this chapter, we have attempted to provide you with some key documents and evidence that you can utilize in the daily care and management of adults, and which will help you to champion this essential aspect of care. The key messages for managing hydration include the following.

- It is a nursing responsibility to identify patients in a clinical environment who are at risk of fluid imbalances (in particular dehydration) and to identify strategies to reduce their risk.

- Nurses have a role in developing local strategies to help improve fluid intake for all patients in the clinical environment.

- The development of expertise in the assessment of fluid/haemodynamics is essential to effective nursing intervention.

- There is a need for robust research that examines the process and outcome of nursing interventions to prevent dehydration and to ensure safe rehydration.

Online Resource Centre

To help you to develop and apply your knowledge and decision-making skills further, we have provided interactive learning resources online at **www.oxfordtextbooks.co.uk/orc/bullock/**

Whilst these are freely available, you will need to use the access codes at the start of the book.

References

Chaudhry, S.J., Wang, Y., Concato, J., *et al.* (2007) Patterns of weight change preceeding hospitalization for heart failure. *Circulation* **116**(4): 1549–54.

Chung, L.H., Chong, S., French, P. (2002) The efficiency of fluid balance charting: an evidence-based management project. *Journal of Nursing Management* **10**: 103–13.

Cook, N.F. (2005) Nurses' perceptions of their role in fluid and electrolyte management. *British Journal of Neuroscience Nursing* **1**(3): 139–46.

Cowen, M., Ugboma, D. (2011) Fluid and electrolyte balance. In C. Brooker, M. Nicol, (eds) *Alexander's Nursing Practice*, 4th edn. Churchill Livingstone: Edinburgh.

Daffurn, K., Hillman, K.M., Bauman, A., *et al.* (1994) Fluid balance charts: do they measure up? *British Journal of Nursing* **3**(16): 816–20.

Department of Health (2010a) *Essence of Care*. http://www.dh.gov.uk/en/Publicationsandstatistics/Publications/Publications-PolicyAndGuidance/DH_119969 (accessed 11 October 2010).

Department of Health (2010b) *The Nursing Roadmap for Quality*. http://www.dh.gov.uk/en/Publicationsandstatistics/Publications/PublicationsPolicyAndGuidance/DH_113450 (accessed 28 March 2011).

Eastwood, G.M. (2006) Evaluating the reliability of recorded fluid balance to approximate body weight change in patients undergoing cardiac surgery. *Heart and Lung* **35**(1): 27–33.

Endacott, R., Jevon, P., Cooper, S. (2009) *Clinical Nursing Skills: Core and Advanced*. Oxford University Press: Oxford.

Hodgkinson, B., Evans, D., Wood J. (2003) Maintaining oral hydration in older adults: a systematic review. *International Journal of Nursing Practice* **9**: S19–S28.

Institute for Innovation and Improvement (2009) *High Impact Actions for Nursing and Midwifery*. http://www.institute.nhs.uk/building_capability/general/high_impact_actions_submissions.html (accessed 11 October 2010).

Johnson, R., Monkhouse, S. (2009) Post-operative fluid and electrolyte balance: alarming results. *Journal of Perioperative Practice* **19**(9): 291–4.

Lobo, D.N., Macafee, D.A., Allison, S.P. (2006) How perioperative fluid balance influences postoperative outcomes. *Best Practice Research Clinical Anaethesiology* **20**: 439–55.

Mentes, J.C., Culp, K. (2003) Reducing hydration linked events in nursing home residents. *Clinical Nursing Research* **12**(3): 210–25.

National Confidential Enquiry into Patient Outcome and Death (NCEPOD) (1999) *Extremes of Age*. NCEPOD: London. http://www.ncepod.org.uk/1999ea.htm (accessed 20 June 2010).

National Confidential Enquiry into Patient Outcome and Death (NCEPOD) (2001) *Changing the Way We Operate*. NCEPOD: London. http://www.ncepod.org.uk/2001cwo.htm (accessed 20 June 2010).

National Confidential Enquiry into Patient Outcome and Death (NCEPOD) (2002) *Functioning as a Team*. NCEPOD: London. **http://www.ncepod.org.uk/2002fat.htm** (accessed 20 June 2010).

National Confidential Enquiry into Patient Outcome and Death (NCEPOD) (2009) *Caring to the End? A Review of the Care of Patients who Died in Hospital within Four Days of Admission*. NCEPOD: London. **http://www.ncepod.org.uk/2009report2/ Downloads/DAH_summary.pdf** (accessed 14 June 2010).

National Institute for Health and Clinical Excellence (NICE) (2003) *Chronic Heart Failure: National Clinical Guideline for Diagnosis and Management in Primary and Secondary Care*. **http://www.nice.org. uk/nicemedia/live/10924/29137/29137.pdf** (accessed 4 July 2010).

National Institute for Health and Clinical Excellence (NICE) (2007) Acutely ill patients in hospital: recognition of and response to acute illness in adults in hospital. NICE Clinical Guideline 50. (CG50) **http://www.nice.org.uk/nicemedia/ live/11810/35950/35950.pdf** (accessed 3 October 2010).

National Patient Safety Agency (NPSA) (2007) Safer care for the acutely ill patient: learning from untoward incidents. **http:// www.nrls.npsa.nhs.uk/resources/?entryid45=59828** (accessed 3 October 2010).

Nursing and Midwifery Council (NMC) (2010) *Record Keeping: Standards for Nursing and Midwives*. **http://www.nmc-uk.org/ Documents/Guidance/nmcGuidanceRecordKeeping GuidanceforNursesandMidwives.pdf** (accessed 7 October 2011).

Pocock, G., Richards, C.D. (2009) *The Human Body: An Introduction for the Biomedical and Health Sciences*. Oxford: Oxford University Press.

Powell-Tuck, J., Gosling, P., Lobo, D.N., *et al.* (2006) British Consensus Guidelines on Intravenous Fluid Therapy for Adult Surgical Patients. **http://www.library.nhs.uk/GuidelinesFinder/View Resource.aspx?resID=299532** (accessed 28 June 2010).

Reid, J., Robb, E., Stone, D., *et al.* (2004) Improving the monitoring and assessment of fluid balance. *Nursing Times*, **100**(20): 36–9.

Renal Association (2007) Complications of chronic kidney disease. **http://www.renal.org/Clinical/GuidelinesSection/ ComplicationsofCKD.aspx** (accessed 3 July 2010).

Royal College of Nursing (2005) Clinical Guidelines for Peri-operative fasting in Adults and Children. **http://www.rcn.org.uk/data/ assets/pdffile/0009/78678/002800.pdf** (accessed 4 July 2010).

Royal College of Nursing, National Patient Safety Agency (2007) Hospital Hydration Best Practice Toolkit. **www.rcn.org.uk/ newsevents/campaigns/nutritionnow/tools_and_resources/ hydration#Download** (accessed 4 July 2010).

Wakefield, B.J., Mentes, J., Homan, J.E., *et al.* (2009) Post-admission dehydration: risk factors, indicators and outcomes. *Rehabilitation Nursing* **34**(5): 209–16.

White, M.M., Dowie-Esquival, J., Caldwell, M.A. (2010) Improving heart failure symptom recognition: a diary analysis. *Journal of Cardiovascular Nursing* **25**(1): 7–12.

World Health Organization (2011) Guidelines for drinking water quality, 4th edn. **http://www.who.int/water_sanitation_ health/publications/2011/dwq_guidelines/en/index.html** (accessed 7 October 2011).

20 *Managing* Hygiene

David Voegeli

Introduction

This chapter addresses the fundamental nursing role in managing hygiene. The ability to maintain personal and oral hygiene forms some of the activities of living that everyone undertakes every day, but which are often taken for granted until a deterioration in a person's physical or mental state, such as illness or ageing, prevents individuals from meeting these needs independently. Being able to assess the need for nursing intervention accurately, and to deliver appropriate evidence-based care, requires considerable skill. It draws on many of the core competencies of professional nursing, such as observation, communication, and clinical decision-making. Therefore it is inappropriate that, in a majority of care settings, these activities are often delegated by the registered nurse to those with the least experience. It is important to remember that, registered nurses retain professional accountability for the quality and effectiveness of the interventions provided or delegated to the patients under their care. Increasingly, this fundamental aspect of care is viewed as an overall indicator of the quality of the care provided.

Understanding the importance of hygiene

Assisting individuals to maintain their personal hygiene needs promotes comfort, safety, well-being, and dignity, and also plays an important part in the prevention of infection. It is also an important aspect of many religions, such as the ritual washing performed by Muslims before prayer. Indeed Young (1991) suggested that cleanliness is a basic human right rather than a luxury.

There has been criticism over the past decade that aspects of nursing care relating to the maintenance of patient hygiene have become neglected, and the Healthcare Commission (2007) reported that 30% of complaints received against UK hospitals related to issues of personal care and dignity, including:

- patients being left in soiled clothing or bedding;
- hygiene needs not being met (patients not being washed or mouthcare given);
- hair and nails not being cared for.

In response to these criticisms, both the Nursing and Midwifery Council (NMC) and the Department of Health (DH) worked to improve the quality of personal care provided by nurses. This is evidenced by the mandatory requirement to demonstrate proficiency in meeting the personal hygiene needs of individuals as part of the Essential Skills Clusters for pre-registration nursing programmes in the UK and the development of a specific set of quality benchmarks for personal hygiene care as part of the Essence of Care (Department of Health, 2010) best practice guidance.

This chapter focuses on your responsibilities as a nurse, for meeting those vital skin hygiene and oral care needs that maintain skin and oral mucosal integrity. It will consider the evidence-based actions that you should take to provide hygiene and oral care needs that maintain skin and oral mucosal integrity. These actions are presented as key therapeutic nursing interventions that prevent skin breakdown.

Defining personal hygiene care

The link between maintaining patient hygiene and reducing healthcare-associated infection has been established in North America, leading to the development of the concept of interventional patient hygiene (IPH) (Vollman *et al.*, 2005). McGuckin *et al.* (2008) define IPH as a comprehensive evidence-based intervention and measurement model for reducing the bioburden of both the patient and healthcare worker. The components of IPH are hand hygiene, oral care, skin care/antisepsis, and catheter site care.

Oral health has been defined by the Department of Health Strategic Review (2005) as:

> The health of the mouth, teeth and associated structures and their functional viability.

The Essence of Care (Department of Health, 2010) best practice guidelines define personal hygiene care as:

> the physical act of cleansing the body to ensure that the hair, nails, ears, eyes, nose and skin are maintained in an optimum condition. It also includes mouth hygiene which is the effective removal of plaque and debris to ensure the structures and tissues of the mouth are kept in a healthy condition. In addition, personal hygiene includes ensuring the appropriate length of nails and hair.

Skin hygiene

The maintenance of skin hygiene and preventing skin breakdown forms one of the cornerstones of professional nursing care, and constitutes a nursing challenge in every field of practice. This aspect of fundamental care is made more complex by the sheer numbers and variety of patients who are at significant risk of skin breakdown. These include those with chronic inflammatory skin conditions (eczema, psoriasis) through to those with incontinence and patients with reduced mobility who are at risk of pressure damage. The focus of the skin care that you provide will differ, but, whatever the context of care, the main objectives of your interventions can be distilled down to two main goals: the prevention of skin breakdown; or the restoration of skin integrity that has been compromised. This aspect of care can consume vast amounts of nursing time. As a consequence, skin breakdown incidence rates, as in the case of pressure ulcers, have rapidly become viewed as an indicator of the quality of nursing care provided (Department of Health, 2010). Despite the growing acknowledgement of the importance of 'basic' skin and oral hygiene, much nursing practice remains based more on ritual than on firm evidence. This is further complicated by the ever-growing number of skin care products on the market, each with their own claims of efficacy.

Assessing the need for skin hygiene interventions

In many clinical areas, the nursing assessment of patients is still based on an adaptation of an activities of living model, such as that developed by Roper *et al.* (1996). This provides a framework that helps to guide the overall assessment of an individual's nursing needs, and provides a means of integrating the numerous factors that need to be considered. Additional factors to consider are: the age of the patient; his or her cognitive ability/mental capacity; motivation; mobility; infection control risk; and medical condition. Thus careful assessment is needed to ensure that any interventions planned are not only safe for the patient, but also for the nurse, and the recognition that additional assessments may need to be performed, e.g. manual handling. Because the patients in any care setting will have a diverse range of nursing needs, from those who might be 'self-caring' and fully able to meet their hygiene needs to those who are totally dependent on their carer, it is useful to consider particular patient groups who may need specific intervention, as indicated in Theory into practice box 20.1.

Bed bath, immersion bath, or shower?

As part of our daily routines, we all have a preference for either having a daily wash, bath, or shower. These preferences are acknowledged during an initial assessment of nursing need, and wherever possible individuals will be assisted to maintain these 'rituals'. However, if nursing care is being provided in an institutional setting (hospital or nursing home), then several other factors come into play, such as maintenance of privacy and dignity, as well as infection prevention.

Clinical assessment of skin condition

Several tools to guide skin assessment are available, such as those discussed in Chapters 12 Understanding Skin Conditions and 27 Managing the Prevention of Skin Breakdown ➡️. Because each one has often been developed to focus the assessment process on one particular

---

Box 20.1   Patient groups potentially requiring nursing interventions to meet hygiene needs

- Individuals at either end of the age spectrum (very old or very young)
- Individuals with learning disabilities
- Individuals with mental health problems
- Individuals with impaired consciousness
- Individuals with cognitive impairment
- Individuals with physical disabilities
- Individuals undergoing radiotherapy or chemotherapy
- Individuals requiring end-of-life care
- Individuals taking medication that can affect skin or oral health (e.g. anticonvulsants, steroids)

(adapted from Dingwall, 2010)

---

area, the choice can be bewildering. In many cases, these tools have been developed in response to local need, and lack the robustness of properly validated clinical tools. However, they can act as a guide, and can be useful to less-experienced care staff. Providing care to meet an individual's hygiene needs provides the ideal opportunity to assess his or her skin and to identify any actual or potential problems that require further intervention, particularly in those at high risk of developing pressure ulcers or those with incontinence. You should routinely make an assessment of skin condition whenever you are providing care to your patients. Directions for assessing skin condition are given in Figure 20.1.

The management of skin hygiene

The usual recommendation for general skin cleansing continues to be washing with soap and water using a flannel, sponge, or disposable wash cloth, and towel drying either by rubbing or patting (Errser *et al.*, 2005). Whilst this approach may be suitable for meeting general hygiene needs, it does expose the skin to several potentially damaging factors that need to be considered when dealing with individuals with skin breakdown, or who require frequent skin cleansing. This is acknowledged more in North American literature, in which a clear distinction is now made between routine skin cleansing for hygiene reasons and the cleansing offered as part of a skin care protocol for use in situations such as the care of individuals with urinary or faecal incontinence (Bliss *et al.*, 2007; Gray *et al.*, 2007). Thus, helping individuals to feel clean by washing is only part of a skin care protocol, with the other components being drying, moisturizing, replenishing, and protecting. In the following sections, an overview is provided of each of these components.

Washing the skin

Washing removes debris from the skin surface, and soap and water are frequently used together for this purpose because of convenience and perceived cost-effectiveness. Soaps are water-soluble sodium or potassium salts of fatty acids that have been treated with a strong alkali, and act as **surfactants** (Abbas *et al.*, 2004). Additional surfactants, such as sodium lauryl sulphate (SLS), may be added to soap to make it a better wetting agent. However, synthetic surfactants, such as SLS, are known to be potent

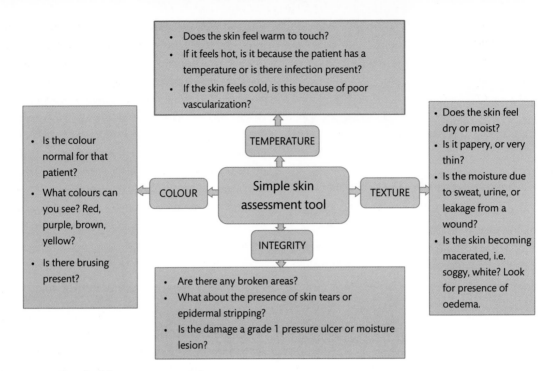

Figure 20.1   Simple skin assessment tool.

Adapted from Newton and Cameron (2003) *Skin Care in Wound Management*. Medical Communications UK: Holsworthy.

skin irritants, and have been shown in research settings to induce **dermatitis** (Held *et al.*, 2001). Further irritation can be caused by the combination of soap and 'hard' water, which produces a precipitate that remains on the surface of the skin if not rinsed off effectively (Timby, 1996). Soaps may also adversely affect the skin by causing the excessive removal of natural oils, precipitating drying of the skin, with these effects being aggravated if the water is too hot (Baillie and Arrowsmith, 2001). Because of its highly alkaline nature, the repeated use of soap may shift the pH of the skin surface, making it more alkaline, thereby negating the protective influence of the acid mantle and upsetting the balance of resident flora on the skin (Korting and Braun-Falco, 1996). This may enhance the risk of skin colonization by potentially pathogenic microorganisms, which may ultimately invade the skin should the barrier function be further disturbed. You should therefore take all of these factors into account when deciding which is the most appropriate approach to cleaning an individual's skin.

Skin cleansers

Skin cleansers provide an alternative means to promote skin hygiene and have recently been extensively reviewed (Ersser *et al.*, 2005; Hodgkinson *et al.*, 2007). Examples commonly found in clinical settings include: Senset (Vernacare); Tena Wash (Tena); Menalind (Hartmann); Attends (Attends Healthcare); Triple care (Smith & Nephew); and Comfortwash and Comfortshield (Sage Products). To add to the confusion, they appear in different forms, some coming as **creams, lotions,** mousses, foams, and others as pre-packed 'wet wipes'. They may reduce some of the adverse effects of soap owing to their chemical composition, and many claim to help to maintain a skin pH level that minimizes barrier disruption. Not surprisingly, because of the claims that these products save nursing time and reduce the incidence of skin breakdown, their use has become more popular, with an increased cost to the NHS (Continence Foundation, 2006). A number of early studies have attempted to compare skin cleansers with soap and water (Reid and Morison, 1994; Dealey, 1995; Whittingham, 1998; Cooper, 2000; Cooper and Gray, 2001). Unfortunately, though, weaknesses in the methodology are common, and these include lack of randomization, small sample sizes, inadequate controls, and poorly defined or inappropriate outcome measures. Thus, whilst there is evidence to support the use of cleansers, the reality is that there is little robust information available to guide practitioners in the exact choice of product or skin care regime, or to determine if one product is more suitable than another under different conditions, e.g. faecal incontinence (Hodgkinson *et al.*, 2007). Thus, any protocols that do exist for skin care tend to be based on anecdotal clinical experience rather than on empirically derived quality evidence. There is clearly a need for further vigorous research in this area to inform quality nursing intervention.

Drying

It is important that the skin is carefully dried after washing, to avoid maceration, undue cooling, and to maintain patient comfort. The capillary action of the towel wicks water away from the surface of the skin. However, the process of towel drying may compound any skin damage occurring during washing by causing direct mechanical injury to the **stratum corneum** (Huh *et al.*, 2002). Ultimately, this may lead to a disruption of the barrier function of the skin. This has been shown to be capable of increasing inflammatory mediator release in the skin, thus increasing the propensity for the skin to break down (Nickoloff and Naidu, 1994). Traditionally, nurses have tended to dry fragile skin by patting rather than rubbing, and this remains a common recommendation (Le Lievre, 2001; Marks, 2001), although a recent study suggests that pat drying with a towel can leave the skin significantly wetter, therefore potentially increasing the risk of overhydration of the stratum corneum, and maceration (Voegeli, 2008). The increased wetness may also expose the skin to a higher risk of friction damage, owing to the wet skin sticking to clothing or bedclothes, although this has yet to be conclusively demonstrated.

Moisturizing and replenishing the skin

The term 'emollient' is commonly used to describe agents that moisturize and increase hydration of the skin. Emollients and **moisturizers** perform similar functions in terms of increasing hydration of the top layer of the epidermis, the stratum corneum. Traditionally, basic emollients, such as petrolatum, have worked by creating an inert barrier over the skin surface, trapping moisture underneath (Holden *et al.*, 2002). Currently used emollients are available in the form of sprays, lotions, creams, and **ointments**. Although the development and formulation of emollients has moved forward, the basic principle remains the same: namely, they are all variations of an oil (lipid) and water emulsion. Technically, these emulsions

may take the form of oil-in-water, or water-in-oil, with oil-in-water emulsions being the commonest (Loden, 2005). Thus, modern emollients can not only help to maintain skin hydration, but can also help to replenish skin barrier lipids. As the formulations become more sophisticated, **emulsifying agents** and surfactants (e.g. cetostearyl alcohol, isopropyl myristate) are commonly added to increase stability and to improve the product by enabling the use of less oil, therefore reducing the overall greasiness of the emollient and making it more acceptable to the patient. It should be noted that there is an increased fire hazard with emollients containing a high paraffin content (Joint Formulary Committee, 2010).

To increase the moisturizing effects of emollients, additional agents known as **humectants** may be added (e.g. propylene glycol, urea, and glycerol). These chemicals attract and absorb water from their surroundings, thus helping to attract water into the stratum corneum when applied topically. The rich mixture of lipid and water makes an ideal breeding ground for bacteria, so in many cases agents to inhibit bacterial growth are also needed (e.g. benzalkonium chloride, hydroxybenzoates). Occasionally, sensitivity to emulsifying agents, preservatives, and other additives may occur, worsening the skin irritation and leading to a **contact dermatitis** (Fan *et al.*, 1999). Often, though, the commonest types of reaction to emollient preparations are sensory, particularly when used on very dry or cracked skin. Lotions and creams may cause a stinging or burning sensation due to the preservatives, and particularly if a humectant, such as urea, is present (Peters, 2005).

As our understanding of skin physiology has increased, so too has the number of emollient preparations available. Many now contain a sophisticated list of ingredients, and span the divide between drugs and cosmetics, leading to confusion when trying to select the most appropriate product (Brown and Butcher, 2005). Although greasier products (ointments) are thought to be more clinically effective, many patients dislike these and find the feel of them, combined with the staining of clothing and bedding that they cause, unacceptable. Preference is generally expressed for rapidly absorbed lotions and creams, particularly if being used on visible parts of the body (Holden *et al.*, 2002).

Surprisingly, despite the acceptance of emollient therapy as one of the mainstays of treatment in dermatology, there remains a lack of high-quality evidence on their effectiveness or an adequate comparison of the various compositions available (Rees, 2002). This rather contentious issue was highlighted in the *Drugs and Therapeutics Bulletin* (DTB, 2007), in which the conclusion was reached that there is no firm evidence to justify the estimated £16 million spent by the NHS on emollient bath additives, sparking considerable debate. Thus, ultimately, it is almost impossible to defend the clinical use of one particular emollient over another. In most cases, the decision of which one to use is largely influenced by patient preference or cost (Ellis *et al.*, 2003). This is a further area in which there is a need for robust research to inform quality nursing interventions.

Protecting the skin

Barrier creams, ointments, and, more recently, films have traditionally been used to protect the skin from damage caused by excessive exposure to water and irritants (e.g. urinary and faecal incontinence). They also have a role to play in preventing skin breakdown around stomas and exudating wounds (Voegeli, 2010). However, they are sometimes confused with emollients, and, although some barrier creams and ointments will have a mildly hydrating effect on the skin, this is not their major action and they should not be substituted for an emollient where one is indicated. Similarly, an emollient should not be substituted for a barrier product, because the two have completely different actions. Basic barrier preparations consist of a lipid/water emulsion base with the addition of metal oxides (e.g. zinc or titanium), which form a thin layer on the surface of the skin to repel potential irritants. The more sophisticated ones often contain a water-repellent silicone-based ingredient such as dimethicone, as well as antiseptic agents such as cetrimide or benzalkonium. Like emollients, there is the potential for some of these ingredients to cause irritation in sensitive individuals, with even innocuous preparations such as zinc and castor oil cream containing arachis (peanut) oil. You should always keep this in mind, particularly if skin irritation appears to worsen when using any preparation.

Advances in polymer science have led to the development of a new generation of products, which allow a thin semi-permeable protective polymer coating to be applied to the skin (e.g. Cavilon™, Skin-Prep™). It would appear that, in some situations, these polymers have an advantage over more conventional products, by saving nursing time and offering greater protection, particularly in the case of protecting peri-wound skin (Schuren *et al.*, 2005). Certainly, these products have grown in popularity, although they remain fairly expensive. Concern has been expressed that the use of barrier products, particularly greasy agents, might 'clog' incontinence pads, leading to pad failure and leakage, a problem that can certainly occur with the overuse of talcum powder. Once again, this is an area that has not been adequately studied; however, Bolton *et al.* (2004) suggest that, if applied sparingly according to manufacturers' instructions, most barrier products are safe to use in combination with incontinence pads and do not significantly affect pad performance. However, this study considered only one make of pad, so these results need to be interpreted with caution, and it remains to be seen whether this is true for all makes of pads.

As with emollients, the range of products that are marketed as barrier products has increased and become more sophisticated; a small range of products that are designed to cleanse, moisturize, and apply a barrier product all in one go has emerged (e.g. Triple Care™, Comfort Shield™). Unfortunately, these products have been developed in the absence of good-quality evidence regarding their effectiveness. There remains a general lack of objective evidence demonstrating the effectiveness of these new products compared with existing products or that highlights which product to use in different circumstances (Hughes, 2002). There is a clear need for further research in this area.

Oral hygiene

Like skin hygiene, oral care forms an essential part of the daily routine and plays a significant role in the maintenance of physical and psychological well-being; it is an area that is often neglected (Miegel and Wachtel, 2009). A guide to oral assessment is given in Figure 20.2. The complications of ineffective or absent oral hygiene measures have been extensively reported (Box 20.2), and range from halitosis (bad breath) through to potentially life-threatening endocarditis and septicaemia (Huskinson and Lloyd, 2009). More recently, effective mouth care has been shown to play a major role in reducing the serious complication of ventilator-associated pneumonia in critically

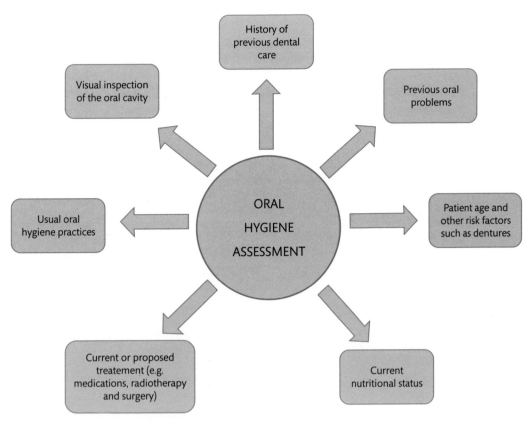

Figure 20.2 **Simple oral hygiene assessment tool.**

<table>
<tr><td>History of previous dental care</td></tr>
<tr><td>Visual inspection of the oral cavity</td><td>Previous oral problems</td></tr>
<tr><td>Usual oral hygiene practices</td><td>ORAL HYGIENE ASSESSMENT</td><td>Patient age and other risk factors such as dentures</td></tr>
<tr><td>Current or proposed treatement (e.g. medications, radiotherapy and surgery)</td><td>Current nutritional status</td></tr>
</table>

Box 20.2 **Potential complications of inadequate oral hygiene**

- Bacteraemia/endocarditis
- Septicaemia
- Respiratory tract infections/ventilator-associated pneumonia
- Xerostomia (dry mouth)
- Halitosis
- Pain and discomfort

ill patients, and forms one of the high-impact interventions recommended for implementation in all critical care areas (National Institute for Health and Clinical Excellence (NICE), 2008). Similarly, there is strong evidence—from two systematic reviews—that good oral hygiene reduces the incidence of respiratory infection in the older patient (Azarpazhooh and Leake, 2006; Sjögren *et al.*, 2008).

The primary functions of the mouth are the chewing of food and communication, both of which involve the lips, tongue, teeth (or dentures), and need adequate levels of saliva (Rawlins and Trueman, 2001). Difficulties with swallowing or eating may make it hard to maintain the mouth's healthy condition, because a build-up of debris can alter oral pH and inadequate dietary intake can reduce salivary flow. In the healthy mouth, the oral mucosa and tongue should be pink and moist, with smooth, moist lips, and clean teeth or well-fitting dentures. Saliva is essential for reducing the risk of oral infections (Malkin, 2009). It has antibacterial properties that help to maintain a healthy balance of normal resident bacteria, which include staphylococci and candida species. Inflammation and infection can occur as a result of reduced salivary flow, leading to the accumulation of plaque at the gum line, which can lead to **gingivitis**, **dental caries**, or **periodontal disease**. The process decalcifies teeth, leaving microscopic crevices that can harbour pathogenic organisms, which can lead to abscess formation (Xavier, 2000). Unfortunately, with the wide variations in uptake of dental care in the UK, it is reasonable to assume that many patients may have pre-existing poor oral health prior to admission. This increases the importance of your role in promoting oral health in the care setting, and ensuring that effective interventions are instigated.

Assessing the need for oral hygiene interventions

The purpose of oral care should be to keep the lips and mucosa soft, clean, intact, and moist. Cleaning the mouth and teeth (including dentures) of food debris and dental plaque should alleviate any discomfort, enhance oral intake, and prevent halitosis (Fitzpatrick, 2000). These activities should also prevent oral infection, although treatment for this may be required (Arkell and Shinnick, 2003). Certain medications and long-term conditions (Table 20.1) can put patients at increased risk of poor oral hygiene, with the very dependent, dysphagic, critically or terminally ill being particularly vulnerable (British Society for Disability and Oral Health, 2000). Similarly, older people may have difficulty managing their own oral care owing to poor dexterity. Additionally, denture wearers are at increased risk of chronic atrophic candidosis (denture stomatitis) because the acrylics used to construct the dentures provide favourable conditions for *Candida albicans* to grow (Arkell and Shinnick, 2003).

Table 20.1 **Factors increasing risk of oral health problems**

Medications	Anticholinergics, diuretics, antihypertensives, antidepressants, antihistamines, opioid-based analgesics, sedatives and tranquillizers, cytotoxics, antiparkinsonian drugs
Nutrition	Deficiency of vitamin A, B, C, zinc, and folic acid Enteral/parenteral feeding
Medical condition	Diabetes mellitus, Parkinson's and other neurological disorders, stroke, dysphagia, osteo/rheumatoid arthritis, dementia, learning disability, respiratory disease

Several oral care assessment tools have been proposed, but, as with skin assessment, evidence on their effectiveness is limited and many have not been adequately tested to determine validity and reliability (Cooley, 2002). Evidence that clinically effective oral care improves outcomes is available (Bowsher *et al.*, 1999), but implementation depends on proper assessment and appropriate staff education (Brady *et al.*, 2006).

Your initial assessment should consist of gathering information on:

- history of previous dental care;
- previous oral problems;
- patient age and other risk factors such as dentures;
- current nutritional status;
- current treatment and any proposed treatment, including medications, radiotherapy, and surgery;
- usual oral hygiene practices;
- visual inspection of the oral cavity.

Oral infections can present as sore, reddened areas, or swelling. Fungal infections (such as *Candida*) often present as creamy white coatings or yellow curd-like mounds that are easily removed (Arkell and Shinnick, 2003). Patients can complain of soreness or difficulty swallowing and are at risk of systemic problems if the infection remains untreated. Figure 20.3 shows thrush (pseudomembranous candidosis) in an elderly patient.

The management of oral hygiene

Frequency

There is a lack of evidence and consensus about the frequency of oral care required to provide maximum benefit for patients (Evans, 2001). However, plaque build-up and gingivitis have been identified after 2–4 days without adequate oral care (Pearson and Hutton, 2002). Adair *et al.* (2001) recommended brushing teeth twice a day, and it is recognized that doing this after every meal reduces the incidence of oral and respiratory infections (Furr *et al.*, 2004). However, brushing the teeth after every meal tends not to be very practical in most acute care settings. Helping patients to maintain twice-daily brushing, as a minimum, would appear to be best practice in line with current British Dental Association

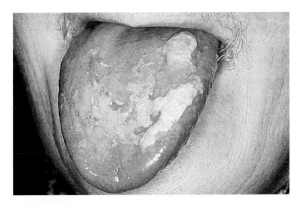

Figure 20.3 **(see Colour Plate 9) Thrush (pseudomembranous candidosis) in an elderly patient.**

Reproduced from Soames and Southam, *Oral Pathology*, with permission from Oxford University Press.

(2009) recommendations. Factors such as dehydration, mouth breathing, and oxygen therapy should increase the frequency of oral care to maintain a patient's comfort and to reduce further risk (Cooley, 2002), and additional care should be given to patients at risk, as previously outlined.

Products

As with personal hygiene care, the choice of what products to use to maintain oral health is difficult due to the large number of products available. Ideally, a soft toothbrush should be used. This will remove plaque and debris from the surfaces and crevices of teeth with minimal gum trauma, as well as allow brushing of the tongue surface (Pearson and Hutton, 2002). An electric toothbrush may be more suitable for individuals with limited dexterity to manage a manual brush or poor technique. They may also be suitable for people whose oral hygiene is difficult to maintain, such as those with learning disabilities (Bernal, 2005). Most recommendations advise the use of a pea-sized amount of toothpaste containing fluoride (British Dental Association, 2009). The use of forceps and gauze to clean the mouth has been shown to be ineffective and may cause damage to the delicate oral tissues (Holmes, 1996). Similarly, the use of foam swabs is ineffective in removing plaque and can present a choking hazard (Pearson and Hutton, 2002).

Mouthwashes may be used to supplement brushing, and are recommended to reduce respiratory complications in the older person and the critically ill (Chlebicki and Safdar, 2007; Scannapieco *et al.*, 2009). Generally, anti-bacterial agents are most effective (e.g. chlorhexidine gluconate, cetylpyridinium chloride), but prolonged use may cause reversible staining of the teeth and adversely affect the natural microorganisms in the oral cavity (Rawlins and Trueman, 2001). They are effective when used a minimum of twice daily (Bowsher *et al.*, 1999); however, they should be used as an adjunct to toothbrushing and not as a replacement (Wise *et al.*, 2008). Other solutions, such as sodium bicarbonate or hydrogen peroxide, may be used to remove debris and dried secretions, although care is needed to ensure that solutions used are not too concentrated, which can damage the tissue of the oral cavity. For this reason, you should use these only following specialist advice, and not for routine oral care.

Special considerations

Particular care needs to be shown when undertaking oral care for an unconscious patient owing to the increased risk of aspiration. In these situations, tooth brushing remains the most effective method; however, the procedure needs to be adapted to reduce risk and to maintain patient safety. Suction equipment may be needed to ensure safe removal of excess liquid, and in the critical care setting specialized suction toothbrushes are available.

Patients who suffer from excessive dry mouth (xerostomia) may require additional measures to maintain moisture and comfort. These range from the use of pineapple pieces to ice chips and artificial saliva (Clay, 2000). It was thought that the proteolytic enzyme ananase, found in pineapple, was responsible for its effect in mouth care, but it is now suggested that this is more likely to be because of a non-specific increase in salivary flow caused by the fruit juice (Ford, 2008). However, care should be taken because acidic substances (such as fruit juices) can rapidly lead to dental caries in those with xerostomia, especially if used for any length of time (Pemberton and Thornhill, 1998). Other effective salivary stimulants include sugar-free chewing gum and mints (Davis, 1997). Some clinical areas may still use glycerine and lemon swabs as moisturizing agents. However, there is a substantial evidence base indicating that these products are detrimental to oral care (Rawlins and Trueman, 2001; Ministry of Health, 2004). These detrimental effects include increasing oral alkalinity, decalcification of teeth, and increased drying of the mouth owing to the osmotic effects of glycerine. You should therefore ensure that these swabs are not used in practice. Dry lips should be moisturized using soft paraffin or lip balm to maintain integrity and function (Cooley, 2002).

Oral care for the patient with dentures needs to be adapted accordingly. Well-fitting dentures are essential for speech and oral intake. There is significant increased risk of infection from poorly fitted dentures, which can irritate the gums and harbour debris, and the use of adhesive denture fixatives can help if the dentures are loose (Fitzpatrick, 2000). Once-daily cleansing with a toothbrush and toothpaste is effective for cleansing dentures. Soaking overnight or when not worn in commercial denture cleaners will also help to prevent infection (Johnson and Chalmers, 2002; de Souza *et al.*, 2009).

Accessing the evidence to inform clinical nursing decisions

As can be seen from the previous sections, there is a growing body of literature from various sources concerning personal hygiene and oral care. Examination of washing practices using soap and water is largely based on literature reviews, drawn from clinical observation, supported by limited experimental (quasi) study evidence and an expert panel source. There is a slightly stronger empirical basis for cleanser use. Overall, the studies comparing skin cleansers with soap and water provide indications that they have therapeutic and economic benefits, especially when combined with an emollient. However, there are common weaknesses in study design, including absent

or unclear reported procedures for randomization, allocation concealment, and loss to follow-up analysis, which limits the robustness and reliability of these conclusions. To date, there are no comprehensive systematic reviews providing clear guidance on the effectiveness of cleansing methods. However, many care settings have developed skin care protocols based on the growing evidence base and a general consensus of clinical opinion. As has already been stated, the evidence surrounding oral hygiene is perhaps clearer and definitive recommendations are available.

In common with many aspects of nursing, the evidence base to support interventions for hygiene and oral care will come from a variety of sources, many from outside the pure nursing literature. The following list highlights reputable journal and web-based sources of information that may be useful when considering the evidence base. However, this list is by no means exhaustive.

Journals

Advances in Skin and Wound Care
British Dental Journal
Journal of Wound Ostomy and Continence Nursing (JWOCN)
Journal of Dental Hygiene
Journal of Wound Care
Journal of Clinical Nursing
Journal of Advanced Nursing
Journal of the American Geriatrics Society
Skin Research and Technology
Skin Physiology and Pharmacology

Web resources

The Cochrane Library **www.thecochranelibrary.com/ view/0/index.html**
Essence of Care (DH) **www.dh.gov.uk/en/Publication- sandstatistics/Publications/PublicationsPolicyAnd- Guidance/DH_119969**
NHS Evidence **www.evidence.nhs.uk/**
NHS Quality Improvement Scotland **www.nhshealth- quality.org**
NMC Essential Skills Clusters **http://standards.nmc-uk. org/Documents/Annexe3_%20ESCs_16092010.pdf**
The British Dental Association **www.bda.org**
British Dental Health Association **www.dentalhealth.org.uk**
British Society for Disability and Oral Health **www.bsdh. org.uk**
British Society of Gerodontology **www.gerodontology.com**

Utilizing evidence-based clinical guidelines

Given the wide range of literature on the subject, it is not surprising that skin and oral care interventions are seen to vary from area to area, even showing considerable variability between clinical areas within the same hospital. In the case of personal hygiene, one way forward is to clearly define what constitutes therapeutic nursing skin care interventions, as opposed to interventions used for general hygiene and social reasons, as is done by nurses in the US. By using this approach, there are some clear guidelines that emerge, and these are formed by a growing evidence base and clinical concensus. These can be utilized to reflect on current practice, and to assist in the development of clinical guidelines and the formulation of skin care protocols. The potential benefits to patients of adopting clear skin care protocols have been highlighted by several studies based both in the UK and North America. Bale *et al.* (2004) reported that the introduction of a protocol for elderly patients with incontinence in a nursing home led to an overall improvement in skin health and integrity. Cole and Nesbitt (2004) and Lyder *et al.* (2002) demonstrated a significant reduction in pressure ulcer incidence rates in both hospital and residential care settings following the implementation of clear skin care protocols. In Cole and Nesbitt's study, the pressure ulcer incidence rate fell from 17.9% to 2% over a 3-year period, and Lyder's group reported a remarkable 87% reduction in incidence rate in one nursing home. These studies demonstrate that small changes in nursing practice, supported by ongoing education, can achieve significant results in terms of improving skin hygiene and health.

Based on the clinical evidence available, and the availability of current guidelines, such as those produced by the American Wound Ostomy and Continence Nurses Society (Wound Ostomy and Continence Nurses Society, 2003), a basic set of guiding principles can be put forward (Box 20.3) These address the basic stages of skin care that have been explored: namely, cleansing, moisturizing, replenishing, and protecting. However, it is up to you to weigh up the evidence concerning individual products before deciding which ones to use for each aspect of your skin care interventions.

The clinical evidence available concerning oral care, and current guidelines, such as those produced by NHS Quality Improvement Scotland (2005) and Heath *et al.* (2011), provide

---

> ### Box 20.3 **General skin care principles**
>
> - **Assess the patient's skin daily**
> - **Cleanse skin when clinically indicated (e.g. soiling) using a pH-balanced cleanser (preferably a no-rinse cleanser)**
> - **Avoid using soap and hot water**
> - **Avoid excessive friction and scrubbing**
> - **Minimize skin exposure to moisture (e.g. incontinence, wound leakage)**
> - **Use a skin barrier product (e.g. cream, ointment, film) to protect vulnerable skin**
> - **Use emollients to maintain skin hydration**
>
> (adapted from Wound Ostomy and Continence Nurses Society, 2003)

some guiding principles for routine daily oral care, and these are illustrated in Box 20.4. These should be used to inform your nursing interventions in oral hygiene.

Measuring the impact of nursing interventions

The principle of measuring both the effectiveness of nursing intervention and the patient's experience of receiving care is one that you should, where possible, facilitate. The NHS Information Centre has supported the development of **Nursing Quality Metrics (NQMs)** that can be used to facilitate quality improvement in patient care and experience **http://signposting.ic.nhs.uk/?k=metrics.**

This recent move within healthcare to be outcome-focused rather than target-driven is a welcome change in policy direction, initiated by Lord Darzi in his review of the NHS, and sustained by the previous and current UK governments. Metrics have been developed for many aspects of nursing care interventions and cover many inpatient areas, regardless of setting. The collection of these types of data helps healthcare organizations to focus on the delivery of safe and effective care, and can be used for local and national benchmarking, as well as for quality improvement.

For further details visit the NHS Information Centre online at **http://www.ic.nhs.uk/,** where you will find details relating to nursing audit tools capturing information on documentation for observations, nutrition, medicines administration, pain management,

Box 20.4 Recommended best practice for daily oral care

Care of lips

- Clean with water-moistened gauze and protect with a lubricant (e.g. white soft paraffin) to reduce risk of dry, cracked lips.

Care of the person with dentures

- Ensure that dentures are marked with the person's name (particularly in long-term care settings).
- Leave dentures out at night if acceptable to the individual.
- Soak plastic dentures in dilute sodium hypochlorite or chlorhexidine solution for dentures with metal parts.
- Clean dentures with individual brush under running water.
- Rinse dentures after meals.
- Use a small quantity of cream/powder fixative if required. Clean off and replace before meals, and clean off last thing at night.

Care of natural teeth

- Clean twice daily and after meals (if possible) with fluoridated toothpaste and a soft toothbrush.
- Provide additional plaque control if required using chlorhexidine mouthwash, spray, or gel.

Care of oral mucosa

- Inspect in a good light.
- Report any unusual appearances.
- Clean with water-moistened foam sponges, 'TePe' special care toothbrush, or baby toothbrush.

Care of the person with xerostomia

- Provide oral lubrication in the form of sips of water or spray or use artificial saliva.

communication, discharge planning, falls, pressure area care, antibiotic prescribing, and infection control.

In determining patient experience of healthcare, NICE has recently published a Quality Standard **http://www.nice.org.uk/** that guides service delivery planning to ensure improvements in patient experience. Further commissioned work by the Department of Health has developed a single measure of patient experience. Supplementing these data is the NHS Survey, which captures patient views relating to ward cleanliness, infection control, staff attitudes, pain management, management of privacy, experience of dignity, nutrition, medicines administration, quality of communication, and discharge. Details can be found online at **http://www.nhssurveys.org/.**

Summary and key messages

- Skin and oral care is an important, yet often neglected, aspect of nursing care.
- Maintaining oral health is fundamental to general health and quality of life.
- Good skin care consists of four aspects: cleansing, hydrating, protecting, and replenishing.
- The range of products and methods available can be confusing.
- There is a lack of robust research evidence about products and skin hygiene approaches to inform

high-quality nursing interventions. More research is required.
- Where they do exist, the adoption of clear evidence-based skin and oral care protocols can have a significant effect on patient outcome.
- Registered nurses should take responsibility for ensuring that all patients in their care receive appropriate, evidence-based skin and oral hygiene interventions, and should closely supervise delegated care.

Online Resource Centre

 To help you to develop and apply your knowledge and decision-making skills further, we have provided interactive learning resources online at **www.oxfordtextbooks.co.uk/orc/bullock/**

Whilst these are freely available, you will need to use the access codes at the start of the book.

References

Abbas, S., Weiss Goldberg, J., Massaro, M. (2004) Personal cleanser technology and clinical performance. *Dermatologic Therapy* **17**: 35–42.

Adair, S.M., Bowen, W.H., Burt, B.A., *et al.* (2001) Recommendations for using fluoride to prevent and control dental caries in the United States. *Mortality and Morbidity Weekly Report* **50**(14): 1–42.

Arkell, S., Shinnick, A. (2003) Update on oral candidosis. *Nursing Times* **99**(48): 52–3.

Azarpazhooh, A., Leake, J.L. (2006) Systematic review of the association between respiratory diseases and oral health. *Journal of Periodontology* **77**: 1465–82.

Baillie, L., Arrowsmith, V. (2001). *Meeting Elimination Needs. Developing Practical Nursing Skills.* Hodder Arnold: London.

Bale, S., Tebble, N., Jones, V., *et al.* (2004) The benefits of implementing a new skin care protocol in nursing homes. *Journal of Tissue Viability* **14**(2): 44–50.

Bernal, C. (2005) Maintenance of oral health in people with learning disabilities. *Nursing Times* **101**(6): 40–2.

Bliss, D.Z., Zehrer, C., Savik, K., *et al.* (2007) An economic evaluation of four skin damage prevention regimens in nursing home residents with incontinence: economics of skin damage prevention. *Journal of Wound, Ostomy & Continence Nursing* **34**(2):143–52.

Bolton, C., Flynn, R., Harvey, E., *et al.* (2004) Assessment of pad clogging. *Journal of Community Nursing* **18**(6): 18–20.

Bowsher, J., Boyle, S., Griffiths, J. (1999) A clinical effectiveness review: a review of research evidenced base for oral care. *Nursing Standard* **13**(37): 31–3.

Brady, M.C., Furlanetto, D., Hunter, R., *et al.* (2006) Staff-led interventions for improving oral hygiene in patients following stroke. *Cochrane Database of Systematic Reviews* Issue 4: Art. No. CD003864. DOI: 10.1002/14651858.CD003864.pub2.

British Dental Association (2009) **www.bda.org** (accessed 11 October 2011).

British Society for Disability and Oral Health (2000) *Guidelines for Oral Health Care for Long-Stay Patients and Residents: Report of BSDH Working Group.* **http://tinyurl.com/oral-healthcare** (accessed 11 October 2011).

Brown, A., Butcher, M. (2005) A guide to emollient therapy. *Nursing Standard* **19**(24): 68–75.

Chlebicki, M.P., Safdar, N. (2007) Topical chlorhexidine for prevention of ventilator-associated pneumonia: a meta-analysis. *Critical Care Medicine* **35**: 595–602.

Clay, M. (2000) Oral health in older people. *Nursing Older People* **12**(7): 21–5.

Cole, L., Nesbitt, C. (2004) A three-year multi-phase pressure ulcer prevalence/incidence study in a regional referral hospital. *Ostomy and Wound Management* **50**(11): 33–40.

Continence Foundation (2006) **www.continence-foundation.org.uk** (accessed 11 October 2011).

Cooley, C. (2002) Oral health: basic or essential care? *Cancer Nursing Practice* **1**(3): 33–9.

Cooper, P. (2000) The use of clinisan in the skin care of the incontinent patient. *British Journal of Nursing* **9**(7): 445–8.

Cooper, P., Gray, D. (2001) Comparison of two patients in care regimens for incontinence. *British Journal of Nursing* **10**(6): 6–20.

Davis, A.N. (1997) The management of xerostomia: a review. *European Journal of Cancer Care* **6**: 209–14.

de Souza, R.F., de Freitas Oliveira Paranhos, H. (2009) Interventions for cleaning dentures in adults. *Cochrane Database of Systematic Reviews* Issue 4: Art. No. CD007395. DOI: 10.1002/14651858.CD007395.pub2.

Dealey, C. (1995) Pressure sores and incontinence: a study evaluating the use of topical agents in skin care. *Journal of Wound Care* **4**(3): 103–5.

Department of Health (2005) Meeting the challenges of oral health for older people: a strategic review. *Gerodontology* **22**(Suppl. 1): 3–48.

Department of Health (2010) *Essence of Care: Benchmarks for the Fundamental Aspects of Care.* Benchmarks for personal hygiene. **http://www.dh.gov.uk/en/publicationsandstatistics/publications/publicationspolicyandguidance/dh_119969** (accessed 11 October 2011).

Dingwall, L. (2010) *Personal Hygiene Care.* Wiley-Blackwell: Chichester.

DTB (2007) Bath emollients for atopic eczema: why use them? *Drug and Therapeutics Bulletin* **45**(10): 73–5.

Ellis, C., Luger, T., Abeck, D., *et al.* (2003) ICCAD II Faculty. International Consensus Conference on Atopic Dermatitis II (ICCAD II): clinical update and current treatment strategies. *British Journal of Dermatology* **148**(Suppl. 63): 3–10.

Ersser, S.J., Getliffe, K., Voegeli, D., *et al.* (2005) A critical review of the inter-relationship between skin vulnerability and urinary incontinence and related nursing intervention. *International Journal of Nursing Studies* **42**: 823–35.

Evans, G. (2001) A rationale for oral care. *Nursing Standard* **15**(43): 33–6.

Fan, W., Kinnunen, T., Niinimake, A. (1991) Skin reactions to glycols used in dermatological and cosmetic vehicles. *American Journal of Contact Dermatitis* **2**: 181–3.

Fitzpatrick, J. (2000) Oral health care needs of dependent older people: responsibilities of nurses and care staff. *Journal of Advanced Nursing* **32**(6): 1325–32.

Ford, S.J. (2008) The importance and provision of oral hygiene in surgical patients. *International Journal of Surgery* **6**: 418–19.

Furr, L.A., Binkley, C.J., McCurren, C., *et al.* (2004) Factors affecting quality of oral care in intensive care units. *Journal of Advanced Nursing* **48**(5): 454–62.

Gray, M., Bliss, D.Z., Doughty, D.B., *et al.* (**2007**) Incontinence-associated dermatitis: a consensus. *Journal of Wound, Ostomy, & Continence Nursing* **34**(1): 45–54.

Healthcare Commission (2007) *State of Healthcare 2007: Improvements and Challenges in Services in England and Wales.* Commission for Healthcare Audit and Inspection: London.

Heath, H., Sturdy, D., Edwards, T., *et al.* (2011) *Promoting Older People's Oral Health.* RCN Publishing: Harrow.

Held, E., Lund, H., Agner, T. (2001) Effects of different moisturizers on SLS-irritated human skin. *Contact Dermatitis* **44**: 229–34.

Hodgkinson, B., Nay, R., Wilson, J. (2007) A systematic review of topical skin care in aged care facilities. *Journal of Clinical Nursing* **16**(1): 129–36.

Holden, C., English, J., Hoare, C., *et al.* (2002) Advised best practice for the use of emollients in eczema and other dry skin conditions. *Journal of Dermatological Treatment* **13**: 103–6.

Holmes, S. (1996) Nursing management of oral care in older patients. *Nursing Times* **92**(9): 37–9.

Hughes, S. (2002) Do continence aids help maintain skin integrity? *Journal of Wound Care* **11**(6): 235–9.

Huh, C.H., Seo, K.I., Kim, S.D., *et al.* (2002) Biophysical changes after mechanical injury of the stratum corneum in normal skin. *Contact Dermatitis* **46**: 24–8.

Huskinson, W., Lloyd, H. (2009) Oral health in hospitalised patients: assessment and hygiene. *Nursing Standard* **23**(36): 43–7.

Johnson, V., Chalmers, J. (2002) *Oral Hygiene Care for Functionally Dependent and Cognitively Impaired Older Adults: Research Dissemination Core.* Iowa City, IA: University of Iowa.

Joint Formulary Committee (2010) *British National Formulary 59.* BMJ Publishing Group Ltd, RPS Publishing: London.

Korting, H.C., Braun-Falco, O. (1996) The effect of detergents on skin pH and its consequences. *Clinics in Dermatology* **14**: 23–7.

Le Lievre, S. (2001) The management and prevention of incontinence dermatitis. *British Journal of Community Nursing* **6**(4): 180–5.

Loden, M. (2005) The clinical benefit of moisturizers. *Journal of the European Academy of Dermatology and Venereology* **19**: 672–88.

Lyder, C.H., Shannon, R., Empleo-Frazier, O., *et al.* (2002) A comprehensive program to prevent pressure ulcers in long-term care: exploring costs and outcomes. *Ostomy and Wound Management* **48**(4): 52–62.

Malkin, B. (2009) The importance of patients' oral health and nurses' role in assessing and maintaining it. *Nursing Times* **105**(17): 19–23.

Marks, R. (2001) *Sophisticated Emollients,* 2nd edn. Georg Thieme Verlag: Stuttgart.

McGuckin, M., Shubin, A., Hujcs, M. (2008) Interventional patient hygiene model: infection control and nursing share responsibility for patient safety. *American Journal of Infection Control* **36**: 59–62.

Miegel, K., Wachtel, T. (2009) Improving the oral health of older people in long-term residential care: a review of the literature. *International Journal of Older People Nursing* **4**(2): 97–113.

Ministry of Health (2004) *Nursing Management of Oral Hygiene.* Ministry of Health: Singapore.

National Institute for Health and Clinical Excellence (2008) *Technical Patient Safety Solutions for Ventilator-Associated Pneumonia in Adults.* **http://guidance.nice.org.uk/PSG002/ Guidance/pdf/English** (accessed 11 October 2011).

Newton, H., Cameron, J. (2003) *Skin Care in Wound Management.* Medical Communications UK: Holsworthy.

NHS Quality Improvement Scotland (2005) *Best Practice Statement: Working with Dependent Older People to Achieve Good Oral Health.* **www.nhshealthquality.org** (accessed 11 October 2011).

Nickoloff, B.J., Naidu, Y. (1994) Perturbation of epidermal barrier function correlates with irritation of cytokine cascade in human skin. *Journal of the American Academy of Dermatology* **30**: 535–46.

Pearson, L., Hutton, J. (2002) A controlled trial to compare the ability of foam swabs and toothbrushes to remove dental plaque. *Journal of Advanced Nursing* **39**(5): 480–9.

Pemberton, M., Thornhill, M.H. (1998) Simple antiseptic mouthwashes are best for infection. *British Medical Journal* **316**: 1246.

Peters, J. (2005) Exploring the use of emollient therapy in dermatological nursing. *British Journal of Nursing* **14**(9): 494–502.

Rawlins, C.A., Trueman, I.W. (2001) Effective mouth care for seriously ill patients. *Professional Nurse* **16**(4): 1025–8.

Rees, M. (2002) Managing atopic eczema. *Primary Health Care* **12**(8): 27–37.

Reid, J., Morison, M. (1994) Towards a consensus: classification of pressure sores. *Journal of Wound Care* **3**(3): 157–60.

Roper, N., Logan, W.W., Tierney, A.J. (1996) *The Elements of Nursing: A Model for Nursing Based on a Model for Living,* 4th edn. Churchill Livingstone: London.

Scannapieco, F.A., Yu, J., Raghavendran, K., *et al.* (2009) A randomized trial of chlorhexidine gluconate on oral bacterial pathogens in mechanically ventilated patients. *Critical Care* **13**: R117.

Schuren, J., Becker, A., Sibbald, G. (2005) A liquid film-forming acrylate for peri-wound protection: a systematic review and meta-analysis (3M™ Cavilon™ no-sting barrier film). *International Wound Journal* **2**(3): 230–8.

Sjögren, P., Nilsson, E., Forsell, M., *et al.* (2008) A systematic review of the preventative effect of oral hygiene on pneumonia and respiratory tract infection in elderly people in hospitals and nursing homes: effect estimates and methodological quality of randomized controlled trials. *Journal of the American Geriatrics Society* **56**: 2124–30.

Timby, B.K. (1996) *Hygiene. Fundamental Skills and Concepts in Patient Care*, 6th edn. Lippincott Raven: London.

Voegeli, D. (2008) The effect of washing and drying practices on skin barrier function. *Journal of Wound Ostomy and Continence Nursing* **35**(1): 84–90.

Voegeli, D. (2010) Care or harm: exploring essential components of skin care regimens. *British Journal of Nursing* **19**(13): 810–19.

Vollman, K., Garcia, R., Miller, L. (2005) Interventional patient hygiene: proactive (hygiene) strategies to improve patients' outcomes. *AACNNews* **22**: 1–9.

Whittingham, K. (1998) Cleansing regimens for continence care. *Professional Nurse* **14**(3): 167–72.

Wise, M., Cole, J.M., Williams, D.W., *et al.* (2008) Efficacy of oral chlorhexidine in critical care. *Critical Care* **12**: 419.

Wound Ostomy and Continence Nurses Society (2003) Guidelines for prevention and management of pressure ulcers 14. *WOCN Clinical Practice Guideline Series*. WOCN Society: Glenview, IL.

Xavier, G. (2000) The importance of mouth care in preventing infection. *Nursing Standard* **14**(18): 47–51.

Young, L. (1991) The clean fight. *Nursing Standard* **5**(35): 54–5.

21 *Managing* Infection

Jacqui Prieto and Martin Kiernan

> ## Introduction
>
> This chapter addresses the fundamental nursing role and responsibility of preventing the risk of infection in all healthcare settings. Every nurse should possess the knowledge and skills to assess the risk of infection, to select and implement evidence-based strategies to prevention infection, and to review the effectiveness of these to inform any necessary changes in care.

Understanding the importance of infection prevention

Definitions

Healthcare-associated infection (HCAI) is the term used to describe an infection that arises as a result of some exposure to healthcare. Unlike the more traditional terms 'hospital-acquired' or 'nosocomial' infection, this updated term encompasses the range of settings in which healthcare is delivered and from which infections may arise. In recent years, much of the attention on HCAIs has focused on methicillin-resistant *Staphylococcus aureus* (MRSA) and *Clostridium difficile* (*C. difficile*), both of which are closely monitored in acute hospitals and in England as part of a programme of mandatory surveillance (National Audit Office, 2009).

It is important to recognize that HCAIs are caused by a wide variety of microorganisms, for example *Escherichia coli* (*E. coli*), which require equal attention in clinical practice. Because the principles of infection prevention are applicable to all causes of HCAIs, this chapter focuses on these underpinning principles rather than on specific microorganisms of concern. As a nurse, you have a fundamental responsibility for minimizing the risk of infection in all healthcare settings and in the patient's own home by understanding and applying these principles in practice.

Prevalence and incidence of HCAIs

HCAI is a significant problem in all healthcare settings, although much more is known about its prevalence and incidence in hospitals than in other healthcare environments. Prevalence of HCAI is the total number of cases that occur either at a particular time (point prevalence) or over a defined period of time (period prevalence). The UK prevalence surveys, conducted in 2006, estimated that, at any one time, approximately one in eight hospital inpatients has a HCAI (Smyth *et al.*, 2008; Reilly *et al.*, 2008). This figure is comparable with data from inpatient populations in other countries, with reported rates ranging between 3.5% and 9.5% (e.g. European Centre for Disease Prevention and Control, 2008; Gravel *et al.*, 2007; Wu *et al.*, 2005). The survey also found the overall prevalence of MRSA to be 1.15% of the patient population, with MRSA being the causative organism in 15.8% of all HCAIs. In the same survey, the prevalence of *C. difficile* infection was 1.72% of the patient population, with 1.21% considered to be hospital-associated and 0.51% community-associated (Smyth *et al.*, 2008). However, caution is needed when comparing rates of infection in different countries because there are differences in the methods used, including definitions of infection.

In the UK surveys, the commonest types of infection were found to be urinary tract, gastrointestinal, lower respiratory tract, surgical site, skin and soft tissue, and bloodstream infections (Smyth *et al.*, 2008; Reilly *et al.*, 2008). There have been no reported national surveys of the prevalence or incidence of HCAI in settings other than hospitals, so the true rate of HCAI in the population is unknown.

Surveillance programmes that monitor the incidence of HCAI provide a valuable source of information. Incidence is the number of new cases in a defined period within a specific population. In England, the mandatory surveillance system of surgical site infections in orthopaedic surgery measures the incidence of infection among patients undergoing specific kinds of orthopaedic surgery. Since these infections are often identified following the patient's discharge from hospital, the system was recently amended to include patients who are readmitted to hospital with a surgical site infection. This change increased the number of infections detected by 40% overall and by nearly 70% in knee prosthesis (Health Protection Agency, 2009). This is still an underestimate of the true rate because only the most serious infections that require readmission are detected.

Causes of HCAI

An infection occurs when a microorganism or other infectious agent enters an area of the body and starts to multiply. Bacteria can release toxins that are absorbed into the body and result in clinical signs and symptoms of infection. The immune response itself also brings about symptoms of infection. A wide variety of infectious agents are capable of causing infection in humans, including bacteria, viruses, fungi, protozoa, prions, and helminths. HCAIs are most commonly caused by bacteria and viruses. The term 'pathogen' is used to refer to an infectious agent's ability to cause disease to its host. Pathogens do not always cause disease in the host. They may be found at other sites on the body and multiply without producing symptoms. This is known as 'colonization' or 'carriage'.

Infectious agents may enter the body through the normal openings (such as the mouth, nose, eyes, and genitalia), through an open wound or skin lesion, or via any breach in normal defences (such as the skin by various routes, including an invasive device such as an intravascular catheter, urinary catheter, or respiratory device). Factors that affect a person's susceptibility to infection include age, immunity, physical well-being, psychological well-being, hygiene, underlying or chronic diseases or medical conditions, other existing infections, and medical treatments and interventions. The risk of infection developing depends on the balance between **host susceptibility** and the dose and **virulence** (disease-producing ability) of the infectious agent.

Routes of transmission

Infectious agents that cause HCAI may be spread from one person to another by one or more routes of transmission. The three main routes of transmission of HCAI are contact, airborne, and droplet. Other routes, including bloodborne and common vehicle (food and waterborne), are less common in relation to HCAI transmission despite being significant routes of infection transmission within the general population. The contact route is regarded as the commonest route of transmission for HCAI. Contact transmission can occur directly from one person to another, indirectly through a third person such as a healthcare worker, or by contaminated equipment or the environment. The role of hands in contact transmission of infection has long been recognized, and the unwashed hands of healthcare staff are considered to be the most important vehicle or 'vector' of infection in hospitals and other healthcare settings (Pittet *et al.*, 2006). For this reason, effective hand hygiene is regarded as a cornerstone of infection prevention practice, preventing exposure to infectious agents transferred from person to person via the hands. Effective management of invasive devices and procedures is another key principle of infection prevention, minimizing the risk of infectious agents, including those present on the patient him or herself from entering susceptible body sites and causing infection.

The human and social burden and costs of HCAI

HCAIs impose a burden on patients and their carers and on health services, both in the acute and community sectors. For the patient, the experience of infection can involve symptoms ranging from mild discomfort to prolonged or permanent disability and, in some cases, death. Increased length of stay or, in some cases, readmission to hospital may incur considerable costs to the patient, as well as the health service, owing to increased absence from work and the need for more frequent hospital outpatient appointments, admissions, or visits to the GP. In one landmark study, patients who had an HCAI took an average of 1–2 weeks longer to resume normal daily activities than patients without infection (Plowman *et al.*, 1999).

An interview study about patients' experiences of healthcare-associated bloodstream infection revealed inadequacies in communication about HCAI by healthcare staff (Burnett *et al.*, 2010). Patients who had an HCAI were more likely to express little or no confidence in the National Health Service (NHS) and were concerned about the possibility of acquiring infection should they go back into hospital. Studies exploring the patient's experience of being nursed in single-room isolation due to infection while in hospital have identified adverse effects, including extreme boredom, lowered or disturbed mood, and feelings of stigma, along with anxiety about the risk of passing his or her infection to relatives and carers (Madeo, 2001; Newton *et al.*, 2001; Tarzi *et al.*, 2001; Rees *et al.*, 2000). These findings illustrate the key role of nurses and other health professionals in ensuring that patients, relatives, and their carers receive high-quality information about HCAI and identify the needs of patients with HCAI who require isolation while in hospital.

The most recent National Audit Office report on HCAI (NAO, 2009) provides a useful overview of the overall cost of HCAIs. It recognizes the limited information currently available to determine both the economic burden of HCAI and the rate of mortality. Litigation costs are also recognized as a potential direct cost to the NHS, arising when patients or their relatives pursue a legal claim for compensation. The study by Plowman *et al.* (1999) is acknowledged as being the most comprehensive in relation to the economic burden of HCAI, although it is now out-of-date. It found that patients who presented with one or more HCAIs during their inpatient stay incurred costs that were, on average, 2.9 times greater than those for uninfected patients, costing the NHS in England an estimated £1 billion annually.

Key nursing responsibilities and accountability for HCAI

Whilst the prevention of HCAI requires the commitment and cooperation of all healthcare staff, you will play a fundamental role in minimizing infection risks to patients, yourself, and others in acute and community settings. In England and Wales, the Health and Social Care Act 2008 places a legal responsibility upon healthcare organizations to provide a clean environment in which infection risks are minimized. As a nurse, you must take responsibility for maintaining up-to-date knowledge and high standards of clinical practice based on best available evidence, and must expect to take the lead and be accountable for your actions in the key elements of infection prevention identified in Figure 21.1.

In this chapter, the evidence that exists to support you in the delivery of effective, nurse-led interventions to prevent and manage infection is examined. Key issues related to clinical assessment of risk of HCAI and the recognition of symptoms are considered, and an overview of the key infection prevention measures is provided. This is followed by a more detailed focus on three major HCAIs that require nurse-led interventions: catheter-associated urinary tract infection (CAUTI); **intravascular catheter-related bloodstream infection (CRBSI)**; and **surgical site infection (SSI)**.

The nursing role in assessing risk of HCAI

To assess a patient's susceptibility to infection, including HCAI, it is important to consider both intrinsic (patient-related) and extrinsic (treatment-related) risk factors.

Intrinsic factors include:

- the patient's age;
- nutrition and build;
- general health;

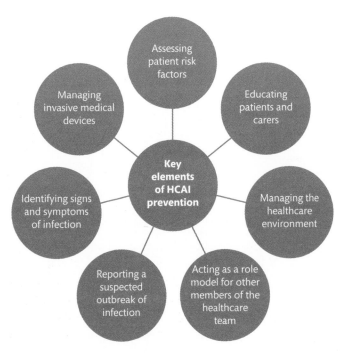

Figure 21.1 Key nurse-led elements of HCAI prevention.

- functional status;
- presence of a wound or skin lesion;
- presence of an underlying disease (e.g. diabetes mellitus, blood and respiratory disorders, cardiopulmonary disease).

Older adults (aged 65 and over) experience greater morbidity and mortality due to infection than younger adults. High *et al.* (2005) identify risk factors for infection relating to the older adult, highlighting the links between age, infection, chronic inflammatory conditions, and reduced functional status (defined as the ability to function independently). The authors emphasize the importance of fully assessing the role that factors such as physical disability, cognitive and emotional impairment, quality of life, and social consequences play in infection risk and outcome. The older adult is less likely to present with the typical signs and symptoms associated with infection, such as a raised temperature, and may instead present with alternative signs, such as a change in cognitive function (e.g. confusion) or complaints of feeling generally unwell.

Extrinsic risk factors for infection include:

- treatment for a condition or disease that affects the immune system (e.g. steroids, cytotoxics);
- antibiotic treatment;
- invasive procedures (e.g. surgery, insertion of an invasive device or implant);

- previous hospitalization or residence in a care home may increase a person's risk of exposure to HCAI, particularly when accommodated in close proximity to other patients or residents with an infectious condition.

There is little published material on the development and use of valid tools to assist nurses in assessing a person's susceptibility to infection. Bowell (1992) developed a risk assessment tool to identify patients at risk of infection, but this has not been validated for routine use. Risk of infection can change significantly from one day to the next, depending on the patient's condition and any treatment or procedures being undertaken. It is therefore important that you assess the patient's risk factors for infection at the start of his or her healthcare treatment and regularly thereafter.

The nursing role in recognizing symptoms of HCAI

The nurse will frequently be the best-placed professional to identify changes in a patient's condition, including obvious and more subtle presentation of infections (symptoms are covered in the next section of the chapter). You are responsible for taking prompt action, including referral to a medical practitioner, collection of a clinical specimen, and,

MICROBIOLOGY REQUEST FORM

Name:	Doctor: *person responsible for the patient*
NHS/Hospital number:	
Age/DoB: Sex: M/F	Location of patient: *for results to be returned*
Type of specimen: *e.g. MSU/CSU/clean-catch urine—never put 'urine' without further specifying how it was collected*	Date and time of collection: *this will show whether prolonged storahas occurred, which may change the nature of the specimenge*
Tests required: *e.g. bacterial culture and sensitivity, specific screening test (e.g. MRSA), virology, mycology, microscopy*	
Source and site of specimen: *e.g. type of wound (chronic/surgical/leg ulcer/IV line site etc) and location on body (especially important if more than one wound is present)*	
Relevant medical history: *this should include symptoms of infection, suspected site of infection, recent overseas/travel and any other information to assist laboratory scientists in identifying the causative organism and determining the tests and methods to use. Please note that 'no significant growth' means that based on the information provided the results are thought to be insignificant.*	
Antimicrobial therapy: *if the patient is receiving antimicrobial therapy this may influence test results, as any antimicrobial present in the specimen may inhibit bacterial growth in the laboratory culture and produce misleadingresults. It is also useful to for the laboratory to be able to see which antibiotics are being used so that sensitivities may be tested.*	
Biohazard label if indicated *(refer to local policy; place label on container and form)*	

Figure 21.2 Sample microbiology request form.

if required, transfer to an isolation facility. When submitting a clinical specimen to the microbiology laboratory for analysis, it is important to collect an adequate amount of the sample being taken, avoiding contamination by other microorganisms while obtaining it. The specimen should be sent promptly to the laboratory or stored appropriately until being sent and must be accompanied by accurate information about the patient's condition to enable laboratory staff to select the appropriate diagnostic tests (Figure 21.2).

Once you think you have identified an infection, it is important to refer to local policies and procedures, those directed towards minimizing the risk of spread of infection to other patients, carers, and healthcare staff. When more than one patient is presenting with similar symptoms of infection that are suggestive of a possible outbreak (e.g. diarrhoea and/or vomiting), you will be responsible for reporting this to the local infection prevention team, assisting with the ongoing investigation, implementing the recommended interventions, and monitoring effectiveness.

The nursing role in preventing HCAI

It is important to recognize that not all HCAIs can be prevented by infection prevention interventions. As already discussed, the risk of infection developing depends on the complex relationship between host susceptibility and the dose and virulence of the infectious agent. However, many risk factors are amenable to preventative interventions, including exposure to an invasive procedure, an invasive device, or to a particular microorganism of concern (e.g. a multidrug-resistant organism). The aim of an infection prevention programme is to decrease infection rates to the irreducible minimum. There are a multitude of evidence-based infection prevention techniques that, when used together, have a demonstrable impact on infection rates.

For example, the potential to reduce intravascular catheter-related bloodstream infections (CRBSI) has been demonstrated by Pronovost *et al.* (2006) in a study involving 103 intensive care units in Michigan, US. Implementation of an intervention comprising five evidence-based procedures—namely, hand hygiene, use of full personal protective equipment (PPE) during catheter insertion, skin preparation using chlorhexidine, avoidance of the femoral insertion site, and removal of unnecessary catheters—resulted in a large and sustained reduction (up to

66%) in rates of CRBSIs during the 18-month study period. This study used a bundle approach, whereby feedback on adherence to the five measures was provided on an 'all or nothing' principle, meaning that implementing four out of the five measures resulted in a score of zero being given.

It is now recognized that successful infection prevention strategies require implementation of a combination of evidence-based interventions. Recently, the grouping of evidence-based interventions into 'care bundles' has been introduced as a means of improving the implementation of best practice in everyday clinical situations. Care bundles have been defined for specific HCAIs and, in particular, catheter-associated bloodstream infections, with emphasis placed on the consistent implementation of all of the interventions, for every patient, all of the time. There are ongoing developments in the field of infection prevention, both in relation to technological advances and specific interventions to minimize risk. In view of this, it is essential for nurses and other healthcare professionals continually to appraise literature on the latest, most effective, and cost-efficient ways in which to prevent infection and to keep up to date with recommended best practice.

The following sections provide an overview of the two key infection prevention measures: standard precautions and aseptic technique.

Standard precautions

A variety of precautions are used to minimize the risk of infection to patients, their carers, and healthcare staff. These precautions are directed towards both recognized and unrecognized sources of infection. 'Standard precautions' apply routinely to all patients, regardless of their diagnosis. They include hand hygiene (Pratt *et al.*, 2007), use of personal protective equipment (Pratt *et al.*, 2007), decontamination of equipment and the healthcare environment (including management of blood and body fluid spillages) (Pratt *et al.*, 2007), respiratory hygiene (Siegel *et al.*, 2007), and safe handling and disposal of linen and waste (including avoidance of sharps injury) (Siegel *et al.*, 2007; Pratt *et al.*, 2007). Additional precautions, known as 'transmission-based precautions', apply to patients with a known or suspected infectious disease or condition, and these may involve additional or increased use of personal protective equipment and increased measures concerning disinfection of reuseable equipment and the environment (Siegel *et al.*, 2007). In the hospital setting, transmission-based

CASE STUDY 21.1 *Clostridium difficile infection*

Mr Brown, a 68-year-old man who suffers from chronic obstructive pulmonary disease (COPD), has been admitted to hospital with a respiratory infection and acute exacerbation of COPD. He is prescribed broad-spectrum antibiotics while awaiting the results of a sputum culture. On the ward, Mr Brown is too short of breath to walk to the toilet, so he uses a commode at the bedside. He is not always offered the opportunity to wash his hands afterwards. Ten days into his hospital stay, Mr Brown develops profuse, watery diarrhoea accompanied by abdominal cramps and an elevated temperature. A stool specimen is sent to the microbiology laboratory for investigation and, 48 hours later, the result is reported as *Clostridium difficile* toxin-positive.

Questions

➤ What factors placed Mr Brown at increased risk of *C. difficile* infection?

➤ What nursing interventions would have minimized the risk of Mr Brown being exposed to *C. difficile*?

➤ How can the risk of transmission of *C. difficile* to other patients on the ward be reduced?

➤ What information would you give Mr Brown about his infection and who should he inform should he experience a relapse of symptoms following discharge from hospital?

precautions may also require the use of a single room to isolate the patient physically. For further information on standard and transmission-based precautions, see Siegel *et al.* (2007).

Aseptic technique

As discussed, a significant proportion of HCAIs arise as a result of an invasive procedure or introduction of an invasive medical device, such as a urinary catheter or intravascular device. These procedures and devices require the use of aseptic techniques to prevent microorganisms from gaining access to susceptible sites on the body, such as surgical wounds and insertion sites of invasive devices. The term 'asepsis' means being free from living, foreign pathogenic microorganisms. Aseptic technique involves preventing direct or indirect microbial contamination of susceptible sites on the body and sterile or 'key parts' of equipment (Rowley *et al.*, 2010). It may be achieved using a variety of methods, which are adapted according to the procedure being undertaken (Rowley *et al.*, 2010).

Complex procedures (e.g. surgery in the operating theatre or insertion of a central venous catheter on a ward) are conducted using maximal sterile barrier precautions, including use of full personal protective equipment, sterile equipment, and a large aseptic field (Rowley *et al.*, 2010). For simple procedures (e.g. changing a simple wound dressing, changing an intravenous fluid administration set, or collecting a catheter specimen of urine), aseptic technique may be achieved by using hand hygiene, sterile equipment, clean gloves, and a non-touch method to avoid contamination of sterile or 'key parts' of equipment, without the need for sterile gloves, a sterile dressing pack, or sterile towel (Rowley *et al.*, 2010). There are many other invasive procedures that require use of an aseptic technique (Dougherty and Lister, 2008). Rowley *et al.* (2010) identify the importance of risk assessment in determining the most appropriate personal protective equipment, hand hygiene method, and aseptic field equipment to use. Effective management of invasive medical devices requires an understanding and application of the principles of aseptic technique. This, along with ongoing monitoring for signs of infection and prompt removal of a medical device when no longer needed, is an important part of the nurse's role, as addressed in more detail below.

Utilizing evidence-based interventions to prevent HCAI

You have an ongoing responsibility to draw on the most up-to-date evidence in supporting your interventions. The next sections of this chapter focus on three major HCAIs commonly encountered when caring for adult patients, which require nurse-led interventions: catheter-associated urinary tract infection (CAUTI); intravascular catheter-related bloodstream infection (CRBSI); and surgical site infection (SSI).

Catheter-associated urinary tract infections (CAUTI)

Urinary catheterization is a very common procedure in acute care, with up to 25% of patients receiving a short-term catheter during their hospital stay (Saint *et al.*, 2000). Less is known about the prevalence of catheter use in non-acute settings, although in one study of UK nursing homes, this was found to be 9% with a range of 0–40% (McNulty *et al.*, 2003).

Risk factors

The duration of catheterization is considered to be the most important risk factor for development of infection (Saint and Chenowith, 2003), yet all too often catheters are left in place for longer than necessary. The rate of bacteriuria (significant growth of bacteria in the urine without symptoms) is thought to be 3–7% per day of catheterization. After 1 month of indwelling catheterization, bacteriuria develops in nearly all patients (Saint, 2000).

Approximately one in five patients with bacteriuria develop a symptomatic infection, and the second commonest cause of healthcare-associated bloodstream infection is thought to be related to the presence of an indwelling urinary catheter (Saint, 2000). The risk of CAUTI is related to the susceptibility of the patient and the intrinsic virulence factors of the infecting organism. It also varies according to the method and duration of catheterization, and the quality of catheter care, factors that are amenable to nurse-led preventative measures.

Prevention strategies

Strategies to prevent CAUTI are directed mainly at short-term catheterization, since no strategy can effectively prevent bacteriuria and CAUTI indefinitely in a person with a long-term catheter (Trautner and Darouiche, 2004).

Box 21.1 Key evidence-based nursing interventions to minimize the risk of CAUTI in the acute care setting

- Consider alternatives to an indwelling catheter, including intermittent catheterization, where appropriate.
- Use portable ultrasound bladder scans to detect residual urine amounts.
- Insert urinary catheters only when necessary for patient care, review daily, and remove as soon as no longer indicated.
- Prior to catheterization, cleanse the urethral meatus using sterile normal saline or antiseptic solution. Thereafter, cleanse daily using soap and water; use of antiseptic solutions is unnecessary.
- Use as small a catheter as possible to allow good drainage, while minimizing urethral trauma.
- Insert catheter using sterile equipment, sterile lubricant, and an aseptic technique, including hand hygiene and use of personal protective equipment.
- Maintain a sterile, continuously closed drainage system and unobstructed urine flow, keeping the drainage bag below the level of the bladder, but above the floor.
- Empty the drainage bag frequently enough to maintain urine flow and prevent reflux, using a separate, clean container for each patient and avoiding contact between the urinary drainage tap and container.

Promoting catheter avoidance has the potential to impact greatly on reducing CAUTI, and the nurse has a key role in achieving this by ensuring that alternatives to an indwelling catheter are considered and discussed with the patient as part of the decision-making process (see Chapter 16 Managing Continence and Elimination ➡).

There is a wealth of published literature on the care of indwelling urinary catheters and the prevention of CAUTI, both in the UK (Pratt *et al.*, 2007; Quality Improvement Scotland, 2004) and overseas (Gould *et al.*, 2010; Hooton *et al.*, 2010; Parker *et al.*, 2009; Willson *et al.*, 2009; Greene *et al.*, 2008; Lo *et al.*, 2008), and a number of 'care bundles' for preventing CAUTI have been developed (e.g. Department of Health, 2010; Curran and Murdoch, 2009; Greene *et al.*, 2008). In a two-part series, Parker *et al.* (2009) and

CASE STUDY 21.2 *The development of sepsis*

Mr Smith, a 53-year-old man with a history of spinal injury, is admitted to hospital with a provisional diagnosis of sepsis with an unknown focus. On admission to hospital, he is extremely unwell and his blood tests demonstrate the likelihood of sepsis (raised white cell count and C-reactive protein). He has been tetraplegic for 12 years following a motorcycle accident and he has a long-term indwelling catheter. On examination, he has two ischial pressure sores that are sloughy and inflamed, and are currently under the management of the community nursing service. He has had the wounds for 3 weeks following a failure in his support cushion that was undetected for a day. Over the past week, he has suffered from a flu-like illness, which has restricted him to bed and his fluid intake has greatly reduced.

Questions

➤ What specimens would you expect to be sent to try to establish the source of Mr Smith's sepsis?

➤ Should specimens be sent before systemic antibiotics are administered?

➤ What is the rationale for sending specimens if treatment with broad-spectrum antibiotics is to be commenced?

➤ How important is it that antibiotics are administered exactly as per the treatment plan and what problems could arise if this plan were not implemented?

➤ Can you describe the risks of antibiotic therapy and give any reasons for prudent use of antibiotics?

Willson *et al.* (2009) presented a comprehensive review of current evidence to support nursing actions for prevention of CAUTI in patients with short- and long-term indwelling catheters. The elements of an evidence-based prevention programme for CAUTI in the acute care setting were defined, including the key nursing interventions featured in national and international guidance. Box 21.1 provides a summary of key evidence-based nursing interventions to minimize the risk of CAUTI in the acute care setting.

Clinical assessment

Clinical diagnosis of CAUTI is not straightforward, because catheterized patients with a UTI usually do not experience the classic symptoms of dysuria, frequency, and urgency. Moreover, other symptoms attributable to CAUTI, including fever and urethral or pelvic pain, may also not manifest (Tambyah and Maki, 2000). There is no evidence that odorous or cloudy urine in a catheterized patient, even when it manifests newly, has clinical significance (Hooton *et al.*, 2010) and urine leukocyte count has been found to have little predictive value in the diagnosis of CAUTI (Tambyah and Maki, 2000). Continuous assessment of the patient with an indwelling catheter is important, because changes in general well-being, such as altered mental state (e.g. onset of confusion) or lethargy, with no other identified cause may be a sign of CAUTI. Catheterized patients should be thoroughly assessed for the source of signs and symptoms before attributing them to the urinary tract (Hooton *et al.*, 2010).

Investigation and treatment

When clinical signs of infection are present, a CAUTI is suspected, and there is a need to treat with systemic antibiotics, you should obtain a urine specimen for microbiological investigation prior to commencing antimicrobial treatment (Hooton *et al.*, 2010). In patients with a short-term indwelling catheter, the specimen should be obtained via the catheter sampling port using an aseptic technique. In patients with a long-term indwelling catheter, it is preferable to replace the catheter and collect a specimen from the freshly placed catheter before initiating antimicrobial therapy (Hooton *et al.*, 2010). Culture specimens should never be obtained from the drainage bag. If the catheter can be removed, a voided midstream urine specimen should be obtained. Ideally, urine specimens should be examined in the laboratory within 2 hours of collection, but they can be refrigerated for up to 24 hours if necessary. Patients requiring antimicrobial treatment for a CAUTI must be closely monitored to ensure resolution of symptoms within the expected time frame, usually within 7 days.

Accessing evidence to inform practice

There are several gaps in the current evidence base relating to urinary catheter care and the prevention of CAUTI (see Chapter 16 Managing Continence ⟶). Further evidence is needed to guide recommendations for long-term urinary catheterization, including the role of newer technologies (e.g. antimicrobial- or antiseptic-impregnated catheters), because there is a lack of agreement about this in the literature. Research on the prevention of biofilm formation on catheters is also needed. Further research is required to determine the optimal aseptic insertion technique for use in acute, long-term, and home settings, including use of antiseptic solution versus sterile saline for meatal cleansing before catheter insertion. A better understanding of the relationship between catheter-associated asymptomatic bacteriuria and CAUTI is needed, particularly whether a reduction in asymptomatic bacteriuria results in a reduction in CAUTI, inappropriate antimicrobial use, or cross-infection (Hooton *et al.*, 2010). The impact of strategies to minimize the use of indwelling urinary catheters on patient outcomes, including use of intermittent catheters in place of indwelling catheters, is an under-researched area.

Intravascular catheter-related bloodstream infections (CRBSI)

Bloodstream infections (BSI) comprise approximately 7% of all HCAIs in the acute care setting (Smyth *et al.*, 2008). They can be severe and life-threatening, with a higher associated mortality rate than most other HCAIs. Intravascular devices represent the single most important cause of healthcare-associated BSI (Maki *et al.*, 2006), since a significant proportion of BSI is related to their use.

Risk factors

The risk of intravascular catheter-related bloodstream infection (CRBSI) is related to the susceptibility of the patient and the intrinsic virulence factors of the infecting organism. It also varies greatly according to the type and intended use of the catheter, the insertion site, the frequency with which the catheter is accessed, the duration of catheter placement, and the quality of catheter care, many of which are amenable to nurse-led preventative measures. Peripheral venous catheters (PVCs) are the devices used most frequently for vascular access. Whilst the associated incidence of bloodstream infections is much lower than for central venous catheters (Maki *et al.*, 2006), the frequency with which PVCs are used means that serious infectious complications contribute considerably to annual morbidity.

The two major sources of CRBSI are colonization of the device and contamination of the fluid administered through the device (Safdar and Maki, 2004). Most CRBSIs are caused by microorganisms that colonize the device, gaining access to the extraluminal or intraluminal surface. For most CRBSIs in short-term devices (PVCs, arterial catheters, and non-cuffed, non-tunnelled central venous devices), the patient's skin is considered to be the most important source of infection (O'Grady *et al.*, 2002), with skin flora gaining access to the bloodstream by migrating extraluminally along the subcutaneous insertion tract at the time of insertion or in the days that follow. Rigorous skin disinfection prior to insertion, use of a sterile dressing, and skin disinfection when changing the dressing are therefore important risk-reducing strategies.

Prevention strategies

Microorganisms, including those on healthcare workers' hands, also gain access to the bloodstream intraluminally through the connecting ports of the catheter. Contamination of the catheter hub contributes substantially to intraluminal colonization of long-term catheters (O'Grady *et al.*, 2002). Adherence to strict aseptic non-touch technique during insertion and subsequent handling of all intravascular devices, and the fluids administered through them, is therefore essential. Microorganisms carried in the bloodstream from remote sources of local infection (e.g. a pneumonia or urinary tract infection) may arrive at the site of the device and cause a CRBSI, representing an additional risk factor in patients with a distant, unrelated infection. The pathogens most frequently associated with CRBSI are Gram-positive bacteria, including *Staphylococcus aureus*, *Staphylococcus epidermidis* and *Enterococcus* species, and Gram-negative

> **Box 21.2   Key evidence-based nursing interventions to minimize the risk of bloodstream infection associated with short-term intravascular catheters in the acute care setting**
>
> General preventative measures
>
> - Insert an intravascular catheter only when necessary for patient care, review daily, and remove as soon as no longer indicated.
> - Disinfect skin rigorously with a single-patient use application of chlorhexidine gluconate 2% in alcohol or aqueous solution prior to insertion and during dressing changes.
> - Select the catheter, insertion technique, and insertion site with the lowest risk of complications for the anticipated type and duration of intravenous therapy.
> - Cover the catheter insertion site using a sterile dressing.
> - Perform hand hygiene, and use clean gloves and an aseptic non-touch technique, or sterile gloves for catheter site care and for accessing the system.
> - Disinfect catheter hubs, needleless connectors, and injection ports before accessing the catheter.
> - Administration sets should be changed immediately after transfusing blood products,
>
> every 24 hours if used for total parenteral nutrition and every 72–96 hours otherwise.
>
> Measures specific to central venous catheters
>
> - Insertion of a central venous catheter should take place in an operating theatre or similar clean environment using hand hygiene, maximal sterile barrier precautions (gown, gloves, drape), and aseptic technique.
> - The subclavian vein is the preferred insertion site for non-tunnelled catheters. The femoral site should be avoided if possible.
> - An antimicrobial-impregnated catheter may be appropriate for patients at high risk for CRBSI.
>
> Measures specific to peripheral venous catheters (PVCs)
>
> - Insertion of PVCs requires hand hygiene, use of a new pair of disposable non-sterile gloves, and an aseptic non-touch technique.
> - Replace in a new site after 72–96 hours or earlier if clinically indicated.

bacteria, including *Klebsiella* species, *Pseudomonas* species, and *Escherichia coli*.

Interventions, including 'care bundles', to reduce the risk of intravascular catheter-related infection have focused predominantly on short-term central venous catheters used in intensive care units (e.g. Guerin *et al.*, 2010; Health Protection Scotland, 2008a; Department of Health, 2007a; Pronovost *et al.*, 2006) and short-term peripheral venous catheters used in acute care settings (Health Protection Scotland, 2008b; Department of Health, 2007b). However, given the infection risk associated with all types of intravascular device (Maki *et al.*, 2006), it is essential that infection prevention measures are applied consistently to all devices in all of the settings in which they are used. Box 21.2 provides a summary of key evidence-based nursing interventions to minimize the risk of CRBSI relating to short-term central and peripheral venous catheters in the acute care setting. More detailed guidance for the prevention of infection in intravascular catheters is available

from a range of sources (APIC, 2009; Bishop *et al.*, 2007; Epic, 2007).

As with all invasive medical devices, intravascular catheters should be used only when necessary and removed as soon as no longer needed. Timely removal or replacement of PVCs is usually a nurse-led intervention as part of best practice. The incidence of thrombophlebitis and bacterial colonization of catheters increases when catheters are left in place for longer than 72 hours (O'Grady *et al.*, 2002). Phlebitis and catheter colonization have been associated with an increased risk for catheter-related infection, and PVCs are therefore commonly removed or replaced at 72–96-hour intervals to reduce the risk of infection and patient discomfort associated with phlebitis (O'Grady *et al.*, 2002). The Visual Infusion Phlebitis (VIP) scale (Jackson, 1998) is an objective scale to measure infusion phlebitis and has been adopted by nurses to support their clinical judgement (Schultz and Gallant, 2005).

Clinical assessment

A definitive diagnosis of CRBSI requires positive percutaneous blood culture results in association with the same microorganism obtained from the catheter tip or catheter-drawn cultures that meet specific culture criteria (Mermel *et al.*, 2009). A localized exit site infection presents with erythema, tenderness, and, occasionally, a discharge at the insertion site. Clinical manifestations of a CRBSI include fever, chills, and/or hypotension with no apparent source of bloodstream infection except for the catheter (Mermel *et al.*, 2009). In clinical practice, it is usual for broad-spectrum intravenous antibiotics to be commenced while awaiting culture results (Bishop *et al.*, 2007). The decision to remove the catheter as part of the treatment of CRBSI is made based on an assessment of the patient and the type and purpose of the catheter. PVCs associated with pain, induration, erythema, or exudate should be removed and any exudate at the insertion site submitted to the microbiology laboratory for culture (Mermel *et al.*, 2009). The risk of CRBSI from such catheters is low (Mermel *et al.*, 2009). Patients requiring antimicrobial treatment for a localized exit site infection or a suspected CRBSI must be closely monitored to ensure resolution of symptoms within the expected time frame.

Accessing evidence to inform practice

Preventing infection related to the use of intravascular devices is a well-researched area and current evidence-based guidance is therefore well defined. Further investigation is needed into the use of needleless connectors because there are reports of increased BSI associated with their use (APIC, 2009). The most appropriate disinfectant to use for disinfecting catheter hubs and injection ports remains controversial, since disinfectants licensed for use on skin are not necessarily suitable for use on IV equipment (APIC, 2009). Research is also needed on the prevention of biofilm formation on catheters and catheter hubs.

Preventing surgical site infections

Surgical site infections (SSIs) are defined as infections occurring within 30 days after a surgical operation (or within 1 year if an implant is left in place after the procedure)

and affecting either the incision or deep tissue at the operation site (Mangram *et al.*, 1999). SSIs comprise at least 14% of all HCAIs in the acute inpatient population (Smyth *et al.*, 2008; Reilly *et al.*, 2008). However, this figure relates only to patients during their hospital admission, so is likely to be a gross underestimate given the increasingly short length of postoperative stay of patients. Surveillance programmes that incorporate follow-up of patients after discharge from hospital provide a much more accurate picture. Data from Scotland (Health Protection Scotland, 2007), collected as part of the Scottish Surveillance of Healthcare Associated Infection Programme (SSHAIP), found that infections occurring after discharge from hospital accounted for approximately 78% of all SSIs in the types of surgery in which post-discharge surveillance was undertaken (Caesarean section and hip arthroplasty).

Risk factors

The risk of SSI varies according to the category of surgical procedure. There are four categories: clean; clean-contaminated; contaminated; and dirty. A clean procedure is one in which no microbial contamination has been encountered and none of the body spaces are entered. A clean-contaminated procedure is one in which the gastrointestinal, respiratory, or urinary tracts are entered under controlled conditions and without contamination occurring. A contaminated procedure is one in which those tracks are entered and contamination does occur. New acute traumatic wounds also fall into the 'contaminated' category. Surgical procedures classed as dirty are those that involve the presence of devitalized or infected tissue at the surgical site at the time of surgery. Clean surgery that does not enter body cavities where organisms are naturally present and in which there is an uncomplicated procedure with no break in aseptic techniques presents very little risk to patients.

There are a number of patient-specific factors that increase the risk of SSI. These factors include excess weight, smoking, diabetes, extremes of age, and poor nutritional status. In the patient undergoing emergency surgery, there is little that can be done to modify these factors. However, in those undergoing planned surgery, you should make every attempt to advise patients of ways in which they can help to reduce the risk of infection: for example, to cease smoking in the immediate preoperative

---

Box 21.3   Key evidence-based nursing interventions to minimize the risk of surgical site infections

Removal of the microorganisms found at the surgical site preoperatively:

- Skin cleansing with recommended antiseptic agent
- Hair removal only if absolutely necessary, as close to the time of surgery as possible and with a single-use disposable clipper

Prevention of multiplication of microorganisms that do gain access to the surgical site:

- Where indicated, ensure that prophylactic antibiotics are given in the hour prior to surgery

Prevention of contamination during the intraoperative period:

- Rigorous aseptic technique

- Use of demonstrably sterile equipment
- Impervious gloves and gowns
- Theatre ventilation maintained to optimal specification

Enhancing the ability of the patient to defend themselves against microorganisms:

- Blood glucose control in diabetic patients
- Maintenance of core body temperature >36.5°C

Protection of the postoperative wound in the immediate postoperative period:

- Appropriate interactive dressing
- Dressing remains intact for 48 hours post-surgery

---

period, to modify their diets to either increase or reduce their intake, and, in patients with diabetes mellitus, to ensure that their condition is well controlled.

Prevention strategies

Recent clinical guidelines for prevention of surgical wound infection have been produced by the National Institute for Health and Clinical Excellence (NICE, 2008). These comprehensive guidelines provide the evidence base underpinning the recommendations for practice and, importantly, give an indication of the strength of the evidence. Practices aimed at reducing the risks of SSI can be divided up into five areas, as presented in Box 21.3.

The evidence for and against many of the preoperative interventions currently recommended is poor and there is a clear need for further research. Some studies have shown the benefit of showering in the immediate preoperative period (Edmiston *et al.*, 2008), and hair removal should be undertaken only when absolutely necessary and never by methods such as shaving, which could damage the skin surface (Tanner *et al.*, 2006). The patient should never be advised to undertake his or her own hair removal before attending for surgery. If hair removal is absolutely necessary, it should be undertaken as close to the time of surgery as possible, using a method that does

not damage the skin surface. If surgical clippers are to be used, the clipper head should be single use and disposable. Preoperative shaving with a razor has been shown to increase the risk of surgical site infection (Court-Brown, 1981). Once in the operating theatre, the skin should be disinfected with an antiseptic agent prior to the incision. Recent studies have indicated that 2% alcoholic chlorhexidine is an extremely effective agent for this purpose (Darouiche *et al.*, 2010).

The timely administration of prophylactic antibiotics in the hour prior to surgery has been shown to reduce the risk of infection significantly in certain categories of high-risk procedure (Classen *et al.*, 1992), as has maintaining core body temperature above 36.5°C (Melling *et al.*, 2001). Patients who arrive in the operating theatre with a temperature lower than 36.5°C should have their surgery deferred until the body temperature reaches this level, unless the surgery is extremely urgent.

Clinical assessment

It is important that you ensure that wounds remain covered with an interactive dressing for at least 48 hours after the surgery to ensure that the wound seals and becomes impervious to microbial contamination. Modern transparent dressings do allow the wound to be visualized without disturbing it, so it is important to check that any discharge drains freely. After 48 hours, any postoperative wound dressing may be removed and the wound exposed. You should immediately report and record any sign of inflammation or discharge from a surgical wound. It is, however, quite normal for wounds to look slightly inflamed as part of the normal healing process, and specimens should not be sent for analysis unless there are clinical signs of infection. Wound drainage devices should be removed at the earliest possible opportunity in the postoperative period and patients should be encouraged to report any problems with the wounds as soon as they occur (Drinkwater *et al.*, 1995). If the patient is to be discharged soon after surgery, it is vital that he or she is given full instructions on how to care for the wound, as well as washing and bathing and whom to contact if he or she has a problem in the post-surgical period. After the wound dressing has been removed at 48 hours, it is quite safe for the patient to take a shower (National Institute for Health and Clinical Excellence (NICE), 2008).

Infected surgical site wounds can be categorized in three ways:

- superficial incisional;
- deep incisional;
- organ/space infections.

Superficial incisional infections are generally mild in nature, with inflammation and occasionally pus being produced. Deep incisional and organ/space infections are more serious, and frequently require hospital admission to be able to treat them. You will have a key role in the detection of SSIs by understanding and observing for the signs of infection. With rapid discharge from hospital following surgery now becoming the norm, there will be an increasing role for nurses working in primary care settings in the assessment of postoperative wounds and the detection of postoperative wound infection.

Accessing evidence to inform practice

Some gaps in the evidence base are summarized in NICE (2008) and Frieden (2010), among which are areas for research that is needed to inform nursing interventions, including:

CASE STUDY 21.3 *Surgical site infection*

Mrs Jones, an 86-year-old resident of a nursing home, has unfortunately fallen and fractured her neck of femur. On admission to hospital, as part of the process by which patients are prepared for surgery, she is screened for methicillin-resistant *Staphylococcus aureus* (MRSA). The following morning, the microbiology laboratory reports that the screen is positive for MRSA. However, Mrs Jones has already been to the operating theatre and has had her surgery. Six days after the surgery, you note there is a discharge coming from her surgical wound. The area around the wound is red and inflamed and, when you take the dressing down, the stitches appear to be tight.

Questions

➤ What factors increased the risk of Mrs Jones being found to be MRSA-positive?

➤ What is the purpose of screening for MRSA?

➤ What are the nurse-led actions to be undertaken when MRSA is detected from a screen?

➤ How could the risk of SSI have been reduced?

➤ How can the risk of transmission of MRSA to other patients on the ward be reduced?

➤ What information would you give Mrs Jones about her MRSA infection?

- the impact of nasal decontamination for all strains of *Staphylococcus aureus*;
- the benefit and cost-effectiveness of different types of post-surgical interactive dressing for reducing the risk of SSI;
- the role of post-surgical wound care in pathogenesis of infection;
- the optimal role of preoperative decolonization strategies.

Accessing the evidence to inform clinical nursing decisions

There is a wealth of resources to support evidence-based nursing practice in relation to HCAI and infection prevention, including the many types of material referred to in this chapter. Clinical practice guidelines bring together the evidence from research and expert opinion. Some of the key sources of national and international evidence-based guidance and a range of care bundles are listed in Table 21.1.

Journal articles are an important source of current material to inform clinical decisions and to stimulate debate about contemporary issues in infection prevention. The main UK-based journals specializing in HCAI and infection prevention issues are the *Journal of Hospital Infection*, the official publication of the Hospital Infection Society, and the *Journal of Infection Prevention*, the official publication of the Infection Prevention Society. Leading international journals include *Infection Control and Hospital Epidemiology*, the official publication of the Society for Healthcare Epidemiology of America, and the *American*

Table 21.1 Sources of evidence on HCAI and infection prevention

Clinical practice guidelines	
Source	**Example**
British Society of Antimicrobial Chemotherapy/Hospital Infection Society/Infection Prevention Society (formerly Infection Control Nurses Association)	Guidelines for the control and prevention of methicillin-resistant *Staphylococcus aureus* (MRSA) in healthcare facilities (2006)
Department of Health (England)	Epic2: National Evidence-Based Guidelines for Preventing Healthcare-Associated Infections in NHS Hospitals in England (2007)
Healthcare Infection Control Practices Advisory Committee (HICPAC), Centers for Disease Control and Prevention (CDC, US)	Guideline for Isolation Precautions: Preventing Transmission of Infectious Agents in Healthcare Settings (2007)
National Institute for Health and Clinical Excellence (NICE)	Surgical Site Infection: Prevention and Treatment of Surgical Site Infection (2008)
Association of Professionals in Infection Control and Epidemiology (APIC)	Guide to the Elimination of *Clostridium difficile* in Healthcare Settings (2008)
Royal College of Nursing	Infection Prevention and Control Minimum Standards (2009)
Society for Healthcare Epidemiology of America (SHEA)	A Compendium of Strategies to Prevent Healthcare-Associated Infections in Acute Care Hospitals (2008)
Care bundles	
Source	**Example**
Department of Health (England)	'High Impact Interventions' to reduce HCAIs
Health Protection Scotland	Care bundles and checklists on HCAI and infection control

> ## Box 21.4 Useful websites
>
> | | |
> |---|---|
> | Association of Professionals in Infection Control and Epidemiology (APIC) | **www.apic.org** |
> | Department of Health (including 'High Impact Interventions') | **www.dh.gov.uk** |
> | Healthcare A2Z | **www.healthcarea2z.org** |
> | Health Protection Scotland | **www.hps.scot.nhs.uk** |
> | Hospital Infection Society | **www.his.org.uk** |
> | Infection Prevention Society | **www.ips.uk.net** |
> | National Institute for Health and Clinical Excellence | **www.nice.org.uk/guidance** |
> | National Resource for Infection Control | **www.nric.org.uk** |
> | Royal College of Nursing | **www.rcn.org.uk** |
> | World Health Organization (including WHO Guidelines on Hand Hygiene in Health Care) | **www.who.int** |

Journal of Infection Control, the official publication of the Association of Professionals in Infection Control and Epidemiology (APIC).

There are some particularly useful websites that provide trustworthy sources of information on HCAI and infection prevention, as listed in Table 21.1. The National Resource for Infection Control (NRIC) hosts an online resource incorporating the National Electronic Library on Infection (NeLI). This provides a comprehensive list of journals relating to infection, current guidance, training resources, and upcoming educational events. Professional associations, including the Infection Prevention Society and the Royal College of Nursing, are also excellent sources of information (see Box 21.4).

Summary and key messages

- Nurses have a vital part to play in protecting patients from avoidable infections, and good practice is integral to good nursing care. Whilst a variety of other healthcare workers will also have their own parts to play in protecting the patient, nurses play a pivotal role in patient safety. No other healthcare workers have as frequent close contact with the patient and so there is a greater opportunity for cross-infection arising from poor practice by nurses than by any other group of staff.

- Nurses must take the lead on the implementation of key evidence-based interventions concerning patient assessment and care, management of invasive devices, and managing risks in the healthcare environment.

- Nurses and other health professionals should ensure that planned improvements in practice are based on careful consideration of the best available evidence. Your infection prevention team can offer expert support with this, and encourage health professionals to question practice to tailor the infection prevention programme to the local context and to identify gaps in evidence.

- Since the majority of research on HCAI and infection prevention is conducted in hospitals and other acute care settings, most evidence-based guidance is directed towards the acute healthcare environment and therefore requires adaptation for use in other settings.

- There is a need for more research to inform nursing interventions to minimize the risk of CAUTI and SSI.

- Nurses must expect to take the lead in practice improvement initiatives, educating patients and carers on HCAIs and how to prevent them, and acting as role models for hand hygiene, aseptic technique, and other key evidence-based interventions, including training and educating clinical colleagues and monitoring standards.

- There is a need to develop HCAI metrics that are sensitive to nursing practice. An example of this was the introduction of a 'High Impact Action for Nurses' by the Chief Nursing Officer of England targeted at reducing urinary tract infection.

Answers to case study questions

Case study 21.1 *Clostridium difficile* infection

➤ Age over 65, broad-spectrum antibiotics, and hospital admission

➤ Hand hygiene by all caring for Mr Brown; ensuring that Mr Brown has an opportunity to cleanse his hands before eating and after using the toilet; ensuring that all antibiotics are given in line with the antimicrobial prescribing guidelines; ensuring that patient care equipment (for example, commodes) are cleaned between patients.

➤ Isolate Mr Brown as soon as he has loose stools and ensure designated toilet facilities; hand hygiene for staff with soap and water whenever entering or leaving Mr Brown's room, even if he has not been touched.

➤ Because he has had a *C. difficile* infection, he is at increased risk of a relapse, and health professionals should be made aware of this, especially if antibiotics are to be considered.

Case study 21.2 The development of sepsis

➤ The development of Sepsis a blood culture, a catheter specimen of urine, and wound swabs from the pressure sores should be sent for analysis.

➤ Specimens should always be sent before antibiotics are administered unless the patient is *in extremis*.

➤ When the results of the analyses are known, the broad-spectrum treatment can be switched to more focused and specific therapy.

➤ It is vital that therapeutic levels of the antibiotics are maintained if the treatment is to be effective. Failure to adhere to the treatment plan may result in the treatment being ineffective owing to subtherapeutic levels of the drug.

➤ Any antibiotic disturbs the microbial ecology of the patient and the environment. Risks include the development of resistant organisms and potential side effects, which could include anaphylaxis if the patient is allergic, other drug reactions, and Clostridium difficile infection.

Case study 21.3 Surgical site infection

➤ Nursing and residential home residency is a risk factor for MRSA carriage, as is previous hospital admission.

➤ Screening allows measures such as topical suppression with antiseptic lotions and nasal cream to reduce risk, and ensures that effective antimicrobial prophylaxis is given for the surgical procedure.

➤ Inform the medical staff responsible for the patient; isolate the patient in a single room with contact precautions and liaise with the Infection prevention and control team.

➤ If surgery is carried out before the results of a screen are known, a risk assessment for potential MRSA carriage should be done.

➤ Mrs Jones should be isolated in a single room and contact precautions instigated. Follow-up screening of other patients may be indicated, and the infection prevention and control team should be contacted for advice.

➤ That she has an infection with a bacterium that is more difficult to treat and she will require a course of antibiotics. She should be advised not to interfere with wound dressings and to report any increasing pain to the nurse caring for her.

Online Resource Centre

 To help you to develop and apply your knowledge and decision-making skills further, we have provided interactive learning resources online at **www.oxfordtextbooks.co.uk/orc/bullock/**

Whilst these are freely available, you will need to use the access codes at the start of the book.

References

Association of Professionals in Infection Control (APIC) (2009) Guide to the Elimination of Catheter-Related Bloodstream Infections. **http://www.apic.org/Content/NavigationMenu/PracticeGuidance/APICEliminationGuides/CRBSI_Elimination_Guide_logo.pdf** (accessed 14 October 2011).

Beck, M., Antle, B.J., Berlin, D., *et al.* (2004) Wearing masks in a pediatric hospital: developing practical guidelines. *Canadian Journal of Public Health* **95**(4): 256–7.

Bishop, L., Dougherty, L., Bodenham, A. (2007) Guidelines on the insertion and management of central venous access devices in adults. *International Journal of Laboratory Hematology* **29**: 261–78.

Bowell, B. (1992) A risk to others. *Nursing Times* **88**(4): 38–40.

Burnett, E., Lee, K., Rushmer, R., *et al.* (2010) Healthcare-associated infection and the patient experience: a qualitative study using patient interviews. *Journal of Hospital Infection* **74**: 42–7.

Classen, D.C., Evans, R.S., Pestotnik, S.L., *et al.* (1992) The timing of prophylactic administration of antibiotics and the risk of surgical-wound infection. *New England Journal of Medicine* **326**: 281–6.

Court-Brown, C.H. (1981) Preoperative skin depilation and its effect on postoperative wound infections. *Journal of the Royal College of Surgeons of Edinburgh* **26**: 238–41.

Curran, E., Murdoch, H. (2009) Aiming to reduce catheter-associated urinary tract infections (CAUTI) by adopting a checklist and bundle to achieve sustained system improvements. *Journal of Infection Prevention* **10**(2): 57–61.

Darouiche, R.O., Wall, M.J., Itani, K.M.F., *et al.* (2010) Chlorhexidine-alcohol versus povidone-iodine for surgical-site antisepsis. *New England Journal of Medicine* **362**(1): 18–26.

Department of Health (2007) Saving Lives: High impact intervention No 1. Central venous catheter care bundle. **http://hcai.dh.gov.uk/files/2011/03/2011-03-14-HII-Central-Venous-Catheter-Care-Bundle-FINAL.pdf** (accessed 14 October 2011).

Department of Health (2008) *Health and Social Care Act 2008 Code of Practice for the NHS on the Prevention and Control of Healthcare Associated Infections and Related Guidance.* Department of Health: London.

Department of Health (2010) High Impact Intervention Urinary Catheter Care Bundle. **http://hcai.dh.gov.uk/files/2011/03/Document_-Urinary_Catheter_Care_High_Impact_Intervention_FINAL_100907.pdf** (accessed 17 June 2011).

Dougherty, L., Lister, S. (eds) (2008) *The Royal Marsden Manual of Clinical Nursing Procedures,* 7th edn. Wiley-Blackwell: Oxford.

Drinkwater, C.J., Michael, J.N. (1995) Optimal timing of wound drain removal following total joint arthroplasty. *Journal of Arthroplasty* **10**(2): 185–9.

Edmiston, C., Krepel, C., Seabrook, G., *et al.* (2008) Preoperative shower revisited: can high topical antiseptic levels be achieved on the skin surface before surgical admission? *Journal of the American College of Surgeons* **207**(2): 233–9.

European Centre for Disease Prevention and Control (2008) *Annual Epidemiological Report on Communicable Diseases in Europe.* European Centre for Disease Prevention and Control: Stockholm.

Frieden, T.R. (2010) Maximizing infection prevention in the next decade: defining the unacceptable. *Infection Control and Hospital Epidemiology* **31**(Suppl. 1): 1–3.

Gallant, P., Schultz, A.A. (2006) Evaluation of a visual infusion phlebitis scale for determining appropriate discontinuation of peripheral intravenous catheters. *Journal of Infusion Nursing* **29**(6): 338–45.

Gould, C.V., Umscheid, C.A., Agarwal, R.K., *et al.* (2010) Healthcare Infection Control Practices Advisory Committee (HICPAC) Guideline for prevention of catheter-associated urinary tract infections 2009. *Infection Control and Hospital Epidemiology* **31**: 319–26.

Gravel, D., Matlow, A., Ofner-Agostini, M., *et al.* (2007) A point prevalence survey of health care-associated infections in pediatric populations in major canadian acute care hospitals. *American Journal of Infection Control* **35**: 157–62.

Greene, L., Marx, J., Oriola, S. (2008) Guide to the elimination of catheter-associated urinary tract infections (CAUTIs). Association for Professionals in Infection Control and Epidemiology (APIC). **http://www.premierinc.net/quality-safety/tools-services/safety/safety-share/04-09-downloads/7-CAUTI-Guide.pdf** (accessed 14 October 2011).

Guerin, K., Wagner, J., Rains, K., *et al.* (2010) Reduction in central line-associated bloodstream infections by implementation of a postinsertion care bundle. *American Journal of Infection Control* **38**(6): 430–3.

Health Protection Agency (2009) *Fifth Report of the Mandatory Surveillance of Surgical Site Infection in Orthopaedic Surgery: April 2004 to March 2009.* Health Protection Agency: London.

Health Protection Scotland (2007) *Surveillance of Surgical Site Infection: April 2002 to June 2007*. Scottish Surveillance of Healthcare Associated Infection Programme (SSHAIP). **http://www.documents.hps.scot.nhs.uk/hai/sshaip/publications/ssi/ssi-2007.pdf** (accessed 14 October 2011).

Health Protection Scotland (2008) Central Vascular Catheter Maintenance Care Bundle. **http://www.hps.scot.nhs.uk/haiic/ic/CVCMaintenanceCareBundle.aspx** (accessed 14 October 2011).

High, K., Bradley, S., Loeb, M., *et al.* (2005) A new paradigm for clinical investigation of infectious syndromes in older adults: assessing functional status as a risk factor and outcome measure. *Journal of the American Geriatrics Society* **53**(3): 528–35.

Hooton, T.M., Bradley, S.F., Cardenas, D.D., *et al.* (2010) Diagnosis, prevention and treatment of catheter-associated urinary tract infection in adults: 2009 International Clinical Practice Guidelines from the Infectious Diseases Society of America. *Clinical Infectious Diseases* **50**: 625–63.

Jackson, A. (1998) Infection control: a battle in vein—infusion phlebitis. *Nursing Times* **94**(4): 68–71.

Lo, E., Nicolle, L., Classen, D., *et al.* (2008) Strategies to prevent catheter-associated urinary tract infections in acute care hospitals. *Infection Control and Hospital Epidemiology* **29**(Suppl. 1): S41–S50.

Madeo, M. (2001) Understanding the MRSA experience. *Nursing Times* **97**(30): 36–7.

Maki, D.G., Kluger, D.M., Crnich, C.J. (2006) The risk of bloodstream infection in adults with different intravascular devices: a systematic review of 200 published prospective studies. *Mayo Clinic Proceedings* **81**(9): 1159–71.

Mangram, A. J., Horan, T. C., Pearson, M.L., *et al.* (1999) Guideline for Prevention of Surgical Site Infection, 1999. Centers for Disease Control and Prevention (CDC) Hospital Infection Control Practices Advisory Committee. *American Journal of Infection Control* **27**(2): 97–132; quiz, 133–134; discussion, 196.

McNulty, C., Freeman, E., Smith, G., *et al.* (2003) Prevalence of urinary catheterization in UK nursing homes. *Journal of Hospital Infection* **55**: 119–23.

Melling, A.C., Ali, B., Scott, E.M., *et al.* (2001) Effects of preoperative warming on the incidence of wound infection after clean surgery: a randomised controlled trial. *Lancet* **358**: 876–80. Erratum in: *Lancet* (2002); **359**: 896.

Mermel, L.A., Allon, M., Bouza, E., *et al.* (2009) Clinical practice guidelines for the diagnosis and management of intravascular catheter-related infection: 2009 update by the Infectious Diseases Society of America. *Clinical Infectious Diseases* **49**(1): 1–45.

National Audit Office (2009) *Report by the Comptroller and Auditor General: Reducing Healthcare Associated Infection in Hospitals in England*. NAO: London.

National Institute for Health and Clinical Excellence (NICE) (2008) *Surgical Site Infection: Prevention and Treatment of Surgical Site Infection*. NICE Clinical Guideline 74 (CG74). **www.nice.org.uk/nicemedia/pdf/CG74NICEGuideline.pdf** (accessed 14 October 2011).

Newton, J.T., Constable, D., Senior, V. (2001) Patients' perceptions of methicillin-resistant *Staphylococcus aureus* and source isolation: a qualitative analysis of source-isolated patients. *Journal of Hospital Infection* **48**(4): 275–80.

O'Grady, N.P., Alexander, M., Dellinger, E.P., *et al.* (2002) Guidelines for the prevention of intravascular catheter-related infections. *Paediatrics* **110**(5): 1–24.

Parker, D., Callan, L., Thompson, D.L., *et al.* (2009) Nursing interventions to reduce the risk of catheter-associated urinary tract infection. Part 1: Catheter selection. *Journal of Wound Ostomy and Continence Nursing* **36**(1): 23–34.

Pittet, D., Allegranzi, B., Sax, H., *et al.* (2006) Evidence-based model for hand transmission during patient care and the role of improved practices. *Lancet Infectious Diseases* **6**(10): 641–52.

Plowman, R., Graves, N., Griffin, M., *et al.* (1999) *The Socio-Economic Burden of Healthcare Associated Infection*. PHLS: London.

Pratt, R.J., Pellowe, C.M., Wilson, J.A., *et al.* (2007) Epic2: National evidence-based guidelines for preventing healthcare-associated infections in NHS hospitals in England. *Journal of Hospital Infection* **65**: S1–S64. **http://www.epic.tvu.ac.uk/PDF%20Files/epic2/epic2-final.pdf** (accessed 14 October 2011).

Pronovost, P., Needham, D., Berenholtz, S., *et al.* (2006) An intervention to decrease catheter-related bloodstream infections in the ICU. *New England Journal of Medicine* **355**(26): 2725–32.

Quality Improvement Scotland (2004) *Best Practice Statement: Urinary Catheterisation and Catheter Care*. NHS Quality Improvement Scotland: Edinburgh.

Rees, J., Davies, H., Birchall, C., *et al.* (2000) Psychological effects of source isolation nursing (2): patient satisfaction. *Nursing Standard* **14**: 32–6.

Reilly, J., Stewart, S., Allardice, G.A., *et al.* (2008) Results from the Scottish national HAI prevalence survey. *Journal of Hospital Infection* **69**: 62–8.

Rowley, S., Clare, S., Macqueen, S., *et al.* (2010) ANTT v2: An updated practice framework for aseptic technique. *British Journal of Nursing (Intravenous Supplement)* **19**(5): S5–S11.

Safdar, N., Maki, D.G. (2004) The pathogenesis of catheter-related bloodstream infection with noncuffed short-term central venous catheters. *Intensive Care Medicine* **30**: 62–7.

Saint, S. (2000) Clinical and economic consequences of nosocomial catheter related bacteriuria. *American Journal of Infection Control* **28**: 68–75.

Saint, S., Chenowith, C.E. (2003) Biofilms and catheter-associated urinary tract infections. *Infectious Diseases Clinics of North America* **17**: 411–32.

Saint, S., Wiese, J., Amory, J.K., *et al.* (2000) Are physicians aware of which of their patients have indwelling urinary catheters? *American Journal of Medicine* **109**: 476–80.

Siegel, J., Rhinehart, E., Jackson, M., *et al.* and the Healthcare Infection Control Practices Advisory Committee (2007) *Guideline for Isolation Precautions: Preventing Transmission of Infectious Agents in Healthcare Settings*. **http://www.cdc.gov/ncidod/dhqp/pdf/isolation2007.pdf** (accessed 14 October 2011).

Smyth, E.T.M., McIlvenny, G., Enstone, J.E., *et al.* on behalf of the Hospital Infection Society Prevalence Survey Steering Group (2008) Four country healthcare associated infection prevalence survey 2006: overview of the results. *Journal of Hospital Infection* **69** (3): 230–48.

Tambyah, P.A., Maki, D.G. (2000) Catheter-associated urinary tract infection is rarely symptomatic. *Archives of Internal Medicine* **160**: 678–82.

Tanner, J., Woodings, D., Moncaster, K. (2006) Preoperative hair removal to reduce surgical site infection. *Cochrane Database of Systematic Reviews* Issue 3: Art. No. CD004122.

Tantipong, H., Morkchareonpong, C. Jaiyindee, S., *et al.* (2008). Randomized controlled trial and meta-analysis of oral decontamination with 2% chlorhexidine solution for the prevention of ventilator-associated pneumonia. *Infection Control and Hospital Epidemiology* **29**(2): 131–6.

Tarzi, S., Kennedy, P., Stone, S., *et al.* (2001) Methicillin-resistant *Staphylococcus aureus*: psychological impact of hospitalization and isolation in an older adult population. *Journal of Hospital Infection* **49**(4): 250–4.

Trautner, B.W., Darouiche, R.O. (2004) Role of biofilm in catheter-associated urinary tract infection. *American Journal of Infection Control* **32**: 177–83.

Willson, M., Wilde, M., Webb, M.L., *et al.* (2009) Nursing interventions to reduce the risk of catheter associated urinary tract infection. Part 2: Staff education, monitoring and care techniques. *Journal of Wound Ostomy and Continence Nursing* **36**(2): 137–54.

Wu, A., Ren, N., Wen, X., *et al.* (2005) One day prevalence survey of nosocomial infection in 159 hospitals. *Chinese Journal of Infection Control.* **http://en.cnki.com.cn/Article_en/ CJFDTOTAL-GRKZ200501004.htm** (abstract accessed 14 October 2011).

22 *Managing* Medicines

Anne Baileff, Jan Davis, and Nicola Davey

Introduction

The management of medicines is a fundamental component of contemporary nursing care and a pervasive form of therapeutic intervention in healthcare (Medicines Partnership, 2002). In this chapter, we will focus on the skills and underpinning knowledge that you need to enable you to undertake an in-depth assessment of an individual's use of medication, and how you can work in partnership with him or her to optimize safe, effective use, regardless of care setting. We will not address factors associated with the scheduled administration of medicines undertaken (for example, during the traditional ward drug round), although the principles articulated in this chapter are transferable. Likewise, the principles of good medicine management are also applicable to all of the chapters in this book on core conditions and health needs ⬅➡.

Understanding the importance of managing medicines

Medicines are used to promote health, and to prevent, control, and treat disease. However, they are potent substances. All have side effects, and many interact adversely, not only with other medicines, but also with common fruit, vegetables, and food products. Ethnicity, race, age, weight, and gender can also affect an individual's response to a specific medicine.

Public access to medicines has increased hugely in the past decade, and prescriptive authority is no longer the sole right of medical practitioners. Nurses, pharmacists, physiotherapists, podiatrists, optometrists, and radiographers are now all able to prescribe a wide range of drugs. Patient group directions enable nurses and other health professionals to supply and administer drugs to patients without referral to a doctor, and medicines are increasingly available without prescription to purchase over the counter from a number of retail outlets and over the Internet.

Defining medicines management

At the outset, it is clearly important to understand what we mean by 'medicines management'; you will then appreciate the extent of your responsibilities and the skills that you need for competent practice. Medicines management is a complex subject and there have been several attempts to define it.

The Audit Commission (2001: 5) defines it as:

the entire way that medicines are selected, procured, delivered, prescribed, administered and reviewed to optimise the contribution that medicines make to producing informed and desired outcomes of patient care.

The National Prescribing Centre (2002: 5) defines it as:

A system of processes and behaviours that determines how medicines are used by patients and by the NHS. Effective medicines management will place the patient as the primary focus, thus delivering better targeted care and better informed individuals.

Medicines and Healthcare products Regulatory Authority (MHRA, 2004, cited by the Nursing and Midwifery Council, 2007: 5) defines it as:

The clinical, cost effective and safe use of medicines to ensure patients get the maximum benefit from the medicines they need, while at the same time minimising potential harm.

While these most commonly used definitions are very similar, each includes a factor that the others do not, and all of the factors in each are important. Therefore we suggest the following amalgamated definition as applied to nursing practice:

Medicines management encompasses the entire way in which nurses select, procure, provide, prescribe, supply, administer, and review a patient's medicines. Optimal medicines management enables patients to get the maximum benefit from the medicines they need. This is achieved through concordance and teamwork, by placing the patient as the primary focus, and by ensuring that nursing interventions are cost-effective, and that any associated risks are identified, communicated, and carefully managed.

It is this definition that will be used to inform the content of this chapter. Having defined what we mean by medicines management, we will now consider how medicines are accessed and used by the adult population in the UK, and the associated problems. You will then understand what issues you need to address in your assessment of individual patients.

Scale of medicines use and associated problems in the UK

Research undertaken on behalf of the Medicines Partnership Programme and the Medicines and Healthcare Products Regulatory Agency (MHRA) provides some insight into medicines use in those over 15 years of age (Ipsos MORI, 2004; 2006). Results suggest that around 70% of the adult population regularly take prescribed medication, that over 30% are long-term users of a prescribed medicine, and that similar numbers regularly purchase medicines over the counter (OTC). Unsurprisingly, the prevalence of medicines use is greater in older adults. It is estimated that 80% of those over the age of 75 take at least one prescribed medicine and that 36% are taking four or more. Polypharmacy, defined as the use of five or more drugs by an individual, is prevalent in more than 10% of those aged 65 years or over living in the community in the UK (Gorard, 2006). This is important because the ageing process affects the body's capacity to handle drugs, and consequently there is an increased risk of interactions, adverse drug reactions, and iatrogenesis in older people (Department of Health (DH), 2001).

Herbal medicines

It is estimated that 35% of British adults regularly use herbal medicines. It is of some concern that, of these, a significant number of people do not appear to know that herbal medicines can adversely interact with conventional medicines. Neither would they divulge their use of a herbal medicine to a health professional unless asked, even if they were to believe it was the cause of a health problem they were experiencing (Medicines and Healthcare products Regulatory Agency (MHRA), 2009).

Over-the-counter medicines

While the availability of OTC medicines offers a convenient and cost-effective way in which the public can access simple medicines, it is not without its problems. The results of a study conducted in Northern Ireland (Wazaify *et al.*, 2005) suggest that over 25% of those regularly taking prescribed medicines are also taking OTC products. Many may be unaware of the risk of adverse interactions between OTC medication and those that are prescribed. Furthermore, prolonged use of OTC products may delay or mask the diagnosis of serious illness, and overuse of products can also cause significant health problems. For example, non-steroidal anti-inflammatory drugs are implicated in gastric ulceration, and prolonged use of codeine-based analgesics in chronic daily headache.

Prescription-only medicines

Members of the public are increasingly able to obtain prescription-only medicines (POM) without a prescription via the Internet from individuals who are not qualified health professionals (Medicines and Healthcare products Regulatory Agency (MHRA), 2010) although data on the extent of this practice are not readily available.

Recreational drug use

Others may be using drugs for recreational purposes. Statistics on drug misuse for 2008–09 showed that 10.1% of adults had used one or more illicit drug within that year. Of those, 3.7% had used class A drugs (class A drugs include drugs such as ecstasy, LSD, heroin, and cocaine) and 7.9% had used cannabis (a class B drug); cannabis was the type of drug most likely to be used by adults (The Health and Social Care Information Centre, 2009). Data are not available for those over the age of 59. It is not unreasonable to suggest that these individuals may be unlikely to disclose this to a health professional for fear of reprimand.

Clearly, there exists a very real risk of individuals inadvertently compromising their health through the uninformed use of medicines. It is therefore essential that your assessments of patients include a sensitive detailed enquiry about all aspects of medicines use, including prescription, OTC, alternative/complementary therapies, Internet-acquired products, and illicit substances.

Financial cost of medicines use

Overall annual expenditure on medicines in the NHS in England is in excess of £12.3 billion annually, approximately 10% of the total NHS budget, with an acute care/primary care split of about 30/70%, respectively. Between 2008 and 2009, the cost of medicines rose overall by 5.6%, and that rise is likely to continue as more medicines are developed and individuals live for longer (National Institute for Health and Clinical Excellence (NICE), 2009; The NHS Information Centre, Prescribing and Primary Care Services, 2010).

Unfortunately, large quantities of medicines are prescribed and dispensed, but never taken by the individual for whom they are intended. The term used to describe this behaviour is 'non-adherence', and the financial cost is huge: an estimated £300 million annually (York Health Economics Consortium and School of Pharmacy, University of London, 2010). However, the real cost of non-adherence is difficult to quantify and includes not only the financial costs to the NHS and society related to loss of productivity and increased healthcare demand, but also the cost to the individual because of loss of earnings and poor disease control (Horne *et al.*, 2005).

Once equipped with a good understanding of non-adherence, you will be in a strong position to identify potential problems, to intervene to minimize these, and thereby to improve cost-effectiveness.

Problems associated with non-adherence

Understanding adherence and non-adherence

A number of terms are used within the literature to discuss and debate the factors that influence whether patients take their medicines as prescribed. The most commonly used terms are 'compliance', 'concordance', and 'adherence'. It is helpful to understand the differences and similarities of these terms, and the arguments for and against their use before we discuss the problems associated with non-adherence (Table 22.1).

Table 22.1 Defining terms

Compliance	The degree or extent of conformity to the recommendations about day-to-day treatment, including timing, dosage, and frequency (Cramer *et al.*, 2008)
Concordance	A partnership approach to interactions about medicines between healthcare professionals and patients (Latter, 2010: 107)
Adherence	The extent to which the patient's action matches the agreed recommendations (National Institute for Health and Clinical Excellence, 2009: 4)

It can be seen that compliance and adherence are similar, and both relate to the act of medicine-taking. However, the term 'compliance with medication' is sometimes seen to suggest an element of enforcement in which the patient acts in accordance with a wish or command, and so the use of this term is declining.

Medicines concordance is different. It is about a partnership process within which it is implicit that the prescriber and patient come to an agreement about the medication regimen that should be followed. Non-concordance suggests that there is a failure in the interaction between the professional and patient (Bell *et al.*, 2007).

Adherence is defined as 'Persistence in a practice or tenet; steady observance or maintenance' (Oxford English Dictionary, 2011). It is not a judgemental term and is therefore argued to be less controversial than the term compliance. It is more closely related to the perseverance that patients need to stick to a medicines regime (Aronson, 2007). Horne *et al.* (2005) also supports the use of the term, and argues that good communication and support are essential for patients to achieve it. In this sense, adherence recognizes the patient–professional relationship as integral to the patient's medicine-taking behaviour and therefore includes concordance.

The impact of non-adherence

The prevalence of non-adherence with prescribed medicine is estimated to be as much as 30–50% in developed countries, such as the UK, but higher in the developing world (World Health Organization, 2003). Non-adherence is a complex issue and is known to have a significantly detrimental impact on the course of many diseases. For example, non-adherence is thought to affect between 40% and 60% of individuals who have ulcerative colitis, and is associated with a five times greater risk of relapse (Kane *et al.*, 2001; 2003; Shale and Riley, 2003). Significant non-adherence has also been identified in individuals with diabetes. Ho *et al.* (2006), in a large retrospective cohort study (11,532 patients with diabetes), found that non-adherence was associated with adverse health outcomes. Similar findings were identified in non-adherent patients with coronary artery disease (Ho *et al.*, 2008).

Patients with mental health problems may be at greater risk of non-adherence, with rates ranging from 10% to 60% (Lingham and Scott, 2002). Patients treated for depression have been found to become increasingly non-adherent over time, with up to 10% of patients failing to collect their prescribed drugs, 30% stopping within 1 month, and 60% by 3 months. The negative impact of mental health problems on an individual's ability to acknowledge the requirement to take medication, and a fear of, or experience of, adverse effects have been shown to be predictors of non-adherence. Comorbid alcohol and substance misuse have also been implicated (Lingham and Scott, 2002).

What is clear is that non-adherence is common across many patient illness groups.

Having explored the scale of medicines use and associated issues, particularly those related to non-adherence, you will be beginning to appreciate some of the issues that you will need to address in your assessment of patients. Before we go on to discuss the assessment process, it is worth spending some time looking at the scope of nursing roles in medicines management, and the legislative and professional frameworks that govern these.

Nursing roles and accountability in medicines management

Expanded nursing roles

Nursing roles in medicines management are expanding and developing all of the time. Increasing numbers of nurses have prescriptive authority, and are permitted in law to prescribe medicines to patients. The scope of a nurse's prescriptive authority is dependent on his or her prescribing qualification. Registered nurse independent/supplementary prescribers (NIPs) (of whom in spring 2010 there were over 19,000 nationally: Latter *et al.*, 2011) are able to prescribe any medicine for any medical condition. There are, however, some restrictions to the controlled drugs that they may prescribe, the conditions for which they may be prescribed, and the route of administration. Research to date demonstrates that the prescribing decisions made by these nurses are clinically appropriate and safe. There is also evidence that patients value the improved access to prescribed medicines that nurse prescribing affords (Latter *et al.*, 2005; 2007). Community practitioner nurse prescribers mainly occupy community nursing or health visiting roles and are able to prescribe only from a limited community practitioner formulary.

Legal and professional frameworks

The practice of medicines management is supported by robust legal and professional frameworks. These frameworks have been designed and implemented to protect the public and to maintain safety. Practising within them therefore provides some assurance of safe practice.

As a nurse, you are required to apply the principles of the Nursing and Midwifery Council (NMC) Code: Standards of Conduct Performance and Ethics for Nurses and Midwives (NMC, 2008) when working with medicines, and to comply with the Standards for Medicines Management (NMC, 2007). Additionally, those nurses with prescriptive authority are required to practise according to the NMC Standards of Proficiency for Nurse and Midwife Prescribers (NMC, 2006). All three documents are comprehensive, with the standards expected of nurses clearly articulated.

This section will therefore focus on aspects of legislation and regulation related to an aspect of medicines management with which nurses are often less familiar, but in which they frequently participate—that is, the legislative framework that governs advice to individuals to purchase and use over-the-counter medicines. We will then move on to consider briefly the regulation of controlled drugs and recent changes introduced in response to the findings of the Shipman Inquiry.

Legislation and regulation of over-the-counter medicines

There are a number of areas of clinical practice, including, but not exclusively, emergency care, community nursing, and primary care, in which nurses need to advise patients about the use of over-the-counter medicines to manage, for example, simple ailments or pain. This is an aspect of practice that is not referred to in any detail in the NMC Standards for Medicines Management, but is common practice nonetheless. To practise safely in this area requires knowledge of how the prescription, administration, and supply of medicines is regulated.

Classification of medicinal products

The legal ability to supply medicines is based on the classification of medicinal products, of which there are three: general sale (GSL); pharmacy (P); and prescription-only

(POM). General sale list (GSL) medicines can be bought in a number of retail outlets, e.g. a supermarket, and are sold without the supervision of a pharmacist; typical examples include small packs of paracetamol and ibuprofen. Pharmacy (P) medicines can be obtained only from a pharmacy, and the sale must be supervised by a pharmacist—an example being the emergency contraceptive pill. Prescription-only medicines (POM) must be prescribed by a health professional with prescriptive authority, e.g. a doctor or nurse independent/supplementary prescriber, or be the subject of a patient group direction.

Manufacturer's authorization

Before a medicine can be sold in the UK, it must have been issued with a licence from the MHRA; this is referred to as a **manufacturer's authorization (MA)** (previously referred to as a product licence). The MA states the indication, form, dose, route of administration, and age group of patient for which the drug is licensed; it can, to some extent, be considered a guarantee of safety, and places liability on the manufacturer for adverse effects arising from the use of the drug. The scope of the MA is described in the summary of product characteristics (SPC) for each specific drug. When a drug is used outside any of these parameters, the use is referred to as being 'off licence' or 'off label'. While this is common practice in a number of fields of clinical practice for legitimate reasons, e.g. diazepam is administered rectally to treat febrile convulsions in infants, but is not licensed for use in children under the age of 1, it is not without risk. Firstly, the drug may be being used in a way for which its efficacy and risks have not been formally assessed by the MHRA; secondly, when prescribing, supplying, or advising the use of a medicine outside the MA, the full liability may well be transferred from the drug company to the clinician if the patient suffers an adverse reaction.

Variance in availability

It is important to appreciate that a significant number of drugs are available both as GSL and POM medicines, but in different licensed forms and under different trade names. To illustrate: ibuprofen is available as both a GSL and POM medicine. When sold as a GSL medicine, the SPC (reflecting the MA) states that the recommended dose is 200–400 mg three times a day to a maximum of 1,200 mg in 24 hours; however, when prescribed as a POM, the recommended dose increases to 1,200–1,800 mg daily in divided doses, not exceeding 2,400 mg in 24 hours, and again this reflects the MA. This is a good example of how the different MAs reflect the risks associated with different applications. In the case of ibuprofen, the risks associated with the drug are greater in higher doses. The use of the drug therefore needs to be carefully monitored by an experienced clinician such as a nurse independent/supplementary prescriber, and hence it is available only as a POM in these circumstances.

Risks

Clearly, this is a more complex area of practice than is initially apparent. However, once you understand the legislative framework that governs OTC medicines, practising within it is relatively straightforward.

Another high-risk area is that related to the supply and administration of controlled drugs. While it is beyond the scope of this chapter to cover this aspect of medicines management in depth, it is important to consider some more recent changes to this aspect of practice.

Controlled drugs

Following the fourth report of the Shipman Inquiry, there has been a renewed focus on the governance arrangements for how controlled drugs are obtained, stored, supplied, recorded, monitored, and safely disposed of. This has resulted in changes in legislation that have an impact on nursing practice; these are included in the NMC Standards of Medicines Management (NMC, 2007). These changes require all healthcare providers to have standard operating procedures (SOPs) for the management and handling of controlled drugs. It is therefore imperative that you familiarize yourself with the SOP of the organization for which you work and comply with these.

Working with controlled drugs in the community is a particularly high-risk area of practice and therefore needs to be managed carefully. Lone working is common, controlled drugs are frequently stored in the patient's own home, and nurses are not infrequently required to collect prescribed controlled drugs from the pharmacy on behalf of the patient. Before working in the community, we would recommend that you familiarize yourself with *The Guide to Good Practice in the Management of Controlled Drugs in Primary Care (England)* (National Prescribing Centre, 2009). This guide comprehensively addresses all aspects of working with controlled drugs, and chapters 13–15 and 19 are particularly relevant for nurses because they cover the recommendations for community nursing, palliative care, care homes, and out-of-hours services.

Having reviewed the professional standards with which you need to comply when managing medicines, we are now in a good position to examine how you should conduct a nursing assessment of an individual's use of medication.

Key nursing responsibilities in supporting use of medicines

In previous sections, we have identified a number of factors related to medicines use that impact on safety and effectiveness. We have suggested that if these factors are identified as issues at the point of assessment, you will be able to work with the patient to identify strategies to enhance his or her use of medication.

Undertaking a medicines management assessment

From the outset, it is important to be clear what you want to achieve through a medicines management assessment. Your aim is to identify what medicines the patient is taking, the effectiveness of these, and any potential safety issues. To achieve this, the assessment can be divided into three stages, as follows.

1. **The interview**—to include:

   - Current use of medication (prescribed, OTC, herbal, homeopathic, shared, and illicit)
   - Experience of taking medicines, including:
     — adverse drug reactions (side effects/allergies) or interactions, both perceived and actual
     — symptom control (subjective effectiveness)
   - Adherence to prescribed medicines, including the patient's:
     — views, beliefs, and expectations about his or her medicines
     — depth of understanding about how his or her medicines work and why he or she is taking them
   - Frequency of therapeutic drug monitoring (when indicated)

2. **The summary**—summarizing back to the patient what you have understood from the information that he or she has provided
3. **The objective assessment of effectiveness**—undertaking any observations and/or examinations that are indicated

We will now explore each of these components in some depth

The interview

Assessing current use of prescribed medicines

Many of those who have long-term conditions, or who are older, struggle to recall the names of the medicines they are taking or why they are taking them. Therefore the simplest way in which to obtain the information you need is to ask the patient to show you all of the medicines he or she is taking and to go through each individually; this is relatively straightforward in the community, more difficult in hospital settings, and rarely immediately possible for unplanned admissions to hospital. If it is not possible to see the medicines, enquire whether the person has a repeat prescription form with him or her; often people keep this in their purse or wallet. You could also contact the patient's GP; it is a simple task for the reception staff to fax a copy of the patient's medicine regimen to a secure fax in a clinic or ward setting. While this is more difficult outside normal working hours, some GPs now participate in a computerized shared clinical data repository to which hospitals have access and which could provide you with the information that you need. If none of these options is available to you, you will need to write down in the patient's own words what he or she is taking: for example, 'a small white water tablet in the morning for high blood pressure'. It is essential that you do not guess or make suggestions to the patient to prompt him or her, because many medicines have similar names and this could lead to inaccurate information being documented and unsafe clinical decisions being made. To make it easy, ask patient what he or she takes at specific times of the day, i.e. the morning, lunchtime, evening and bedtime, and any other times in between.

Assessing current use of non-prescribed products

Once you have achieved a clear picture of what the patient is being prescribed, you then need to explore other aspects of medicines use. This includes obtaining an understanding of what other medicines/substances the patient is taking, why he or she is taking them, and what he or she hopes to achieve from so doing.

As established previously, while patients may freely give you information about their use of conventional over-the-counter medicines, they may be less willing to tell you about their use of homeopathic or herbal products, and even less comfortable about disclosing illicit drug use because of fear of reproach. However, this information may prove crucial in determining the effectiveness of the patient's prescribed medicines and revealing any safety issues related to drug interactions, so it is important to pursue this line of enquiry. The questions in Box 22.1 will help you to explore these areas.

Finally, it is important to discern whether the patient is using anyone else's medicines. This is not uncommon and, for example, family members often share inhalers and prescribed analgesia. Again, this will require sensitive enquiry using a similar approach to that given above.

Assessing experience and adherence in medicines use

Once you have established what medicines the patient is taking, you then to need to gain an understanding of his is her experiences of taking those medicines, including actual and perceived side effects and benefits. Enquiry about adherence to prescribed/advised medication should also be undertaken at this time, including both intentional and unintentional non-adherence.

The World Health Organization (2003) highlights five interacting dimensions of non-adherence: social and economic factors; healthcare team and system-related factors; condition-related factors; therapy-related factors;

Box 22.1 Suggested questions to explore use of non-prescribed products

Question: Many people believe that herbal or homeopathic products can be helpful in treating diseases and ailments, but sometimes health problems can occur when they are used in conjunction with prescribed medicines. Can you tell me what herbal or homeopathic medicines you use?

Question: Some people use recreational substances, or 'street drugs', to help them relax or to manage their pain; again, these can interact with prescribed medicines. Have you ever taken any of these?

Table 22.2 Potential reasons for intentional and unintentional non-adherence

Intentional non-adherence	Unintentional non-adherence
Decision to omit doses owing to: • adverse effects of medication • interferes with lifestyle • failure to understand the benefits Beliefs: • incomplete understanding of the nature of the illness and treatment • influences of prior experiences of taking medication • influences from experiences of family and friends • influenced by factors of culture, education, social circumstances • fears and anxieties—concern and risks of medication outweigh perceived benefits	Poor communication by health professional, resulting in: • difficulty understanding instructions • lack of information being given to understand treatment regime fully Forgetfulness or poor recall Inability to pay for treatment Complexity of regime resulting in: • medication being taken at the wrong time • taking incorrect doses—too many or too few or complete omissions Difficulties accessing medicines owing to: • difficulties obtaining supply • repeat prescription failures • difficulties using device • inability to open packaging • poor labelling with limited instructions on when to take

and patient-related factors. It then discusses intervention strategies for each of these dimensions. It is important to address these dimensions during the assessment. Table 22.2 outlines the reasons for intentional and unintentional non-adherence, and includes factors from each of the five dimensions, all of which you will need to explore.

You can achieve an understanding of all of the issues presented in Table 22.2 by approaching each topic in a matter-of-fact way, so that no blame or judgement is apportioned. Explaining why you are asking will encourage the patient to give honest answers (National Institute for Health and Clinical Excellence, 2009). Using non-judgemental statements such as 'Sometimes patients miss taking their medication . . .' followed by questions such as 'How often do you miss taking your medicine?' will give the patient the opportunity to respond in an open and frank way.

A crucial factor in determining if, how, and when an individual takes his or her medication is his or her beliefs about it (Horne and Weinman, 1999; Britten *et al.*, 2000). There is evidence to suggest that providing the patient with an opportunity to discuss beliefs about both his or her illness and his or her medicines may improve adherence (Stevenson *et al.*, 2004). The mnemonic PIECE will help you to structure the questioning in this area, as illustrated

in Figure 22.1. The questions in Box 22.2 may help you to elicit the information you need in these areas.

Assessing the need for therapeutic drug monitoring

Therapeutic drug monitoring is an important component of medicines management, because some drugs are toxic at certain levels or in certain physiological circumstances, while others are effective only at specific levels of concentration. It is important that you familiarize yourself with the drugs that commonly require regular monitoring, e.g. lithium, digoxin, and warfarin. You also need to be aware of those that may have an adverse effect on renal function, such as angiotensin-converting enzyme inhibitors, or on liver function, such as the lipid-lowering drug simvastatin. You should enquire during the assessment about how frequently patients taking such drugs are monitored and when the last measurement was made.

The summary

Summarizing back to a patient is an important component of any consultation. It is important that you feed back to the patient the key points you have understood from the information you have been given. This provides the patient with an opportunity both to correct any misunderstanding and to discuss any other aspects of medicines use that have not been addressed. It is good practice

P	Patient Perspectives
I	**Ideas**: about their illness and their understanding about how their medicines work.
E	**Experiences/Effects** of taking medication: Ask about any problems e.g. are there any difficulties obtaining their supplies; does taking the medicines interfere in any way with their lifestyle; is there any difficulty opening containers or swallowing medication; do they think their medication is working effectively to manage their illness and ask if they experiencing any side effects.
C	**Concerns**: ask about any particular worries a patient may have about taking their medication. Remember if a patient has heightened concerns and does not believe medication is effective then they are at high risk of non adherence.
E	**Explore**: medicines adherence with the patient. Has the patient missed taking any medication, would they like to stop their medication or have thought about stopping. Ask if they ever taken more medication than that which is prescribed.

Figure 22.1 PIECE—patient perspectives (developed from a seminal consultation model).

Reproduced from Pendleton, D., Schofield, T., Tate, P., Havelock, P., *The Consultation: An Approach to Learning and Teaching*, with permission from Oxford University Press.

not to restrict this to the end of the interview, but to summarize and feed back aspects of information throughout the consultation.

The objective assessment of effectiveness: observation and examination

You will often need to gain an objective assessment of the effectiveness of prescribed medicine, e.g. the blood pressure of a patient with hypertension, the peak flow rate of a patient with asthma, or the blood sugar in a patient with diabetes. This should be undertaken on completion of the interview.

Many of the above elements are included in the 'medicines use review' model. This model has long been advocated by the pharmacy profession as a robust framework for comprehensively considering all aspects of medicines use (National Prescribing Centre, 2008).

Once you have gathered this information, you will be able to identify what, if any, interventions are indicated to maximize the effectiveness of medicines usage.

Interventions to improve safety, effectiveness, and adherence

Once you have obtained and documented the information provided from the patient, you need to analyse this to identify any further issues related to safety or effectiveness.

This can be achieved by referring to the *British National Formulary* (BNF) and the summary of product characteristics of the prescribed and over-the-counter medicines being used; both are easily available electronically and will enable you to identify possible side effects, interactions, special monitoring requirements, and adjustments necessary because of age or disease. It is important that you understand how to use the BNF properly; this can be achieved very simply by reading the relevant opening chapters of the formulary.

The use of the Screening Tool of Older Peoples Potentially Inappropriate Prescriptions (STOPP), and the Screening Tool to Alert (doctors/prescribers) to Right Treatment (START) may be valuable in enabling you to identify potentially inappropriate medications that are being prescribed for an older person, or medicines that are indicated, but are not currently being prescribed. Although these tools have been predominantly utilized in the acute setting, they are transferable to community settings, and the validity and reliability of each has been tested (O'Mahony *et al.*, 2010).

If you are concerned that a patient's use of herbal or illicit substances may be interacting with his or her prescribed medicines, the regional drug information service for the area in which you are working will be able to provide you with the information you need. The contact details for the service are always provided inside the front cover of the current BNF. Alternatively, *Stockley's Herbal Medicines Interactions* (Williamson *et al.*, 2009) is a useful resource.

Box 22.2 Suggested questions to elicit patient perspectives

Ideas: How are you feeling about your [name of illness]?

Do you feel it is being managed well?

Sometimes it can be difficult to remember how your medicines help you. Can you tell me what you think your medicines are for?

Experiences/effects: Sometimes patients have difficulties with their medication. How are you getting on with them?

Do you believe your medicines are effective?

Sometimes patients develop side effects from their medication. Have you noticed any side effects?

Concerns: Sometimes patients worry about taking their medication. How do you feel about taking them?

Is there anything specific that might be worrying you about your medicines?

Explore: Sometimes patients miss taking their medication. Have you missed taking any medicines in the past week?

How happy are you to continue with taking your medicines?

Are there any medicines that you have thought about stopping?

Have you ever taken more medication than was prescribed?

Have you ever taken anyone else's medicines?

The outcome of your analysis could identify the need for any of the following interventions:

- interventions to improve safety;
- interventions to improve effectiveness;
- interventions to improve adherence;
- advice to self-medicate.

Interventions to improve safety and effectiveness

Interventions to improve safety or effectiveness are indicated if, as part of your assessment, you identify a potential drug/drug interaction (e.g. aspirin and warfarin), a drug/disease interaction (e.g. atenolol and asthma), insufficient

therapeutic drug monitoring (e.g. digoxin levels), or medicines use that does not reflect current national or local evidence-based guidelines or best practice. If you do identify these, you will need to inform a medical or non-medical prescriber and discuss your concerns with them. This should be done within a timescale that reflects the potential seriousness of the issue you have identified. It is important that you do *not* attempt to make any changes to a patient's medication without reference to a prescriber.

Interventions to improve adherence

There is a plethora of research into interventions to improve concordance and adherence in long-term health problems, and the consensus is that it is a complex area requiring multiple approaches and that there is no one solution. A Cochrane review (Haynes *et al.*, 2008) has found that even with improvements to adherence there are not always corresponding improvements in clinical outcomes. The findings from this review highlight that no one intervention is more effective than the others. However, for short-term treatments, the provision of written information, personal telephone calls, and counselling has been shown to be somewhat effective (Haynes *et al.*, 2008). In long-term care, the diversity and complexity of interventions to improve adherence made it difficult for the reviewers to make generalizations about which strategies worked better than others; those that appeared to have some impact were family therapy, psychological therapy, and crisis intervention. Unfortunately, even the most effective interventions did not result in large increases in adherence rates or improved treatment outcomes (Haynes *et al.*, 2008).

It is clear from the evidence that adherence is not just patient-related; the complexity of healthcare systems can also have a negative impact on adherence. This can be illustrated by this simplistic example. If the length of an appointment is insufficient, and clinicians are unable to address adherence issues within the time allocated, then, unless this is addressed, improvements to adherence levels will be limited (World Health Organization, 2003). Remember that one of your nursing responsibilities is to evaluate care and to act as a change agent to lead service improvement initiatives and to enhance care outcomes (Nursing and Midwifery Council, 2010). This applies equally to medicines management as to other areas of healthcare.

When working with patients to improve adherence, the National Institute for Health and Clinical Excellence

> **Box 22.3   Five interventions to increase adherence (NICE, 2009)**
>
> Determine whether the patient is intentionally or unintentionally non-adherent, and discuss relevant beliefs and concerns (intentional non-adherence) and/or practical problems of taking his or her medicines (unintentional non-adherence).
>
> Address any beliefs or concerns the patient has about his or her medicines.
>
> Only use interventions to overcome practical problems if there is a specific need, e.g.:
>
> - Suggesting that patients record their medicine-taking
> - Encouraging patients to monitor their condition
> - Simplifying the dosing regimen
> - Using alternative packaging
> - Using a multicompartment medicines system
>
> If the patient is concerned about side effects:
>
> - Discuss these alongside the potential benefits and long-term effects; ascertain how the patient would like to deal with side effects
> - Consider adjusting the dosage, switching to another medicine, and other strategies such as changing the timing of medicines
>
> Ask if prescription costs are a problem and consider options for reducing costs.

(NICE) provides pragmatic evidence-based guidance (NICE, 2009). Firstly, any intervention to support adherence should be discussed with the patient; it should considered on a case-by-case basis and, as we have stressed earlier, should address the concerns and needs of individual patients. The Institute then identifies the five interventions outlined in Box 22.3 that, if implemented, have the potential to increase adherence (NICE, 2009). It is sensible to follow this guidance.

Advising patients to self-medicate

As a result of your assessment, you may decide that the patient would benefit from taking medicines, e.g. simple analgesia, that are easily available over the counter, and that this would be the most cost-effective option. When so doing, you need to be cognizant of the fact that many

OTC medicines have significant side effects and can interact with prescribed or other OTC medicines. Arguably, the knowledge and skills that you need to be able to safely advise a patient about the use of OTC medicines are the same as those needed to prescribe that medicine, and include knowledge of both the patient and the product.

The use of the mnemonic EASE (National Prescribing Centre, 1999) has long been used in prescribing and could be applied equally well when making decisions about OTC medicines, as follows.

E   how **E**ffective is the product?
A   is it **A**ppropriate for this patient?
S   how **S**afe is it?
E   is the product cost-**E**ffective?

Table 22.3 (see page 389) illustrates the breadth and depth of knowledge you require to practise safely with OTC medicines.

While much of this information can be obtained during the patient interview/assessment, and other drug-specific aspects from the *British National Formulary* and the summary of product characteristic, it is clear that you still need a sound underpinning knowledge of applied pharmacology to be able to practise safely in this area. It is imperative therefore that, as a student, you *always* refer to a registered practitioner before advising a patient about the use of OTC medicines. Once registered, in every instance, you should carefully consider whether you have the necessary knowledge and skills to advise patients safely. If in any doubt, you should either refer to a prescriber or direct the patient to a retail pharmacist who will be able to assist them.

Case study 22.1 (see page 390) illustrates the range and depth of information you need to be able to practise safely in this area. It reinforces the position that all of your interventions should be based on robust evidence and/or best practice. We will now go on to discuss where you can access the evidence to inform your medicines management and what you need to consider when evaluating that evidence.

Accessing the evidence to inform clinical decisions

In healthcare, despite having developed an extensive evidence base for many drug treatments and interventions, there is often a delay of many years between establishing

Table 22.3 **What you need to know for safe over-the-counter (OTC) practice**

Patient/product knowledge	Why the factors are important
Efficacy of the medicine in the circumstances being advised	The NMC Code states that you must ensure any advice you give is evidence-based if you are suggesting the use of healthcare products or services.
Age	The ability to metabolize and excrete drugs slows with age. As a result, drug action may be prolonged, and adaptations of the drug dose and regimen may be required to prevent toxicity.
Interactions (current medication: prescribed, OTC, and complementary)	Two or more drugs given at the same time may interact. The interaction may be antagonistic (one drug stops or slows the effect of the other) or synergistic (one drug enhances the effect of the other).
Pregnancy	Many medicines are contraindicated in pregnancy because they adversely affect the developing fetus.
Breastfeeding	Some drugs can reach levels in the breast milk that are toxic to the infant.
Comorbidities/contraindications	Any disease state that affects the absorption, distribution, metabolism, or excretion of medicines can result in prolonged effect and sometimes toxicity. The use of some drugs is contraindicated in certain diseases because they have the potential to increase the severity of symptoms.
Allergies and sensitivity	Individuals may be sensitive or allergic to certain drugs or drug groups.
Dose, regimen	Drugs are effective only if given in therapeutic doses at certain intervals. If the dose or regimen is incorrect, there is a risk of either ineffectiveness or toxicity.
Side effects	Few medicines are without side effects. Patients need to be aware of these so that they can: • make an informed choice about whether they wish to take the medicine; • manage the side effects; • recognize when to seek advice.
Scope of manufacturers authorization for GSL or P use	As discussed above

the evidence and its reliable translation into clinical practice. This is in part because the ways of working in healthcare do not make it easy to change and to embed new practice. Access to the evidence base is just one reason for the delay, and one that you will need to overcome to practise safely.

Information and communication technology offers opportunities to access evidence more easily, and there are a number of excellent easy-to-access resources that provide information about evidence-based medicines management interventions.

• The Map of Medicine (Map of Medicine, 2011) offers one of the most comprehensive and easily accessible routes to the evidence base. Algorithms describe typical clinical pathways and include up-to-date referencing and a summary of the evidence base for pharmacological treatments and interventions.

• The National Electronic Library for Medicines (NeLM, 2010) is a database covering published studies, alerts, and guidance on both drugs and disease, with an active news feed facility to bring you up-to-date information as it is published.

• The National Institute for Health and Clinical Excellence is a key reference source for NeLM, providing technology appraisals on the costs and benefits of new and existing treatments, as well as clinical guidelines. It also offers an active news feed service.

CASE STUDY 22.1 *Vignette*

James is a healthy 25-year-old engineer who has attended the emergency department one morning where you are working as a student nurse.

He complains of tripping over a kerb the night before and has a painful ankle, causing him to limp. There are no other reported injuries.

He is seen, assessed, and diagnosed with an acute mild ankle sprain. He asks you to recommend something to help relieve his pain.

The emergency department does have a patient group direction for paracetamol and ibuprofen.

- What do you need to consider in his medicines assessment and about your professional accountability before you give any advice?
  As a student nurse, are you able to supply and administer using a patient group direction?

Clue:

- Think about James' age and past medical history.
- Refer to the *Code of Conduct* (NMC, 2008) and the *Standards for Medicines Management* (NMC, 2007).

Points to consider

James is 25 years old and healthy. Because he is healthy and young, it is less likely that he will be taking regular prescribed medication. A good medication history will elicit any current medication—either prescribed, OTC, herbal, or recreational drugs.

James should be asked about any allergies or sensitivities to any previously taken medication.

What might you consider to be an effective mild analgesic?

James could consider himself 'healthy', but have, or have a past history of, asthma. Specific questioning to identify a history of asthma is important if you were thinking that ibuprofen might be suitable to

recommend as a mild analgesic to buy OTC. The WHO analgesic pain ladder recommends non-opioid analgesia, e.g. paracetamol, ibuprofen, or aspirin, for mild pain.

Ibuprofen, although commonly used as a mild analgesic and easily bought from chemists and supermarkets, has many drug interactions and potential side effects, e.g. a small proportion of people with asthma will react to ibuprofen and aspirin, causing an exacerbation of their asthma symptoms.

As a student, you must recognize and stay within the limits of your competence (NMC, 2010: 15). Recommending OTC medication without full knowledge of its side effects, interactions, and an understanding of how age-related factors, disease, and ethnicity affects the absorption, metabolism, and excretion of those drugs would mean that you were acting outside of your professional code and could put the patient's safety at risk.

After considering the above points and your professional accountability, what advice should you give?

Can you supply and administer a mild analgesic under patient group direction? As a student nurse, it is essential that you do not recommend any OTC medication, but refer to a registered nurse, ideally a prescriber, to give advice to James. Even though the medication is freely available, you are accountable for any advice you may give (NMC, 2008). A good alternative is to recommend that he seek the advice of a pharmacist at the local chemist.

You are unable to supply and administer as a student nurse using a patient group direction (NMC, 2007: 18).

What alternative pain relief advice could you offer? Non-pharmacological management of pain is an option. However, you must ensure that any advice you give is evidence-based (NMC, 2008).

- The National Prescribing Centre, also hosted by NICE, publishes the medicines bulletin MeRec, which contains concise, evidence-based information about medicines and prescribing issues; this is a vital intelligence source for prescribers and healthcare providers on newly launched medicines and their place in therapy and, in the case of more established drug treatments, the results of meta-analysis studies.

- PRODIGY (formerly CKS) also falls under the NICE umbrella of NHS Evidence information sources. These provide essential information for healthcare professionals working in primary and first-contact care. They are particularly useful when dealing with medicines with risk profiles that require routine monitoring, such as drug levels, U&Es, creatinine levels or other laboratory tests; they also describe the symptoms of toxicity and treatment regimens where appropriate.

- The Cochrane Library provides easy-to-access systematic reviews, including a significant number that relate to drug therapy and medicines management.

- When searching for evidence related to aspects of medicines management, it would be prudent to utilize the Excerpta Medica database (EMBASE), which is a major biomedical and pharmaceutical database and includes journals from the following fields: drug research; pharmacology; pharmaceutics; toxicology; and clinical and experimental human medicine.

Box 22.4 Useful links

The Map of Medicine: **http://www.mapofmedicine. com/**

National Electronic Library for Medicine: **http:// www.nelm.nhs.uk/en/**

National Institute for Health and Clinical Excellence: **http://www.nice.org.uk/**

The National Prescribing Centre: **http://www.npc. co.uk/**

Clinical Knowledge Summaries (CKS): **http://www. cks.nhs.uk/home**

The Cochrane Library: **http://www. thecochranelibrary.com/view/0/index.html**

How to evaluate the evidence

Results of medicines-related research are often described in terms of numbers needed to treat (NNT) and numbers needed to harm (NNH), and it is therefore important that you understand what these terms mean and how they are calculated. To calculate the NNT for one person to benefit from taking a drug, you need to know the absolute risk reduction (ARR), i.e. the difference in the control event rate in a group of people taking a placebo and the experimental event rate in a matched group taking the drug. The NNT is the reciprocal of the absolute risk reduction.

The NNH shows how many people would need to be treated with the drug in order for one person to experience the harmful effect. To calculate the NNH, you subtract the control event rate from the experimental event rate, where the event is the adverse effect or unwanted harm. This gives the absolute risk increase (ARI), the reciprocal of which gives the NNH. NNT and NNH are both demonstrated well in an e-learning module from the University of Nottingham (University of Nottingham, 2007).

It is also important to appreciate that the results of large studies may be statistically significant without being clinically important, and that small studies may fail to identify clinically important benefits owing to a lack of statistical power. It is important that you understand the difference between statistical significance and clinical significance. The latter requires a change in something that matters to the patient. A study may generate results that are statistically significant, but this might relate to issues that are of trivial concern and benefit to the patient in his or her everyday life.

Future research

Throughout this chapter, we have referred to research and best practice to inform our discussion and guidance. It is clear, however, that there are areas in which we still need to undertake more research to help us to understand peoples' behaviour in relation to the use of medicines.

1. With the exception of teenage patients, there is little research, if any, that describes individuals' use of the Internet to access medicines and why they choose this route.

2. Non-adherence is a complex subject and, despite a significant body of research, we still do not fully understand which interventions to improve adherence will be successful.

3. Nurses' roles in managing medicines continue to grow. While research to date tells us that nurses are safe prescribers, we are yet to find at whether they are more or less successful than other health professional groups in working with patients in terms of health to improve outcomes.

Summary and key messages

In this chapter, we have explored the concept of medicines management, the implications of increased public access to medicines, and the important issue of adherence. We have looked at the changing roles of nurses in medicines management, and the knowledge and skills necessary to conduct an in-depth assessment of an individual's use of medicines. In so doing, we have provided you with a framework to support your assessment and management of individuals—one that is aimed at improving safety and clinical effectiveness, and which focuses on patients' experience of medicines use.

Medicines are potent substances; very few are without side effects and most have the potential to interact with other medicines and substances.

- When undertaking a patient assessment, you should aim to identify all of the medicines that he or she is taking. This should include gathering information about the use of prescribed medicines, those purchased over the counter and/or via the Internet, herbal and homeopathic products, medicines intended for someone else, and illicit substances.

- Understanding the patient's experience of medicines use, his or her views, beliefs, and concerns, is fundamental to optimizing adherence.

- Interventions should be aimed at improving safety, effectiveness, and adherence, and should be undertaken in partnership with the patient and a professional with prescriptive authority.

Online Resource Centre

 To help you to develop and apply your knowledge and decision-making skills further, we have provided interactive learning resources online at **www.oxfordtextbooks.co.uk/orc/bullock/**

Whilst these are freely available, you will need to use the access codes at the start of the book.

References

Aronson, J. K. (2007) Editors' view: compliance, concordance, adherence. *British Journal of Clinical Pharmacology* **63**(4): 383–4.

Audit Commission (2001) *A Spoonful of Sugar: Medicines Management in NHS Hospitals*. Audit Commission: London.

Bell, J.S., Airaksinen M.S., Lyles, A., *et al.* (2007) Concordance is not synonymous with compliance or adherence. *British Journal of Clinical Pharmacology* **64**(5): 710–13.

Britten, N., Stevenson, F.A., Barry C.A., *et al.* (2000) Misunderstandings in prescribing decisions in general practice: qualitative study. *British Medical Journal* **320**: 484–8.

Cochrane Library (2011). **http://www.thecochranelibrary.com/view/0/index.html** (accessed 19 March 2011).

Cramer, J.A., Roy, A., Burrell, A., *et al.* (2008) Medication compliance and persistence: terminology and definitions. *Value in Health* **11**(1): 44–7.

Department of Health (2001) *National Service Framework for Older People*. Department of Health: London.

Gorard, D.A. (2006) Escalating polypharmacy. *Quarterly Journal of Medicine* **99**(11): 797–800. **http://qjmed.oxfordjournals.org/content/99/11/797.full.pdf+html** (accessed 19 March 2011).

Haynes, R.B., Ackloo, E., Sahota, N., *et al.* (2008) Interventions for enhancing medication adherence. *Cochrane Database of Systematic Reviews* Issue 2: Art. No. CD000011. DOI: 10.1002/14651858. CD000011. pub3.

Health and Social Care Information Centre (2009) *Statistics on Drug Misuse: England, 2009*. The NHS Information Centre for Health and Social Care: London.

Ho, P.M., Magid, D.J., Shetterly, S.M., *et al.* (2008) Medication non-adherence is associated with a broad range of adverse outcomes in patients with coronary artery disease. *American Heart Journal* **155**(4): 772–9.

Ho, P.M., Rumsfeld, J.S., Masoudi, F.A., *et al.* (2006) Effect of medication non-adherence on hospitalization and mortality among patients with diabetes mellitus. *Archives of Internal Medicine* **166**: 1836–41.

Horne, R., Weinman, J. (1999) Patients' beliefs about prescribed medicines and their role in adherence to treatment in chronic physical illness. *Journal of Psychosomatic Research* **47**(6): 555–67.

Horne, R., Weinman, J., Barber, N., *et al.* (2005) *Concordance, Adherence and Compliance in Medicine Taking: Report for the National Coordinating Centre for NHS Service Delivery and Organization R & D (NCCSDO)*. **http://www.sdo.lshtm.ac.uk/files/project/76-final-report.pdf** (accessed 24 October 2010).

Ipsos MORI (2004) *The Public and Prescribed Medicines: Social Research*. **http://www.mori-eire.com/researchpublications/researcharchive/670/The-Public-And-Prescribed-Medicines.aspx** (accessed 17 March 2011).

Ipsos MORI (2006) *The Risks and Benefits of Medicines and Medical Devices, Social Research*. **http://www.mori-eire.com/default.aspx** (accessed 17 March 2011).

Kane, S.V., Cohen, R.D., Aikens, J.E., *et al.* (2001) Prevalence of nonadherence with maintenance mesalamine in quiescent ulcerative colitis. *American Journal of Gastroenterology* **96**(10): 2929–33.

Kane, S.V. Huo, D., Aikens, J., *et al.* (2003) Medication non adherence and the outcomes of patients with quiescent ulcerative colitis. *American Journal of Medicine* **114**(1): 39–43., pp.107–18

Latter, S. (2010) Promoting concordance in prescribing interactions. In M. Courtney, M. Griffiths (eds) *Independent and Supplementary Prescribing: An Essential Guide*, 2nd edn. University Press Cambridge: Cambridge, pp.107–18.

Latter, S., Blenkinsopp, A., Smith, A., *et al.* (2011) *Evaluation of Nurse and Pharmacist Independent Prescribing*. Faculty of Health Sciences, University of Southampton; School of Pharmacy, Keele University on behalf of Department of Health: Southampton Keele.

Lingham, R., Scott, J. (2002) Treatment non-adherence in affective disorders. *Acta Psychiatrica Scandinavica* **105**(3): 164–72.

Map of Medicine (2011) **http://www.mapofmedicine.com/evidence/map/index.html** (accessed 19 March 2011).

Medicines and Healthcare Products Regulatory Agency (MHRA) (2009) Public perceptions of herbal medicines. *Drug Safety Update* **2**(8): 11.

Medicines and Healthcare Products Regulatory Agency (MHRA) (2010) Risks of buying medicines over the Internet. Safety Information. **http://www.mhra.gov.uk**

Medicines Partnership (2008) *Room for Review: A Guide to Medication Review—The Agenda for Patients, Practitioners and Managers*. Medicines Partnership: London.

National Electronic Library for Medicines (2011). **http://www.nelm.nhs.uk/en/** (accessed 19 March 2011).

National Institute for Health and Clinical Excellence (2009) *Medicines Adherence Involving Patients in Decisions about Prescribed Medicines and Supporting Adherence*. National Institute for Health and Clinical Excellence: London.

National Institute for Health and Clinical Excellence (2009) **http://www.nice.org.uk/** (accessed 19 March 2011).

National Prescribing Centre (1999) Signposts for prescribing nurses: general principles of good prescribing. *Prescribing Nurse Bulletin* **1**(1): 1–4.

National Prescribing Centre (2002) *Modernising Medicines Management: A Guide to Achieving Benefits for Patients, Professionals and the NHS (Book 1)*. National Prescribing Centre: Liverpool. **http://www.npc.nhs.uk/developing_systems/intro/resources/library_good_practice_guide_mmmbook1_2002.pdf** (accessed 17 March 2011).

National Prescribing Centre (2008) *A Guide to Medication Review*. **http://www.npc.co.uk/review_medicines/intro/resources/agtmr_web1.pdf** (accessed 4 November 2011).

National Prescribing Centre (2009) *A Guide to Good Practice in the Management of Controlled Drugs in Primary Care (England)*. **http://www.npc.nhs.uk/controlled_drugs/resources/controlled_drugs_third_edition.pdf** (accessed 3 June 2011).

NHS Information Centre, Prescribing and Primary Care Services (2010) *Hospital Prescribing, England: 2009*. The NHS Information Centre for Health and Social Care: London.

NHS PRODIGY (2011). **www.prodigy.clarity.co.uk** (accessed 9 January 2012).

Nursing and Midwifery Council (NMC) (2006) *Standards of Proficiency for Nurse and Midwife Prescribers*. Nursing and Midwifery Council: London.

Nursing and Midwifery Council (NMC) (2007) *Standards for Medicines Management*. Nursing and Midwifery Council: London.

Nursing and Midwifery Council (NMC) (2008) *The Code: Standards of Conduct, Performance and Ethics for Nurses and Midwives.* Nursing and Midwifery Council: London.

Nursing and Midwifery Council (NMC) (2010) *Standards for Preregistration Nursing Education.* Nursing and Midwifery Council: London.

O'Mahoney, D., Gallagher, P., Ryan, C., *et al.* (2010) STOPP & START criteria: a new approach to determining inappropriate prescribing in old age. *European Geriatric Medicine* **1**: 45–51.

Oxford English Dictionary (2011) **http://www.oed.com:80/ Entry/2328** (accessed 27 March 2011).

Pendleton, D., Schofield, T., Tate, P., *et al.* (1984) *The Consultation: An Approach to Learning and Teaching.* Oxford University Press: Oxford.

Shale, M.J., Riley, S.A. (2003) Studies of compliance with delayed-release mesalazine therapy in patients with inflammatory bowel disease. *Alimentary Pharmacology and Therapeutics* **18**: 191–8.

Stevenson, F.A., Cox, K., Britten, N., *et al.* (2004) A systematic review of the research on communication between patients and health care professionals about medicines: the consequences for concordance. *Health Expectations* **7**: 235–45.

University of Nottingham School of Nursing and Academic Division of Midwifery (2007) *RLO: Numbers Needed to Treat (NNT) and Numbers Needed to Harm (NNH).* **http://sonet. nottingham.ac.uk/rlos/ebp/nnt_nnh/index.html** (accessed 19 March 2011).

Wazaify, M., Shields, E., Hughes, C.M., *et al.* (2005) Societal perspectives on over-the-counter (OTC) medicines. *Family Practice* **22**(2): 170–6.

Williamson, E.M., Driver, S., Baxter, K. (eds) (2009) *Stockley's Herbal Medicines Interactions.* Pharmaceutical Press: London.

World Health Organization (2003) *Adherence to Long-term Therapies: Evidence for Action.* World Health Organization: Geneva.

York Health Economics Consortium, School of Pharmacy University of London (2010) *Evaluation of the Scale Causes and Costs of Waste Medicines.* **http://www.pharmacy. ac.uk/fileadmin/documents/News/Evaluation_of_NHS_ Medicines_Waste__web_publication_version.pdf** (accessed 4 November 2011).

23 *Managing* Mobility

Nicky Hayes and Julie Whitney

> ## Introduction
>
> This chapter addresses the fundamental nursing role in the management of mobility. Every nurse should possess the knowledge and skills to assess mobility needs, to select and implement evidence-based strategies to maintain mobility or assist mobility, and to review the effectiveness of these to inform any necessary changes in care.

Understanding the importance of mobility

Defining mobility

Mobility is the ability to move around independently. The most readily recognizable component of mobility is locomotion—the ability to walk. It includes transition from one position to another, which is necessary to allow walking to be incorporated into functional activities. Examples of transitions are moving from sitting to standing and from standing to lying down. Virtually all bodily systems are required for safe and effective mobility (see Figure 23.1).

Maintaining mobility and good health

Maintaining higher levels of physical activity has been associated with reduced mortality and morbidity from many common diseases (Gregg *et al.*, 2003). People with higher levels of physical activity are less likely to suffer or die from cardiovascular disease (Kesaniemi *et al.*, 2001), have reduced risk of all types of stroke (Wendel-Vos *et al.*, 2004a; 2004b), gain less weight, are less likely to develop type 2 diabetes, breast or colon cancer, osteoarthritis, osteoporosis, falls, and depression (Kesaniemi *et al.*, 2001; Thune and Furberg, 2001). Beneficial effects on cognition have also been documented, the most physically active having 20% lower risk of cognitive decline (Weuve *et al.*, 2004; Yaffe *et al.*, 2001). Maintaining good physical activity levels is associated with generalized well-being, and improved physical function, ability to perform activities of daily living, and walking distance. An active person is less likely to be disabled and is more likely to be independent. There is a lower incidence of depression in people who remain active, and physical activity is known to reduce the symptoms of clinical depression (Kesaniemi *et al.*, 2001). For these reasons, it is important for nurses to promote the benefits of appropriate physical activity as part of their health promotion role.

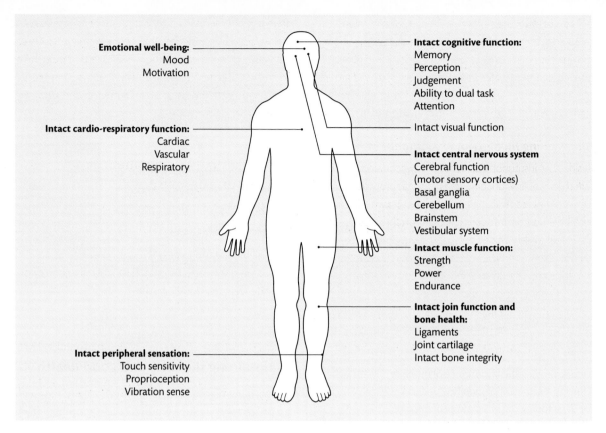

Figure 23.1 What is required for safe and effective mobility?

Exercise for those with no health problems

The American College of Sports Medicine and the American Heart Association recommends levels of physical activity required to maintain good health (Box 23.1).

Exercise for those with chronic conditions

People with chronic health conditions require more specific exercise routines both to ensure the exercise is appropriate to their condition and to encourage good adherence. If achieved, this is effective in improving health and function in coronary heart disease (Fletcher *et al.*, 2001; Pollock *et al.*, 2000; Thompson *et al.*, 2003), chronic obstructive airways disease (Pauwels *et al.*, 2001), diabetes (Sigal *et al.*, 2004), obesity (US Preventive Services Task Force, 2003), peripheral vascular disease (McDermott *et al.*, 2006), osteoporosis (Going *et al.*, 2003), falls (Gillespie *et al.*, 2009), and arthritis (American College of Rheumatology Subcommittee on Osteoarthritis Guidelines, 2000; American Geriatrics Society, 2001).

Box 23.1 ACSM and AHA recommendations on physical activity

- People aged over 18 should undertake at least 20 minutes of vigorous aerobic exercise three times a week or 30 minutes of moderate aerobic exercise five times a week (Nelson *et al.*, 2007; Haskell *et al.*, 2007).
- Aerobic exercise is exercise that increases heart rate and respiratory rate, such as running, jogging, or brisk walking.
- Women aged >55 and men >45 with risk factors for coronary heart disease should be screened prior to starting vigorous exercise.

Maintaining mobility during hospital admission

All patients admitted to hospital should undergo a nursing assessment of mobility and falls risk. Referral to physiotherapy should be made when a person has new or significant

Labels within Figure 23.1:

Emotional well-being:
Mood
Motivation

Intact cardio-respiratory function:
Cardiac
Vascular
Respiratory

Intact peripheral sensation:
Touch sensitivity
Proprioception
Vibration sense

Intact cognitive function:
Memory
Perception
Judgement
Ability to dual task
Attention

Intact visual function

Intact central nervous system
Cerebral function
(motor sensory cortices)
Basal ganglia
Cerebellum
Brainstem
Vestibular system

Intact muscle function:
Strength
Power
Endurance

Intact join function and bone health:
Ligaments
Joint cartilage
Intact bone integrity

difficulties with their mobility. Nurses have a role in the maintenance of mobility throughout an admission by making sure that patients who are able to do so get out of bed regularly and walk to the toilet, day room, and around the ward. Maintaining mobility while in hospital is likely to lead to shorter length of stay and better long-term health.

Maintaining mobility in institutional care

Residents in institutional care should be encouraged to maintain their mobility function with regular appropriate activity. This could include walking rather than using a wheelchair and often even outdoor mobility. It is important to assess each individual to determine the level of supervision required for each mobility task. This assessment should be continuous, but take into account declines in mobility associated with new or progressive causes of mobility impairment or acute illness. Any acute changes must be investigated promptly, including medical referral as appropriate, because they could be caused by musculoskeletal problems, stroke, or infection.

Nursing assessment of mobility function

Assessment of mobility provides information about current and premorbid mobility function and causes of mobility impairment, activity limitation, and loss of social participation. This information is crucial for the application of person-centred, evidence-based interventions.

Mobility assessment is not in itself an intervention; it is a means to providing patient-specific, evidence-based interventions. Therefore, information on the level of mobility, changes in mobility, and the reasons for these changes (whether physiological or psychosocial) should be used to develop a care plan to address the issues identified. The aim is to allow patients to achieve their optimum mobility function and independence, while minimizing the risk of falls and complications of immobility. A mobility assessment is an ideal time to provide appropriate information about healthy lifestyles and exercise requirements.

Assessment of mobility should be undertaken with minimal discomfort while respecting the person's dignity. It is important to consider the safety of both patients and staff because mobility assessment poses a moving and handling risk (covered later in this chapter). The person's verbal consent for this process must be obtained. If the patient lacks mental capacity to consent to the assessment (for example, because he or she is unconscious or has advanced dementia), then assessment should take place if it is deemed to be in the patient's 'best interests' (see Chapter 7 Understanding Dementia and Chapter 17 Managing Delirium and Confusion ➡).

Making a clinical assessment of a person's mobility

1. Take a history
2. Observe and examine
3. Undertake clinical testing
4. Analyse information collected to set goals/delivery of evidence-based interventions

Taking a history

The history identifies the person's premorbid mobility level, as well as the nature of any current problem. A good history identifies the duration and course of any impairment, plus any contributory factors such as concurrent acute illness, previous injuries, or long-term conditions. It should be used to enhance and complement the physical assessment to identify problems, set goals, and plan discharges.

Table 23.1 shows the types of questions that should be asked.

THEORY INTO PRACTICE 23.1
Multidisciplinary teamworking

When working in the multidisciplinary team, interpreting clinical assessments from other health professionals will complement and enhance your own assessment. A good recent medical or therapy history can be a key source of information, allowing you to adapt your questions and observations.

Use open questions and simple language to maximize the information obtained. If the history obtained is poor, information from other reliable sources should be sought, e.g. from formal or informal carers, from health records, or by contacting the patient's care home or community health or social care professionals. It is helpful to phrase questions positively, asking the person what his or her aim is and what he or she feels might be needed to achieve it (Table 23.1).

Table 23.1 Assessment questions and rationale

Question	Rationale
Have you any problems with your mobility, e.g. walking, getting in or out of bed, sitting or standing? How far can you walk or move?	Identifies extent of the person's current and normal levels of mobility to inform care plan, rehabilitation, and moving and handling requirements
How long have you had this problem? Has it got worse recently?	Identifies whether it is acute or chronic, because it may need a different treatment and care approach as a result
Do you use any aids or equipment, such as a walking stick, wheelchair, or adaptations at home? Do you need help from another person?	Establishes aids or equipment the person needs, if they are appropriate, and if in hospital ensures that these are kept with patient or supplied
Does anything make it more difficult to move? Does anything make it easier to move?	Identifies strategies such as (analgesic) medication or non-pharmacological approaches, and incorporates these into the care plan
Do you experience discomfort if you move or are moved? Describe the discomfort—does anything make it worse or better?	Identifies any pain or discomfort and strategies such as (analgesic) medication or non-pharmacological approaches, and incorporates into moving and handling risk assessment
Do you get short of breath on moving?	This may suggest a cardiac or respiratory condition for which medical advice should be sought
What medications are you taking? (Include both prescription medications and those obtained elsewhere)	A review of medication reveals treatment for chronic diseases that the patient may fail to mention, e.g. chronic pain, anxiety/depression, movement disorders, and epilepsy Particular attention should be paid to the use of psychotropic medications (hypnotics/anxiolytics and antipsychotic medications) owing to the possible side effects—notably, increased risk of falls (Thapa *et al.*, 1995)
Have you fallen lately?	Important for falls prevention because previous falls are a risk factor for further falls (Nevitt *et al.*, 1989)
Do you feel giddy on rising from bed or chair?	Identifies possible orthostatic hypotension (see Table 23.4 for more information on assessment and treatment)
Any eyesight problems that affect your mobility?	Vision impacts on mobility and interventions can improve vision (cataract surgery/adequate spectacles)
Any bone, joint, ligament, tendon, muscle, or nerve problems?	Identifies any obvious contributory factors owing to medical conditions that may need further investigation/management
Any illnesses or conditions in the past that have affected your mobility, such as stroke or arthritis? Have you had any treatment or rehabilitation for this?	Helps to decide whether further rehabilitation is required

Observation and examination

It is possible to learn a lot about the person's mobility just by observing him or her entering the room, sitting in a chair, or lying on a bed/trolley. Any obvious abnormalities of movement and injuries should be noted. The location of attachments (such as intravenous lines, oxygen tubing, and feeding or nasogastric tubes) will be important when it comes to planning how to allow the person to move comfortably and safely. Weightbearing status should be established before observing ability to stand/walk. This is primarily to avoid injury if unable to stand unsupported; in some orthopaedic cases, full

Table 23.2 Observations and examinations

Observation	Rationale
Posture and positioning (note the position: sitting, lying, or standing)	To determine whether the person has adequate sitting or standing balance and any obvious limb or trunk deformities, such as kyphosis (abnormal curving of the spine) or contracture
Examine the limbs and joints for: deformity, redness or swelling of joints, weakness (see Box 23.2 for grading), altered muscle tone (measured by moving the limb throughout range and detecting resistance that is not caused by soft-tissue shortening) NB. When moving the limb passively, observe the patient very carefully for signs of pain or discomfort and stop the movement if this occurs.	Suggestive of: contractures or previous fractures; arthritis, gout, infection; pain, disuse, arthritis, neurological conditions; spasticity (velocity-dependent resistance of a muscle to stretch), rigidity (resistance of muscle at any velocity), or hypotonia (flaccidity or low tone) (reduced muscle activity) caused by various conditions affecting the central and peripheral nervous systems
Examine for loss of range of motion (assess by asking the patient to move the limbs actively throughout available range)	Suggestive of: contracture, arthritis, immobility (e.g. post fracture) If any of the above are noted, compare to the opposite limb
Walking and balance: if the patient is able to walk, note excessive slowness, step length, and symmetry (is equal amount of time spent stepping each leg?) Can the patient stand without support?	Particular walking patterns are suggestive of particular pathology (e.g. shuffling gait = Parkinsonism) Merely stating whether gait is steady or not is a good indicator of balance function (Mathias *et al.*, 1986) Poor balance and unsteady gait are risk factors for falls (Dargent-Molina *et al.*, 1996; Clark *et al.*, 1993)
Non-verbal signs of discomfort or pain, such as grimacing, twisting, flinching	Patients with communication difficulties, such as stroke, dementia, or reduced level of consciousness, may communicate pain only through non-verbal responses
Orthotic devices, such as sole inserts, dressings, and support garments	It is important to ensure that they are fitted correctly and do not impede mobility
Skin (examine for lesions, such as pressure sores, wounds, bruising, fragile skin)	Necessary to: prevent further damage due to immobility; take care when assisting with mobility NB. Unexplained injuries on a vulnerable adult should be further investigated following local vulnerable adult protocols
Feet (examine the health and condition of the feet for ulcers, joint problems, corns, or poor foot care)	Foot problems may contribute to the person's ability to mobilize Referral to podiatry services may be necessary if a patient cannot manage his or her own foot care

weightbearing on an unstable fracture may cause further harm.

The extent of physical examination required will differ: for a frail older patient, an extensive examination is likely to be necessary, as compared to an ambulant young adult. Table 23.2 gives details of mobility observations and examinations.

Clinical tests

Clinical tests will establish an individual's position when considering known normal values and provide a baseline against which to measure progress during rehabilitation.

Tests are routinely performed by physiotherapists or occupational therapists. However, you can carry out tests, including those described in Table 23.3, without needing access to specialist equipment or therapy facilities.

Collation of the information collected to inform goal-setting and delivery of evidence-based interventions

Once the clinical assessment is complete and information collated to form a comprehensive analysis of mobility, individualized patient goals should be agreed with the patient and interprofessional team. The agreed intervention

Box 23.2 Muscle power grading

0. No movement
1. Muscle flicker or twitch, but no visible movement
2. Movement possible, but not against gravity (test in horizontal plane)
3. Movement possible against gravity, but not against resistance provided by the examiner
4. Movement against resistance, but weaker than normal
5. Normal power

(Medical Research Council, 1981)

programme should then commence, with a focus on achieving these goals.

Understanding the importance of impaired mobility

Definition of impaired mobility

Impaired mobility can be defined as a temporary or permanent loss of mobility function. How a mobility problem progresses varies depending on the underlying disease processes, the effects of rehabilitation programmes, and the process of degeneration and ageing.

Mobility disorders range from those that cause minimal disruption with a full and productive life maintained,

Table 23.3 Clinical tests

Test	Procedure	Rationale and interpretation	Implication
Chair rise test (Csuka and McCarty, 1985)	The patient sits in a standard height straight-backed chair with his or her feet flat on the floor and arms crossed over his or her chest. Ask him or her to stand up without using his or her arms. Graded 4 = able, 3 = able but uses arms, 2 = able with assistance, and 1 = unable	This test provides an indication of ability to undertake a basic mobility function and relates to lower limb muscle strength, general mobility function, and falls risk (Guralnik *et al.*, 1994)	Inability to stand from a chair seriously limits independent mobility and suggests that a rehabilitation programme, and/or adaptations are required. NB. If a person cannot get out of a chair and is living at home, a review of care requirements is vital
Berg balance scale (Berg *et al.*, 1992)	Measures performance on 14 observable tasks common to everyday life (maximum score 56)	A score of <44 suggests balance impairment, which increases the risk of falls and difficulties with activities of daily living	Strategies for falls prevention are indicated, such as balance exercise. More in-depth assessment for causes of the balance impairment by a physiotherapist may be indicated
Timed up and go (TUAG) (Podsialdo and Richardson, 1991)	Measures the time taken to stand up from a standard height chair, walk 3 metres, return to the chair, and sit down	Normal TUAG time for people aged >65 is <12 seconds (Bischoff *et al.*, 2003). Those with TUAG of >15 seconds are at increased risk of falls (Whitney *et al.*, 2005) and taking >20 seconds indicates functional impairment (Podsialdo and Richardson, 1991)	Consider more in-depth assessment to determine underlying cause of poor performance. May benefit from rehabilitation or exercise programme

to severe disruption with complete dependence on others for even basic functions. Mobility problems can affect people of all ages and can be short term (e.g. an injury such as a fracture) or chronic (such as the impairment remaining following a stroke). Chronic mobility problems may remain static or, by the nature of the primary pathology, be progressive (e.g. Parkinson's disease). When working with patients with impaired mobility, consider:

- body structure and function;
- activity limitation;
- social participation.

Understanding mobility impairment in the context of all these areas will aid provision of holistic, patient-centred care (World Health Organization, 2010a).

Prevalence of impaired mobility

The prevalence of impaired mobility increases with age and affects a large proportion of the population. Around 10% of people aged over 18 report 'some' mobility difficulty in activities such as walking, climbing stairs, or standing (Iezzoni *et al.*, 2001). The incidence is higher in older people, ranging between 16% and 18% (Spiers *et al.*, 2005; Melzer *et al.*, 2005; Mottram *et al.*, 2008), and around one-third of people aged over 65 will experience a decline in mobility over a 4-year period (Guralnik *et al.*, 1993). Those with chronic conditions, pain in the hip, knee, or back, hip fracture, depression, or poor vision are at greater risk of developing mobility difficulties (Melzer *et al.*, 2005; Mottram *et al.*, 2008; Guralnik *et al.*, 1993).

Burden of impaired mobility

There are very little data on the cost of reduced mobility to health and social services, and to the economy in general. Indicative costs can be inferred from the costs of social care service provision to people with disability: £15.3 million was spent on adult care in England between 2006 and 2007. Of this, £8 million was spent on older people, split between residential care and domiciliary and day care services (The NHS Information Centre, 2009). When mobility limitations are less severe, ability to maintain employment or be involved in social or sporting activities remain important considerations, affecting both mood and quality of life.

Morbidity

Causes of mobility impairments include the following.

- Musculoskeletal system—injury or disease affecting bones, joints, ligaments, muscles, or tendons results in pain, stiffness, weakness, or inability to weightbear
- Neurological system—injury or disease to the neurological system affecting brain, spinal cord, peripheral nerves, or neuromuscular junction functions, with symptoms including weakness, stiffness (spasticity/rigidity), sensory loss, coordination problems, balance defects, cognitive, and perception difficulties
- Cardiac and respiratory systems—symptoms include poor exercise tolerance, pain, shortness of breath (dyspnoea), and skeletal muscle weakness

Prolonged bed rest is another common cause of impaired mobility, and may occur after surgery, trauma, or critical illness, resulting in muscle weakness, reduced exercise tolerance, and contractures.

THEORY INTO PRACTICE 23.2
Useful Internet resources

Healthtalkonline has some interesting patient stories about impaired mobility caused by motor neurone disease, which you can watch online at **http://www.healthtalkonline.org/Nerves_and_brain/motorneuronedisease/Topic/3439/** (accessed April 2010).

The effect of ageing on mobility

Ageing is associated with physiological changes, including loss of muscle mass, strength, and power, a reduction in bone density, and degenerative changes to joint cartilage. It also affects the central and peripheral nervous systems, with loss of neurons, reduction in some neurotransmitters, and slower nerve conduction times (Knight and Nigam, 2008a; b). The individual consequence of these changes is variable. Older people at higher risk of developing mobility problems, particularly after certain events such as surgery, trauma, illness, or a fall, can be described using the term 'frail'. Frailty has been defined as a combination of muscle weakness, weight loss, slow walking speed, fatigue, and reduced activity levels. Frail older adults have a higher risk of developing disability, being hospitalized, and have higher mortality rates (Walston *et al.*, 2006).

Acute immobility

Acute immobility occurs as a result of prolonged bed rest following serious medical illness, or after surgery or trauma. Complications include:

- musculoskeletal—muscle weakness (half strength lost within 3–5 weeks), loss of joint flexibility, contractures, and reduction in bone mineral density (30–60% loss in 12 weeks) (Dittmer and Teasell, 1993);
- cardiovascular—venous thromboembolism (deep vein thrombosis), orthostatic hypotension;
- respiratory—respiratory tract infections, pneumonia;
- skin—breakdown leading to pressure sores;
- other—constipation, mood and cognitive decline.

Evidence-based nursing management of the patient with impaired mobility

Nurses work in partnership with older patients, their relatives and other members of the interprofessional team, including local falls teams where relevant, and use referral to community and primary care staff to ensure personalised and ongoing interventions that meet the patient's mobility needs and his or her needs and preferences regarding interventions to reduce the risk of falls.

Best practice statement from *Promoting Mobility and Preventing Falls* (Bridges *et al.*, 2009)

Your role in managing the patient with impaired mobility is based on your assessment, with major responsibility for moving and handling, ensuring safe mobility, falls prevention, rehabilitation, and understanding aids provided and adaptations that may be required.

Manual handling

Patients with mobility difficulties often need assistance to move. Manual handling legislation came into place to protect workers from the risk of injury. The Manual Handling Operation Regulations 1992, as amenda apply to handling of loads by human effort, and apply to the moving and handling of patients (HMSO, 1992; 2002).

When handling is not necessary, it should be avoided. Where no other option exists, risk assessment should be undertaken. Generic risk assessments are available for routine activities. Risk assessment should consider:

- the task (i.e. a particular transfer);
- the individual (the handler);
- the load (usually the patient);
- the environment.

Following risk assessment, appropriate management of risk includes training in handling techniques, use of handling aids, use of lifting aids such as hoists, and ensuring adequate staff resources to deal with handling issues (Chartered Society of Physiotherapy, 2008).

Figures 23.2a–f show aids that can be used to assist with manoeuvres on and off the bed. These usually involve levers or handles that allow the user to pull into a sitting position or move in bed.

If a person has difficulty standing up from a chair, in the first instance raising the height of the chair may make it easier; if this problem does not significantly improve with rehabilitation, a chair riser is a solution in some cases. If a person cannot get out of a chair, he or she will also have difficulties toileting, and aids to assist getting on and off the toilet may be required. Equipment for these situations is shown in Figures 23.3a–c.

Ensuring safe mobility

Individuals with poor mobility and balance will be at risk of falls and injury while they are moving around. It is important for you to consider how to maximize safety while not compromising a person's rights to move around as he or she wishes. Wandering and reduced awareness of safety and abilities is indicative of cognitive impairment. This impairment may be acute in cases of delirium or chronic as a result of dementia. The general consensus in UK practice is that physical restraint should not be used and chemical restraint avoided unless there is potential danger to the individual or others. Pragmatic ways of reducing the risk of falls from unsafe mobility include orientating patients

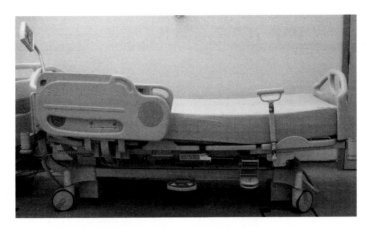

Figure 23.2a **Mobility handles.**

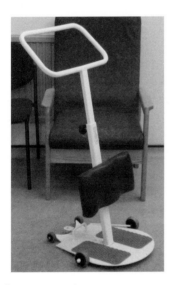

Figure 23.2b Rota stand.

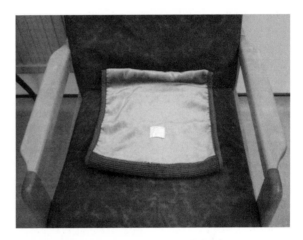

Figure 23.2c **One-way glide anti-slide sheet.**

to their environments, closer supervision (including the use of movement sensors to alert staff), and rehabilitation to improve balance and mobility. Remember, you are required to follow the Mental Capacity Act 2005 and, if necessary, the Deprivation of Liberty Safeguards (England and Wales, or equivalent legislation in Scotland) before considering imposing any restrictions that are considered necessary to ensure the person's safety.

Falls prevention

Each year, around one-third of people aged >65 years will have a fall, defined as 'an event where a person comes to rest on the ground, floor or lower level' (Lamb *et al.*,

2005), and around 10% of falls will result in some injury, the most significant being hip fracture (see Chapter 3 Understanding Bone Conditions ⮕) (Campbell *et al.*, 1990; Tinetti *et al.*, 1988). Falling results in loss of confidence and fear of further falls, leading to restriction in activity and decline in function and independence (Vellas *et al.*, 1987). This cycle of decline may result in many older people entering a state of frailty.

Falls are not random events; they can be predicted by analysing individuals for known 'risk factors'. There are many risk factors for falling, including increased age, a history of previous falls, fear of falling, problems with walking and balance, visual or sensory impairment, muscle weakness, previous stroke, Parkinson's disease, or cognitive impairment and taking multiple medications, in particular psychotropic

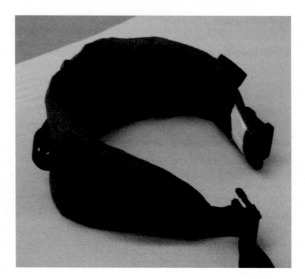

Figure 23.2d   Handling belt.

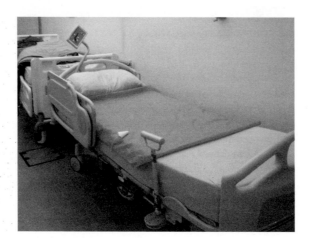

Figure 23.2e   Sliding sheet.

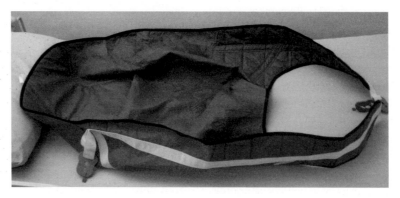

Figure 23.2f   Hoist sling.

(a)

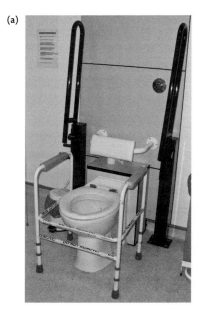

(b)

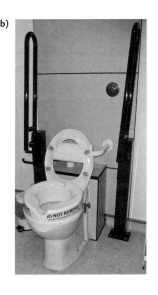

(c)

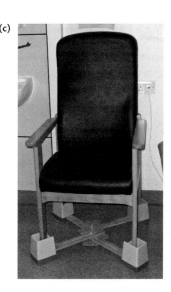

Figure 23.3 (a) Toilet surround; (b) Raised toilet seat; (c) Chair raiser.

medications (Campbell *et al.*, 1989; Lord and Clark, 1996; Lord *et al.*, 1991; 1992; 2003; 2007; Lord and Dayhew, 2001; Tinetti, 1986; 1987; Tinetti *et al.*, 1986; 1988; 1995a, b).

Multifactorial interventions, when interventions are targeted to identified risk factors, appear to reduce the number of falls (Gillespie *et al.*, 2009). Effective single interventions include vitamin D supplementation for those with low vitamin D levels (Gillespie *et al.*, 2009), withdrawal of psychotropic medications (Campbell *et al.*, 1999), medical staff and patient education on medication and falls with medication review (Pit *et al.*, 2007), cardiac pacemakers for those with cardio-inhibitory carotid sinus syndrome (Kenny *et al.*, 2001), cataract surgery (Harwood *et al.*, 2005), home safety assessment for those with severe visual impairment (Campbell *et al.*, 2005), environmental assessment and intervention for those at high risk of falls (Gillespie *et al.*, 2009), wearing shoes with non-slip soles in winter (Gillespie *et al.*, 2009), and exercise (Gillespie *et al.*, 2009). A recent review of exercise for falls prevention (Sherrington *et al.*, 2008) found that a programme of exercise consisting of high-intensity balance training with a dose of more than 50 hours (equivalent to exercising twice a week for 6 months) is required to reduce falls.

Table 23.4 provides information on how to address falls risk factors with appropriate evidence-based interventions.

Rehabilitation

Research suggests that, historically, the role of the nurse in rehabilitation has been underrecognized and underutilized, with therapists being seen as the 'experts' (O'Connor, 1993; Waters and Luker, 1996), and the nursing curriculum failing to address the knowledge and skills required to realize nursing's potential in this area adequately (Nolan and Nolan, 1999). The concept and process of rehabilitation as a 24-hour, patient-centred approach suggests that, in contemporary practice, the nursing role is integral to successful outcomes.

The World Health Organization's definition of rehabilitation is:

> A process aimed at enabling people with disabilities to reach and maintain their optimal physical, sensory, intellectual, psychological and social functional levels. Rehabilitation provides disabled people with the tools they need to attain independence and self-determination. (World Health Organization, 2010b)

Rehabilitation is not a passive process that happens to a patient; it requires active participation. Therefore motivating patients to take up and adhere to their programmes is a vital component of the process. Those with acute mobility problems, such as a new stroke or fracture, will usually require a period of rehabilitation with the aim

Table 23.4 **Falls prevention interventions**

Risk factor	Suggested intervention

Mobility/function:
  Impaired walking
  Impaired sit to stand
  Impaired standing balance
  Reduced physical activity
	Exercise: high-intensity balance training at least twice a week for at least 6 months*
	Provision of walking aids

Sensorimotor: Impaired vision	Eye examination, correct spectacle prescription, cataract surgery if indicated*
Impaired peripheral sensation	Medical examination to detect reversible causes (vitamin B12 deficiency, glucose control in diabetics), correct footwear, advice on dealing with impairment sensation = turn the lights on at night when getting up; look at feet when walking on uneven ground
Impaired muscle strength	Exercise: strength training*
Slow reaction times	Exercise: high-intensity balance training at least twice a week for at least 6 months*
Medical conditions	Optimal management of medical conditions
Environment/function	Home hazard reduction* Provision of equipment* Advice and information* (Effective if provided by occupational therapist to those at high risk of falls)
Medication	Medication review* Withdrawal of psychotropic medication* Vitamin D for those with low levels* Avoidance of polypharmacy where possible Avoidance of drugs such as diuretics, which can predispose to hypotension and therefore falls
Fear of falling	Exercise: high-intensity balance training at least twice a week for at least 6 months*
Causes of syncope: Orthostatic hypotension (see Box 23.3 for how to test)	Medication review, fluid therapy, support stockings, behavioural changes (stand up slowly, do ankle pump exercises)
Carotid sinus hypersensitivity	Cardiac pacemaker*, medication Medication or pacemaker
Arrhythmias Vasovagal syndrome and postprandial hypotension	Medication review, fluid therapy, support stockings, behavioural changes (avoid standing still for long periods or avoid large meals/standing after eating, do ankle pump exercises)

*Effective in randomized controlled single intervention trials.

of regaining as much previous function as possible. Those with chronic mobility problems, such as those caused by arthritis or Parkinson's disease, may require periods of rehabilitation as part of the disease management process.

Rehabilitation will always start with an assessment, as previously described, and encompass all areas of the WHO classification of functioning, disability, and health. At the impairment level, biological functioning should be addressed to ensure that, wherever possible, the causes of impaired mobility can be identified and treated directly. Medical management of other conditions that may affect rehabilitation outcomes should also be optimized. Understanding the person's problems as they apply to each individual in terms of his or her activity limitation and social participation is also an essential part of rehabilitation (World Health Organization, 2010a).

Box 23.3 **Measuring lying/standing blood pressure**

Procedure

The first measurement should be taken after at least 5 minutes lying supine. Ask the patient to stand up and measure the blood pressure with the arm at heart height 1 minute and 3 minutes after standing up. If pressure dropped on standing, measurement should continue every 3 minutes until normal or lying pressure is restored.

Interpretation of results

Orthostatic hypotension is defined as a systolic fall of >20 mmHg or to less than 90 mmHg, or a diastolic fall >10 mmHg within 3 minutes of standing up (Brignole *et al.*, 2001).

Implications

Orthostatic hypotension may be a cause of dizziness or syncope (fainting) and could contribute to falls. Patients with the condition should be referred for medical investigation.

The rehabilitation process involves management of relevant medical conditions, and a programme of activity aimed at improving muscle strength, walking, balance, fitness, and skill in functional activities. In addition to this, it may involve provision of aids and adaptations to optimize function, or even to prevent loss of function.

During and at the end of rehabilitation interventions, some form of evaluation should take place to measure progress and outcome. These range from measures of simple functions such as walking ability, to measures of quality of life or achievement of goals.

The rehabilitation team will usually include physiotherapists, occupational therapists, speech therapists, counsellors, and psychologists, working alongside nurses and doctors.

Aids and adaptations required

Walking aids

These range from a single walking stick to be used only when outdoors to the use of a walking frame for walking at all times. Walking aids will usually be prescribed by a physiotherapist. The indications for the more common walking aids are described in Table 23.5. When considering prescription of walking aids, it is important to consider the risks and benefits of introducing a new aid: for example, starting to use a walking frame will encourage reliance on the arms for balance.

Wheelchairs

These may be prescribed for outdoor use to cover long distances or for all mobility tasks (i.e. a complete spinal cord injury). Wheelchairs can be self-propelled, whereby a person moves using his or her arms to propel the wheels, or attendant-propelled, whereby the chair requires another fit and mobile person to push it. People who have very poor sitting balance and cannot safely sit in a normal chair may be provided with a specialist wheelchair that has been designed to support them in a safe sitting position. Wheelchairs should be prescribed by an appropriately qualified professional to optimize comfort and safety.

Measuring the impact of nursing interventions

The principle of measuring both the effectiveness of nursing intervention and the patient's experience of receiving care is one that you should, where possible, facilitate. The NHS Information Centre has supported the development of Nursing Quality Metrics (NQMs), which can be used to facilitate quality improvement in patient care and experience **http://signposting.ic.nhs.uk/?k=metrics**.

This recent move within healthcare to be outcome-focused rather than target-driven is a welcome change in policy direction, initiated by Lord Darzi in his review of the NHS, and sustained by the previous and current UK governments. Metrics have been developed for many aspects of nursing care interventions and cover many inpatient areas, regardless of setting. The collection of these types of data helps healthcare organizations to focus on the delivery of safe and effective care, and can be used for local and national benchmarking, as well as for quality improvement.

For further details, visit the NHS Information Centre online at **http://www.ic.nhs.uk/**, where you will find

Table 23.5 Walking aids

Aid	Indication	Things to check	Considerations
Walking stick	Pain in lower limb(s), weakness in lower limb(s), unsteadiness/poor balance, sensory impairment, poor exercise tolerance	Correct height = the elbow relaxed (bent no more than 15°) with aid on the floor while standing up straight That there is no damage to any part of the aid, including the handle That the ferrule (the rubber end) is present and not worn	If a person has pain or deformity in the hands, using a stick may be difficult or painful. There are sticks with handles designed to minimize discomfort that may be used.
Crutches	Usually a temporary measure used to reduce weight taken through a lower limb while recovering from injury or surgery	Correct height (as above) Ensure correct weightbearing status after orthopaedic injury or surgery That there is no damage to any part of the aid, including the handle That the ferrules (the rubber ends) are present and not worn	Weightbearing status: non-weightbearing = no weight to be taken through the affected leg; touch weightbearing = the affected leg can touch the ground but not take weight; partial weightbearing = some weight to be taken through the affected leg; full weightbearing = the affected leg can take weight normally
Walking frames	Any of the indications for stick or crutches when they do not provide adequate support	Correct height = the elbow should be only slightly flexed (around 15°) with aid on the floor while standing up straight That the ferrules (the rubber ends) are present and not worn	Frames can have two wheels at the front or no wheels. Wheels on the frame mean that it does not need to be picked up to move forward; so there will not a moment at which there will be lack of support and potential loss of balance. These frames are not designed for outdoor mobility.

Table 23.5 *(continued)*

Aid	Indication	Things to check	Considerations
Wheeled walking frames	When a walking frame is required for use outdoors	Correct height = the elbow should be only slightly flexed (around 15°) with aid on the floor while standing up straight That there is no damage to any part of the aid, including the handle, the wheels/tyres, and brakes	Most of these models have brakes that need to be used to control the motion of the frame.
Tripod/quadripod	When a walking frame is required, but cannot be used because of impaired function in one arm	Correct height = the elbow should be only slightly flexed (around 15°) with aid on the floor while standing up straight That there is no damage to any part of the aid, including the handle That the ferrules (the rubber ends) are present and not worn	May produce asymmetry when moving, which could cause muscle imbalance and upper limb and back pain.

details relating to nursing audit tools capturing information on documentation for observations, nutrition, medicines administration, pain management, communication, discharge planning, falls, pressure area care, antibiotic prescribing, and infection control.

In determining patient experience of healthcare, NICE has recently published a Quality Standard http://www.nice.org.uk/ that guides service delivery planning to ensure improvements in patient experience. Further commissioned work by the Department of Health has developed a single measure of patient experience. Supplementing these data is the NHS Survey, which captures patient views relating to ward cleanliness, infection control, staff attitudes, pain management, management of privacy, experience of dignity, nutrition, medicines administration, quality of communication,

and discharge. Details can be found online at http://www.nhssurveys.org/.

Accessing the evidence to inform clinical decisions

How to find the evidence

There is a large body of evidence of different levels within healthcare literature relating to mobility impairments and related problems such as falls. Systematic reviews are rigorously evaluated reviews of research and are published in sources including the Cochrane Library (http://www.thecochranelibrary.com/view/0/index.html). These identify the best-quality evidence available, and in doing so may reveal the gaps that exist in rigorous evaluation of the effectiveness of interventions—at the time of writing, a classic area being prevention of falls in hospital, in which relatively few randomized controlled trials have been published. In these cases, we also need to look at sources of national guidance, which draw together other levels of evidence. For example, at the time of writing, useful sources of guidance include the National Patient Safety Agency's report *Slips Trips and Falls in Hospital* (Healy and Scobie, 2007) and the best practice statement on promoting mobility and preventing falls in hospital *Best Practice for Older People in Acute Care Settings* (Bridges *et al.*, 2009; see Figure 4). NICE carries both topic-specific and general evidence guidance **http://www.nice.org.uk/**, and general searches can be made using NHS Evidence **http://www.evidence.nhs.uk/**.

Summary and key messages

Good mobility is dependent on effective functioning of all bodily systems, and problems with mobility arise for varying reasons. Mobility problems affect people through every age group, from childhood to old age, but reduced mobility is highly prevalent in older people, and places a burden on health and social services. Nurses have contact with patients through the whole spectrum of medical disorders, as well as the healthy population, and are therefore in an ideal position to promote physical activity and be involved in managing those with mobility impairments. To do this effectively involves in-depth assessment of mobility function, including assessment of falls risk, to target appropriate evidence-based interventions to the problems identified. The research evidence available on this subject is limited, although there is sufficient research evidence to be able to promote increased physical activity levels and to implement effective falls prevention interventions. Therefore some of the content of this chapter provides pragmatic 'best practice' advice.

Online Resource Centre

 To help you to develop and apply your knowledge and decision-making skills further, we have provided interactive learning resources online at **www.oxfordtextbooks.co.uk/orc/bullock/**.

Whilst these are freely available, you will need to use the access codes at the start of the book.

References

American College of Rheumatology Subcommittee on Osteoarthritis Guidelines (2000) Recommendations for the medical management of osteoarthritis of the hip and knee: 2000 update. *Arthritis & Rheumatism* **43**: 1905–15.

American Geriatrics Society (2001) Exercise prescription for older adults with osteoarthritis pain: consensus practice recommendations. *Journal of the American Geriatrics Society* **49**: 808–23.

Berg, K.O., Wood-Dauphinee, S.L., Williams, J.I., *et al.* (1992) Measuring balance in the elderly: validation of an instrument. *Canadian Journal of Public Health* **83**: S7–11.

Bischoff, H.A., Stahelin, H.B., Monsch, A.U., *et al.* (2003) Identifying a cut-off point for normal mobility: a comparison of the timed 'up and go' test in community-dwelling and institutionalised elderly women. *Age and Ageing* **32**: 315–20.

Bridges, J., Flatley, M., Meyer, J., *et al.* (2009) *Best Practice for Older People in Acute Care Settings (BPOP)*. Guidance for Nurses. RCN Publishing Company: London.

Brignole, M., Alboni, P., Benditt, D., *et al.* (2001) Guidelines on management (diagnosis and treatment) of syncope. *European Heart Journal* **22**: 1256–306.

Campbell, A.J., Borrie, M.J., Spears, G.F. (1989) Risk factors for falls in a community-based prospective study of people 70 years and older. *Journal of Gerontology* **44**: M112–17.

Campbell, A.J., Borrie, M.J., Spears, G.F., *et al.* (1990) Circumstances and consequences of falls experienced by a community population 70 years and over during a prospective study. *Age and Ageing* **19**: 136–41.

Campbell, A.J., Robertson, M.C., Gardner, M.M., *et al.* (1999) Psychotropic medication withdrawal and a home-based exercise program to prevent falls: a randomized, controlled trial. *Journal of the American Geriatrics Society* **47**: 850–3.

Campbell, A.J., Robertson, M.C., Grow, S.J.L., *et al.* (2005) Randomised controlled trial of prevention of falls in people aged 75 with severe visual impairment: the VIP trial. *British Medical Journal* **331**: 817–20.

Chartered Society of Physiotherapy (2008) *Guidance on Manual Handling in Physiotherapy*. Chartered Society of Physiotherapy: London.

Clark, R.D., Lord, S.R., Webster, I.W. (1993) Clinical parameters associated with falls in an elderly population. *Gerontology* **39**: 117–23.

Csuka, M., McCarty, D.J. (1985) Simple method for measurement of lower extremity muscle strength. *American Journal of Medicine* **78**: 77–81.

Dargent-Molina, P., Favier, F., Grandjean, H., *et al.* (1996) Fall-related factors and risk of hip fracture: the EPIDOS prospective study. *Lancet* **348**: 145–9.

Dittmer, D.K., Teasell, R. (1993) Complications of immobilization and bed rest. Part 1: Musculoskeletal and cardiovascular complications. *Canadian Family Physician* **39**: 1428–32, 1435–7.

Fletcher, G.F., Balady, G.J., Amsterdam, E.A., *et al.* (2001) Exercise standards for testing and training: a statement for healthcare professionals from the American Heart Association. *Circulation* **104**: 1694–740.

Gillespie, L.D., Robertson, M.C., Gillespie, W.J., *et al.* (2009) Interventions for preventing falls in older people living in the community. *Cochrane Database of Systematic Review* Isssue 2: Art. No. CD007146. DOI: 10.1002/14651858.CD007146.pub2.

Going, S., Lohman, T., Houtkooper, L., *et al.* (2003) Effects of exercise on bone mineral density in calcium-replete postmenopausal women with and without hormone replacement therapy. *Osteoporosis International* **14**: 637–43.

Gregg, E.W., Cauley, J.A., Stone, K., *et al.* (2003) Relationship of changes in physical activity and mortality among older women. *Journal of the American Medical Association* **289**: 2379–86.

Guralnik, J.M., Lacroix, A.Z., Abbott, R.D., *et al.* (1993) Maintaining mobility in late life. I. Demographic characteristics and chronic conditions. *American Journal of Epidemiology* **137**: 845–57.

Guralnik, J.M., Simonsick, E., Ferrucci, L., *et al.* (1994) A short physical performance battery assessing lower extremity function: association with self-reported disability and prediction of mortality and nursing home admission. *Journal of Gerontology* **49**: M85–94.

Harwood, R.H., Foss, A.J.E., Osborn, F., *et al.* (2005) Falls and health status in elderly women following first eye cataract surgery: a randomised controlled trial. *British Journal Ophthalmology* **89**: 53–9.

Haskell, W.L., Lee, I.M., Pate, R.R., *et al.* (2007) Physical activity and public health: updated recommendation for adults from the American College of Sports Medicine and the American Heart Association. *Medicine & Science in Sports & Exercise* **39**: 1423–34.

Healy, F., Scobie, S. (2007) *Slips Trips and Falls in Hospital: Third Report from the Patient Safety Observatory*. National Patient Safety Agency: London.

HM Stationery Office (1992) *Manual Handling Operation Regulations*. HMSO: London.

HM Stationery Office (2002) *Manual Handling Operations Regulations*. HMSO: London.

Iezzoni, L.I., Mccarthy, E.P., Davis, R.B., *et al.* (2001) Mobility difficulties are not only a problem of old age. *Journal of General Internal Medicine* **16**: 235–43.

Kenny, R.A.M., Richardson, D.A., Steen, N., *et al.* (2001) Carotid sinus syndrome: a modifiable risk factor for nonaccidental falls in older adults (SAFE PACE). *Journal of the American College of Cardiology* **38**: 1491–6.

Kesaniemi, Y.K., Danforth, E., Jr., Jensen, M.D., *et al.* (2001) Dose-response issues concerning physical activity and health: an evidence-based symposium. *Medicine & Science in Sports & Exercise* **33**: S351–8.

Knight, J., Nigam, Y. (2008a) Exploring the anatomy and physiology of ageing: Part 5–the nervous system. *Nursing Times* **104**: 18–19.

Knight, J., Nigam, Y. (2008b) Exploring the anatomy and physiology of ageing: Part 10–muscles and bone. *Nursing Times* **104**: 22–3.

Lamb, S.E.D, Jorstad-Stein, E.C.M., Hauer, K.P., *et al.* and Prevention of Falls Network Europe and Outcomes Consensus (2005) Development of a common outcome data set for fall injury prevention trials: the Prevention of Falls Network Europe consensus. *Journal of the American Geriatrics Society* **53**(9): 1618–22.

Lord, S.R., Clark, R.D. (1996) Simple physiological and clinical tests for the accurate prediction of falling in older people. *Gerontology* **42**: 199–203.

Lord, S.R., Clark, R.D., Webster, I.W. (1991) Physiological factors associated with falls in an elderly population. *Journal of the American Geriatrics Society* **39**: 1194–200.

Lord, S.R., Dayhew, J. (2001) Visual risk factors for falls in older people. *Journal of the American Geriatrics Society* **49**: 508–12.

Lord, S.R., March, L.M., Cameron, I.D., *et al.* (2003) Differing risk factors for falls in nursing home and intermediate-care residents who can and cannot stand unaided. *Journal of the American Geriatrics Society* **51**: 1645–50.

Lord, S.R., McLean, D., Stathers, G. (1992) Physiological factors associated with injurious falls in older people living in the community. *Gerontology* **38**: 338–46.

Lord, S.R., Sherrington, C., Menz, H.B., Close, J. (2007) *Falls in Older People: Risk Factors and Strategies for Prevention.* Cambridge University Press: Cambridge.

Mathias, S., Nayak, U.S.L., Isaacs, B. (1986) Balance in elderly patients: the 'Get-up and Go' test. *Archives of Phsyical Medicine and Rehabilitation* **67**: 387–9.

McDermott, M.M., Liu, K., Ferrucci, L., *et al.* (2006) Physical performance in peripheral arterial disease: a slower rate of decline in patients who walk more. *Annals of Internal Medicine* **144**: 10–20.

Medical Research Council (1981) *Aids to the Examination of the Peripheral Nervous System.* Memorandum No. 45. HMSO: London.

Melzer, D., Gardener, E., Guralnik, J.M. (2005) Mobility disability in the middle-aged: cross-sectional associations in the English Longitudinal Study of Ageing. *Age and Ageing* **34**: 594–602.

Mottram, S., Peat, G., Thomas, E., *et al.* (2008) Patterns of pain and mobility limitation in older people: cross-sectional findings from a population survey of 18,497 adults aged 50 years and over. *Quality of Life Research* **17**: 529–39.

Nelson, M.E., Rejeski, W.J., Blair, S.N., *et al.* (2007) Physical activity and public health in older adults: recommendation from the American College of Sports Medicine and the American Heart Association. *Medicine & Science in Sports & Exercise* **39**: 1435–45.

Nevitt, M.C., Cummings, S.R., Kidd, S., *et al.* (1989) Risk factors for recurrent nonsyncopal falls: a prospective study. *Journal of the American Medical Association* **261**: 2663–8.

NHS Information Centre, Social Care Statistics (2009) Personal social services expenditure and unit costs England, 2007–8. http://www.ic.nhs.uk/ (accessed April 2010).

Nolan, M., Nolan, J. (1999) Rehabilitation, chronic illness and disability: the missing elements in nurse education. *Journal of Advanced Nursing* **29**: 958–66.

O'Connor, S.E. (1993) Nursing and rehabilitation: the interventions of nurses in stroke patient care. *Journal of Clinical Nursing* **2**: 29–34.

Pauwels, R.A., Buist, A.S., Calverley, P.M.A., *et al.* (2001) Global strategy for the diagnosis, management, and prevention of chronic obstructive pulmonary disease: NHLBI/WHO Global Initiative for chronic obstructive lung disease (GOLD) workshop summary. *American Journal of Respiratory and Critical Care Medicine* **163**: 1256–76.

Pit, S.W., Byles, J.E., Henry, D.A., *et al.* (2007) A quality use of medicines program for general practitioners and older people: a cluster randomised controlled trial. *Medical Journal of Australia* **187**: 23–30.

Podsialdo, D., Richardson, S. (1991) The timed 'up & go': a test of basic functional mobility for frail elderly persons. *Journal of the American Geriatrics Society* **39**: 142–8.

Pollock, M.L., Franklin, B.A., Balady, G.J., *et al.* (2000) Resistance exercise in individuals with and without cardiovascular disease: benefits, rationale, safety, and prescription and advisory from the Committee on Exercise, Rehabilitation, and Prevention, Council on Clinical Cardiology, American Heart Association. *Circulation* **101**: 828–33.

Sherrington, C., Whitney, J.C., Lord, S.R., *et al.* (2008) Effective exercise for the prevention of falls: a systematic review and meta-analysis. *Journal of the American Geriatrics Society* **56**: 2234–43.

Sigal, R.J., Kenny, G.P., Wasserman, D.H., *et al.* (2004) Physical activity/exercise and type 2 diabetes. *Diabetes Care* **27**: 2518–39.

Spiers, N.A., Matthews, R.J., Jagger, C., *et al.* (2005) Diseases and impairments as risk factors for onset of disability in the older population in England and Wales: findings from the Medical Research Council Cognitive Function and Ageing Study. *Journals of Gerontology Series A: Biological Sciences and Medical Sciences* **60**: 248–54.

Thapa, P.B., Gideon, P., Fought, R.L., *et al.* (1995) Psychotropic drugs and risk of recurrent falls in ambulatory nursing home residents. *American Journal of Epidemiology* **142**: 202–11.

Thompson, P.D., Buchner, D., Pina, I.L., *et al.* (2003) Exercise and physical activity in the prevention and treatment of atherosclerotic cardiovascular disease: a statement from the council on clinical cardiology (subcommittee on exercise, rehabilitation, and prevention) and the council on nutrition, physical activity, and metabolism (Subcommittee on Physical Activity). *Circulation* **107**: 3109–16.

Thune, I., Furberg, A.-S. (2001) Physical activity and cancer risk: dose-response and cancer, all sites and site-specific. *Medicine & Science in Sports & Exercise* **33**: S530–S550.

Tinetti, M.E. (1986) Performance-oriented assessment of mobility problems in elderly patients. *Journal of the American Geriatrics Society* **34**: 119–26.

Tinetti, M.E. (1987) Factors associated with serious injury during falls by ambulatory nursing home residents. *Journal of the American Geriatrics Society* **35**: 644–8.

Tinetti, M.E., Doucette, J., Claus, E., *et al.* (1995a) Risk factors for serious injury during falls by older persons in the community. *Journal of the American Geriatrics Society* **43**: 1214–21.

Tinetti, M.E., Doucette, J.T., Claus, E. B. (1995b) The contribution of predisposing and situational risk factors to serious fall injuries. *Journal of the American Geriatrics Society* **43**: 1207–13.

Tinetti, M.E., Speechley, M., Ginter, S.F. (1988) Risk factors for falls among elderly persons living in the community. *New England Journal of Medicine,* **319**: 1701–7.

Tinetti, M.E., Williams, T.F., Mayewski, R. (1986) Fall risk index for elderly patients based on number of chronic disabilities *American Journal of Medicine* **80**: 429–34.

US Preventive Services Task Force (2003) Screening for obesity in adults: recommendations and rationale. *Annals of Internal Medicine* **139**: 930–2.

Vellas, B., Cayla, F., Bocquet, H., *et al.* (1987) Prospective study of restriction of activity in old people after falls. *Age and Ageing* **16**: 189–93.

Walston, J., Hadley, E.C., Ferrucci, L., *et al.* (2006) Research agenda for frailty in older adults: toward a better understanding of physiology and etiology: summary from the American Geriatrics Society/National Institute on Aging Research Conference on Frailty in Older Adults. *Journal of the American Geriatric Society* **54**: 991–1001.

Waters, K.R., Luker, K.A. (1996) Staff perspectives on the role of the nurse in rehabilitation wards for elderly people. *Journal of Clinical Nursing* **5**: 105–14.

Wendel-Vos, G., Schuit, A., Feskens, E., *et al.* (2004a) Physical activity and stroke: a meta-analysis of observational data. *International Journal of Epidemiology* **33**: 787–98.

Wendel-Vos, G.C., Schuit, A.J., Feskens, E.J., *et al.* (2004b) Physical activity and stroke: a meta-analysis of observational data. *International Journal of Epidemiology* **33**: 787–98.

Weuve, J., Kang, J.H., Manson, J.E., *et al.* (2004) Physical activity, including walking, and cognitive function in older women. *Journal of the American Medical Association* **292**: 1454–61.

Whitney, J.C., Lord, S.R., Close, J.C.T. (2005) Streamlining assessment and intervention in a falls clinic using the timed up and go test and physiological profile assessments. *Age and Ageing,* **34**: 567–71.

World Health Organization (2010a) *International Classification of Functioning, Disability and Health* (ICF). **http://www.who.int/classifications/icf/en/** (accessed April 2010).

World Health Organization (2010b) *Rehabilitation.* **http://www.who.int/topics/rehabilitation/en/** (accessed 15 April 2010).

Yaffe, K., Barnes, D., Nevitt, M., *et al.* (2001) A prospective study of physical activity and cognitive decline in elderly women: women who walk. *Archives of Internal Medicine* **161**: 1703–8.

24 *Managing* Nutrition

Sue Green

Introduction

This chapter addresses the essential nursing responsibility to ensure that adequate nutritional care is offered to all patients, whether in hospital or community-based settings. To provide appropriate nutritional care to patients or clients, nurses must have a good knowledge and understanding of the principles of human nutrition, and be able to deliver nutritional support that is informed by current clinical guidelines and up-to-date evidence, as well as to evaluate that care.

Understanding the importance of nutrition

Healthcare organizations have a duty to ensure that patients and clients receive high-quality nutritional care. The Council of Europe (2003) has published guidelines on food and nutritional care in hospitals, and a recent Europe-wide campaign has been launched to improve nutritional care in all types of care facility (Ljungqvist *et al.*, 2010). A European strategy to address obesity has also been launched (Commission of the European Communities, 2007). In England, the Care Quality Commission (CQC,

2010), which regulates care settings, has set national standards concerning nutrition.

The provision of high-quality nutritional care involves a range of services and requires a multidisciplinary team approach. As a nurse, your role within the multidisciplinary team is fundamental in ensuring the delivery of appropriate nutritional care. In the UK, this is clearly identified by the incorporation of 'Nutrition and Fluid Management' within the Essential Skills Clusters for pre-registration nursing education (Nursing and Midwifery Council, 2010).

Defining nutrition and malnutrition

Human nutrition is the study of nutrients and their effect on health, and the processes by which individuals obtain nutrients and use them for growth, metabolism, and repair. The term 'human nutrition' therefore incorporates many aspects of behaviour and physiology. The way in which the body obtains, ingests, digests, absorbs, and metabolizes nutrients is described in core anatomy and physiology textbooks (for example, Marieb and Hoehn, 2010), and it is important that a good knowledge and understanding of these processes is gained before considering the nursing management of nutritional care. This chapter considers the principles of human nutrition that underpin the nursing management of nutritional care and focuses on the key nursing interventions that you should be able to provide with confidence.

The amount and type of nutrients that a person obtains influences his or her 'nutritional status'. Nutritional status can be defined as the physiological and psychological state of a person caused by the balance between intake and use of nutrients. A person who consumes sufficient nutrients for his or her bodily needs is said to have good nutritional status. Consuming too little or too much of a nutrient, or range of nutrients, results in malnutrition. Nurses have a responsibility to take an active lead in supporting patients to achieve a good nutritional status.

The body requires a range of nutrients and water in appropriate amounts to function optimally. Nutrients are used to provide structural materials that form the body, enable metabolic processes to take place, and provide energy for the cells to function.

Malnutrition can be divided into two subcategories: undernutrition and overnutrition. Undernutrition is the term used to describe the condition that results from a lack of nutrients. Changes that can be observed in patients with undernutrition are illustrated in Figure 24.1. Conversely, overnutrition is used to describe the condition that results from an excess of nutrients. Obesity and protein-energy malnutrition are considered in some detail in this chapter, because you will be frequently involved in the management of people with these conditions. Obesity is caused when an individual's intake of energy-providing nutrients exceeds his or her energy expenditure. Protein-energy malnutrition is caused by a deficiency of protein and other energy-providing nutrients, and is often referred to as 'malnutrition' in the literature. Table 24.1 shows how body mass index (weight (kg)/height (m²)) (BMI) is used to classify those adults who are underweight, overweight, and obese. Patients or clients with conditions treated by a specific type of diet (such as renal or coeliac disease) and conditions caused by a deficiency or an excess of specific nutrients (such as iron deficiency anaemia) are generally managed by a dietitian or medical doctor, although the registered nurse may play a key role in screening and assessment, appropriate referral, and planned interventions.

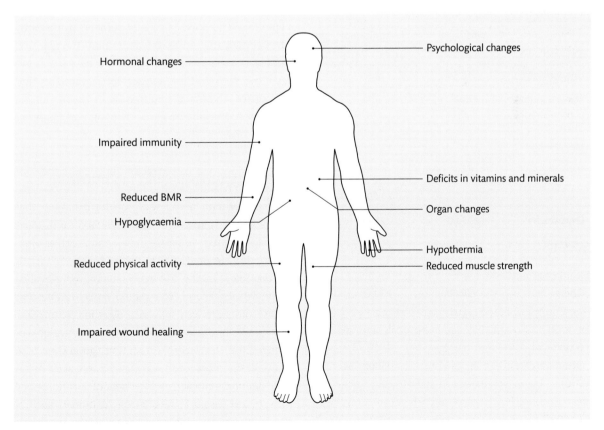

Figure 24.1   Changes associated with undernutrition.
BMR, Basal metabolic rate.

The prevalence of obesity and protein-energy malnutrition

Malnutrition is a major global health problem (WHO, 2010). The prevalence of obesity in Europe varies from country to country, but is reported to have reached epidemic proportions (Berghöfer *et al.*, 2008). In England in 2009, almost a quarter of adults (22% of men and 24% of women) were classified as obese (NHS Information Centre, 2011). Whilst undernutrition is relatively uncommon in most developed countries, a substantial proportion of individuals in healthcare settings experience it (Lean and Wiseman, 2008), and it is estimated that more than 3 million people in the UK are living at high risk of malnutrition (BAPEN, 2009). Groups at risk of undernutrition include those of a low socio-economic status, older adults, those who are institutionalized, and those with a long-term health condition (Brownie, 2006; Salva *et al.*, 2009).

Older adults are more at risk of undernutrition because they are more likely to be institutionalized, to experience physiological changes associated with ageing, to have a long-term condition, and to take medication, all of which can affect nutritional intake. Institutionalized people are more likely to be older, and they may have little influence over their food intake and the amount of time they spend exposed to sunlight. Long-term conditions can affect nutrient intake by reducing an individual's food intake, his or her capacity to absorb nutrients, or influencing his or his metabolism.

The causes of obesity and protein-energy malnutrition

Essentially, a person becomes obese or loses weight because he or she consumes either more or less energy than his or her body requires; however, the reasons why he or she does so are multifactorial and can be both psychosocial and physiological. It is useful to consider each step of the acquisition and use of nutrients by the body when considering causes of malnutrition. The type and amount of food available is influenced by cultural and economic factors. These include food availability and accessibility, and income. Individuals requiring nursing care may not be able to eat a range of food in appropriate quantities. They may be unconscious or have their normal eating behaviour altered as a result of ill-health, genetic or acquired factors, or because they opt to eat an unhealthy diet. It is therefore your responsibility to ensure that normal food-seeking behaviour that is absent or inappropriate is compensated for in some way. This may require simple intervention such as offering appropriate utensils, ensuring that palatable foods are available, assisting the patient to eat, or providing healthy eating advice. You should remain aware that disease processes may influence digestion, absorption, and metabolism, resulting in fewer nutrients available or changed nutrient usage. For example, patients with an illness such as cancer can experience cachexia, a metabolic syndrome characterized by loss of appetite, skeletal muscle, and weight (Evans, 2010). Treatments such as chemotherapy for cancer may also result in changes in consumption and metabolism.

Table 24.1 The international classification of adults that are underweight, overweight, and obese according to BMI

Classification	BMI (kg/m^2)	
	Principal cut-off points	Additional cut-off points
Underweight	**<18.50**	**<18.50**
Severe thinness	<16.00	<16.00
Moderate thinness	16.00–16.99	16.00–16.99
Mild thinness	17.00–18.49	17.00–18.49
Normal range	**18.50–24.99**	**18.50–22.99**
		23.00–24.99
Overweight	**≥25.00**	**≥25.00**
Pre-obese	25.00–29.99	25.00–27.49
		27.50–29.99
Obese	**≥30.00**	**≥30.00**
Obese class I	30.00–34.99	30.00–32.49
		32.50–34.99
Obese class II	35.00–39.99	35.00–37.49
		37.50–39.99
Obese class III	≥40.00	≥40.00

Source: WHO, 2010

There is research evidence that supports the existence of a genetic component to the development of obesity (National Obesity Forum, 2009). Generally, several chromosomal locations are implicated, although, in some rare cases, a single gene disorder may result in obesity, e.g. Prader–Willi syndrome. However, individuals with the genetic propensity to become obese can become obese only in an environment that promotes obesity.

The human and social burden and costs of malnutrition

Malnutrition is costly both in terms of the social economy and the burden on individuals. Morbidity, mortality, and healthcare costs are higher for those that are malnourished. Undernutrition is associated with poor recovery from illness and surgery (Stratton *et al.*, 2003), and can lead to the development of other conditions that threaten life. The economic cost of undernutrition in the UK is estimated at £13 billion a year (BAPEN, 2009), and this is likely to rise as the population ages and the prevalence of long-term conditions increases.

Comorbidities associated with obesity include type 2 diabetes, coronary heart disease, hypertension, various cancers, and osteoarthritis (National Institute for Health and Clinical Excellence (NICE), 2006a). The World Health Organization (WHO, 2010) estimated that 2–8% of health costs and 10–13% of deaths in different parts of Europe are linked to obesity. The annual economic cost of obesity in the UK has been estimated at £2.3 billion (Department of Health, 2008b), and human costs include poor health, social exclusion, and discrimination.

Nursing responsibilities and accountability for meeting nutritional needs

As a nurse, you are responsible for helping patients in your care to obtain an appropriate range of nutrients in appropriate amounts. You should be able to identify those at risk of malnutrition to develop, deliver, and evaluate appropriate plans of care, and to refer your patients to other healthcare professionals or services as required. The

Nursing and Midwifery Council (NMC) (2010) states that a newly registered nurse should be able to:

- assess and monitor nutritional status and, in partnership, formulate an effective plan of care;
- assist with choosing a diet that provides an adequate nutritional and fluid intake;
- assist in creating an environment that is conducive to eating and drinking;
- ensure that those unable to take food by mouth receive adequate fluid and nutrition to meet their needs.

You also have a responsibility for ensuring that unregistered healthcare staff and lay carers are supported and prepared to give appropriate nutritional care.

Key nursing responsibilities in nutritional care

As a nurse, you have a responsibility to monitor patients' nutritional status, and to plan and deliver appropriate nutritional care. This involves careful and regular screening and assessment, assisting patients to access an appropriate diet, whether orally or parentally, and promoting a conducive environment to maximize good nutrition.

Screening and clinical assessment of nutrition

It is essential that you are able to identify individuals in your care who are malnourished so that you can give appropriate nutritional support (National Institute for Health and Clinical Excellence (NICE), 2006b). A number of UK publications (Nursing and Midwifery Practice Development Unit, 2002; NICE, 2006b) recommend that nutritional screening and assessment should be undertaken when patients are admitted to care settings, and that screening should be repeated weekly for inpatients or more frequently if there is clinical concern. If screening indicates that a patient is at risk of malnutrition, then an assessment of nutritional status should be undertaken. Whilst nurses are essential to the screening process, nutritional status may be assessed by a range of healthcare professionals, including nurses, depending on the type of problem identified at screening.

The majority of patients will need to be referred to a dietitian if undernutrition is suspected or if they are required to follow a therapeutic diet (such as gluten-free or low potassium). Referral to another healthcare professional such as an occupational therapist may be required.

The four principal methods that you can utilize to screen or assess nutritional status are: dietary history and intake; clinical examination; anthropometric measures; and biochemical tests.

Taking a dietary history

A basic assessment of dietary history and intake will enable you to determine the risk and potential causes of obesity and undernutrition, as well as dietary habits, food preferences, and economic factors influencing food intake. Each patient should be asked about his or her appetite, food intake, bowel activity, use of supplements, and any other issues that may be important—for example, dietary adherence. Patients or clients on a restrictive diet such as a renal diet can find it very difficult to adhere to their dietary regime. Recording food intake using a food chart or food diary can be a useful way of identifying quantity and type of food and fluid intake. Asking a person to recall what he or she has eaten over the previous day, or to describe what he or she generally eats, are also useful ways of assessing dietary intake.

A food frequency checklist can be used to record how often particular types of food are eaten, giving an indication of dietary quality. This method is generally used in research and by dietitians rather than by nurses in the clinical setting, although some screening and assessment tools may incorporate some aspects of this approach (Vellas *et al.*, 2006). Reported intakes of food may not represent a person's habitual diet because intake of food over the time of recording may change owing to scrutiny of the diet or misreporting (Patterson and Pietinen, 2004).

Clinical examination

A general clinical examination undertaken on patients on admission to care can highlight nutritional concerns, and should include observation and assessment of the following factors:

- general appetite;
- ability to taste and smell;

- mouth and denture condition;
- activity level;
- general appearance, fit of clothes, condition of hair, skin, and eyes;
- medication use;
- alcohol use.

These can give you an indication of nutritional status and possible causes of poor nutritional intake or obesity. You should also assess functional ability to eat and physical or emotional and cognitive factors that might impair the process of eating. The impact of the patient's medical condition or medications and treatment on intake, digestion, and absorption of nutrients should be factored in (Mason, 2010; White, 2010). Finally, if written dietary advice is required, then literacy level, ability to read the language in which any advice is written, and any visual impairment need to be considered.

Using anthropometric measures

You can use simple anthropometric measures to screen and assess nutritional status. The most basic measure of these is body weight. Patients should be weighed carefully on admission if there is cause for concern about nutritional status and periodically thereafter to identify any subsequent changes. Percentage weight change can be calculated using the equation:

$$\% \text{ Weight loss/gain} = \frac{\text{Usual weight} - \text{Current weight (kg)}}{\text{Usual weight(kg)}} \times 100$$

A loss of 10% in the previous 3 months is suggestive of malnutrition. BMI provides a more accurate assessment of the degree to which a person is underweight or overweight than weight alone because it considers weight in relation to height. However, it is important to remember that BMI must be considered in the context of an individual's circumstances. A long-distance runner will be likely to have a low BMI, but be fit and healthy, whereas a person with extensive oedema is likely to have a BMI that does not reflect his or her muscle and fat mass. It is also possible for an obese person to be undernourished. Therefore, relying solely on BMI as an indicator may result in an obese person not being provided with appropriate nutritional support.

The correct clinical procedure for assessing a patient's weight and height is shown in Dougherty and Lister (2008). Height can sometimes be difficult to determine, due to factors such as spine curvature and inability to stand, in which case an estimation of height can be made using a proxy measure, such as ulnar length (Elia, 2003). There are limitations in the use of weight as a measure of nutritional status. Body weight changes with dehydration, oedema, and tumour growth and weight, and may therefore not reject nutritional status. When using BMI with older people, the resulting plan and interventions need to be carefully considered, because a BMI of 24–29 can be considered healthy in older people aged 70 years and over (The Scottish Government, 2009).

Waist circumference can be used to screen for cardiovascular risk in primary care. This measure assesses the amount of fat located in the abdominal region. Men with a waist circumference greater than 102 cm and women with a waist circumference of more than 88 cm should be advised that weight reduction would be beneficial (Lean *et al.*, 1995). Other measures, including skin fold measures and bioimpedance to assess fat mass or muscle mass of a person, may be used in specialist units after training in their use.

Biochemical testing

Biochemical tests are frequently used in conjunction with other tests to assess nutritional status. Nitrogen balance can be estimated from urine output, and gives an indication of intake and excretion of protein. If protein is used by the body without being replaced by dietary intake, a person will become malnourished. Levels of serum albumin and other body proteins can also be used to assess protein status, although the interpretation of these needs to be carefully considered because they vary in response to illness and treatment independent of nutritional status (Banh, 2006). Levels of vitamins and minerals in the body may be measured, and will give an indication of nutritional status. Some frequently used measures include electrolyte and haemoglobin levels. The interpretation of the results of biochemical tests in relation to nutritional status is complex because disease state will influence the level of many vitamins and minerals. For this reason, biochemical tests are generally not used to screen for malnutrition, but may be used by the multidisciplinary team as part of a nutritional assessment.

The use of nutritional screening tools

Many tools have been developed that enable registered nurses to screen patients for undernutrition (Green and Watson, 2005; 2006). These tools typically consist of a number of questions concerning risk factors for malnutrition that, when considered together, give an overall risk of malnutrition. Tools used by registered nurses should be quick, valid, and reliable. The National Institute for Health and Clinical Excellence (NICE) (2006b) highlights the Malnutrition Universal Screening Tool (MUST) (BAPEN, 2006) as being suitable for use. This tool has been developed to identify risk of protein-energy malnutrition and is reported to be simple, valid, and reliable (Elia, 2003). Of the many other tools available, few have been rigorously tested in terms of validity and reliability (Green and Watson, 2005; 2006).

As outlined previously, careful nutritional screening and assessment will enable identification of the patient's or client's nutritional needs so that appropriate interventions can be planned and goals set.

Nursing management of nutritional interventions

Nurses have responsibility for supporting both patients who are obese and those who are at risk of undernourishment to access appropriate nutrition. The following sections of this chapter outline the key elements of effective interventions across this spectrum of need.

Supporting overweight and obese patients

A number of national bodies have produced evidence-based guidance and resources to guide the management of overweight and obese patients (Department of Health 2006; Scottish Intercollegiate Guidelines Network (SIGN), 2010). Many primary care areas have developed local obesity care pathways that ensure that services are aligned with local needs and that provision is equitable with other areas. The development of a clearly defined provision can also facilitate monitoring and evaluation of services offered. Obesity care pathways highlight the need for a number of approaches to the management of obesity, all of which are based on the principle of ensuring that energy intake is lower than energy expenditure. The approaches are normally arranged in tiers or stages and increase in resource intensity. The first tier or stage may be managed by the registered nurse working in primary care and is discussed in more detail below. The subsequent tiers or stages generally involve multicomponent weight management programmes and specialist multidisciplinary weight management interventions (Pheasant and Enock, 2010).

Promoting healthy eating and behavioural change

Your initial assessment of the client/patient should follow the National Institute for Health and Clinical Excellence (NICE, 2006a) guidelines and cover weight history, willingness to change, and screening for eating disorder. You should highlight to the patient or client the health benefits associated with sustained weight loss (Logue *et al.*, 2010) and agree an individual plan of care with goals. NICE (2006a) recommends interventions that involve behaviour change to increase physical activity level, improve eating behaviour, and reduce energy intake. A diet that follows healthy eating advice and contains 600 kilocalories (kcal) fewer than the person needs to stay the same weight, or reduces energy intake by lowering the fat content, should be recommended (NICE, 2006a). A recent review by Bray (2008) suggests that there is little evidence to support the use of a diet of any particular macronutrient composition (e.g. high fat, high carbohydrate) for weight loss. There are a vast range of published weight loss diets that advocate various types and combinations of food.

Low-energy (1,000–1,600-kcal) diets may be followed, but are less likely to be nutritionally complete. Very low-energy diets (lower than 1,000 kcal a day) may be useful in the short term (NICE, 2006a), but should be used only for a limited period of time by people with obesity who have tried other forms of weight loss. A diet of lower than 600 kcal/day must be undertaken only under clinical supervision (NICE, 2006a). Very low-energy diets are increasing in popularity and can be effective in promoting weight loss (Hankey, 2010); however, they are severely restrictive and have been associated with a number of side effects. NICE (2006a) does not recommend the use of very restrictive and nutritionally incomplete diets because they may be detrimental to the health.

It is important that you work in partnership with patients to identify which dietary management approach best suits their needs and lifestyle, although there is little evidence concerning the most effective way of delivering dietary advice (Logue *et al.*, 2010).

Behavioural change

People with obesity need to change or modify their behaviours to change their diet and activity levels. Behavioural interventions for adults include strategies such as self-monitoring of behaviour and progress, stimulus control, problem-solving, cognitive restructuring (modifying thoughts), reinforcement of changes, and dealing with weight regain (NICE, 2006a). Behavioural change to modify eating behaviour can be supported by individual or group counselling sessions (Bray, 2008). Some people may find that the support gained from a reputable 'slimming club' is helpful (Truby *et al.*, 2006). The effectiveness of weight loss services provided in primary care compared with that of commercial providers has not been well evaluated (Jolly *et al.*, 2010).

Physical activity

Physical activity may be most useful in helping patients/clients maintain weight loss (Bray, 2008). NICE (2006a) suggests that people who have been obese and lost weight may need to do 60 to 90 minutes of moderate activity per day. The term 'activity' is preferred to the term 'exercise' because an 'activity' is easier to incorporate within the daily routine, e.g. walking rather than taking the bus.

For the average person, 30 minutes (or more) of moderate intensity physical activity on 5 or more days of the week, either as one session or several sessions of 10 minutes or more, should be undertaken (NICE, 2006a). Some people will be unable to achieve the required level of physical activity owing to a medical condition, and they should be advised to consult their general practitioner for advice and may be referred to an exercise on prescription scheme.

Pharmacological management and surgical interventions

Currently in the UK, medication that can be used in the management of obesity blocks intestinal lipase, thereby reducing fat absorption. This can be prescribed or supplied by pharmacists provided that certain criteria are met. Management of obesity by surgical procedures in accordance with NICE (2006a) is considered to be effective in maintaining weight loss (Office of Health Economics, 2010; Bray, 2008). Bariatric surgery and other invasive interventions for obesity include a number of approaches. These generally focus on reducing the amount of food that can be tolerated in the stomach and/or the amount of nutrients that can be absorbed in the small intestine. The size of the stomach can be reduced by the use of a balloon in the lumen of the stomach (gastric balloon), constriction by a band (gastric band) or staples (gastric stapling) externally, or removal of a portion of the stomach (sleeve gastrectomy). The surgeon may consider a gastric bypass procedure appropriate, in which the size of the stomach is reduced and part of the small intestine bypassed, thus reducing the absorptive area. Surgical methods are constantly evaluated and new methods of controlling obesity are being developed. For example, a new method that avoids the need for surgery is a gastrointestinal barrier device placed by endoscope that reduces absorption from the small intestine (Schouten *et al.*, 2010).

Surgical and other invasive interventions can be carried out by NHS or private providers. Providers must have a specialist team of surgeons and other clinicians who are appropriately trained and qualified, and who provide aftercare. An invasive intervention is not a quick fix and patients/clients need expert dietetic, psychological, and medical aftercare. There are risks associated with surgery for obesity (Padwal *et al.*, 2011) and some patients or clients may not be accepted for surgical treatment. A person may be required by the specialist team to lose weight prior to surgery (for example, 5% of body weight) to reduce the risks associated with surgery, such as operation duration (Becouarn *et al.*, 2010). The specialist team will assess the patient's/client's risks and benefits of having a surgical or invasive intervention and identify which approach is most appropriate. However, patients/clients may ask you for information and advice concerning surgery for obesity prior to referral to the specialist team, and it is important that up-to-date and relevant information is given.

A person who has obesity and loses weight is always at risk of regaining the weight lost, and the evidence for the effectiveness of interventions that support maintenance of weight loss is limited (Logue *et al.*, 2010). Even patients or clients who have undergone a surgical procedure may be at risk of gaining weight (Júnior *et al.*, 2011).

Managing undernutrition

There are various approaches to the management of undernutrition; these range from the non-invasive and non-intensive provision of food in an appropriate environment to having nutrients delivered directly into the bloodstream. Any nutritional support provided to the undernourished patient must be introduced gradually and the patient closely monitored to avoid the development of refeeding syndrome (Mehanna *et al.*, 2008). Refeeding syndrome is a serious condition that occurs when malnourished people experience changes in the extracellular and intracellular fluid and electrolyte levels as a result of receiving nutritional support. Patients should always be offered a diet that is appropriate for their needs, taking into account preferences, cultural needs, prescribed diets, and required food textures.

THEORY INTO PRACTICE 24.1
How do we know how much of a particular nutrient a person requires?

In the UK, the term 'dietary reference value' (DRV) is used to describe how much of a nutrient different groups of healthy people require. Review the British Nutrition Foundation web page on nutrient requirements and recommendations (http://www.nutrition.org.uk/nutritionscience/nutrients/nutrient-requirements) to help you to understand the concept of DRVs. It is difficult to determine exactly how much of a nutrient a person requires when he or she is unwell. Sometimes, it may be more than required in health owing to loss and increased use, and sometimes less as a result of lower activity levels or use of nutrients. Generally, therefore, nutrient requirements in ill-health are estimated by a healthcare practitioner specializing in nutritional care, such as a dietitian.

Providing nutrition for those able to take food orally

To prevent as well as to treat malnutrition, it is important that you ensure that the environment is appropriate for eating and drinking for all patients. This aspect of nursing management is most relevant to patients who are cared for in institutional settings, although if you are visiting patients in their own homes, you should also consider environmental factors that can affect the quantity and quality of dietary intake. A recent review has suggested that creating an environment that encourages institutionalized older adults to eat can lead to improved nutritional status and quality of life (Nieuwenhuizen *et al.*, 2010). There are various strategies that can be used to promote dietary intake. These include improving the choice of food, improving the mealtime environment, and ensuring that the individual is able or supported to eat.

In hospitals or care homes, it would be your responsibility to ensure access to drinks, meals, and snacks regularly over a 24-hour period.

Environment

You should also consider the setting in which individuals will be eating. Obnoxious sounds, sights, and smells that are sometimes encountered in institutions have the potential to reduce appetite. The introduction of 'protected mealtimes' is currently being promoted in the NHS (Age UK, 2010), so that mealtimes are not interrupted by routine ward activities and non-emergency procedures such as blood tests. There is some evidence that a home-style approach at mealtimes using interventions such as tablecloths and settings to improve ambience, food choice at the table, and staff engagement can improve nutritional intake (Nijs *et al.*, 2006), although the effectiveness of the individual components of such interventions is not well evaluated.

It is also important to ensure that the patient is ready to eat and drink. This involves attending to elimination needs prior to serving food, offering facilities to wash hands, ensuring that mouth condition is appropriate for eating, making sure that pain and nausea are well controlled, and checking that the table from which the food is eaten is clean and uncluttered. Assistance with eating must always be provided if required (Hogston and Marjoram, 2010).

Maximizing nutritional intake

If the patient is able to swallow sufficient quantities safely, initially the use of nutrient-dense 'normal' meals and snacks should be promoted. The nutrient density of a meal can be increased by adding high nutrient density foods to the meal or making the food with higher nutrient

density components: for example, porridge can be made with full fat milk, and sugar and cream added on serving. There is some evidence that this can increase nutritional intake, although generally by only a small amount (Nieuwenhuizen *et al.*, 2010).

Promoting a diet that contains a variety of foods and the promotion of frequent eating may also increase food intake (Nieuwenhuizen *et al.*, 2010). Following this, oral nutritional food supplements in milk, yoghurt, juice, or dessert form should be offered because there is good evidence that they are effective in improving nutritional status (Milne *et al.*, 2009; Nieuwenhuizen *et al.*, 2010). It is important to offer supplements at the appropriate temperature (i.e. warm or chilled) in the patient's preferred glass or cup to maximize palatability. Offering a variety of supplements with different sensory characteristics (appearance, flavour, texture, consistency, and composition) is thought to increase intake more than when only one type of supplement is used (Nieuwenhuizen *et al.*, 2010).

Manufacturers have recently developed a number of new products to maximize nutritional intake. These include a fortified ice cream that can be dispensed via a machine in the clinical area and fortified thickened drinks for people with **dysphagia**.

People with dysphagia may be prescribed a modified texture diet (often termed a 'puree diet') following assessment by the speech and language therapist. This type of diet facilitates swallowing for people who, as a result of an anatomical or physiological disorder, have difficulty in manipulating food in the mouth and/or swallowing (**deglutition**). People who are prescribed this type of diet are at risk of receiving a poorer quality diet and of malnutrition, although it is not clear whether this is because of the nutritional adequacy of the diet or as a direct result of the condition (Foley *et al.*, 2009; Wright *et al.*, 2005). The registered nurse needs to ensure that patients/clients are referred for assessment by the speech and language therapist if dysphagia is suspected to avoid the risk of aspiration, and that any dietary and fluid modifications prescribed are incorporated into their plans of care. Relatives and carers need to be informed of the importance of adherence to the prescribed modified diet. It is important that the presentation and palatability of the food is considered carefully to promote nutritional intake.

Reflecting on mealtime care and documentation

In your clinical environment, observe the meal-time activities at one mealtime for a group of patients. Reflect on what you observe and review relevant documentation (e.g. care plans and food charts) in relation to the mealtime.

Did each patient receive support to prepare for his or her meal, such as assistance in handwashing and removing food wrappings, as required?

Are there ways in which the environment could be improved to enhance the patients' experience of mealtime?

Was food intake documented for patients at risk of malnutrition?

Providing nutrition for those unable to take food orally

If a person is unable to consume enough orally, then you will need to manage nutritional support via a tube. If the gut is functional and accessible, then enteral nutrition may be given; if not, then parenteral nutrition may be appropriate. Enteral nutrition can be given via a tube that travels through the nose into the stomach (nasogastric tube) and occasionally the small intestine (nasoduodenal/nasojejunal tube). If longer term enteral nutrition is required, then it can be delivered via a tube that traverses the abdominal wall into the stomach (radiologically inserted gastrostomy and percutaneously endoscopically inserted gastrostomy) and, more rarely, the small intestine (jejunostomy). Parenteral nutrition is used when the gut is unable to provide nutrients to the body and is delivered by a dedicated intravascular line.

Enteral nutrition

The care of the patient receiving enteral nutrition via a tube is an important part of a nursing role. The feed type is usually prescribed by a dietitian, but all other aspects of the delivery of the feed are generally managed by a nurse. You should therefore be confident and competent in the insertion and removal of nasogastric tubes. These proce-dures are shown in detail in Dougherty and Lister (2008).

However, unless you have had specialized training, you should not attempt to insert nasogastric tubes in patients with basal skull fractures, maxillofacial disorders, oesopha-geal disorders, and those who have undergone maxillo-facial or oesophageal surgery, because the route to the stomach may be distorted (Higgins, 2005). Generally, fine-bore tubes (6–8 FG) are used for the administration of enteral nutrition. Before the tube is used to give any fluid, it is essential that the position of the tube is checked to ensure that the tip is placed in the stomach. The National Patient Safety Agency highlights that harm to patients has occurred as a result of feed being infused into the res-piratory tract; this risk increases when nasogastric tubes are inserted at night and when X-rays taken to check the placement of the tube have been misinterpreted (NPSA, 2011). It has developed a decision-making tool to use when checking nasogastric tube placement.

Caring for a person with a nasogastric and gastrostomy tube in situ includes the following key components:

- maintaining the patency and position of the tube;
- administering food, fluids, and medication;
- ensuring that the tube does not cause tissue damage (such as pressure ulcers);
- providing or encouraging oral and nasal hygiene;
- providing psychological support and monitoring the patient's condition.

Most clinical areas have developed guidelines outlining in detail the care of patients with enteral tubes. These guide-lines are usually informed by published evidence-based guidelines and available research; however, due to a pau-city of research, some aspects of care are supported by expert consensus rather than research findings (Depart-ment of Health, 2010).

Feed given via an enteral tube can be administered as a bolus, intermittently, overnight, or continuously (Howard, 2009). If not given as a bolus, the feed should be administered via a pump designed for the delivery of enteral nutrition to ensure delivery of the appropriate rate and volume. In the UK, feeds are usually made by the manufacturers in ready-to-hang bags to reduce the risk of infection. Medication can be delivered via the enteral feeding tube, but the pharmacist should be consulted to ensure that preparations are suitable for administration in this way and water should be used to flush the tube before and after each medication type. Syringes that are not compatible with intravenous system use, such as a bladder-tipped syringe or enteral syringe, must be used with enteral tubes.

A number of nutritional algorithms have been developed for use in intensive care settings because initiation of feeding may be delayed owing to availability of a dietitian, compromised feed absorption (because of the physiological effects of critical illness on gastrointestinal tract function), and interruptions caused by treatments. The use of an evidence-based algorithm has been suggested to assist nurses to improve the provision of nutritional support and efficiency of care by reducing practice variation (Binnekade, 2004).

Complications of enteral feeding by tube include: gastrointestinal disturbances such as infection, diarrhoea, constipation, and abdominal distension; line-associated complications such as tube removal and blockage; and metabolic complications such as fluid overload. Barrett *et al.* (2008) highlight that diarrhoea and abdominal distension are common complications of enteral feeding by tube, which can be managed by identifying the cause, where possible, and altering the method of delivery or the type of formula delivered. These authors propose that the development of an algorithm can assist management of gastrointestinal complications (Barrett *et al.*, 2008). There is evidence to suggest that enteral feeds are often not delivered according to prescription owing to frequent interruptions of the feed (O'Meara *et al.*, 2008). The use of a nasal bridle with a nasoenteral feeding tube may be part of the solution to this because it can prevent dislodgement of the tube (Gunn *et al.*, 2008; Beavan *et al.*, 2010).

Parenteral nutrition

This is used when the gut is unable to provide nutrients to the body, and macronutrients and micronutrients in solution are delivered directly into the bloodstream. As a rule, this is commenced in a critical or acute care setting. Patients can receive all or part of their nutritional requirements via parenteral nutrition, depending on whether some nutrition is given enterally. Current European guidelines suggest that critically ill patients who are not expected to receive nutritional input within 3 days should be considered for parenteral nutrition within 24–48 hours if enteral nutrition is contraindicated. Because this type of

nutritional support is intensive and invasive, a nutrition support team or clinicians with expertise in parenteral nutrition should be involved at the start because there is some evidence that this reduces the risk of complications (Singer *et al.*, 2009). In the UK, registered nurses are generally required as part of hospital protocol to undertake post-registration training prior to managing parenteral nutrition owing to the high risk of complications developing. Complications include: problems with the line, such as fracture and infection; problems associated with the metabolic consequences of the body dealing with the infusion of nutrients that bypass the safety mechanisms of the gastrointestinal tract; and problems associated with infection.

Parenteral nutrition is given via a dedicated line or lumen, peripherally in the short term and if the solution is low in osmolarity (and, therefore, does not irritate the vein), and centrally in the long term and for feeds of higher osmolarity and volume (Singer *et al.*, 2009). A volumetric pump is used to deliver the feed infusion to avoid the risk of overinfusion or underinfusion and associated complications. In the UK, generally all of the nutrients are placed in one bag in a controlled environment in pharmacy or by the manufacturers, and the bag is delivered over 24 to 48 hours to reduce the risk of administration errors and microbial contamination of the solution by more frequent bag changes. The infusion is generally given continuously in those that are unwell and cyclically in long-term delivery to enable the person to fit the feed administration with his or her lifestyle. Because of the high risk of complications, close monitoring of the patient's condition is essential (NICE, 2006b). This includes careful monitoring of blood glucose level, particularly in the critically ill, because higher glucose levels (glucose greater than 10 mmol/l) have been associated with poor clinical outcomes (Singer *et al.*, 2009). Whilst the provision of parenteral nutrition is usually seen as a complex clinical intervention, patients can be discharged home with parenteral nutrition in progress: for example, in Scotland in 2006, a total of 53 patients received parenteral nutrition at home (Hallum *et al.*, 2010). Even when people receive parenteral nutrition at home, they must still be closely monitored to detect potential or existing complications. There is some evidence to suggest that monitoring of patients receiving parenteral nutrition at home does not follow recommendations outlined by NICE (2006b), although this has been shown not to impact on the rate of complications (Hallum *et al.*, 2010).

Patients receiving enteral and parenteral nutritional support via tube can manage their own nutritional support if physically and mentally able. Patients in the community can be supported to self-manage by their carer, dietetics team, home care nutrition company, district nursing team, or nutrition nurse specialists. It is difficult to truly appreciate the experience of the person who has to receive nutritional support via tube for an extended period of time. Informing patients or clients of support groups that exist, such as PINNT (Patients on Intravenous and Nasogastric Nutrition **http://www.pinnt.co.uk/ index.htm**) can enable them to gain the support that they need to be able to adapt to life receiving nutrients via a tube.

THEORY INTO PRACTICE 24.3
Undernutrition and nutritional support

Mrs J has been admitted to your care following surgery for a fracture. Her BMI is 18 kg/m². She reports that she has lost a lot of weight over the past 3 months, and she has eaten little over the past 2 weeks.

- Of what syndrome is she at risk?
- How would you manage her nutritional care?

See **http://guidance.nice.org.uk/CG32/Guidance/ pdf/English**

Accessing and evaluating the evidence to inform clinical nursing decisions

The literature informing the evidence base for nutritional care originates from a wide range of disciplines including biology, sociology, psychology, dietetics, and medicine, as well as nursing. In addition, there is a great deal of 'grey literature', such as manufacturer's information concerning devices and products. Some published research is variable in quality and generalizability. For example, many papers have reported the development of nutritional screening tools, but they do not clearly demonstrate that the tool presented is valid or reliable in different practice areas (Green and Watson, 2005). In addition, many aspects of nutritional care that are relevant to nursing care have not been rigorously tested: for example, the use of volunteers to assist patients to eat (Green *et al.*, 2011). A variety of clinical interventions involving nutrition are supported by the lower levels of the hierarchy of evidence formed from experience and 'common sense': for example, assisting someone to eat who is not able to eat without assistance is likely to result in improved nutritional intake. For these reasons, whenever possible you should access national clinical guidelines, which summarize relevant literature and present a consensus of expert opinion which you can use in your clinical practice. There are a number of important publications that guide the way in which healthcare professionals should provide nutritional care in the UK. The clinical guidelines produced by the National Institute for Health and Clinical Excellence concerning the management of obesity and nutrition support (NICE 2006a, 2006b) are essential reading. Specific guidelines concerning screening and assessing eating disorders (NICE, 2004) are also available. The Department of Health produces a number of documents that aim to enhance the nutritional care of patients. A publication entitled *Healthy Weight, Healthy Lives: A toolkit for developing local strategies* (DH, 2008) has also been developed in the UK.

If clinical guidelines on a particular nutritional topic do not exist, then you will need to search for appropriate literature in a variety of databases, for example MEDLINE, EMBase, and PubMed. Other sources of information can also be used, such as up-to-date books aimed at healthcare professionals and professional body, government or learned society websites. There is an enormous amount of information concerning nutrition on the Internet and in the media. The information available can be contradictory and not based on sound evidence. Currently, the title 'nutritionist' is unregulated by a professional body in the UK, and therefore individuals with limited knowledge and level of proficiency in nutritional care can give individuals advice on a commercial basis. Patients should therefore be advised to adhere to guidelines given by a registered dietitian or other healthcare professional competent to give nutritional advice or treatment.

Box 24.1 Sources of EBN

National Institute for Clinical Excellence clinical guidelines

Department of Health documents such as *Healthy Weight, Healthy Lives: A toolkit for developing local strategies* (2008)

Databases including:
- MEDLINE
- EMBase
- PubMed

Measuring the impact of nursing interventions

The principle of measuring both the effectiveness of nursing interventions and the patient's experience of receiving care is one that you should, where possible, facilitate. The NHS Information Centre has supported the development of Nursing Quality Metrics (NQMs), which can be used to facilitate quality improvement in patient care and experience **http://signposting.ic.nhs.uk/?k=metrics.**

This recent move within healthcare to be outcome-focused rather than target-driven is a welcome change in policy direction, initiated by Lord Darzi in his review of the NHS, and sustained by the previous and current UK governments. Metrics have been developed for many aspects of nursing care interventions and cover many inpatient areas, regardless of setting. The collection of these types of data helps healthcare organizations to focus on the delivery of safe and effective care, and can be used for local and national benchmarking, as well as for quality improvement.

For further details, visit the NHS Information Centre online at **http://www.ic.nhs.uk/**, where you will find details relating to nursing audit tools capturing information on documentation for observations, nutrition, medicines administration, pain management, communication, discharge planning, falls, pressure area care, antibiotic prescribing, and infection control.

In determining patient experience of healthcare, NICE has recently published a Quality Standard **http://www.nice.org.uk** that guides service delivery planning to ensure improvements in patient experience. Further commissioned work by the Department of Health has developed a single measure of patient experience. Supplementing

these data is the NHS Survey, which captures patient views relating to ward cleanliness, infection control, staff attitudes, pain management, management of privacy, experience of dignity, nutrition, medicines administration, quality of communication, and discharge. Details can be found online at **http://www.nhssurveys.org/.**

Key evidence gaps and challenges

Overall, there is limited available vigorous research on the nursing management of many common nursing interventions related to nutritional support. As highlighted above, clinical guidelines are often informed by a general consensus of opinion. An example of this is that there is little evidence to support the best way in which to give medication via an enteral tube despite this being an intervention undertaken by a large number of nurses each day (Phillips and Nay, 2008). A recent review outlined that there is a lack of evidence of the effect of nutritional care (defined as any care provided with the aim of maximizing food intake, such as nutrition screening, assistance with menu selection, preparation of patients for their meals, provision of feeding assistance, and food service) and calls for more research to determine the cost-effectiveness of interventions (Weekes *et al.*, 2009).

There is more available evidence for the best strategies for the management of obesity (indeed the obesity care pathways developed by primary care trusts in the UK are normally based upon this), but there is limited evidence to guide the nursing role in the management of obesity. More research is needed to identify effective nurse-led strategies to support those trying to manage their weight, particularly interventions delivered in the community by, for example, a practice nurse.

Challenges in delivering evidence-based nursing intervention

Some practice areas may not have the resources available to implement appropriate interventions: for example, there is some evidence that a home-style dining environment promotes food intake and quality of life in nursing home residents (Nijs *et al.*, 2006), but space to provide this may not be available. In some areas, services may be limited. A further example is an appropriately structured nutrition support team can improve patient safety, reduce cost, and decrease inappropriate use of parenteral nutrition (Sriram *et al.*, 2010), but some areas do not have such a team.

Malnutrition is generally considered to be preventable (Stratton, 2007). However, it must be noted that intervention may not always be appropriate. Patient choice and clinical condition need to be factored in when considering the prevention of malnutrition. Appetite and weight loss is often experienced at the end of life, and weight loss can be a natural consequence of the process of dying rather than a direct cause. Aggressive nutritional support is not appropriate at the end of life. Instead, measures should be taken to promote the patient's preferences and comfort. Often, difficult clinical situations can present when it is difficult to decide what type of nutritional support is appropriate. The Royal College of Physicians has published a guide to practical care for use in such situations (Royal College of Physicians, 2010).

This chapter has focused on the delivery of nutritional care to individual patients or clients, but, as a nurse, you may also need to act at an organizational level to ensure that appropriate nutritional care is delivered. Organizational activities include the development of policy, procedures, and audit, and fall within the scope of clinical governance. You may also need to contribute to the nutritional education of co-workers and lay carers. Education is seen as an important factor in addressing the problem of malnutrition (Elia and Russell, 2009). If your practice involves contact with many patients or clients with nutritional care needs, you may wish to specialize in nutritional care following registration, and undertake training and education to develop the extended knowledge and skills required (NNNG, 2010).

Summary and key messages

- Malnutrition is one of the most commonly encountered conditions in nursing practice, and embraces the conditions of obesity and undernutrition.

- Malnutrition is caused by a variety of factors, and results in significant morbidity and mortality.

- It is a nursing responsibility to ensure that good nutritional care is delivered so that the nutritional needs of patients and clients are met.

- It is a key nursing responsibility to screen and assess a patient's nutritional status on admission to care, and to develop, with other members of the healthcare team, an appropriate plan of care that is evaluated regularly.

- There is some evidence about the most effective nursing interventions when working with people to promote weight loss, facilitate oral food intake, and manage nutritional therapy via tube.

- The evidence base informing good nutritional care is expanding, but more research relating to nurse-led aspects of care is required.

Online Resource Centre

 To help you to develop and apply your knowledge and decision-making skills further, we have provided interactive learning resources online at **www.oxfordtextbooks.co.uk/orc/bullock/**

Whilst these are freely available, you will need to use the access codes at the start of the book.

References

Age UK (2010) *Still Hungry to be Heard.* Age UK: London.

Banh, L. (2004) Serum proteins as markers of nutrition: what are we treating? *Practical Gastroenterology,* October: 46–64.

BAPEN (2006) *The 'MUST' Toolkit.* BAPEN: Redditch. **http://www.bapen.org.uk/musttoolkit.html** (accessed 13 October 2011).

BAPEN (2009) *Combating Malnutrition: Recommendations for Action.* BAPEN: Redditch.

Barrett, J.S., Shepherd, S.J., Gibson, P.R. (2008) Strategies to manage gastrointestinal symptoms complicating enteral feeding. *Journal of Enteral and Parenteral Nutrition* **33**: 21–6.

Beavan, J., Conroy, S.P., Harwood, R., *et al.* (2010) Does looped nasogastric tube feeding improve nutritional delivery for patients with dysphagia after acute stroke? A randomised controlled trial. *Age and Ageing* **39**(5): 624–30.

Becouarn, G., Topart, P., Ritz, P. (2010) Weight loss prior to bariatric surgery is not a pre-requisite of excess weight loss outcomes in obese patients. *Obesity Surgery* **20**(5): 574–7.

Berghöfer, A., Pischon, T., Reinhold, T., *et al.* (2008) Obesity prevalence from a European perspective: a systematic review. *BMC Public Health* **5**(8): 200.

Binnekade, J.M. (2004) Commentary. *Evidence-Based Nursing* **7**: 89.

Bray, G.A. (2008) Lifestyle and pharmacological approaches to weight loss: efficacy and safety. *Journal of Clinical Endocrinology & Metabolism* **93**(11 Suppl. 1): s81–s88.

Brownie, S. (2006) Why are elderly individuals at risk of nutritional deficiency? *International Journal of Nursing Practice* **12**: 110–18.

Care Quality Commission (2010) *The Essential Standards.* **http://www.cqc.org.uk/usingcareservices/essentialstandardsofqualityandsafety.cfm** (accessed 13 October 2011).

Commission of the European Communities (2007) *A Strategy for Europe on Nutrition, Overweight and Obesity-Related Health Issues.* Commission of the European Communities: Brussels.

Council of Europe (2003) Resolution ResAP(2003)3 on food and nutritional care in hospitals. **https://wcd.coe.int/ViewDoc.jsp?id=85747** (accessed 23 December 2010).

Department of Health (2006) *Obesity Care Pathway and Your Weight Your Health.* Department of Health: London.

Department of Health (2008a) *Healthy Weight, Healthy Lives: A Toolkit for Developing Local Strategies.* Department of Health: London.

Department of Health (2008b) *Healthy Weight, Healthy Lives: A Cross-Government Strategy for England.* Department of Health: London.

Department of Health (2010) *Essence of Care.* HMSO: London.

Dougherty, L., Lister, S. (2008) *The Royal Marsden Hospital Manual of Clinical Nursing Procedures.* Wiley-Blackwell: Oxford.

Elia, M. (2003) *The 'MUST' Report.* BAPEN: Redditch.

Elia, M., Russell, C. (2009) *Combating Malnutrition: Recommendations for Action—Executive Summary.* British Association for Parenteral and Enteral Nutrition: Redditch.

Evans, W.J. (2010) Skeletal muscle loss, cachexia, sarcopenia and inactivity. *American Journal of Clinical Nutrition* **91**(4): 1123S–7S.

Foley, N.C., Martin, R.E., Salter, K.L., *et.al.* (2009) A review of the relationship between dysphagia and malnutrition following stroke. *Journal of Rehabilitation Medicine* **41**(9): 707–13.

Green, S.M., Watson, R. (2005) Nutritional screening and assessment tools for use by nurses: literature review. *Journal of Advanced Nursing* **50**(1): 69–83.

Green, S.M., Watson, R. (2006) Nutritional screening and assessment tools for use by nurses: literature review. *Journal of Advanced Nursing* **54**(4): 477–90.

Gunn, S.R., Early, B.J., Zenati, M.S., *et.al.* (2008) Use of a nasal bridle prevents accidental nasoenteral feeding tube removal. *Journal of Parenteral and Enteral Nutrition* **33**(1): 50–4.

Hallum, N.S., Baxter, J.P., O'Reilly, D., *et al.* (2010) Home parenteral nutrition in Scotland: frequency of monitoring, adequacy of review and consequence for complication rates. *Nutrition* **26**(11–12): 1139–45.

Hankey, C.R. (2010). Session 3: management of obesity weight-loss interventions in the treatment of obesity. *Proceedings of the Nutrition Society* **69**: 34–8.

Higgins, D. (2005) Nasogastric tube insertion. *Nursing Times* **101**(37): 28.

Hogston, R., Marjoram, B. (eds) (2010) *Foundations of Nursing Practice: Leading the Way,* 4th edn. Palgrave Macmillan: Basingstoke.

Howard, P. (2009) Basics in clinical nutrition: administration of enteral tube feeds. *e-SPEN, the European e-Journal of Clinical Nutrition and Metabolism* **4**(4): e170–71.

Jolly, K., Daley, A., Adab, P., *et al.* (2010) A randomised controlled trial to compare a range of commercial or primary care led weight reduction programmes with a minimal intervention control for weight loss in obesity: the Lighten Up trial. *BMC Public Health* **10**: 439.

Júnior, W.S., do Amaral, J.L., Nonino-Borges, C.B. (2011) Factors related to weight loss up to 4 years after bariatric surgery. *Obesity Surgery,* 21 April. [Epub ahead of print].

Lean, M., Wiseman, M. (2008) Malnutrition in hospitals. *British Medical Journal* **336**: 290.

Lean, M.E.J., Han, T.S., Morrison, C.E. (1995) Waist circumference as a measure for indicating need for weight management. *British Medical Journal* **311**: 158.

Ljungqvist, O., van Gossum, A., Sanz, M.L., *et.al.* (2010) The European fight against malnutrition. *Clinical Nutrition* **29**(2):149–50.

Logue, J., Thompson, L., Romanes, F., *et al.* (2010) Management of obesity: summary of SIGN guideline. *British Medical Journal* **340**: c154.

Marieb, E.N., Hoehn, K. (2010) *Human Anatomy and Physiology,* 8th edn. Benjamin-Cummings Pub: San Francisco.

Mason, P. (2010) Symposium 8: drugs and nutrition—important drug–nutrient interactions. *Proceedings of the Nutrition Society* **69**: 551–7.

Mehanna, H.M., Moledina, J., Travis, J. (2008) Refeeding syndrome: what it is, and how to prevent and treat it. *British Medical Journal* **336**: 1495–8.

Milne, A.C., Potter, J., Vivanti, A., *et.al.* (2009) Protein and energy supplementation in elderly people at risk from malnutrition.

Cochrane Database of Systematic Reviews, Issue 2: Art. No. CD003288. DOI: 10.1002/14651858. CD003288. pub3.

National Institute for Health and Clinical Excellence (NICE) (2006a) *Obesity: The Prevention, Identification, Assessment & Management of Overweight & Obesity in Adults & Children.* NICE: London. **http://www.nice.org.uk/guidance/index. jsp?action=byID&o=11000** (accessed 23 December 2010).

National Institute for Health and Clinical Excellence (NICE) (2006b) *Nutrition Support in Adults.* NICE: London. **http:// www.nice.org.uk/page.aspx?o=cg032#summary** (accessed 23 December 2010).

National Nurses Nutrition Group (NNNG) (2010) *A Competency Framework for Nutrition Nurse Specialists.* **http://www.nnng. org/Links/NNNG%20&%20BAPEN%20Correspondence/ NNNG%20Competencies%20first%20Edition%202010.pdf** (accessed 22 June 2011).

National Obesity Forum (2009) Health professionals page. **http:// www.nationalobesityforum.org.uk/index.php/healthcare-professionals.html** (accessed 13 October 2011).

National Patient Safety Agency (2011) *Reducing the Harm Caused by Misplaced Nasogastric Feeding Tubes in Adults, Children and Infants.* NPSA: London. **http://www.nrls.npsa.nhs.uk/ resources/?entryid45=129640** (accessed 13 October 2011).

NHS Information Centre (2011) Statistics on obesity, physical activity and diet: England, 2011. The Health and Social Care Information Centre: Leeds.

Nieuwenhuizen, W.F., Weenen, H., Rigby, P., *et.al.* (2010) Older adults and patients in need of nutritional support: review of current treatment options and factors influencing nutritional intake. *Clinical Nutrition* 29(2):160–9.

Nijs, K.A.N.D., De Graf, C., Siebelink, E., *et al.* (2006) Effect of family-style meals on energy intake and risk of malnutrition in Dutch nursing home residents: a randomised controlled trial. *Journal of Gerontology Series A: Biological Sciences and Medical Sciences* 61A: 935–42.

Nursing and Midwifery Council (NMC) (2010) Standards for Pre-registration Nursing Education, Annexe 3. Nursing and Midwifery Council: London.

Nursing and Midwifery Practice Development Unit (2002) *Nutrition: Assessment and Referral in the Care of Adults in Hospital.* NMPDU: London.

Office of Health Economics (2010) *Shedding the Pounds: Obesity Management, NICE Guidance and Bariatric Surgery in England.* Office of Health Economics: London.

O'Meara, D., Mireles-Cabodevila, E., Frame, F., *et al.* (2008) Evaluation of delivery of enteral nutrition in critically ill patients receiving mechanical ventilation. *American Journal of Critical Care* 17: 53–61.

Padwal, R., Klarenbach, S., Wiebe, N., *et al.* (2011) Bariatric surgery: a systematic review and network meta-analysis of randomized trials. *Obesity Reviews* 12(8): 602–21

Patterson, R.E., Pietinen, P. (2004) Assessment of nutritional status in individuals and populations. In: M.J. Gibney, B.M. Margetts, Kearnery, *et.al.* (eds) *Public Health Nutrition.* Blackwell Publishing: Oxford. pp. 66–82

Pheasant, H., Enock, K. (2010) *Obesity Care Pathway Support Package.* Public Health Action Support Team: Gerrards Cross.

Phillips, N.M., Nay, R. (2008) A systematic review of nursing administration of medication via enteral tubes in adults. *Journal of Clinical Nursing* 17(17): 2257–65.

Royal College of Physicians (2010) *Oral Feeding Difficulties and Dilemmas.* RCP: London.

Salva, A., Coll-Planas, L., Bruce, S. and the Task Force on Nutrition and Ageing of the IAGG and the IANA (2009) Nutritional assessment of residents in long-term care facilities (LTCFS): recommendations of the task force on nutrition and ageing of the IAGG European region and the IANA. *Journal of Nutrition, Health and Aging* 13(6): 475–83.

Schouten, R., Rijs, C.S., Bouvy, N.D., *et al.* (2010) A multicentre, randomized efficacy study of the EndoBarrier Gastrointestinal Liner for presurgical weight loss prior to bariatric surgery. *Annals of Surgery* 251(2): 236–43.

Scottish Government (2009) *Older People Living in the Community—Nutritional Needs, Barriers and Interventions: A Literature Review.* **http://www.scotland.gov.uk/ Publications/2009/12/07102032/6** (accessed 13 October 2011).

Scottish Intercollegiate Guidelines Network (SIGN) (2010) *Management of Obesity. A National Clinical Guideline.* Scottish Intercollegiate Guidelines Network: Edinburgh.

Singer, P., Berger, M.M., Van den Berghe, G., *et al.* (2009) ESPEN guidelines on parenteral nutrition: intensive care. *Clinical Nutrition* 28(4): 387–400.

Sriram, K., Cyriac, T., Fogg, L.F. (2010) Effect of nutritional support team restructuring on the use of parenteral nutrition. *Nutrition* 26(7–8): 735–9.

Stratton, R.J. (2007) Malnutrition: another health inequality. *Proceedings of the Nutrition Society* 66(4): 522–9.

Stratton, R.J., Green, C.J., Elia, M. (2003) *Disease Related Malnutrition.* CABI Publishing: Washington.

Truby, H., deLooy, A., Fox, K.R., *et al.* (2006) Randomised controlled trial of four commercial weight loss programmes in the UK: initial findings from the BBC 'diet trials'. *British Medical Journal* 332: 1309–14.

Vellas, B., Villars, H., Abellan, G., *et al.* (2006) Overview of the MNA: its history and challenges. *Journal of Nutrition Health and Aging* 10(6): 456–63.

Weekes, C.E., Spiro, A., Baldwin, C., *et al.* (2009) A review of the evidence for the impact of improving nutritional care on nutritional and clinical outcomes and cost. *Journal of Human Nutrition and Dietetics* 22(4): 324–35.

White, R. (2010) Symposium 8: drugs and nutrition. *Proceedings of the Nutrition Society* 69: 558–64.

WHO Europe (2010) Obesity. **http://www.euro.who.int/en/ what-we-do/health-topics/diseases-and-conditions/obesity** (accessed 13 October 2011).

Wright, L., Cotter, D., Hickson, M., *et.al.* (2005) Comparison of energy and protein intakes of older people consuming a texture modified diet with a normal hospital diet. *Journal of Human Nutrition and Dietetics* 18(3): 213–19.

25 *Managing* Pain

Nick Allcock and Ruth Day

Introduction

This chapter aims to provide you with the knowledge to be able to take an evidence-based approach to the nursing management of people who are experiencing pain. As a practising nurse, pain will be something that many of your patients will experience; however, one individual's pain may be very different from another person's. Pain can vary depending on the circumstances in which it is experienced and the individual characteristics of the person experiencing it. Understanding someone's pain experience is therefore challenging because you cannot see someone's pain or easily judge how bad it is, what it feels like, or how it affects him or her. This chapter provides you with knowledge and skills to recognize, assess, and manage the patient's experience of pain effectively with evidence-based strategies.

Understanding the importance of managing pain

Defining pain

The variability of the experience of pain makes defining pain difficult. Pain is something that we have all experienced at some point in our lives and therefore, through these experiences, we have developed an understanding of what we consider to be pain. One of the most widely accepted definitions is that of the International Association for the Study of Pain (IASP), which defines pain as:

> An unpleasant sensory and emotional experience associated with actual or potential tissue damage, or described in terms of such damage. (Merskey and Bogduk, 1994)

Although this definition is often quoted, the difficulty in defining pain is illustrated by the fact that the IASP added a note (go to **http://www.iasp-pain.org/** and search for 'pain definitions') to highlight the individual nature of pain and the fact that pain is a sensory experience with an emotional component. The individual nature of pain is also highlighted by another commonly used definition:

> Pain is whatever the experiencing person says it is and happens whenever he/she says it does. (McCaffery, 1972)

This definition highlights the fact that pain is an individual experience and that measuring pain objectively is difficult. Therefore asking the person and actively listening to the self-report of the experience is the best way in which to understand another person's pain. A common criticism of McCaffery's definition is that some people cannot say what they are experiencing. McCaffery argued that people can also communicate through body language and facial expressions, and it is important to use all of the possible ways in which pain can be communicated. However, describing pain is not always easy because it is a complex combination of sensory, emotional, and behavioural factors.

> **THEORY INTO PRACTICE 25.1**
> **How would you describe pain?**
>
> Think about the last time you experienced pain: how would you describe it? What words would you use?

Categories of pain

Although pain is normally unpleasant, it does have a protective role in making us aware that we are experiencing something that is potentially damaging. In the relatively rare circumstances in which someone is unable to feel pain, this can result in people harming themselves. For example, researchers identified a 10-year-old child in Pakistan who was well known to the medical service after regularly performing 'street theatre' (Cox *et al.*, 2006). He placed knives through his arms and walked on burning coals owing to an inherited inability to experience pain; sadly, he died before seeing his 14th birthday, after jumping off a house roof. It is therefore important to distinguish between different types of pain. Pain has been divided into acute, chronic, or persistent pain (more recently, this is sometimes referred to as non-acute pain), and cancer-related pain.

Acute pain is pain of (recent) sudden onset and (probably) limited duration, usually associated with an injury or disease. Acute pain includes postoperative pain and pain associated with trauma such as fractures. Although often of limited duration, acute pain can have a range of negative emotional effects, as well as physical effects on respiratory, circulatory, and endocrine systems. Poorly controlled acute pain may increase the likelihood of an individual developing chronic pain (Allcock, 2000).

Chronic or persistent pain is defined as pain that persists beyond the time at which healing would be expected to have been complete, or that is associated with disease in which healing does not take place. Some definitions also refer to pain that persists beyond 3 months (e.g. Merskey and Bogduk, 1994). It is important to note that chronic pain can sometimes exist in patients with no evidence of tissue damage.

Cancer pain is pain that is caused by or related to cancer or the treatment of cancer. For further discussion of cancer mechanisms, refer to Chapter 4 Understanding Cancer ⟹.

Acute and chronic pain may be regarded as a continuum; however, it is important to take into account the very different approaches that may be needed to treat these different types of pain. Similar interventions may be used, but the approach to pain management, the way in which they are applied, and the aims of the interventions may be very different in acute and chronic pain. For example, in acute pain, treatment may be aimed at preventing or quickly addressing and reducing a patient's pain as much as possible. In contrast, the aim of care with chronic pain may be more appropriately focused at maintaining function and ability to maintain a quality of life.

Prevalence and epidemiological profile of pain

Data show that patients in hospitals experience unnecessary pain. The Care Quality Commission inpatient survey of 2008 identified that 66% of patients reported being in pain during their stay, a figure that has changed little over the past 5 years. Despite this, 72% of patients reported that hospital staff did everything they could to help to control the pain. Although pain is often associated with postoperative care, it is also common in medical patients, with 52% of patients on medical wards reporting pain. Of these, 20% reported severe pain and 12% unbearable pain (Dix, 2004).

Similar findings have been reported in the US, where approximately 80% of patients experienced acute moderate, severe, or extreme pain after surgery. Almost 25% of patients who received pain medications experienced adverse effects; however, almost 90% of them reported being satisfied with their pain medications (Apfelbaum *et al.*, 2003). However, Dolin *et al.* (2002), in a review of the effectiveness of acute postoperative pain management, suggested that there had been improvement, although UK Audit Commission targets are yet to be met. In a brief reference to postoperative pain in 1997, the Audit Commission proposed a standard that <20% of patients should experience severe pain, which should reduce to <5% by 2002.

Chronic pain is a devastating and widespread problem affecting one in five adults across Europe. Sufferers are affected for an average of 7 years, with one in five suffering for 20 years or more (Breivik *et al.*, 2006). A UK survey in 2005 suggested that pain is experienced every day or most days by one in five (21%) of us, and a further one in four (26%) said they had pain some days (British Pain Society, 2005).

Research has demonstrated that 77% of cancer sufferers report pain attributable to their cancer. Almost one-third of cancer patients have been experiencing pain for more than 12 months and more than half of patients experience pain at least once a day, while almost a quarter of patients who experience moderate to severe pain are not receiving treatment for it (European Association of Palliative Care (EAPC), 2007).

Understanding the pathophysiology of pain

New imaging and experimental techniques have expanded our understanding of pain mechanisms. The processes by which pain is recognized are normally initiated in the periphery and can be divided into four stages: transduction, transmission, perception, and modulation (McCaffery and Pasero, 1999).

Transduction

Most pain occurs in response to (potential) tissue damage that is detected by nerve endings that respond to strong stimuli. The nerve endings are called **nociceptors** and can respond to thermal, mechanical, and chemical stimuli. These are referred to as high-threshold nociceptors. The nociceptors can be stimulated by a range of chemical mediators released from damaged cells, including **prostaglandins**, bradykinin, **serotonin**, substance P, potassium, and histamine.

Transmission

Nociceptors transmit action potentials to the spinal cord along two different types of fibre: A and C fibres.

A fibres: these myelinated fibres conduct at a speed of 12–20 m/s. These fast signals allow us to locate the pain and to respond quickly. A fibres produce localized sharp stinging, pricking pain referred to as fast or first pain.

C fibres: these smaller, unmyelinated fibres are responsible for the delayed slower signals and conduct at a speed of 0.5–2 m/s. They are stimulated in tissue damage such as trauma, surgery, or inflammation. Some C fibres in the skin and viscera are not normally active, or are 'silent', and become active only when inflammatory processes are stimulated. C fibre pain is dull and diffuse, and may be burning or aching in nature, and is referred to as slow or second pain.

The A and C fibres conduct the stimuli from the sensory nerve endings in the periphery to the central nervous system, where they **synapse** in the **dorsal horn** of the spinal cord (Figure 25.1). A fibres and C fibres synapse at different levels in the dorsal horn, and send messages via secondary neurones through three different pathways—the neospinothalamic, paleospinothalamic, and archispinothalamic tracts—which connect to various structures in the central nervous system.

Perception

Once nociceptive signals are transmitted to the central nervous system, fibres connect to a range of structures in the brain that are involved in our perception of these signals as pain, and our affective behavioural and physiological responses to pain (Table 25.1). The complexity of these connections and the range of centres involved illustrate the complex nature of the pain experience and the reasons why pain is such an individual experience.

Modulation

Our increasing understanding of the mechanisms responsible for pain has led to an appreciation of the way in which nociceptive inputs to the central nervous system can be modified at several different stages. The concept of the gate control mechanism of pain first proposed by Melzack and Wall in 1965 suggested that the pain signals arriving in the spinal cord can be blocked by messages from other fibres that respond to touch and pressure (Figure 25.2). Thus, rubbing an area you have just hit can block the pain messages—a mechanism that explains some of the effect of interventions such as massage, and transcutaneous electrical nerve stimulation (TENS) and heat. However, the processes by which pain messages can be modulated also involve descending messages from the brain that can

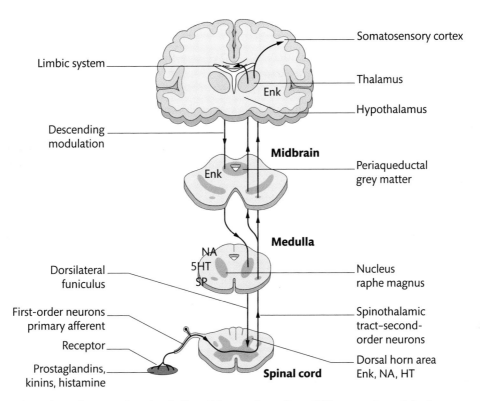

Figure 25.1 The pain pathway. Enk, enkephaline; NA, noradrenaline; 5HT, serotonin or 5-hydroxytryptamine; SP, substance P.

Reprinted from *Rheumatology*, 3rd edn, Hochberg, M.C., Silman, A.J., Smolen, J.S., Weinblatt, M.E., Weisman, M.H., with permission from Elsevier.

Table 25.1 Structures in the brain and their pain-related functions

Structure	Function
Thalamus	Many nuclei within the thalamus are involved in pain pathways; fibres from these nuclei link to a range of structures in the brain
Hypothalamus	Provides the links to the endocrine system; endocrine responses to pain include increases in cortisone, glucagon, growth hormone, and catecholamines
Periaqueductal grey and nucleus raphe magnus	Involved in descending inhibitory systems
Reticular formation	This area of the brain is responsible for our alertness
Cerebral cortex	Pain is interpreted in relation to our past experiences, our culture, understanding, and the context in which the pain occurs
Somatosensory cortex	The area of the brain that allows the recognition of the location and sensory qualities of the pain
Limbic system	A collection of structures that constitute the emotional centre of the brain; this area is responsible for the affective component of the pain, fear, anxiety, and interruption of sleep

inhibit pain (descending inhibitory control) and descending excitatory pathways. The nervous systems that are involved in pain are therefore very adaptable; this is referred to as neuroplasticity. Nociceptive inputs can lead to changes in the way in which signals are processed, leading to an increased sensitivity to pain—a process referred to as sensitization. This can lead to patients experiencing allodynia (pain in response to stimuli that would not normally be painful) and hyperalgesia (excessive pain in response to a normally painful stimulus). These processes help to explain why some chronic pain patients continue to experience pain despite the lack of any identifiable tissue damage.

Types of pain

Neuropathic pain

As well as nociceptive and inflammatory pain mechanisms, pain can result from injury to nerve fibres that may result in abnormal functioning of the nerves. Neuropathic pain has been defined as 'pain initiated or caused by

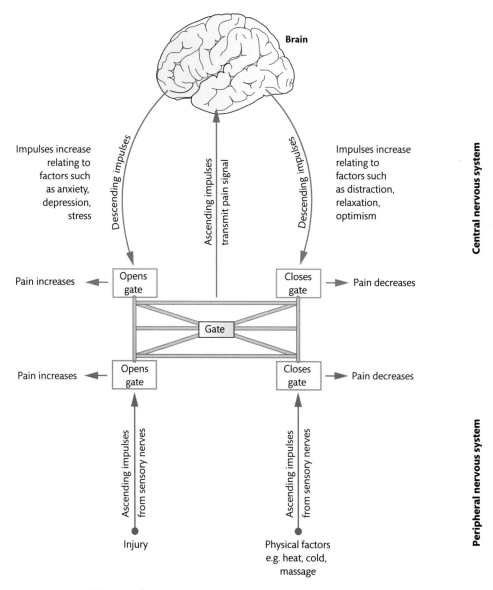

Figure 25.2 Gate control theory of pain.

Reproduced from Doherty and McCallum, *Foundation Clinical Nursing Skills*, by permission of Oxford University Press.

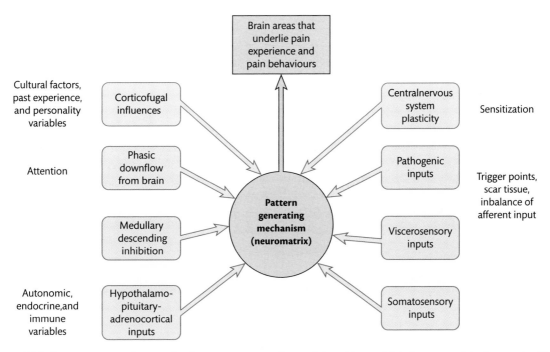

Figure 25.3 Pattern-generating mechanism or neuromatrix modulated by multiple inputs and the internal milieu.

Reproduced from John D. Loeser, Ronald Melzack. Pain: an overview. *Lancet* 1999; 353: 1607–9, by permission of Elsevier.

a primary lesion or dysfunction in the nervous system' (Merskey and Bogduk, 1994; Loeser and Treede, 2008). Damage to nerves from trauma (crushing, surgery) or from medical conditions (diabetes, infection, e.g. shingles) can lead to loss of sensation, but also to pain. This type of pain can result from abnormal functioning of the nerves or disruption to the balance of excitatory and inhibitory pathways. Neuropathic pain is often described in terms such as burning, shooting, and shock—descriptors that have been incorporated into many assessment tools for neuropathic pain (Jensen, 2006).

Visceral pain

There are fewer (<1%) nociceptors in visceral structures (the internal organs) compared with the somatic structures (skin and muscles, as well as in joints, bones, and ligaments). Visceral pain is therefore different in nature from that from somatic structures. Pain from visceral structures is poorly localized and diffuse, and can be referred to other structures that are sometimes at some distance from the source of the pain.

Pain neuromatrix

The complexity of the systems responsible for our experience of pain and the different inputs into the system has been summarized in the concept of a pain neuromatrix (Melzack and Loeser, 1978; Melzack, 1990). Figure 25.3 illustrates the concept of the neuromatrix, illustrating the inputs to the brain structures that process the nociceptive inputs and interpret them as pain.

The human, social, and financial burden of pain

In 2004, the International Association for the Study of Pain and the World Health Organization promoted the Global Day against Pain, suggesting that pain management was a universal human right. Brennan *et al.* (2007) suggest that:

> unreasonable failure to treat pain is viewed worldwide as poor medicine, unethical practice, and an abrogation of a fundamental human right.

Pain has a significant impact on physical, psychological, and social aspects of the sufferer's life. The UK's Chief

---

EVIDENCE BOX 25.1
Acceptance therapy for chronic pain

New approaches to treating chronic pain focus on reducing the distressing and disabling influences of pain as they concern important areas of a patient's life, rather than on reducing pain. In this study, an acceptance-based approach to chronic pain within an interdisciplinary treatment programme was evaluated. Some 108 patients with complex chronic pain conditions completed treatment. The treatment included a number of exposure-based, experiential, and other behaviour change methods focused on increasing:

(a) engagement in daily activity regardless of pain; and

(b) willingness to have pain present without responding to it.

Significant improvements in emotional, social, and physical functioning and healthcare use were demonstrated following treatment, and the majority of these improvements were maintained at 3 months post treatment. Improvements in most outcomes during treatment were correlated with increases in acceptance.

Adapted from McCracken, L.M., Vowles, K.E., Eccleston, C. (2005) Acceptance-based treatment for persons with long standing chronic pain: a preliminary analysis of treatment outcomes in comparison to a waiting phase. *Behaviour Research and Therapy* 43: 1335–46.

Medical Officer (2009) suggested that chronic pain appears to be more common now than it was 40 years ago, and that chronic pain has a major impact on people's lives, causing sleeplessness and depression, and interfering with normal physical and social functioning (also see Evidence box 25.1). Over 40% of chronic pain sufferers say that their pain impacts on everyday activities, from lifting and carrying to taking exercise and sleeping. Despite advances in the management of chronic pain, many chronic pain patients still suffer unnecessarily owing to inadequate evaluation, assessment, monitoring, and treatment (Breivik *et al.*, 2006). In the UK, of those suffering from chronic pain, 25% had lost their jobs and 24% had been diagnosed with depression. Chronic and recurrent pain can therefore have a significant impact on an individual's self-worth (Morley, 2008).

Nursing responsibility for pain management

Acute pain has a significant impact on a range of physiological responses associated with injury. Pain can contribute to protein catabolism, raised free fatty acid levels (lipolysis), hyperglycaemia, and changes in water and electrolyte balance (Wu and Liu, 2008; Carli and Schricker, 2009). These responses can also lead to cardiovascular effects from increased sympathetic activity, and a range of

effects on coagulation, respiration, and immune function (Wu and Liu, 2008). Many of these changes are contrary to promoting tissue healing and recovery, and potentially leave the patient at increased risk of complications. Acute pain can also lead to a range of psychological effects, including anxiety, inability to sleep, demoralization, a feeling of helplessness, loss of control, and inability to think and interact with others (Cousins *et al.*, 2004). Unrelieved acute pain may also be a contributing factor in the development of chronic pain (Perkins and Kehlet, 2000).

The impact of both acute and chronic pain on the individual can therefore be significant. The cost of unrelieved pain across Europe is huge, with pain accounting for an estimated 500 million lost working days every year; this costs the European economy at least €34 billion (Breivik *et al.*, 2006).

Nurses play an important role in the multidisciplinary team approach that is required for effective pain management. In the UK, since the report on pain after surgery, most hospitals have introduced acute pain services (APS) with the responsibility to manage pain, as well as service development training, audit, and research. There is still a lot of variation in the structure and operation of APS; however, nurses play a key role in these services.

Nurses also play an important role working with other healthcare professionals, including medical specialists, pharmacists, psychologists, physiotherapists, and occupational therapists to manage chronic pain conditions

CASE STUDY 25.1 *Janet Allcock, aged 73, retired healthcare worker and housewife living in Eastbourne*

'It's very hard for me to actually give you a time when the pain started because it has been from various causes. When I look back, the arthritis must have started at least 20 years ago in that I used to have quite bad neck pain—which of course one puts down to lying awkwardly or being in a draught or something like that, but gradually you realise it's because of wear and tear. It's a pain that varies from a stabbing, like a hot knife going through a joint, to something like a continual pressure that [makes] you want to try and move the joint and get rid of it, but it just doesn't go; and on some days it's a continual dull ache. And together with the pain, depending on the severity, goes the depression, because I do find it's a very depressing illness. I think what worries me the most about pain is how it takes over and becomes the centre of your life. The rest of your life revolves around the amount of pain you've got. Whether you can go out with your family or go on an outing or just go to the shops depends on the amount of pain and what effect it's having on you at that moment in time. Nobody really wants to know or discuss [your pain] to any length. And that's quite difficult because your life tends to revolve around pain and yet, at the same time, it's not something that's seen as being something you can talk too much about. This is why I use the word "lonely", and I think pain can make you feel lonely because you feel that you're the only one who is suffering and can cope with it, and that is a lonely experience'.

(The full case study and others can be found in Kumar and Allcock (2008) *Pain in Older People: Reflections and experiences from an older person's perspective*, Help the Aged. Available on the Age UK website at **http://www.ageuk.org.uk/documents/en-gb/for-professionals/research/pain%20in%20older%20people%20%282008%29_pro.pdf?dtrk=true.**

both in secondary and primary care. Many nurses have developed innovative services (Carr *et al.*, 2010) and are involved in delivering complementary therapies; however, there is still a need to make pain management a greater priority (Taylor and Stanbury, 2009).

Clinical assessment of pain

Whilst all members of the healthcare team have a responsibility to assess a patient's pain, it could be argued that nurses have a pivotal role, undertaking pain assessment alongside the monitoring of other vital signs (temperature, pulse, blood pressure, and respirations). The Chronic Pain Policy Coalition has spearheaded a campaign in the UK to establish pain as the '5th Vital Sign'® (CPPC, 2007). Accurate assessment and measurement of pain is necessary in diagnosing the cause of the pain, choosing a method of pain relief, and evaluating its effectiveness.

Sometimes, the cause of the pain may seem obvious, such as after surgery, but it is good nursing practice not to assume that this is so and to ask the patient directly. Case Study 25.2 shows the importance of this.

What needs to be assessed?

Undertaking a pain assessment needs a structured approach to include a number of elements (Table 25.2). The frequency of assessment will vary. In acute pain, the intensity of the pain may be assessed every 15 minutes in the first hour after surgery. In long-standing pain, assessment may occur formally only at outpatient appointments, but more aspects of the experience of pain, will be explored.

The results of the assessment should be documented in the patient's notes so that all healthcare professionals are aware of the issues, treatment, and related outcomes.

Pain should be assessed both when the patient is at rest (static) and during movement (dynamic or functional). In acute pain, for example after surgery, pain may be controlled at rest, but may be so severe on movement that the patient is unable to undertake physiotherapy exercises. In such cases, the pain causes a lack of function that may lead to unwanted outcomes. In chronic pain, the efficacy of an intervention is frequently assessed by an improvement in function: is the patient able to walk further, engage in work, household tasks, sleep better, or cope with other activities of living?

Assessing pain is part of the nurse's skill in many nursing situations. Chapter 28 Managing Wounds ⟶ indicates the need for good pain assessment in the management of wounds; it is also an important part of procedural management (Chapter 26 Managing Perioperative Care ⟶). In palliative care, pain assessment is a part of the assessment of the whole person, including spiritual and family aspects (see Chapter 4 Understanding Cancer ⟶ for further exploration of this). Visit the Online Resource Centre where you will find a role play exercise to complete with your colleagues @ .

What pain assessment tool should you use?

Measurement and assessment of pain should be based on the patient's own report of his or her pain; studies have shown that the correlation of the patient's report and the nurse's assessment is poor. Nurses frequently underestimate patients' pain (Zalon, 1993; Sloman *et al.*, 2005; Cox, 2009).

Using a validated pain assessment tool is good nursing practice, and the City of Hope website provides updated information on a wide variety of pain assessment tools

---

CASE STUDY 25.2
Assessing pain

Mr K was admitted to the vascular ward following a below-knee amputation of his right leg. He had an epidural in progress. When asked, he rated his pain as 8/10 and getting worse. Initially, it was thought that his epidural was ineffective, but, on further investigation, it transpired that his severe pain was from a long-standing upper back problem for which he used a TENS machine. This was applied and his pain reduced to his normal levels.

Table 25.2 Elements of a pain assessment

Site of pain	Location of the pain (verbal description, pointing it out, drawing on a body map) (Note that pain may be present in multiple areas.)
What caused it?	Trauma, surgery, unknown
Character of the pain	These descriptors may be sensory (sharp, throbbing, shooting) or affective (exhausting, sickening)
Intensity of the pain	Needs to be assessed at rest and on movement. Does it alter during the day? Is it continuous or intermittent? What is the worst it has been and the best?
Effect of the pain on activities of daily living	Does the pain interfere with activities such as walking or coughing? Is it disturbing the patient's sleep?
Treatment	What is the current treatment and is it effective?
Other symptoms	For example, does the pain make the patient feel sick?
Relevant medical history	For example, underlying painful conditions and previous treatment
Enquire about other factors that may influence treatment	Beliefs about the cause of the pain; pain management preferences; previously used coping strategies; any anxiety or depression

(http://prc.coh.org/pain_assessment.asp). Because pain can occur in many different situations, the use of assessment tools needs to be appropriate to the context. Pain specialist nurses can be a useful resource if you are unsure about the appropriateness of tools.

Sometimes, it is impossible to obtain a reliable self-report of pain and in these circumstances it is even more important to use a validated assessment tool. There are pain assessment tools available for young children (Franck *et al.*, 2000), critical care patients (Puntillo *et al.*, 1997; Géli-nas *et al.*, 2006), and people with impaired cognition (see http://prc.coh.org/PAIN-NOA.htm for a range of tools). Sometimes, hearing or language difficulties make pain assessment challenging; the British Pain Society provides a pain assessment tool in various languages.

A variety of pain assessment tools are available, many of which are available online. Some tools are best used in the acute setting" some in chronic pain, and some for particular patient groups.

Unidimensional tools

Unidimensional tools measure intensity, which is only one aspect of pain, but usually the simplest and most frequently used measure.

1. The verbal rating scale (VRS) uses words to describe the intensity of pain. Terms such as 'none', 'mild', 'moderate', and 'severe' are used (Moore *et al.*, 2003). This scale is quick and easy to use, and is particularly useful when a simple approach is needed, such as with elderly patients or people with mild cognitive impairment (Closs *et al.*, 2004).

2. The numerical rating scale (NRS) asks the patient to apply a number to the intensity of his or her pain. It can be used verbally or as a written scale. It is important to be aware of the range of these scales because they commonly vary between 0–3, 0–5, 0–10, or even 0–100. Zero (0) indicates no pain, and the higher the number, the worse the pain. When using these scales, it must be clear what the denominator is, because a pain score of 3 may indicate severe pain (in a 0–3 scale) or mild pain (in a 0–10 score).

3. The visual analogue scale (VAS) comprises a printed 10 cm line with words anchoring either end. Usually, the left-hand end is anchored with a descriptor such as 'no pain' and the right-hand end with 'worst pain possible'. The patient is asked to mark a point along the line indicating the amount of pain that he or she has.

Table 25.3 Unidimensional pain rating scales

VRS	No pain	Mild	Moderate	Severe
NRS (0–3)	0	1	2	3
NRS (0–10)	0	1–3	4–6	7–10
VAS (0–100 mm)	0–5	5–44	45–74	75+

Source: (Based on Aubrun *et al.*, 2003; Brevik *et al.*, 2000)

There has been shown to be good correlation across these various unidimensional pain rating scales, as Table 25.3 shows.

In persistent pain, a unidimensional pain relief scale may be used; rather than measuring the intensity of the pain, it measures the effectiveness of the pain intervention by applying a number to the amount of pain relief obtained.

Multidimensional tools

The main disadvantage of a unidimensional tool is that it reports only one aspect of the pain experience. Sometimes this is adequate: for example, when checking that pain relief medication is effective. However, often other information is needed. The location of the pain can be helpful in identifying the cause and if a patient is experiencing multiple pains. For example, someone having surgery may suffer from arthritis and have joint pain, may have muscle pain caused by positioning during surgery, or may experience pain from drains or other equipment as well as the surgical wound.

Multidimensional tools aim to discover more about the pain than intensity, including the pain's characteristics (what it feels like), its location and temporal features, as well as the impact that the pain has on the patient in areas such as sleep, mood, and function. These tools take longer to complete and, although sometimes used in the acute setting, are more frequently seen in the management of persistent pain.

Two frequently used multidimensional tools are the Brief Pain Inventory (BPI) and the Short Form McGill Pain Questionnaire (SF-MPQ). The BPI is a measurement tool for both the pain and its impact on the life of the patient (covering areas such as sleep, work, and mobility) (Daut *et al.*, 1983). The SF-MPQ (Melzack, 1987) explores the characteristics of the pain with a 10 cm VAS, a 6-point verbal rating score of present pain, and a selection of words describing the characteristics of the pain. A recent adaptation of the tool includes specific descriptors for neuropathic pain (SF_MPQ2; Dworkin *et al.*, 2009; see **http://prc.coh.org/res_inst.asp**).

Psychologically focused pain assessments may be made, reflecting the understanding that pain can impact on both physical function and psychological function.

Using a pain assessment tool does not ensure that a patient experiences good pain management, but good assessment is essential to ensure that appropriate decisions about interventions are made.

Accessing the evidence to inform clinical decisions

The evidence base for pain management is constantly being revised in the light of new laboratory and clinical studies. It is an enormous task to sift through the evidence, therefore it is invaluable to look at a few key areas before making a clinical decision. There are some guidelines on specific areas of pain management in the UK NICE guidelines (mostly chronic pain); the following websites and journals are pain-orientated.

- *Acute Pain Management: Scientific Evidence*, 3rd edn, assesses the current evidence and best practice in acute pain, and is available from **http://www.nhmrc.gov.au/publications/synopses/cp104syn.htm**
- The Cochrane Collaboration has a library of healthcare-related evidence with a substantial number of reviews relating to pain and can be found at **http://www.thecochranelibrary.com/view/0/index.html**
- Bandolier is a website that also provides evidence for interventions in healthcare and hosts the Oxford Pain website: **http://www.medicine.ox.ac.uk/bandolier/**
- **http://www.pain-out.eu/** is the website for PainOut. This is a multinational research project that has the objective of developing benchmarking, a clinical decision support system and a knowledge library to enable clinicians in the management of postoperative pain.
- The journal *PAIN* is published by the International Association for the Study of Pain and there are other well-established pain journals (e.g. *The Clinical Journal of Pain*, *The European Journal of Pain*). In the UK,

the British Pain Society publishes a newsletter and a journal (*Reviews in Pain*) and the RCN also has a pain forum with a newsletter.

- Hospital and trust guidelines should be based on best evidence and should be revised regularly.

Using the evidence base in the nursing management of pain

In nursing a patient with pain, it is important to take a holistic approach to consider the biological, psychological, and social impact of the pain (biopsychosocial); the neuromatrix theory of pain (see Figure 25.3) shows the interplay of these factors in the perception of pain. Although nurses frequently rely on medical interventions in the management of pain (surgery, drugs), there is a large evidence base for the use of psychological interventions and other non-pharmacological strategies.

Relieving pain

Pharmacological approaches

A multimodal approach is taken to the management of pain in acute, persistent, and cancer pain in order to respond to the variety of pain pathways (described above) and the different neurotransmitters involved. Similar medications are seen in all three areas, but the use of them differs. For instance, in acute pain, opiate-naive patients may be exposed to large amounts of opiate-based analgesics for a short period of time; in cancer pain, they may be exposed to gradually increasing amounts of opiate-based medication over a long period of time. To monitor and evaluate pain relief appropriately, you should understand both the medications being used and the way in which they are being used (see Chapter 22 Managing Medicines ➡).

The WHO Pain Ladder (**http://www.who.int/cancer/palliative/painladder/en/**) has been instrumental in challenging clinicians' approaches to acute and persistent pain management. This ladder links the severity of the pain to the medication choice.

Medications used in pain management fall into three groups: non-opioid analgesics; opioid analgesics; and other agents (Table 25.4).

Table 25.4 **Some examples of medications used in pain management**

Non-opioid analgesics	Opioid analgesics	Other agents
Paracetamol	Tramadol	Local anaesthetics (e.g. bupivacaine, lidocaine)
Non-steroidal anti-inflammatory drugs (e.g. ibuprofen, diclofenac, celecoxib)	Codeine	Antidepressants (e.g. amitriptyline)
	Morphine	Anticonvulsants (e.g. gabapentin)
Nefopam	Oxycodone	Ketamine
	Fentanyl	Entonox®

As Chapter 22 ⇒ makes clear, the nurse administering the medication and monitoring its effect should understand what it is expected to do and what the common side effects of the drug are. The *British National Formulary* is a good place to find this information (**www.bnf.org**). Sometimes, these drugs are administered in a technically advanced manner: for instance, via an indwelling epidural catheter or patient-controlled analgesia system. Hospital guidelines will detail the safety of the patient's care environment, observations to be completed, and action to be taken in the event of problems related to particular administration techniques. It is your responsibility to ensure that you understand local policy.

Non-opioid analgesics

Paracetamol

Paracetamol is an effective analgesic, frequently underestimated, and should be the mainstay of any multimodal analgesic approach. It is well tolerated, has few side effects, and can be given via a number of routes. It has been shown to be useful in postoperative pain (Barden *et al.*, 2004a) and as an adjunct to opioids, reducing opioid requirements by 20–30% (Rømsing *et al.*, 2002). It must be given regularly to achieve this effect.

Non-steroidal anti-inflammatory drugs (NSAIDs)

NSAIDs are effective analgesics in acute and chronic pain conditions (Barden *et al.*, 2004b; Roelofs *et al.*, 2010), and can be given with opioids and paracetamol to reduce opioid use postoperatively. Use of an NSAID and paracetamol together improves pain relief (Rømsing *et al.*, 2002). They are an integral part of the concept of multimodal analgesia.

However, NSAIDs do have significant contraindications and side effects, limiting the patients who should use them (consult the BNF). Cyclo-oxygenase-2 selective inhibitors (COX-2 inhibitors) are as effective as NSAIDs and have been developed to overcome some of the side effects of NSAIDs. COX-2 inhibitors do show fewer side effects than traditional NSAIDs, but there is evidence that some patients have a greater risk of cardiovascular events when using some COX-2 inhibitors (Roelofs *et al.*, 2010).

Opioid analgesics

For managing severe to moderate pain, opioids in conjunction with non-opioids are the drugs of choice (Macintyre *et al.*, 2010). Although the action of the drugs and side effects are similar, they are divided into two groups: weak (e.g. codeine) and strong (e.g. morphine, fentanyl). Opioids can be given by many routes, but it is important to remember that the side effects are the same whichever route is used. Monitoring for life-threatening side effects (e.g. respiratory depression) is often undertaken routinely when a technically advanced delivery system (e.g. intravenous patient-controlled analgesia system, or PCA) is used, but not when the same drug is administered orally.

Dosages of opioids vary depending on the route and the specific drug. Titrating the effective dose for a specific patient can be challenging. In acute pain, the best predictor of opiate use in adults is age, with older patients requiring less (Macintyre and Jarvis, 1996). However, individual requirements may vary up to tenfold. In cancer pain, large doses of opiates may be used, but the time period for titration is usually greater and treatment is started with smaller doses. The use of strong opioids in persistent pain is widespread, and is the subject of much debate. Evidence shows that long-term opiate use can have deleterious effects to the immune and neuroendocrine systems, as well as involve the development of tolerance and escalation of doses (The British Pain Society, 2010b).

Further information on the use of specific opioids in pain management can be found in the *British National Formualry*, Macintyre and Ready (2001), and Stannard and Booth (1998).

Other agents

The transmission and perception of pain is complex, and involves neuronal pathways that are not affected by traditional analgesics. For example, neuropathic pain is often not responsive to usual medications, and so anticonvulsants (e.g. gabapentin) and antidepressants (e.g. amitriptyline) are used. Nitrous oxide and oxygen (Entonox®) is an inhalation agent that can be used for short painful procedures during which a quick onset of pain relief is needed (Macintyre *et al.*, 2010).

Non-pharmacological approaches

It is helpful to consider non-pharmacological strategies within a biopsychosocial framework. The list in Table 25.5 is by no means exhaustive and there are many approaches that individual patients will have found useful. A challenge is that many of these strategies do not have a robust evidence base because they do not easily lend themselves to testing in a double-blind randomized controlled trial. There is much debate about the efficacy of many of these approaches and how much of their effect is due to a placebo effect. However, the nature of the placebo effect in pain is itself complex and is beginning to be seen in a more positive light (Colloca and Benedetti, 2005).

Use of these strategies involves a wide range of healthcare professionals and demonstrates the need for an interdisciplinary approach to pain management. Self-help is also important, particularly in chronic pain, and the Expert Patient Programme (**http://www.expertpatients.co.uk/**) provides a good resource.

Preventing the problem of pain

When possible, pain should be anticipated. For patients with planned admissions for elective surgery, a plan for postoperative pain management should begin at pre-assessment. A growing number of elective patients present with long-standing pain conditions and need extra consideration in planning pain relief. Written provision of

Table 25.5 Table of some non-pharmacological strategies for pain management

Method of pain relief	Examples
Physical	Position of the injured part
	Exercise
	Acupuncture
	TENS
	Heat/ice packs
	Desensitization
Psychological	Information and explanation
	Cognitive behavioural therapy
	Hypnosis
	Focusing
	Distraction/relaxation
Social	Adaptation of environment
	Involvement of relatives and friends
	Awareness of cultural differences

individual guidance for their pain management helps to coordinate all involved in their treatment.

Movement frequently causes an exacerbation of pain, and employing a pain management strategy prior to this can improve function in all types of pain. Some painful nursing procedures are planned (e.g. dressing changes) and it is good practice to give pain relief prior to these (e.g. Entonox®).

Chronic pain following surgery is common (Kehlet *et al.*, 2006), and consideration should be given to both pre-emptive and preventative analgesic interventions. An example would be the use of a preoperative dose of gabapentin and the use of ketamine postoperatively (Macintyre *et al.*, 2010).

Taking analgesics regularly, in anticipation of the pain returning, will speed up patients' recovery. The provision of effective pain management is basic to the provision of enhanced recovery from surgical techniques (Kehlet, 2009). In chronic pain, the use of pacing and goal-setting aims to prevent the distress of the pain and its interference with daily life (The British Pain Society, 2010a).

Nurses have a key role to play in the prevention of pain, providing information about the many strategies that are available. Most hospitals have a pain service (acute, chronic, or combined) with a variety of specialists. They are happy to provide advice and practical help when challenges in pain management are anticipated.

Evaluating the impact of nursing interventions for pain

In adopting best practice, nurses should regularly assess whether patients are experiencing pain and how interventions implemented have affected the level of pain experienced. Information about how to do this has been given in previous sections.

Each hospital or trust with a chronic or acute pain service should audit the impact of the service on the experience of its patients. It can be difficult to measure the impact of interventions for pain, but patients should be satisfied that all is being done to try to manage their pain.

The Department of Health published a new benchmark for the prevention and management of pain in 2010. Benchmarks aim to support localized quality improvement and therefore can be used to measure pain assessment and management services. The benchmarking process aims to help practitioners to take a structured approach to sharing and comparing practice, enabling them to identify best practice and to develop action plans to remedy poor practice.

Pain is also audited nationally by the Care Quality Commission in its survey of the experiences of inpatients. Recent information can be obtained via its website at **www.cqc.org.uk** and searching for the 'inpatient survey.'

Sources of evidence-based nursing

To stay up to date in this field, please look at the sources of evidence described at the end of the chapter.

Summary and key messages

Nurses have a key role as members of the interdisciplinary team in the assessment, management, and prevention of pain. Pain, and the response to it, is an individual experience. Pain may be acute, persistent, or related to cancer, or a combination of these. When assessing pain, the use of a validated pain assessment tool is recommended and the choice of tool determined by the patient (e.g. a child, or someone unable to communicate, or able adult). In most cases, a self-report tool will be the best choice.

Where possible, pain should be anticipated and treated in a multimodal manner by an interdisciplinary team supported by a specialist service. In acute pain following major surgery, a multimodal analgesic approach is appropriate (paracetamol, NSAID, and opiate), along with simple non-pharmacological strategies (e.g. positioning, ice pack). With persistent pain, there may be a greater emphasis on non-pharmacological approaches (e.g. cognitive behavioural therapy, goal-setting), with the use of common analgesics and other adjunctive medications (e.g. antidepressants). The multimodal approach reflects the complex pathways through which pain is perceived.

Nurses need to consider pain management as the fifth vital sign, which should be documented and evaluated.

Online Resource Centre

 To help you to develop and apply your knowledge and decision-making skills further, we have provided interactive learning resources online at **www.oxfordtextbooks.co.uk/orc/bullock/**

Whilst these are freely available, you will need to use the access codes at the start of the book.

References

Allcock, N. (2000) Physiological rationale for early pain management. *Professional Nurse* **15**(6): 395–7.

Apfelbaum, J.L., Chen, C., Mehta, S.S., *et al.* (2003) Postoperative pain experience: results from a national survey suggest postoperative pain continues to be undermanaged. *Anesthesia & Analgesia* **97**(2): 534–40.

Aubrun, F., Langeron, O., Quesnel, C., *et al.* (2003) Relationship between measurement of pain using visual analog score and morphine requirements during postoperative intravenous morphine titration. *Anesthesiology* **98**: 1415–21.

Audit Commission (1997) *Anaesthesia Under Examination.* Audit Commission: London.

Barden, J., Edwards, J., Moore, R.A., *et al.* (2004a) Single dose oral paracetamol (acetaminophen) for postoperative pain. *Cochrane Database of Systematic Reviews* Issue 1: Art. No. CD004602. DOI: 10.1002/14651858.CD004602. pub2.

Barden, J., Edwards, J., Moore, R.A., *et al.* (2004b) Single dose oral diclofenac for postoperative pain in adults. *Cochrane Database of Systematic Reviews* Issue 2: Art. No. CD004768. DOI: 10.1002/14651858.CD004768.

Breivik, E.K., Björnsson, G.A., Skovlund, E. (2000) A comparison of pain rating scales by sampling from clinical trial data. *Clinical Journal of Pain* **16**: 22–8.

Breivik, H., Collett, B., Ventafridda, V., *et al.* (2006) Survey of chronic pain in Europe: prevalence, impact on daily life, and treatment. *European Journal of Pain* **10**(4): 287–333.

Brennan, F., Carr, D.B., Cousins, M. (2007) Pain management: a fundamental human right. *Anaesthesia and Analgesia* **105**(1): 205–21.

British Pain Society (2005) NOP Pain Poll. **http://www.britishpainsociety.org/full_report.pdf** (accessed 12 October 2011).

British Pain Society (2010a) Understanding and managing pain: information for patients. **http://www.britishpainsociety.org/book_understanding_pain.pdf** (accessed 13 October 2010).

British Pain Society (2010b) Opioids for persistent pain: good practice. **http://www.britishpainsociety.org/pub_professional.htm#opioids** (accessed 13 October 2010).

Care Quality Comission (2008) Survey of adult inpatients: National NHS patient survey programme. **http://www.cqc.org.uk/_db/_documents/National_results_for_each_question,_with_comparisons_to_previous_years_and_identifying_changes_that_are_statistically_significant.pdf** (accessed 16 March 2010).

Carli, F., Schricker, T. (2009) Modification of metabolic response to surgery by neural blockade. In M.J. Cousins, P.O. Bridenbaugh, D. Carr, *et al.* (eds) *Neural Blockade in Clinical Anesthesia and Pain Medicine*, 4th edn. Lippincott, Wolters Kluwer, Lippincott Williams & Wilkins: Philadelphia, PA, pp. 133–43.

Carr, E., Layzell, M., Christensen, M. (2010) *Advancing Nursing Practice in Pain Management.* Blackwell: Oxford.

Chief Medical Officer (2008) Pain: Breaking through the barrier. 150 years of the Annual Report of the Chief Medical Officer: On the state of public health. Department of Health. Available From **http://www.dh.gov.uk/en/Publicationsandstatistics/Publications/AnnualReports/DH_096206** (accessed 20 December 2011)

Chronic Pain Policy Coalition (CPPC) (2007) Policy document. **http://www.paincoalition.org.uk/cppc/campaign** (accessed 2 April 2010).

Closs, S.J., Barr, B., Briggs, M., *et al.* (2004) A comparison of five pain assessment scales for nursing home residents with varying degrees of cognitive impairment. *Journal of Pain and Symptom Management* **27**: 196–205.

Colloca, L., Benedetti, F. (2005) Placebos and painkillers: is mind as real as matter? *Nature Reviews Neuroscience* **6**: 545–52.

Cousins, M.J., Brennan, F., Carr, D.B. (2004) Pain relief: a universal human right. *Pain* **112**(1–2): 1–4.

Cox, F. (ed.) (2009) *Perioperative Pain Management.* Wiley-Blackwell: Chichester.

Cox, J.J., Reimann, F., Adeline, K., *et al.* (2006) An SCN9A channelopathy causes congenital inability to experience pain. *Nature* **444**: 894–8.

Daut, R.L., Cleeland, C.S., Flanery, R.C. (1983) Development of the Wisconsin Brief Pain Questionnaire to assess pain in cancer and other diseases. *Pain* **17**: 197–210.

Department of Health (2009) *Essence of Care: A Consultation on a New Benchmark for Pain.* **http://www.dh.gov.uk/en/Consultations/Liveconsultations/DH_103064** (accessed 10 April 2010).

Department of Health (2010) *Benchmarks for the Prevention and Management of Pain.* **http://www.dh.gov.uk/prod_consum_dh/groups/dh_digitalassets/@dh/@en/@ps/documents/digitalasset/dh_119977.pdf** (accessed 13 October 2010).

Dix, P. (2004) Pain on medical wards in a district general hospital. *British Journal of Anaesthesia* **92**(2): 235–7.

Dolin, S., Cashman, J.N., Bland, J.M., *et al.* (2002) Effectiveness of acute postoperative pain management: I. Evidence from published data. *British Journal of Anaesthesia* **89**: 409–23.

Dworkin, R.H., Turk, D.C., Revicki, D.A., *et al.* (2009) Development and initial validation of an expanded and revised version of the Short-Form McGill Pain Questionnaire (SF-MPQ2). *Pain* **144**: 35–42.

European Association of Palliative Care (EAPC) (2007) The European Pain in Cancer survey (EPIC). **http://www.paineurope.com/index.php?q=en/book_page/epic_survey** (accessed 25 March 2010).

Franck, L.S., Smith Greenberg, C., Stevens, B. (2000) Pain assessment in infants and children. *Pediatric Clinics of North America* **47**(3): 487–512.

Gélinas, C., Fillion, L., Puntillo, K.A., *et al.* (2006) Validation of the critical-care pain observation tool in adult patients. *American Journal of Critical Care* **15**: 420–7.

Jensen, M.P. (2006) Review of measures of neuropathic pain. *Current Pain and Headache Reports* **10**: 159–66.

Kehlet, H. (2009) Multimodal approach to postoperative recovery. *Current Opinion in Critical Care* **15**: 355–8.

Kehlet, H., Jensen, T.S., Woolf, C.J. (2006) Persistent postsurgical pain: risk factors and prevention. *Lancet* **367**: 1618–35.

Loeser, J.D., Treede, R.D. (2008) The Kyoto protocol of IASP Basic Pain Terminology. *Pain* **137**(3): 473–7.

Macintyre, P.E., Jarvis, D.A. (1996) Age is the best predictor of postoperative morphine requirements. *Pain* **64**: 357–64.

Macintyre, P.E., Ready, B.R. (2001) *Acute Pain Management: A Practical Guide,* 2nd edn. Saunders: London.

Macintyre, P.E., Scott D.A. Schug, S.A., *et al.* APM:SE Working Group of the Australian and New Zealand College of Anaesthetists and Faculty of Pain Medicine (2010) *Acute Pain Management: Scientific Evidence,* 3rd edn. ANZCA & FPC: Melbourne.

McCaffery, M. (1972) *Nursing Management of the Patient in Pain.* Lippincott: Philadelphia, PA.

McCaffery, M., Pasero, C. (1999) *Pain: Clinical Manual.* St.Louis MO, Mosby,

McCracken, L.M., Vowles, K.E., Eccleston, C. (2005) Acceptance-based treatment for persons with complex, long standing chronic pain: a preliminary analysis of treatment outcome in comparison to a waiting phase. *Behaviour Research and Therapy* **43**: 1335–46.

Melzack, R. (1987) The Short-Form McGill Pain Questionnaire. *Pain* **30**: 191–7.

Melzack, R. (1990) Phantom limbs and the concept of a neuromatrix. *Trends in Neuroscience* **13**: 88–92.

Melzack, R., Loeser, J.D. (1978) Phantom body pain in paraplegics: evidence for a central 'pattern generating mechanism' for pain. *Pain* **4**: 195–210.

Melzack, R., Wall, P.D. (1965) Pain mechanisms: a new theory. *Science* **19**: 971–9.

Merskey H., Bogduk, N. (eds) (1994) Part III: pain terms, a current list with definitions and notes on usage. *Classification of Chronic Pain,* 2nd edn. IASP Task Force on Taxonomy, IASP Press: Seattle, pp. 209–14.

Moore, A., Edwards, J., Barden, J., *et al.* (2003) *Bandolier's Little Book of Pain.* Oxford University Press: Oxford.

Morley, S. (2008) Psychology of pain. *British Journal of Anaesthesia* **101**(1): 25–31.

Perkins, F.M., Kehlet, H. (2000) Chronic pain as an outcome of surgery: a review of predictive factors. *Anesthesiology* **93**: 1123–33.

Puntillo, K., Miaskowski, C., Kehrle, K., *et al.* (1997) Relationship between behavioral and physiological indicators of pain, critical care patients' self-reports of pain, and opioid administration. *Critical Care Medicine* **25**(7): 1159–66.

Roelofs, P.D.D.M., Deyo, R.A., Koes, B.W., *et al.* (2010) Non-steroidal anti-inflammatory drugs for low back pain. http://www.mrw. interscience.wiley.com/cochrane/clsysrev/articles/CD000396/ frame.html (accesssed 8 April 2010).

Rømsing, J., Møiniche, S., Dahl, J.B. (2002) Rectal and parenteral paracetamol, and paracetamol in combination with NSAIDs, for postoperative analgesia. *British Journal of Anaesthesia* **88**: 215–26.

Sloman, R., Rosen, G., Rom, M., *et al.* (2005) Nurses' assessment of pain in surgical patients. *Journal of Advanced Nursing* **52**(2): 125–32.

Stannard, C.F., Booth, S. (1998) *Churchill's Pocket Book of Pain.* Churchill Livingstone: Edinburgh.

Taylor, A., Stanbury, L. (2009) A review of postoperative pain management and the challenges. *Current Anaesthesia and Critical Care* **20**: 188–94

Wu, C.L., Liu, S.S. (2008) Neural blockade: impact on outcome. In M.J. Cousins, P.O. Bridenbaugh, D. Carr, *et al.* (eds) *Neural Blockade in Clinical Anesthesia and Pain Medicine,* 4th edn. Wolters Kluwer, Lippincott, Williams & Wilkins: Philadelphia, PA, pp.144–59.

Zalon, M.L. (1993) Nurses' assessment of postoperative patients' pain. *Pain* **54**: 329–34.

26 *Managing* Perioperative Care

Jane Jackson

> ## Introduction
>
> This chapter focuses on the preparation and care of adult patients undergoing elective surgery, the associated challenges, and supporting evidence in providing safe and effective care. A key principle is the identification of relevant health issues and optimizing comorbidities prior to admission for surgery, which will minimize cancellations on the day of surgery. Informed consent, patient education, and teamworking all contribute to effective care and efficient service delivery.

Understanding the patient's health needs

To provide the optimum healthcare, it is essential that the health professional has a full understanding of the patient's physical and psychological health and social history, allowing tailored care to be shaped and implemented. It is important that the patient understands the associated risks and benefits of planned treatment.

Patients often present for elective surgery with comorbidities. In optimizing the treatment, it is possible to prevent negative consequences related to planned care, and to increase the patient's understanding of these so that he or she they can make an informed choice. Gathering information prior to admission is important because patients are often anxious on the day of surgery, and medication/anaesthetic agents can render them unable to provide clear decisions relating to treatment. This is commonly referred to as the preoperative assessment (POA), but is probably better referred to as patient preparation.

Definition of patient preparation

Patient preparation is the process by which a patient's health status is identified and comorbidities made known to the relevant healthcare professionals. The healthcare professional will interpret the information, decide on additional investigations and examinations, and then determine the risk factors associated with the patient's health and the anticipated anaesthetic and surgical intervention. The patient must be informed of the risk and benefits and be provided with sufficient information to ensure an informed choice.

Integral to patient preparation is the anticipation of potential outcomes, including length of hospitalization, ability to complete activities of daily living, and discharge planning. The process will involve the patient and his or her carer(s) and all healthcare professionals appropriate to the individual patient in primary and secondary care. It may be that, at the end of the patient preparation stage, the patient decides not to proceed with surgery.

Timing of patient preparation is dependent upon the patient's requirements—whether he or she is expecting surgery within the week or may have several weeks to wait. In many healthcare settings, assessment is completed at the time the decision is made to treat; in others, the patient preparation is just 1 week prior to admission, in sufficient time that his or her healthcare needs are addressed and optimized prior to admission.

Who requires patient preparation?

All patients due for admission to hospital will benefit from preparation prior to arrival. For those patients who have either no comorbidities or comorbidities that are well controlled, the patient preparation may be a simple checklist prior to the patient receiving an admission date. For others, failure to identify patient health status accurately and lack of coordination between healthcare professionals to address patient needs in advance of admission will result in poor patient experience on admission, and may be detrimental to the patient outcome, increasing mortality.

Preparation will include identification of psychological and social needs, identification of physical needs, medication requirements, and provision of information regarding general health, as well as pending procedure/investigation. It is the responsibility of the nurse in patient preparation to address all aspects of daily living and to identify observations that differ from the normal values or comorbidities that will need optimization prior to admission. The experienced nurse working in patient preparation will follow up any such referrals and ensure that the areas of concern have been fully investigated and action taken to optimize the patient's health.

For some patients, a specific focus may be required: for instance, a vulnerable patient may have specific needs that involve multiple agencies in primary and secondary care (Box 26.1).

Human and social burden and costs

Admission to secondary care for elective surgery has many demands and can be an anxious time for the patient and his or her dependants. The patient needs to be psychologically prepared for the surgical intervention and its ramifications during the perioperative period, as well as post immediate recovery; this is most important when the surgery may result in potential lifelong changes to lifestyle. Considered preparation prior to admission for surgery will

---

Box 26.1 **Patients with learning disability and patient preparation**

For the patient who has learning needs, the preparation for admission is especially important—it is the opportunity for trust to build between the patient, the carer, and the surgical team. The incidence of learning disability (LD) within the general population is estimated to be 2% (Emerson and Hatton, 2008) (four people in every 1,000 with severe learning disability, and 20 in the mild to moderate category).

The 10-year strategy *Carers at the Heart of the 21st Century Families and Communities* (Department of Health, 2008) expects carers to be partners in diagnosis and discharge planning alongside care and adult care service staff. Patients with learning disabilities may not be able to express their needs as readily as other patients, e.g. their pain needs will need to be discussed on an individual basis, with input from the carer and the pain specialist nurse, and a health action plan may be used. People with learning disabilities have a range of abilities, but all will need clear explanations in plain language with the use of diagrams or signing. See **www.easyhealth.org.uk**.

The patient should be assessed in a single examination room by the professional team. If possible, any blood tests, ECG, etc. should be taken by the nurse in the patient's room. Special consideration should be given to cardiovascular and respiratory systems, and, when a physical disability is also present, specific checks for clear airway access should be performed. An ECG will identify any cardiac conduction abnormalities, and the patient should be assessed by the anaesthetist at the earliest opportunity. Where possible, the patient should receive his or her care in an environment where the carer can accompany them, and where a few 'home comforts' can be positioned. Post surgery, if the patient shows distress caused by any wound covering, drains, or infusions, these should be well secured and left for the minimum time possible, and the patient returned to his or her usual routine/environment as soon as is practical.

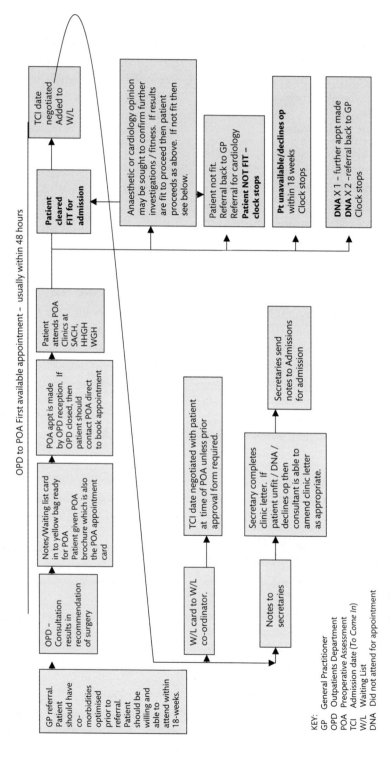

Figure 26.1 Outpatient to waiting list process.

Developed by West Hertfordshire NHS Trust. Reproduced with permission.

provide support and reassurance that the patient's personal needs are being identified and addressed.

In the 2004 NHS Improvement Plan, the Department of Health encouraged health professionals to treat patients within a timely manner. Within a single outpatient appointment, the patient may expect to have his or her outpatient consultation, preoperative assessment, and pathology investigations completed. An example of the process is given in Figure 26.1.

Enhanced recovery programme

Enhanced recovery, developed in early 2000 by Professor Henrik Kehlet in Copenhagen, challenged what had hitherto been the traditional surgical pathway, and an alternative process was put in place that is reinforced by a strong interprofessional teamwork, resulting in a considerably reduced length of secondary care admission.

Following a trial at 12 NHS trusts during 2009–2010, the programme received its national launch in 2010, and an implementation guide was introduced (Department of Health, 2010). The enhanced recovery programme improves patient experience, challenging previous interventions such that, through minimally invasive techniques, optimal fluid management, and patient-centred care, the patient is ready for discharge earlier. This improves the patient experience, and reduces the length of hospitalization, and waiting times (Figure 26.2).

Morbidity

Cardiovascular disease, respiratory disease, diabetes, obesity, smoking, alcoholism (**www.statistics.gov.uk** 2010), mental health, and cancers account for the majority of morbidities that are addressed within patient preparation. For example, a patient with cardiovascular disease will require care with regard to fluid replacement. It is essential to maintain normal fluid volume rather than overhydrate the patient, which would increase the workload of the cardiovascular system and result in complications for the patient (pulmonary oedema).

Smoking

Smoking is to be discouraged for all patients due for admission for elective surgery, because it is associated with local wound complications, as well as respiratory and cardiac complications. To gain maximum benefit from smoking cessation, patients should cease 8 weeks prior to surgery

with the intention of quitting for good (Department of Health, 2009). Nicotine clears from the body after 48 hours; after 3–9 months of smoking cessation, lung function is increased by up to 10%. This is particularly useful for the patient due to undergo surgical procedures with general anaesthetic, and when oxygen demand will be increased around wound healing. See NICE Public Health Guidance No. 10 (February 2008), as well as **www.nhs.uk/smokefree.**

Healthcare-acquired infections

National targets and clinical guidelines are evidence-based and, provided that they are implemented correctly, will deliver improved patient care. Healthcare-associated infections (HCAI) are continually monitored, and *Saving Lives: Reducing Infection, Delivering Clean and Safe Care* (Department of Health, 2007) recommends best practice to reduce infection rates—in particular the infections, including methicillin-resistant *Staphylococcus aureus* (MRSA) and *Clostridium difficile*. In 2010, the Department of Health launched a national health promotion to share best practice in reduction of HCAIs.

Saving Lives interventions look specifically at:

- central venous catheter care;
- peripheral intravenous cannula care;
- renal dialysis catheter care;
- prevention of surgical site infection;
- care for ventilated patients/tracheostomies;
- urinary catheter care;
- reducing risk of *Clostridium difficile*.

The bare-below-the-elbow campaign has seen the dissemination of Saving Lives interventions to all professionals and to the user of the healthcare provider—the patients and their relatives. The use of hand gel, soap and water washing, and bare-below-the-elbows should now be a part of every patient's experience in healthcare sector.

Surgical site infections

Neither the health professional nor the patient expects to see infection within the wound of an elective operation; however, for a variety of reasons, infections do occur and are associated with extended hospital stay and, in some cases, mortality. It is important that we identify infections at an early stage and that prompt treatment begins. According to the National Institute for Health and Clinical

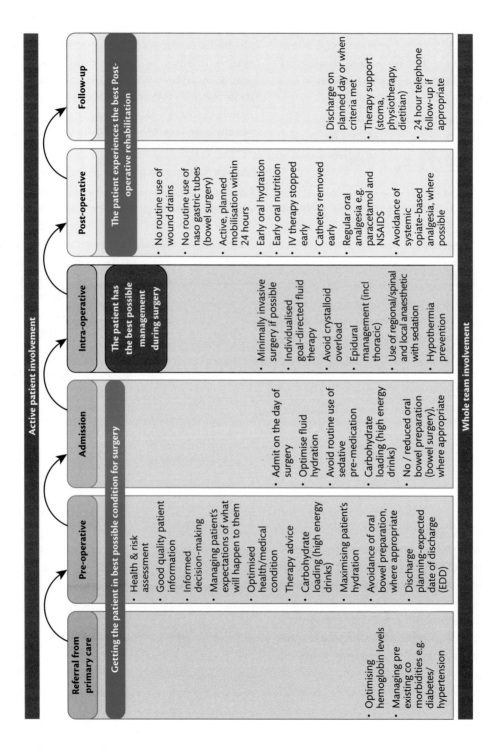

Figure 26.2 The enhanced recovery pathway.

Reproduced from *Delivering Enhanced Recovery: Helping Patients to Get Better After Surgery* (Department of Health, 2010).

CASE STUDY 26.1 *Musculo skeletal enhanced recovery*

Mrs A attends her general practitioner (GP) complaining of pain in the hip, reduced mobility, difficulty and pain on bending. The GP recommends referral to an orthopaedic surgeon.

At consultation, Mrs A is examined and radiology confirms that the patient requires a hip replacement. This is discussed and the patient agrees to surgery.

Following patient preparation, Mrs A attends joint school, an educational session on the procedure and aftercare, at which the procedure and aftercare are discussed by the interprofessional team.

Mrs A arrives on the ward for hip replacement fasted, and sees the anaesthetist and surgeon. The anaesthetic may be a spinal anaesthetic with an infiltration of local anaesthetic or femoral block. In the recovery area, the patient will be encouraged to sit up, maintained with a temperature at or above 36.5°C, and oral fluids encouraged. Physiotherapy exercises may begin in recovery.

On return to the ward area, Mrs A was able to drink as desired, and had her intravenous infusion discontinued as soon as she was tolerating fluids. That same afternoon, Mrs A was out of bed mobilizing. Pain relief was maintained throughout the hospital stay, with oral analgesia as soon as appropriate.

Medication required for discharge was dispensed from the pharmacy and, once Mrs A achieved the discharge criteria, she was discharged. The discharge criteria include: medical review that the patient is medically fit for discharge; medication prepared for discharge; physiotherapist and occupational therapist discharge criteria met; normal diet and fluids; pain well controlled; observations within normal limits; wound site clean and dry; any home care support in place; contact numbers provided in case of need.

Mrs A received a follow-up telephone call 24 hours post discharge to check on progress.

Excellence (NICE), 'surgical site infections comprise up to 20% of all healthcare-associated infections. At least 5% of patients undergoing surgery develop a surgical site infection' (NICE, 2008). The recommendations from NICE are split into three phases: preoperative, intraoperative, and postoperative. During the preoperative phase, hair removal should only be completed if absolutely necessary and single-use electric clippers should be used on the day of surgery. Antibiotic prophylaxis should be used when undertaking surgery for prosthetic implant, or where the wound is contaminated, but not for routine clean, non-prosthetic surgery.

The intraoperative care involves preparing the surgical site immediately before incision using an aqueous or alcohol-based solution. Post surgery, the wound should be covered with an interactive dressing.

During the postoperative phase, the role of the surgical site infection and tissue viability nurse are crucial in providing expertise. The Health Protection Agency introduced a monitoring programme for infections acquired in hospitals, with data being collated nationally to calculate rates of wound infection for different types of operation. Continual audit of postoperative wounds, e.g. post joint replacement, provides the opportunity to identify trends of infection, and to implement a change in practice that will reduce the recurrence of further infection.

Creutzfeldt-Jakob disease (vCJD)

Creutzfeldt-Jakob disease (CJD) is a rare brain disorder that affects about 1 in 1 million people each year. Variant CJD (vCJD) is a form of this disease, and results in the build-up in the brain of abnormal proteins called prions. There is no known treatment or cure for CJD or vCJD and there is no known blood test to identify the disease–it can only be confirmed at post mortem. In 2006, the Department of Health Clinical Governance Advisory Group reported that every patient due to undergo elective surgery should be asked if he or she has ever been informed that he or she is at risk of vCJD. There is no blood test to check if a patient is infected with vCJD.

The abnormal prion protein that causes vCJD cannot be eradicated from surgical instruments, so it is essential that patients are identified as being potentially infected prior to any surgical intervention, so that disposable instruments can be used. Where this is not an option, instruments need to be isolated for sole use on the particular patient. For more details, see *Transmissible Spongiform Encephalopathy Agents: Safe Working and the Prevention of Infection: Annex J* (Department of Health, 2006; revised 2011).

Nursing responsibility and accountability for managing perioperative care

Prior to surgery, the nurse is responsible for history-taking (collecting information), recording observations, undertaking investigations, identifying and communicating comorbidities to all relevant healthcare professionals, and determining overall health status. Throughout the perioperative period, the nurse will monitor progress and deterioration through accurate observation, recording and reporting changes, and alerting the team to the potential need for intervention. The nurse is responsible for managing perioperative fasting, hydration, and pain, as well the prevention of deep vein thrombosis and pulmonary embolism. Working alongside the interprofessional team, the nurse will recognize and manage the challenges that health issues such as obesity can cause, contribute to discharge planning, and follow the criteria for correct site surgery.

Skills for effective patient interview

Competent history-taking skills are essential to patient safety; the health professional is responsible for gaining the appropriate training and experience to enable competency and confidence in history-taking, examination, and appropriate ordering of investigations. The Department of Health White Paper (July 2010) *No Decision About Me Without Me* should be at the centre of all healthcare decision-making.

The information will be used to identify changes in condition and to anticipate potential reactions to treatment. The information must be recorded clearly on the patient's records in chronological order, dated, timed, and signed, and must provide a true record of events with clarity such that another person reading the notes will have a clear understanding of the information discussed and decisions made.

Always commence any interview by introducing yourself. Clearly give your name and position, explain the reason for the meeting, and ask for consent. It is disrespectful to address the patient or his or her relative by a first name without permission.

Patient identification should be checked with the patient's full name, date of birth, and NHS number against relevant healthcare records. It is the responsibility of each nurse and all health professionals to ensure that they identify the patient on each occasion that they undertake observations, record changes to treatment or events, or administer medication. When undertaking an interview, it is important to consider the following:

- environment;
- interview objectives;
- medication and allergies;
- habits.

Environment

It may be appropriate to include relatives/carers, so be certain to provide sufficient space for their attendance. Ensure that the environment is appropriate for the need, providing chairs/examination couch/wheelchair access as appropriate. Provide a room that is private and minimize interruptions; this provides privacy for the patient, and maintains confidentiality and dignity when conducting examinations or discussing sensitive information.

If examination is required, ensure that access to equipment is made in advance to ensure that the health professional has no cause to leave the room during the examination.

History-taking objectives

Before commencing an interview, be clear on the objectives. What is it that you wish to ask or achieve? Consider the questions that you will need to ask and offer the patient the opportunity to provide additional information. Interviews usually start with open questions, which require detailed answers. Closed questions—which require direct answers—can then be used to check facts. Box 26.2 shows the typical questions that would be asked at patient preparation regarding medical and surgical history.

Medication and allergies

The role of the nurse with regard to medication and allergies is to ensure that a full and accurate record is made of the name of prescribed medication (no abbreviations), dose, and frequency. If possible, obtain this information from the prescription supplied from the community dispensary.

Certain drugs may need to be stopped prior to admission for elective surgery, e.g. warfarin—local protocol will apply. The patient must be advised of this need and provided with written information.

The patient should be asked if he or she takes any 'over the counter' medication (e.g. tablets or ointments purchased without prescription). It should be noted that herbal remedies and multivitamins should be stopped for 2 weeks prior to admission because the limited evidence available has indicated a link to reduced clotting and some, such as St John's wort, can reduce the effectiveness of prescribed drugs.

Allergies to medications, foods, inhaled substances, or skin contact should be established, recording the allergy along with the reaction that is caused. This information about the effect of the allergy provides the healthcare professionals with valuable knowledge to enable them to make decisions on which antibiotics to administer and to be alert for a severe allergic reaction to any administered drugs.

Habits/social history

The interviewer should identify patient habits with respect to drug abuse, smoking, and alcohol misuse. The duration of misuse, the quantity, and the type of misuse are pertinent to patient safety, and the professional has a duty to provide patients with advice on cessation of drug abuse and smoking prior to admission, and on keeping alcohol intake to within the recommended daily allowance of 2–3 units for women and 3–4 units for men. Beyond this, patients should be offered referral for ongoing support in primary care. Drugs, smoking, and alcohol are all addictive and will alter the patient's physiological state; they will also have an adverse affect on the patient's ability to recover from anaesthesia and wound healing.

Observations

In addition to obtaining a history from the patient, the nurse working in patient preparation will undertake baseline observations to identify the current physical health of the patient. It is the responsibility of the nurse or health professional undertaking these to ensure accuracy both in completing and in recording the findings, including the date and time of any observations or examination. Changes to the patient's baseline observations can then be attributed to medication or treatments during the course of his or her care.

Typical observations to be undertaken at the time of patient preparation and after surgery are as follows.

- **Functional capacity**, e.g. shuttle test—recording the patient's ability to walk up a flight of stairs and the number of pillows that they use at night will help the anaesthetist to have a clear understanding of the patient's functional capacity.
- **Body mass index (BMI)**—this may be used by the medical team to determine the quantity of drugs that the patient requires. It also gives the nurse an opportunity to discuss healthy eating.
- **Skin pallor**—is he or she jaundiced, anaemic, or cyanosed?
- **Radial pulse rate**—is the pulse regular or irregular? If irregular, ensure that the blood pressure is recorded using a manual sphygmomanometer to elicit accurate systolic and diastolic reading, and an ECG should also be recordeds.
- **Blood pressure**—is the reading within normal values?
- **Respiratory rate**—is the reading within normal values? The respiratory rate is an important observation and should be recorded in the patient preparation stage so that the baseline reading is available post surgery. Does the patient have a cough? If so, is the cough productive? If it is, what colour is the sputum? This should trigger the nurse to request a sputum sample for microbiology culture and sensitivity.
- **Pulse oximetry**—this should be undertaken to identify the patient's oxygen saturation on air—or on oxygen if the patient is taking oxygen at the time. NB Pulse oximetry is reliant upon a good capillary bloodflow to the peripheries. Readings less than normal (less than 95% in the person with normal haemoglobin levels; Schultz, 2001) should immediately be reported to the senior nurse or doctor.
- **Physical examination**—this should be carried out by a senior nurse or doctor, and may include chest auscultation or abdominal examination.

Box 26.2 Past Medical History Checklist

Medical history – DO YOU CURRENTLY HAVE OR HAVE YOU EVER BEEN DIAGNOSED WITH:

	YES	NO	Date diagnosed:
Heart disease (including pacemaker)	☐	☐	
MI (heart attack)	☐	☐	
Hypertension (high blood pressure)	☐	☐	
Angina (chest pain)	☐	☐	
DVT/PE (blood clots)	☐	☐	

	YES	NO	Controlled by:
Stroke (CVA/TIA)	☐	☐	Diet ☐ Tablets ☐ Insulin ☐
Diabetes type 1/2	☐	☐	
Epilepsy	☐	☐	
Jaundice	☐	☐	
Gastric acidity, hiatus hernia,	☐	☐	
Irritable bowel	☐	☐	
Kidney disease	☐	☐	

	YES	NO	Type:
Arthritis	☐	☐	Osteo ☐ Rheumatoid ☐
Asthma	☐	☐	Peak Flow L/min (If less than 360 to see RGN)
Chronic respiratory disease	☐	☐	Peak Flow L/min (If less than 360 to see RGN)
Thyroid disorders			
Sickle cell status (if relevant)	N/A ☐	Positive ☐	Carrier ☐ Negative ☐

			Yes	No
Have you ever been notified that you are at risk of CJD or vCJD for public health purposes?				

	Yes	No
Female patients:		
Are you currently pregnant?	☐	☐
Is there a possibility that you may be pregnant?	☐	☐
All patients:		
Do you have any other health conditions?	☐	☐

If yes, please write below:

(continued)

Box 26.2 *(continued)*

Previous operations		
Date/Year Approximate	Operation	Hospital

Previous anaesthetic problems for patient or relatives

Investigations

The National Confidential Enquiry into Patient Outcome and Death report *Adding Insult to Injury* (NCEPOD, 2009) stresses that all emergency admissions must be prioritized and performed routinely as good practice. Key findings of the report showed that 33% of patients had inadequate basic clinical examination/simple laboratory tests. Subsequently, because investigations such as urinalysis were not performed or observations recorded, it was not possible to monitor and communicate changes promptly to enable prompt treatment to minimize deterioration.

The National Institute for Health and Clinical Excellence produced Preoperative Investigations Clinical Guideline No. 3 (NICE, 2003) **http://www.nice.org.uk/ CG003.** Investigations may be indicated depending upon the age of the patient, his or her comorbidities, and the procedure to be undertaken. The NICE guide should also be considered alongside the Department of Health 2010 guide *Helping the Patient to get Better Sooner after Surgery*. The Association of Anaesthetists of Great Britain and Ireland (AAGBI) *Safety Guideline: Preoperative Assessment and Patient Preparation* (AAGBI, 2010) should be applied, and the HSC2002/009 *Better Blood Transfusion:Appropriate Use of Blood* (**www.dh.gov.**

uk/en/publicationsandstatistics) expects trusts to manage preoperative anaemia effectively with the intention of limiting blood transfusion.

Investigations should be appropriate to patient need, and should provide information that will enhance care. It is the responsibility of the nurse and junior doctor to ensure that results and/or actions of all investigations should be checked and acted upon in a timely manner.

Electrocardiograph (ECG): local policy may differ, but the nurse working in patient preparation may be required to undertake an ECG on patients due to undergo major surgery. This should be dated and timed, and should be clearly labelled with the patient's details and then shown to the senior nurse and/or doctor. If the patient is experiencing any discomfort or chest pain at the time of the recording, then this should be recorded on the top of the tracing because this provides additional information for the professional interpreting the ECG.

Microbiology: all patients will have MRSA microbiology swabs taken to ascertain their MRSA status. Patients who show a positive result to MRSA will require decolonization treatment prior to admission.

Urine analysis: urine analysis should be routinely undertaken to check for leukocytes, protein, glucose, and blood. Patients with a urine infection should have a

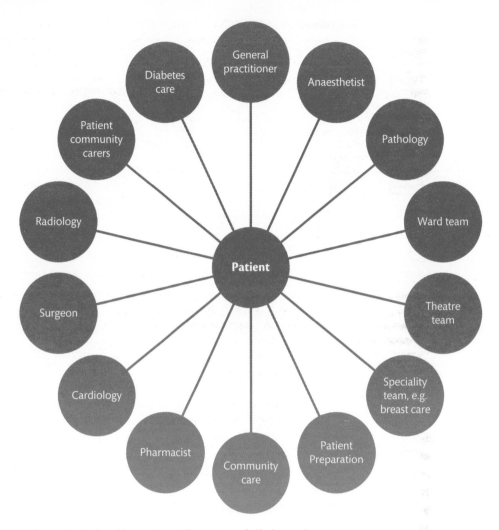

Figure 26.3 **The patient should remain at the centre of all planned care.**

midstream urinary sample sent to microbiology for micro-scopy, culture, and sensitivity, and, if found, any infection treated. If glucosuria is identified in a patient attending preparation clinics, this should always be followed up by a random and fasting glucose level, and bloods for LFT, U&E, and HbA1c. If the patient is not known to have diabetes, the GP should be advised of the finding so that this can be monitored and investigated to determine the cause of the glucosuria.

Optimization of health

For some patients, their comorbidities may be such that, despite medication and other treatments, their condition

remains poor. It is the responsibility of the nurse or doctor in patient preparation to identify these patients and to bring them to the attention of the consultant anaesthet-ist and/or surgeon. This will provide time before admis-sion for further investigations and referral. Considering the detailed patient history, the experienced nurse and junior doctor will ensure that all relevant healthcare pro-fessionals—in both primary and secondary care—are alerted to the patient's requirements. Support mecha-nisms, including community care, can be put into place to provide appropriate care for the patient before, during, and after the operation (Figure 26.3).

For all patients, the decision to proceed will be taken on admission and after examination by the anaesthetist

Table 26.1 American Society of Anesthesiologists scoring system

ASA 1	Healthy adult, no health concerns
ASA 2	A patient with mild systemic disease that is controlled with/without medication
ASA 3	A patient with severe incapacitating disease that limits activity, but is not life-threatening
ASA 4	A patient with incapacitating disease that is a constant threat to life
ASA 5	A moribund patient who is not expected to survive 24 hours with or without an operation

and the surgeon. If the patient's health has not been sufficiently optimized, then the surgery may be postponed and, without discharge arrangements being in place, the patient will be unable to return home when medically fit.

Determine overall health status for patient preparation

On completion of the interview, summarize the past history, current history, medications, observations, and examination. It is common practice then to determine the patient's ASA status. In 1963, the American Society of Anesthesiologists devised a score system (Table 26.1), the outcome of which would provide an approximation of the patient's health status. The adult patient who had no health issues other than the reason for surgery would be given a score of ASA 1, whilst the patient with multiple comorbidities that give a constant threat to his or her life—for example, uncontrollable hypertension despite medication—would be scored as ASA 4.

Interprofessional teamwork and patient preparation

Professionals are responsible to their own governing body: the General Medical Council (GMC; **www.gmc-uk.org**) and the Nursing and Midwifery Council (NMC; **www.nmc-uk.org.**). In all professions, the role provided by each professional has some degree of overlap, thereby providing the ability for good understanding of issues and a basis for effective communication. Doctors and nurses work in close proximity, each professional being accountable for keeping within his or her professional codes of conduct, and for delivering and committing expertise to benefit patient care. The importance of effective teamworking has emerged over the past decade, with particular focus on human factors incorporating individual characteristics and skills, group skills, and safety issues (Flin and Maran, 2004; Baker *et al.*, 2005). The team ethos and approach in patient preparation is key to ensuring positive outcomes and reducing errors at the start of the patient journey.

Assessment of patients in advance of admission provides the opportunity to plan theatre lists and ward workload. The NHS Institute provides useful quality improvement tools focused on how to get this aspect of the patient admission right—preoperative assessment and planning (POA) is seen as key to optimizing patient health (National Health Institute for Health and Improvement, 2008, **www.institute.nhs.uk/ quality_and_service_improvement_tools_for_the_nhs. html**). Useful links on individual aspects of preoperative planning can be found on producing patient information, did not arrive forms (DNAs), cancelled operations, and discharge planning here: **http://www.institute.nhs.uk/ quality_and_service_improvement_tools/quality_and_ service_improvement_tools/pre-operative_assessment_ and_planning.html.**

Use the service improvement tools available from the NHS Institute to facilitate your understanding of effective planning and communication. There are also examples of effective practice available to explore.

Pharmacist role in patient preparation

The pharmacist within assessment will advise the team and the patient on medication interactions, and on medication to stop or start prior to admission. Patients may be taking over-the-counter preparations that may react adversely with prescribed medication/anaesthetic drugs, so the pharmacist can advise on the risks and, where necessary, the need to stop these preparations prior to admission. The independent prescriber can write up the drug chart for admission and, in some circumstances, make arrangements to anticipate the tablets that a patient may require to take home post discharge. Once the patient is admitted, the pharmacist team visits the patient in the ward area and ensures that the medication plan continues as expected.

Consultant anaesthetist in patient preparation

During surgical preparation, the patient who has multiple comorbidities may see the anaesthetist. The anaesthetist is able to guide the specially trained nurse in patient preparation and to request appropriate investigations prior to the admission. Where the patient is at high risk of adverse events, the anaesthetist will assess the patient in a preadmission clinic and discuss the risks of surgery/anaesthetic. It may be appropriate that the patient has a cardiopulmonary test to determine his or her oxygen/carbon dioxide uptake when exercising, which is an indicator of how he or she will be during the anaesthetic and perioperative period.

This interprofessional teamworking is the essence of patient preparation and patient safety.

Observations and national early warning score

Observations recorded at patient preparation are the baseline observations from which changes will be measured. The nurse will monitor progress and deterioration through accurate observation, record and report changes, and alert the team to the potential need for intervention.

The use of the World Health Organization surgical checklist (WHO, 2009a) and the NEWS (national early warning score) observations charts were devised to support and improve patient safety. The World Health Organization (WHO, 2009b) Guidelines for Safe Surgery recognize that patient safety is compromised by human error. The checklist (Figure 26.4) is designed to be completed at multiple stages in the patient's pathway: prior to leaving the ward environment, in the anaesthetic room, and in the operating room. The checklist is completed by two or more individuals simultaneously to ensure that there is open communication. This challenges behaviour and provides clear unambiguous checks with which to confirm the following: patient identity; site of surgery; minimizing the risks of high blood loss; methods to minimize surgical site infection; minimizing the risks of inaccurate or inappropriate administration of medication.

When the NEWS chart is applied, deviations from the baseline observations can be easily identified, prompting an increase in the rate of observations and escalation of changes to senior team members **www.hse.ie/go/nationalearlywarningscore.**

No surgical intervention is without risks, and each surgical nurse must be on the alert for the signs of respiratory distress, deep vein thrombosis, pulmonary embolism, wound drainage, wound infection, and postoperative confusion. The patient who has a poor mental score test prior to anaesthetic is more likely to have postoperative confusion than the person who has little or no cognitive impairment (National Institute for Health and Clinical Excellence (NICE), 2010). Ensure that the patient and his or her relatives are aware of this so that the confused state does not become alarming in the immediate postoperative period.

Following any procedure, patients may experience pain. This should be addressed swiftly and by the most appropriate method for the individual patient. The nurse specialist for acute pain will provide advice for the patient in your care. Pain is stressful for the patient and limits patient activity, and, in turn, this restricted mobility may be a predisposing factor to chest infection or deep vein thrombosis (see Chapter 25 Managing Pain ➡).

Postoperative nausea and vomiting can be minimized if it is identified in advance of theatre that a patient has had a similar experience following a previous anaesthetic; this will pre-empt the need for antiemetics.

Nil by mouth

In 2005, UK clinical practice guidelines were launched for perioperative fasting in adults and children (RCN, 2005; Smith *et al.*, 2011). These evidence-based guidelines addressed the need to maintain patient safety by reducing the chance of aspiration pneumonitis at induction of anaesthesia, whilst maintaining patient comfort and hydration. Elective surgical adult patients are able to drink water up to 2 hours prior to induction: solid food, including milk, milk products, and sweets, should be ceased 6 hours prior to anaesthesia. Children are as above; those breastfeeding may have breast milk up to 4 hours prior to anaesthesia.

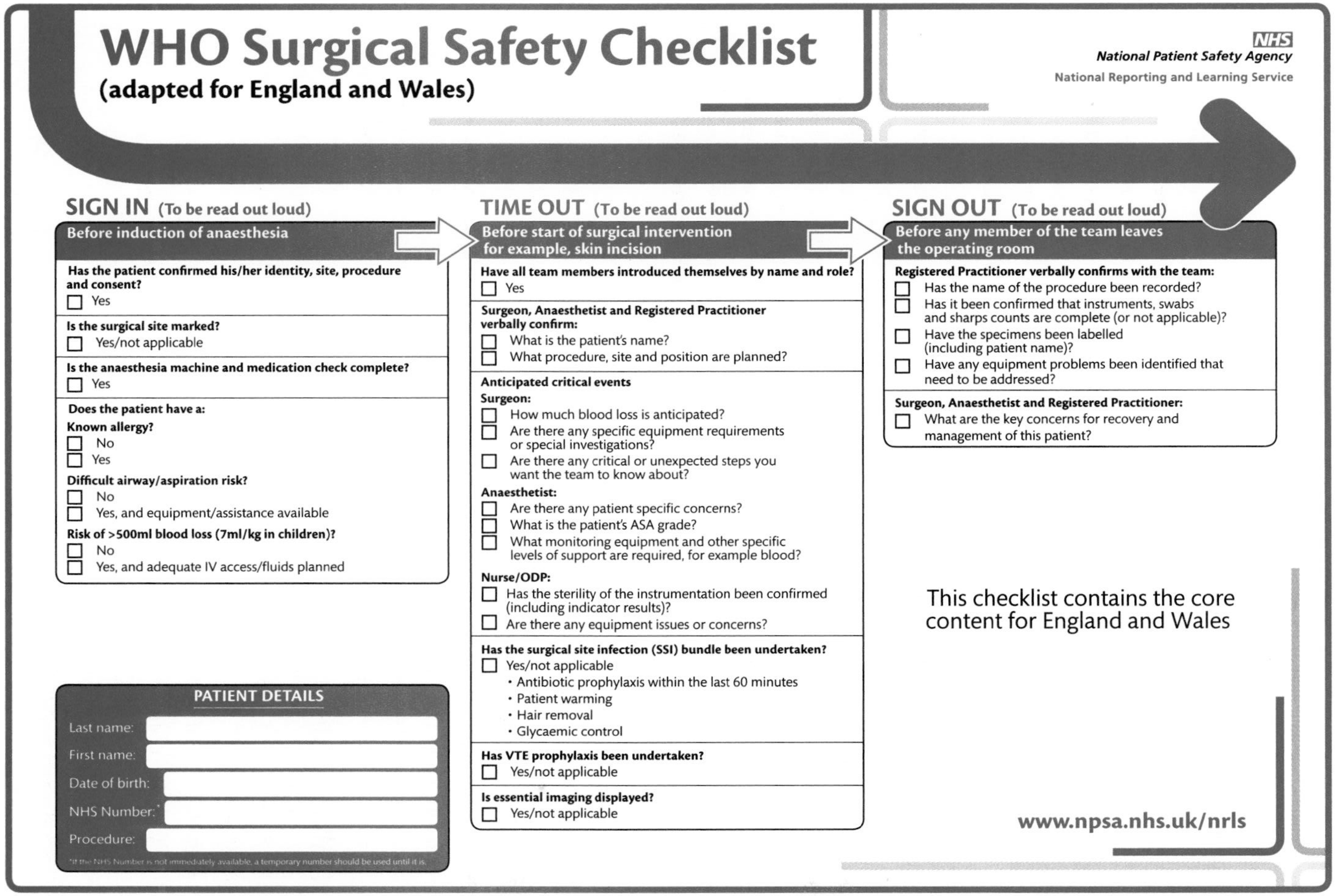

WHO Surgical Safety Checklist
(adapted for England and Wales)

NHS
National Patient Safety Agency
National Reporting and Learning Service

SIGN IN (To be read out loud)

Before induction of anaesthesia

Has the patient confirmed his/her identity, site, procedure and consent?
☐ Yes

Is the surgical site marked?
☐ Yes/not applicable

Is the anaesthesia machine and medication check complete?
☐ Yes

Does the patient have a:
Known allergy?
☐ No
☐ Yes
Difficult airway/aspiration risk?
☐ No
☐ Yes, and equipment/assistance available
Risk of >500ml blood loss (7ml/kg in children)?
☐ No
☐ Yes, and adequate IV access/fluids planned

PATIENT DETAILS
Last name:
First name:
Date of birth:
NHS Number:*
Procedure:
*If the NHS Number is not immediately available, a temporary number should be used until it is.

TIME OUT (To be read out loud)

Before start of surgical intervention for example, skin incision

Have all team members introduced themselves by name and role?
☐ Yes

Surgeon, Anaesthetist and Registered Practitioner verbally confirm:
☐ What is the patient's name?
☐ What procedure, site and position are planned?

Anticipated critical events
Surgeon:
☐ How much blood loss is anticipated?
☐ Are there any specific equipment requirements or special investigations?
☐ Are there any critical or unexpected steps you want the team to know about?
Anaesthetist:
☐ Are there any patient specific concerns?
☐ What is the patient's ASA grade?
☐ What monitoring equipment and other specific levels of support are required, for example blood?
Nurse/ODP:
☐ Has the sterility of the instrumentation been confirmed (including indicator results)?
☐ Are there any equipment issues or concerns?

Has the surgical site infection (SSI) bundle been undertaken?
☐ Yes/not applicable
- Antibiotic prophylaxis within the last 60 minutes
- Patient warming
- Hair removal
- Glycaemic control

Has VTE prophylaxis been undertaken?
☐ Yes/not applicable

Is essential imaging displayed?
☐ Yes/not applicable

SIGN OUT (To be read out loud)

Before any member of the team leaves the operating room

Registered Practitioner verbally confirms with the team:
☐ Has the name of the procedure been recorded?
☐ Has it been confirmed that instruments, swabs and sharps counts are complete (or not applicable)?
☐ Have the specimens been labelled (including patient name)?
☐ Have any equipment problems been identified that need to be addressed?

Surgeon, Anaesthetist and Registered Practitioner:
☐ What are the key concerns for recovery and management of this patient?

This checklist contains the core content for England and Wales

www.npsa.nhs.uk/nrls

Figure 26.4 Safe surgery checklist.

Box 26.3 Specific surgical risk factors for VTE

- Major surgery
- Pelvic or lower limb surgery
- Significant blood loss
- Use of a tourniquet
- Increased risk with age
- Obesity
- Dehydration
- Immobilization
- Hormone treatment
- Malignancy

The patient will have his or her hydration maintained during the perioperative period by intravenous fluids, but oral fluids should resume as soon as possible provided that there are no contraindications. With the enhanced recovery programme, patients are encouraged to drink high-protein fluids up to 2 hours prior to surgery—including major bowel resection—and, unless contraindicated by the surgery, will be encouraged to resume drinking the high-protein fluids immediately post surgery in the recovery ward area. Follow-up studies in more than 400 patients showed no difference in gastric fluid or pH at induction of anaesthesia between those who drank and those who fasted from midnight, nor did the volume ingested (50–1,200 ml) influence the residual volume in the stomach. This is not surprising because clear liquids empty within 2 hours. Gastric contents after that time consist of gastric secretions and swallowed saliva, as in patients who fast from midnight (see Chapter 19 Managing Hydration ➡️).

Venous thromboembolism

The definition of a thrombosis is a formation of thrombi within the lumen of the vessels that make up the deep venous system. Three separate components (known as Virchow's triad) can contribute to this—changes in the blood vessel walls (e.g. atherosclerosis), hypercoagualability of blood (e.g. dehydration), and stasis. The thrombosis can occur in the distal veins in the calf or to proximal veins—such as the popliteal or femoral veins. Some 80% of deep venous thromboses (DVTs) are clinically silent, most being identified following fatal pulmonary embolism (Sandler and Martin, 1989).

With pulmonary embolism, the postoperative patient complains of sudden chest pain, sudden onset **dyspnoea**, **cyanosis**, and occasionally **haemoptysis**. Most deaths from

a pulmonary embolism occur within 30 minutes of the acute event (Donaldson *et al.*, 1962), and this is generally caused by pulmonary hypertension with right ventricular failure owing to a large clot lodging in the right ventricle.

The symptoms of a DVT include pain or tenderness over the area, swelling, and local heat. There may be **erythema** associated with the vessel wall damage. The majority (80%) of DVTs, however, are asymptomatic. Prevention is crucial if the health profession is to reduce the number of deaths from pulmonary embolism and the number of long-term health problems resulting from DVT.

From 1 June 2010, it is mandatory to have a documented risk assessment for every patient admitted to hospital, adhering to the criteria as set by the NICE Clinical Guidance No. 92. (See Venous Thromboembolism Risk Assessment form—Department of Health Gateway Reference 10278. The form can be downloaded from **http://www.kingsthrombosiscentre.org.uk**. See also Scottish Intercollegiate Guideline Network (SIGN) guidelines on prevention and management of venous thromboembolism.)

Each patient should be provided with verbal and written information about prevention of DVT, information on the signs and symptoms, and what action to take should he or she have concerns. Also see Chapter 23 Managing Mobility ➡️ .

Discharge planning

When facilitated effectively, discharge planning can lead to containing costs and improving patient outcomes (Shepherd *et al.*, 2010). Key to this is determining the appropriate time in the individual's care, with forward planning and notice so that the provision of essential services can be organized.

The importance of good discharge planning is highlighted by a number of useful high-quality resources, which can be found at:

- Royal College of Nursing, 2004 **http://www.rcn.org.uk/_data/assets/pdf_file/0011/78509/001376.pdf**
- NHS Institute 2008 **http://www.institute.nhs.uk/quality_and_service_improvement_tools/quality_and_service_improvement_tools/discharge_planning.html**

With 40% of surgical patients being elderly, it is imperative that good discharge planning takes into consideration health and social care needs. Patients with home care prior to admission should be encouraged to make their own arrangements to stop and restart the care on the dates provided by the secondary care provider. Those patients who have no prior arrangements, but for whom it is anticipated that care will be required following surgery, should have the required documentation completed at the patient preparation appointment. This can then be filed in the notes and faxed to the appropriate care department on the morning of admission. Social care support usually takes 48 hours to arrange.

Criteria for correct site surgery

The National Patient Safety Agency (NPSA) and the Royal College of Surgeons remain committed to the promotion of correct site surgery. Rather than leave the decision as to the site of surgery (e.g. right or left side, arm or leg) to one individual, the NPSA concluded that multiple checks should be made along the patient's surgical pathway.

The NPSA is a body that monitors incidents and near misses. Safer surgery can be improved through better understanding of incidents, and the reporting and learning system has been devised to be anonymous and, as such, supports the commitment of the health professional to report incidents such that they can be collated and guidance developed to minimize further occurrences. This is then implemented across the NHS. The surgical safety checklist gives a minimum number of checks that are required prior to induction, before skin incision, and before the patient leaves the operating room. Contained on a single page, the checks are made with a minimum of two interprofessionals and are designed to ensure that basic safety checks are made to confirm that equipment is functional, that emergency equipment is available, and that there is careful anticipation of patient potential concerns from the perspective of the surgeon, anaesthetist, and nursing team.

Obesity and surgery

Surgery and anaesthetics are not without risks, and there are additional risks when the obese patient requires surgery.

Body mass index (BMI) is the term used to describe the height/weight ratio of an adult. BMI is the ratio of weight in kilograms to height in metres squared, and provides a more accurate measure of obesity or overweight than weight alone (National Cancer Institute Factsheet, 2004). Obesity is the medical term given when the BMI is 30 or more (National Audit Office, 2001). A BMI of 40 or more is considered morbidly obese, i.e. presenting a real threat to

health. It should be noted that there are exceptions, notably a person who, perhaps through sport, is very muscular and may have a BMI greater than 25.

Some 50% of patients with a BMI of >40, and 100% of those whose BMI is >70, have sleep apnoea. In February 2001, the National Audit office issued *Tackling Obesity in England* and *Statistics on Obesity, Physical Activity and Diet England: 2010* (NHS Information Centre, 2010; **http://www. ic.nhs.uk/webfiles/publications/003_Health_Lifestyles/ opad11/Statistics_on_Obesity_Physical_Activity_and_ Diet_England_2011_revised_Aug11.pdf**). This noted that there are 30,000 deaths per annum associated with obesity, and details the trends within the English population on diet and exercise on obesity and obesity management. Also see Chapter 24 Managing Nutrition ⊙.

Implications of obesity for surgery

Obese patients have a reduced functional residual capacity, resulting in airway closure and desaturation in the supine position, as well as rapid desaturation if difficulty is encountered at intubation. Careful respiratory history is essential, looking for a SpO^2 of ≥96% on air—as per the AAGBI guidelines published June 2007, Perioperative management of the morbidly obese patient.

Cardiovascular disease is common in obese patients—particular attention will be given to hypertension, ischaemic heart disease, and to heart failure. Ascertaining exercise tolerance will reveal the patient's current ability. Morbidly obese patients have a high incidence of diabetes; all should have random and fasting blood glucose. Patients with gastro-oesophageal reflux may be candidates for prescribing antacid prophylaxis.

Prior to surgery, it is important that health professionals identify and assess the obese patient, outline treatment options, and monitor and audit their weight management. An example of an obesity care pathway can be found in Figure 26.5 and more detail can be found on the National Obesity Forum website: **http://www.nationalobesityforum.org.uk/index.php/lifestyle/adults_/ obesity-care-pathway/25-care-pathway-a-toolkit.html**.

Preventing problems

With patient preparation for surgery, nursing objectives are to identify patient health status, to advise on expected length of hospitalization, and to ensure that all comorbidities are optimized prior to admission for surgery, preventing patient harm and minimizing cancellations on the day of admission.

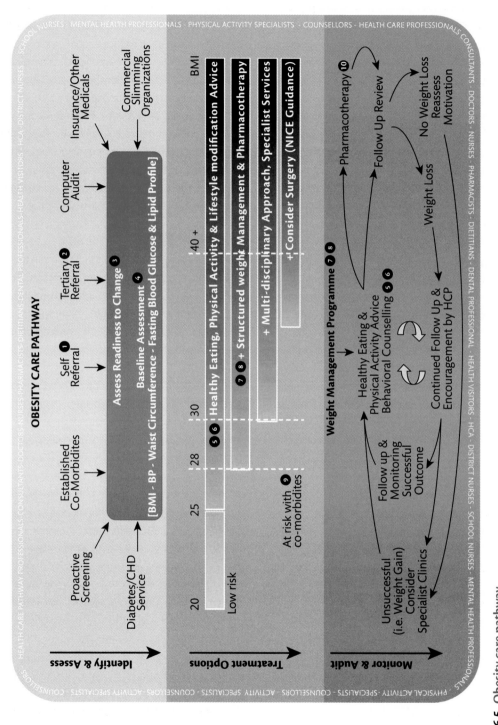

Figure 26.5 Obesity care pathway.

The assessor must communicate specific patient requirements to the appropriate person(s), e.g. MRSA-positive, risk of vCJD, or latex allergy. Whilst the number of patients requiring additional communication is small, a mechanism needs to be identified within the healthcare setting to ensure that the waiting list coordinators, ward manager, theatre manager, and theatre team are fully aware of this need.

Patient preparation for admission and perioperative nursing care provides a base for all levels of nursing professionals, from healthcare assistants through to consultant nurse. You can read more about the role of the nursing team in perioperative care on the Online Resource Centre ⓦ.

Accessing the evidence to inform clinical decisions

Several evidence-based tools have been mentioned in this chapter. Go online, find, and read the following documents:

- NICE Preoperative Investigations No. 3
- NICE Reducing the Risks of Venous Thromboembolism No. 92
- SIGN Guidelines on Prevention and Management of Venous Thromboembolism
- NPSA Correct Site Surgery Checklist
- WHO Surgical Safety Checklist
- NEWS
- Waterlow Chart
- Nutrition Score

Information on medical history for each patient will be included on the GP referral letter and in the patient case notes, and can be obtained from the patient and his or her relatives. The physiotherapist, occupational therapist, and other allied professionals will also keep a record of their interventions. All of the data provide evidence from which intervention can and will be planned. The ongoing care of the patient on admission will be recorded in the notes and transferred to the next professional by the written record as well as verbally. Communication is key for safe patient care.

Challenges in delivering evidence-based nursing

There are several factors in patient preparation that can be challenging. In particular are those associated with assessing patients who present to the nurse with their health history, much of which may not have been documented previously. It is the responsibility at patient preparation to refer all abnormal results and patients with comorbidities to a senior nurse, and for the senior nurse/house officer to determine the relevance of this information and whether further investigations, evidence, and/or action is required to mitigate the risk that the comorbidity may present to the expected surgery.

The nurse working within the division of surgery will need to demonstrate high-level communication skills to enable effective communication with the wide health professional team in primary and secondary care across many environments and specialties. Daily, the nurse will work with pharmacists and anaesthetists to convey information regarding his or her patient caseload accurately. The nurse will be expected to work outside the surgical specialty, obtaining information from medical specialties such as cardiology or endocrinology. He or she will then accurately interpret this information and reflect this in the care plan for the surgical admission, working with the waiting list coordinators, planning the admission for the patient, negotiating dates for surgery, and planning operating lists.

Measuring the impact of nursing interventions

Effective patient preparation should result in the patient being admitted on the day of his or her operation and proceeding as planned with the surgery. Patients have their surgery cancelled for a variety of reasons, some of which are out of their control and others of which are a direct result of their becoming unfit for surgery between preparation and admission, such as developing a chest infection or becoming pregnant.

Patients might also have their operations cancelled on the day of surgery owing to issues that should have been identified by a healthcare provider during the patient preparation, such as the patient having a cardiac condition that was not identified on the ECG, a poorly controlled diabetic, or an anaemic patient who should have received intervention prior to admission.

By monitoring the number of patients who completed their surgery, the number of assessments, and the number cancelled due to omissions at the time of patient preparation, it is possible to work out the percentage of patients cancelled because of poor preparation.

PROMs

On 12 April 2009, the Department of Health introduced Patient Reported Outcome Measures (PROMs). Patients due to undergo hip or knee replacement, groin hernia repair, or varicose vein surgery are invited to complete a patient questionnaire prior to surgery, to identify their perception of the quality of life, pain, and restrictions of daily living. The completion of the form is not compulsory and a few patients may be unable or reluctant to complete it. The Department of Health has set targets for completion of each of these procedures. Three months after surgery, the general surgical patients receive a follow-up questionnaire (6 months later for the orthopaedic patients), which is designed to measure the patient's perception post surgery. An independent company then produces a comparison of the two questionnaires, and the information is delivered back to the strategic healthcare commissioners and the healthcare providers. This principle will be expanded to include other aspects of patient care and additional procedures.

Go to **http://www.ic.nhs.uk/statistics-and-data-collections/hospital-care/patient-reported-outcome-measures-proms**

Summary and key messages

- Communication is key throughout the whole interprofessional team, in both primary and secondary care. Unless there is clear communication with everyone involved in a patient's admission episode, then key concerns may not receive the full attention that they deserve.

- Communication with the patient and his or her relatives is important so that the patient and, where appropriate, his or her relatives are provided with information that allows informed choice regarding any treatment.

- Consent must be informed and valid. Check that the patient has received all relevant information in a format that he or she can understand, and that he or she has been given the opportunity to discuss any concerns. Where patients lack capacity to reach a decision, ensure that the correct process is followed to safeguard the patient's care.

- Accurate, concise history recording is key to provide clarity and a summary of comorbidities, their duration, and current status. It is from this concise information that treatment will be planned and implemented.

- Investigations and tests must be appropriate to the patient; tests should be necessary for the patient's treatment, and must be checked and prompt action taken and recorded on the findings.

- Observations must be accurate and appropriately reported onwards. Comparisons will be made with baseline observations and will affect the treatment regime.

- High-quality patient care is the right of every patient. This can be achieved through interprofessional teamwork that supports evidence-based practice, maintains accuracy, and undergoes continual audit and development.

Online Resource Centre

 To help you to develop and apply your knowledge and decision-making skills further, we have provided interactive learning resources online at **www.oxfordtextbooks.co.uk/orc/bullock/**

Whilst these are freely available, you will need to use the access codes at the start of the book.

References

Association of Anaesthetists of Great Britain and Ireland (AAGBI) (2010) *Pre-operative Assessment and Patient Preparation:The Role of the Anaesthetist*, 2nd edn. AAGBI: London.

Baker, D.P., Gustafson, S., Beaubien, J.M., *et al.* (2005) Medical team training programs in health care. *Advances in Patient Safety: From Research to Implementation, Vol. 4.* Agency for Healthcare Research and Quality: Rockville, MD.

Department of Health (2007) *Saving Lives: Reducing Infection, Delivering Clean and Safe Care.* Department of Health: London.

Department of Health (2008). Carers at the heart of 21st century families and communities: a caring system on your side, a life of your own. Gateway reference 9971. **http://www.dh.gov.uk/en/ Publicationsandstatistics/Publications/PublicationsPolicy- AndGuidance/DH_085345** (accessed 23 December 2011).

Department of Health (2010) *Delivering Enhanced Recovery: Helping Patients to get Better Sooner after Surgery.* Department of Health: London.

Department of Health ACDP TSE Risk Management Subgroup (2006, updated January 2011) Annex J. vCJD assessment to be carried out before surgery and endoscopy to identify patients with, or at risk of CJD or vCJD. Department of Health: London.

Emerson, E., and Hatton, C. (2008) *Estimating Future Need for Adult Social Care Services for People with Learning Disabilities in England.* Lancaster: Centre for Disability Research, Lancaster University.

Flin, R., Maran, N. (2004) Identifying and training non-technical skills for teams in acute medicine. *Quality and Safety in Health Care*, **13**: (Suppl. 1): i80–i84.

Health Protection Agency Surgical Site Infection Surveillance Scheme (SSISS) **www.hpa.org.uk** (accessed 23 December 2011)

National Audit Office (2001) *Tackling Obesity in England.* NAO: London.

National Audit Office (2010) *Statistics on Obesity, Physical Activity and Diet: England, 2011.* **http://www.ic.nhs.uk/webfiles/ publications/003_Health_Lifestyles/opad11/Statistics_ on_Obesity_Physical_Activity_and_Diet_England_2011_ revised_Aug11.pdf** (accessed 26 March 2012).

National Cancer Institute (2004) Factsheet: Obesity and Cancer—Questions and Answer. National Cancer Institute: London.

National Confidential Enquiry into Patient Outcome and Death (NCEPOD) (2009) *Adding Insult to Injury.* NCEPOD: London.

National Institute for Health and Clinical Excellence (NICE) (2003) *The use of routine preoperative tests for elective surgery.* NICE Clinical Guideline 3 (CG3). **http://www.nice.org.uk/CG003** (accessed 26 March 2012).

National Institute for Health and Clinical Excellence (NICE) (2008a) *Surgical Site Infection.* NICE Clinical Guideline 94 (CG94). NICE: London.

National Institute for Health and Clinical Excellence (2008b). Clinical Guideline No. 74 *Surigical Site Iinfections* **http://guidance.nice. org.uk** (accessed 23 December 2011).

National Institute for Health and Clinical Excellence (NICE) (2010). *Delirium.* NICE Clinical Guideline 103 (CG103). NICE: London.

National Health Institute for Health and Improvement (2010) *Discharge Planning.* **http://www.institute.nhs.uk/quality_ and_service_improvement_tools/quality_and_service_ improvement_tools/discharge_planning.html** (accessed 23 December 2011).

National Health Institute for Health and Improvement (2008) *Preoperative Assessment.* **http://www.institute.nhs.uk/ quality_and_service_improvement_tools/quality_and_ service_improvement_tools/pre-operative_assessment_ and_planning.html** (accessed 23 December 2011).

National Obesity Forum Obesity Care pathway (2006) **http:/www. nationalobesityforum.org.uk** (accessed 23 December 2011)

Neasham, J. (1996) Nurse led pre-assessment clinics. *British Journal of Theatre Nursing* **6**(8): 5–6.

NHS Information Centre for Health and Social Care (2010) Statistics on obesity, physical activity and diet: England 2010. **www. ic.nhs.uk/webfiles/publications/opad10/Statistics_on_ Obesity_Physical_Activity_and_Diet_England_2010.pdf/**

Royal College of Nursing (2004) *Discharge Planning: Fact Sheet for Day Surgery.* **http://www.rcn.org.uk/data/assets/pdf_ file/0011/78509/001376.pdf** (accessed 23 December 2011).

Royal College of Nursing (2005) *Preoperative Association, BADS, APA, RCM Perioperative Fasting in Adults and Children.* RCN: London.

Sandler, D.A., Martin, J.F. (1989) Autopsy proven pulmonary embolism in hospital patients: are we detecting enough deep vein thrombosis? Journal of the Royal Society of Medicine **82**: 203–5.

Schutz, S. (2001). Oxygen saturation monitoring with pulse oximetry. In K.K. Carlson, D.J. Lynn-McHale *AACN Procedure manual for critical care, 4th ed*, pp. 129–38. Elsevier: London.

Shepherd, S., McClaren, J., Phillips, O., *et al.* (2010) Discharge planning from hospital to home. *Cochrane Database of Systematic Reviews* Issue: Art. No. CD000313. DOI: 10.1002/14651858. CD000313.pub3. (accessed 23 December 2011).

Smith, I., Krake, P., Murray, I. (2011) Perioperative fasting in adults and children. *European Journal of Anaesthesiology* **28**: 556–69.

World Health Organization (WHO) (2008) Surgical Safety Checklist **http://www.who.int/patientsafety/safesurgery/ss_check- list/en/index.html** (accessed 23 December 2011).

World Health Organization (WHO) (2009) *Safe Surgery Saves Lives.* WHO: Geneva.

27 *Managing* the Prevention of Skin Breakdown

Andrea Nelson

Introduction

This chapter addresses the fundamental role of nurses in the prevention of skin breakdown. Every nurse should possess the knowledge and skills to identify people at risk of skin breakdown, to select and implement strategies to maintain skin integrity, and to review the effectiveness of these to inform any necessary changes in care.

Skin breakdown is associated with long-term conditions such as diabetes, cardiovascular disease, and spinal cord injury, and with acute illnesses that cause mobility restriction such as surgery and severe illness. Diabetes is associated with foot ulcers, cardiovascular disease with leg ulcers, and acute or long-term mobility restriction is associated with pressure ulcers. This chapter focuses on these three categories of skin breakdown and illuminates the key responsibilities carried by nurses in each of these areas.

The first section of this chapter provides detailed guidance on the nursing management of pressure ulcer prevention. This is followed by a subsidiary section on the prevention of diabetic foot ulcers. The final section provides a short overview of the nursing role in preventing or managing venous ulceration.

Understanding the importance of the prevention of skin breakdown

Definitions

Pressure ulcers, which are also called pressure sores, bed sores, and decubitus ulcers, have been defined as:

> localized injury to the skin and/or underlying tissue usually over a bony prominence, as a result of pressure, or pressure in combination with shear. (European Pressure Ulcer Advisory Panel and National Pressure Ulcer Advisory Panel, 2010)

Pressure ulcers may present as persistent redness (where the skin is damaged, but not yet broken), blisters, shallow sores, or necrotic wounds extending to the muscle and bone.

An 'avoidable pressure ulcer' is one that developed and the provider of care did not do one of the following:

- evaluate the person's clinical condition and pressure ulcer risk factors;
- plan and implement interventions consistent with the person's needs and goals, and recognize standards of practice;
- monitor and evaluate the impact of the interventions; or
- revise the interventions as appropriate.

(Department of Health England, 2011)

An 'unavoidable pressure ulcer' is one that developed even though the provider of the care had:

- evaluated the person's clinical condition and pressure ulcer risk factors;
- planned and implemented interventions consistent with the person's needs and goals, and recognized standards of practice;
- monitored and evaluated the impact of the interventions; and
- revised the approaches as appropriate; or
- the individual refused to adhere to prevention strategies in spite of education of the consequences of non-adherence.

(Department of Health England, 2011)

Diabetic foot ulcers are a specific form of pressure ulceration in people with diabetes. Alterations in foot architecture, as well as neuropathic and ischaemic changes, can result in skin damage and ulceration.

Venous leg ulcers are areas of skin loss between the knee and the heel secondary to chronic venous insufficiency. If a wound on the leg fails to heal within 6 weeks, then it is deemed to be a 'leg ulcer'. The majority of leg ulcers are secondary to vascular insufficiency, with venous ulcers being the commonest, followed by arterial ulcers. Their management may be complicated by the presence of both arterial and venous disease (mixed arterial–venous ulcers).

The prevention of pressure ulcers

Pressure ulcers are a significant problem in all healthcare settings. Up to 25% of people in Canadian hospitals (Hurd and Posnett, 2009) and 18% in European hospitals (EPUAP survey, 2007) were found to have pressure ulcers. The majority of these were superficial: for example, 57% of those seen in one survey (Tannen *et al.*, 2006) had no skin break and 28% were shallow sores. Severe pressure ulcers, although rarer, are recorded as 'clinical incidents' and investigated to learn how they might be prevented in future.

The vast majority of pressure ulcers are avoidable; they have occurred because risk assessment, intervention (e.g. equipment provision, nursing care, patient education), monitoring of skin condition, or revision of care plans in light of changes in the condition or skin health were inadequate. Health services are now using the number of avoidable pressure ulcers as an indicator of the quality of nursing care. The number of unavoidable pressure ulcers can only be determined if there is accurate recording of all stages of care planning, actions taken, and monitoring of effect, with any revisions made in the light of changes in skin health or patient general condition. This means that your responsibility is not only to be engaged in pressure ulcer prevention, but also to record all elements of the nursing care plan accurately so that healthcare providers can identify when ulcers developed *in spite of* adequate care (i.e. they were unavoidable). Careful audit can help nurses to identify where they need to improve the systems of care in pressure ulcer prevention, because these complications can be devastating to patients.

The human and economic costs of pressure ulcers

The human impact of pressure ulcers has been investigated using interviews and surveys designed to measure 'health-related quality of life'. A systematic review of such studies (Gorecki *et al.*, 2009) described the major physical, psychological, and social effects that pressure ulcers had on patients. Having an ulcer reduces an individual's ability to get out and about, to go shopping, and to perform activities of daily living. The pain from pressure ulcers affects appetite, and makes it difficult to get comfortable sitting or lying down. Pressure ulcers also affect social life due to the pain and smell. Some people reported no longer being able to sleep with their partner owing to the difficulties in positioning themselves in bed and needing to move frequently. Pain is common and has been described as 'constant' and 'punishing'. Having a pressure ulcer is costly because of time required off work, frequent laundry of clothes and bedding (after ulcers leaked), and prescriptions for dressings, antibiotics, etc. Psychological impacts include low mood, anger, frustration, anxiety, depression, and hopelessness. Some patients become angry, as they feel their ulcer could have been avoided if health professionals had acted when they first reported discomfort. Patients report that pressure ulcers affect friends and family and their relationships/sociability, making the patient more dependent on their family for help. There is also a conflict between patients' needs and good nursing management. For example, patients want to sleep through the night, whereas the care plan calls for frequent repositioning.

Between 1% (Severens *et al.*, 2002) and 4% (Bennett *et al.*, 2004) of the healthcare budget is used on pressure ulcer prevention and treatment. One UK estimate makes pressure ulcers the most costly wound to the UK NHS. Posnett and Franks (2008) estimate that they cost between £1.8 and £2.6 billion per year in the NHS, and much of this will be in nursing time.

Risk factors for pressure ulceration

There are a number of intrinsic (patient-related) and extrinsic (environment-related) factors that increase the risk of tissue damage (Table 27.1). The extrinsic factors are the damaging forces that act on the body; the intrinsic factors are those that affect the body's response to these forces. Studies have identified the characteristics that people who develop pressure ulcers have in common. The risk of developing an ulcer may be associated with factors that are correlated, such as being older and being incontinent.

Table 27.1 Factors associated with pressure ulcer development

The likely intrinsic factors associated with pressure ulcers	The likely extrinsic factors that increase the risk of pressure ulcers
Immobility	Pressure
Incontinence	Shear
Malnutrition	Friction
Decreased sensation	Moisture
Altered mental status	Chemical irritants
Poor circulation	

Recognizing extrinsic risk factors of pressure, friction, and shear

When the skin is compressed or stretched, the skin arterioles and venules can become occluded. You can see the effect of pressure by holding a glass firmly–the skin is paler where it is compressed between your bones and the glass (see Figure 27.1). If the skin is compressed for only a short period of time, when the pressure is released the skin is reperfused with arterial blood, venous blood is drained away, and there is no damage. The reperfusion makes the skin flush red when the pressure is released (this 'blanching hyperaemia' becomes paler when pressed as the blood vessels are intact). Prolonged pressure means that the skin receives insufficient arterial blood supply and that waste products from skin metabolism accumulate, while local tissues are deprived of oxygen (they become anoxic). When the blood supply resumes, white blood cells react to the anoxia in the local environment by releasing the chemical triggers for inflammation and the resultant chemical cascade can lead to cell damage and death. This may result in damage to the small blood vessels so that, when you touch the reddened skin, the skin does not turn pale (blanche) as it should do. This *persistent* redness is called 'non-blanching erythema', and is a sign that the skin has already been damaged and that urgent action is required to prevent this damage (which at this stage is reversible) from progressing to open ulceration.

Pressure acts in a perpendicular orientation to the skin, whereas shear and friction both act parallel to the skin. Hess (2004) notes that shear is the force *within the skin layers* when the skeleton is moving in one direction (e.g. down the bed) and the upper layers of skin are tending to move in the opposite direction (staying in contact with the sheets). The layers between the skin and skeleton is deformed due to shear, and this reduces the blood supply. Ultimately, this may lead to ischaemia, cellular death, and skin breakdown. Friction exists where two surfaces move across one another, or

are about to move. For example, friction is the force exerted when skin moves across a surface such as sheets, or if the skin is rubbed: friction therefore acts *at the surface*. The forces on the person in bed are illustrated in Figure 27.2.

The development of pressure ulcers

Pressure ulcers do not occur every time the skin is under pressure. Skin can withstand the following without damage:

● High pressure for a short period of time; **or**

● Low pressure for a long time.

Healthy people move to relieve pressure simply through small, frequent, often imperceptible, movements. If the frequency is limited, however, injury can result. The 'critical' combination of pressure and duration will vary between patients, and over time, according to how well their skin is perfused, their response to reperfusion injury, and their general level of health or vulnerability. It is important to keep the following formula in mind at all times.

Pressure ulcer = Magnitude of pressure × Duration of pressure

The key to the nursing management of pressure ulcer prevention is to reduce the amount of pressure on the body (magnitude), and/or the time for which the pressure is acting on each area of skin (duration). There is no 'safe' pressure or time that applies to everyone. Hence you will need to adopt a personalized approach to reducing pressure magnitude and duration. Regular, careful clinical assessment of the skin will confirm whether a pressure ulcer prevention plan is effective.

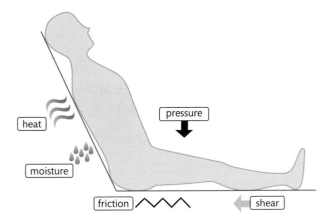

Figure 27.1 **The effect of pressure on skin perfusion. (Note the blanching at the fingertip caused by pressing skin against glass).**

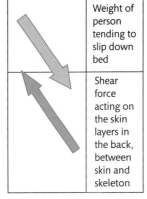

Figure 27.2 **Forces acting on a person in bed.**

Nursing responsibilities and accountability for pressure ulcer prevention

The overarching principles comprise assessment, communication, action, and review. Ulcer prevention involves ensuring that hydration and nutritional needs of patients are met (see Chapters 19 Managing Hydration and 24 Managing Nutrition ➡), identifying continence problems (see Chapter 16 Managing Continence ➡), and maintaining comfort, dignity, and skin integrity (see Chapter 20 Managing Hygiene ➡).

Clinical assessment of the risk of skin breakdown

Approximately 40 risk assessment tools have been developed to help nurses to identify patients at risk of pressure ulceration (Moore and Cowman, 2008). Not all of these can identify risk accurately and reliably, and they are no substitute for clinical judgement. An example of one widely used tool is the Braden scale, which asks about mobility, activity, nutrition, sensory perception, moisture, and friction and shear (Bergstrom *et al.*, 1987).

If a risk assessment tool is very sensitive, but not specific, it will identify people at risk correctly, but will also identify some people who are not actually at risk as being so, meaning that resources could be wasted. If a risk assessment tool is not sensitive, but is very specific, then it will underpredict risk, identifying people not at risk correctly but missing some people at risk, meaning that people may miss out on the care they need. The ideal risk assessment tool, therefore, has high sensitivity and specificity so that we can trust it won't miss people at risk or waste resources (Box 27.1).

The nurse's responsibilities for assessing risk include the following steps:

- using a validated pressure ulcer risk assessment tool;
- recording assessment findings;
- taking action based on assessment to provide the most appropriate evidence-based interventions;
- evaluating whether the actions have been effective;
- re-evaluating the plan for care and risk assessment as the patient's condition dictates.

It is important to assess the risk to all patients in relation to developing a pressure ulcer, and if a patient already has ulcers, you should assess them according to the principles laid out in Chapter 28 Managing Wounds ➡.

Additionally, you should be aware of ulcer rating systems such as the European Pressure Ulcer Advisory Panel (EPUAP) scale **http://www.epuap.org/grading.html**, which categorizes ulcers as follows.

- Category/Grade 1 damage in the EPUAP scale is non-blanching erythema (persistent redness)
- Category/Grade 2 damage is partial thickness skin loss, i.e. blister or shallow open ulcer with a red/pink wound bed
- Category/Grade 3 damage is full thickness skin loss; subcutaneous fat may be visible, but bone, tendon, or muscle are not exposed
- Category/Grade 4 damage is full thickness tissue loss with exposed tendon, bone, or muscle

The use of a common ulcer rating scale for describing pressure damage across settings helps communication between colleagues when patients move between settings, and helps to ensure that all clinicians are 'speaking the same language' when they describe a pressure ulcer, for example at handover.

Nursing interventions to prevent skin breakdown

You should employ two complementary strategies to reduce the risk of your patients developing a pressure ulcer:

- reducing the extrinsic risk factors (pressure, shear, and friction—both the duration and/or magnitude of these forces)
- improving the body's resilience against the pressure.

Box 27.1 Sensitivity and specificity

The ability of a tool to identify people *at risk* of a condition correctly is 'sensitivity'.

The ability of a tool to identify people who are *not at risk* of a condition correctly is 'specificity'.

Both sensitivity and specificity range from 0% to 100% (a perfect tool is 100% sensitive and 100% specific).

A summary of pressure ulcer prevention strategies can be found in Table 27.2 and each of these strategies is discussed below.

Reducing the magnitude of pressure

Pressure exerted by a body on a point is defined as the weight acting at that point divided by the area at that point able to support the body (Pressure = Force/Area). For example, stiletto heels produce a higher pressure on the floor than trainers because the area of contact is much smaller. You should use this principle to reduce skin interface pressure by increasing the *area of support*. For example, patients in chairs have a smaller contact area to support their body weight than when they are lying flat, hence the risk of pressure ulcers is higher when seated. Figure 27.3 outlines extrinsic factors such as pressure, shear, and friction that can damage the skin.

In addition, you can choose specialist foam or soft fibre mattresses that conform (mould) to the shape of the body and allow the body to 'sink' into them, increasing the skin contact area and reducing pressure. There are also a number of high-tech mattresses that work on this prin-ciple. For example, the air-fluidized bead bed provides a surface that is stable and firm until air is pumped through a reservoir of small ceramic beads, which become fluidized, so that the person 'floats' on the beads: high contact area means low pressure. Similarly, the low air-loss bed has the patient 'floating' on an array of vertical 'semi-permeable pillows', which are inflated by an air source: lying on the soft pillows increases surface area and reduces pressure. The evidence for the effectiveness of pressure ulcer support surfaces can be found in Table 27.3.

Reducing duration of pressure

Repositioning is the key to reducing the duration of deforming forces (pressure, shear, and friction) acting on the skin (see Figure 27.3). If the patient is in a chair, help him or her to stand for a few seconds to allow the skin to reperfuse, or transfer him or her back to bed. For patients in bed, you will need to position the patient in rotation (back, right side, back, left side), to ensure that the pressure on any one area is not sustained for long enough to lead to damage. A repositioning 'clock' can prompt the change in position every few hours and is illustrated in Figure 27.4.

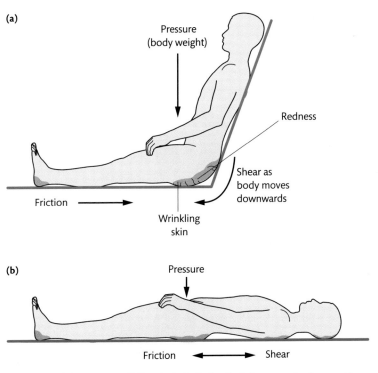

Figure 27.3 **Pressure, shear, and friction: a sliding in (a) chair; (b) lying on a bed or trolley.**

Reproduced from Docherty & McCallum, *Foundation Clinical Nursing Skills*, by permission of Oxford University Press.

Principles: reducing shear

When patients are positioned in a bed or chair, it is easy for them to slip down. If this happens, the upper layers of skin are pulled in the opposite direction to the lower layers of skin, and this causes disruption of the blood supply. To reduce shear, your patient needs to be positioned so that he or she is not prone to slippage. This is difficult if a standard hospital bed or the patient's own bed is being used, because if the patients are propped up with pillows at the back, they will tend to slip simply due to gravity. To counteract this, profiling beds can be used to raise the knees, and this reduces the tendency to slip down.

Maintaining the body's resilience to pressure and shear

As a nurse, you have a responsibility not only to limit the external forces acting upon the skin by reducing pressure, shear, and friction, but also to ensure that the patient has well perfused skin, with the ability to resist skin damage. This means paying attention to skin care to ensure that the skin is kept clean, dry, well moisturized, is not exposed to damaging excesses of moisture such as sweat or urine, and is not damaged by harsh soaps and physical damage during washing or moving and handling (see Chapter 20 Managing Hygiene ➡), and attending to skin hygiene.

The expert nursing care of skin perfusion means paying attention to nutrition and hydration (see Chapters 19 Managing Hydration and 24 Managing Nutrition ➡).

Accessing the evidence base for pressure ulcer prevention strategies

A number of studies have been undertaken to evaluate the relative effectiveness of different preventative interventions for pressure ulcerations. The gold standard research design for such studies is the randomized controlled trial (RCT). Table 27.2 details strategies for avoiding pressure ulcers. A summary of systematic reviews of these studies is provided in Table 27.3. It is also important to look at the impact of such interventions in terms of quality of life, acceptability, and economic cost. Further qualitative and quantitative studies are required to inform these areas. Evidence box 27.1 highlights the evidence gaps in pressure ulcer knowledge.

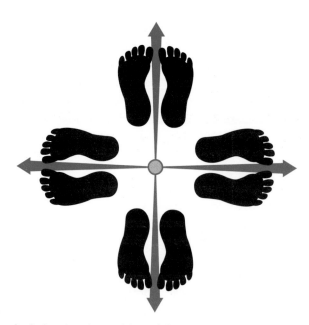

Figure 27.4 **Repositioning clock showing the position of the person at 12, 3, 6, and 9 o'clock.**

Table 27.2 Summary of pressure ulcer prevention strategies

Principle	Interventions	Example
Reduce magnitude of pressure	Provide a conforming mattress/overlay/cushion (for chair/wheelchair)	Specialized foam mattress, medical sheepskin or hollow fibre overlay, low airless mattress, air-fluidized bead bed
Reduce duration of pressure	Reposition person frequently Use an alternating mattress/overlay	Plan repositioning schedule for the day to allow person to be seated during mealtimes and to return to bed between times to relieve pressure on buttocks Reposition person in chair—standing/bed/chair to avoid excessive time in one position Ensure alternating pressure equipment working correctly
Reduce shear	Position patient in bed or chair to prevent slippage	Use a profiling bed Ensure chairs are correct height and depth to prevent slippage
Reduce friction	Avoid sliding patient over sheets Reduce friction during skin care	When moving patient, ensure technique does not drag skin over sheet/transfer equipment Avoid rubbing skin with rough towels or clothes during cleansing and drying—blot skin
Support skin perfusion	Maintain hydration and nutrition Support cardiovascular system	Ensure patient is well hydrated and nourished Ensure blood supply to extremities is adequate
Support skin environment	Maintain clean dry skin Moisturize skin	Inspection of skin at pressure areas to identify dampness due to incontinence, fever, sweat, and skin care to wash, carefully dry

Diabetic foot ulcers

Understanding the importance of the prevention of diabetic foot ulcers

Foot ulcers affect many people with diabetes at some time in their life. They are associated with reduced quality of life, higher costs, and increased mortality and morbidity (Iversen *et al.*, 2009). Around 6% of the people with diabetes in the UK have had a foot ulcer (Williams *et al.*, 2000), with a 15–25% lifetime risk of a foot ulcer (Singh *et al.*, 2005). Diabetic foot ulcers take weeks (often months) to heal, and while they are open they increase the risk of infection of the foot or lower limb (including osteomyelitis) and/or gangrene.

The diabetes community set itself a target to halve the number of foot amputations arising from diabetic foot ulcers within 10 years in the St Vincent Declaration (World Health Organization/IDF Saint Vincent Declaration Working Group, 1990) by reducing the number of people with diabetes developing foot ulcers, and improving care of open ulcers. The responsibility of the nurse is to minimize the risk of foot ulcer development by educating patients about how they can reduce the chances of all complications of diabetes through good diabetic control (see Chapter 9 Understanding Diabetes Mellitus ➡) and good skin care (see Chapter 20 Managing Hygiene ➡), as well as how to identify potential problems with their feet that require prompt attention from their nurse, doctor, or podiatrist, and how to care for their feet.

The human and economic costs of foot ulcers

When people with foot ulcers are compared with a group without ulcers, research has found that foot ulcers are associated with a significantly lower health-related quality of life: for example, in the physical limitations that the ulcer places on mobility and ability to do things around the house as well as general well-being (Ribu *et al.*, 2007). A majority of people with foot ulcers find them painful, and Ribu and colleagues noted that 75% of their patients reported some pain related to their diabetic foot ulcer (Ribu *et al.*, 2006). Foot ulcers require frequent expert dressings and medical treatment (usually from a diabetic foot ulcer clinic in hospital), and Posnett and Franks (2008) estimated that foot ulcers cost the NHS around £300 million per year.

Risk factors for diabetic foot ulceration

Both type 1 diabetes (insulin-dependent diabetes), and type 2 diabetes (non-insulin-dependent diabetes) can lead to significant health problems. Complications of diabetes can affect the feet through a number of intrinsic factors, including:

- changes to foot architecture, leading to increases in plantar pressures;
- reduced sweating, leading to cracked skin;
- poor sensation, leading to increased susceptibility to trauma;
- reduced circulation, leading to reduced ability to heal wounds and fight infection.

These changes, secondary to neuropathy and ischaemic changes, either alone or in combination, predispose the foot to damage and ulceration. The intrinsic and extrinsic factors that contribute to foot ulceration in people with diabetes are summarized below, and illustration of how this knowledge can help to guide you in your care plan is also given.

Foot infections in people with diabetes can be hard to manage because of the impaired arterial supply to the legs, as well as disruption of the immune system, especially of the function of polymorphonuclear leukocytes that accompany diabetes. This means that there is an increased risk of worsening infection, resulting in more damage to the tissues of the foot, including the bones, and extending infection that progresses up the foot or leg and damages more tissues, as well as systemic spread into the bloodstream. Thus, when foot ulcer infection spreads, the treatment may need to include some level of lower extremity amputation (Williams and Airey, 2002), as a leg-saving and ultimately life-saving measure. The vast majority of foot or leg amputations in people with diabetes are preceded by a foot ulcer infection. Amputation is a major operation. It dramatically reduces the quality of life, and is expensive for the patient and the healthcare system. Therefore foot clinics have been established to coordinate and deliver the various elements of foot care to prevent ulceration and amputation. These clinics involve input from a range of health professionals, including nurses.

Causes of diabetic foot ulcers

The intrinsic factors that predispose people to foot ulceration are changes to foot architecture (shape), reduced sweating, and poor sensation, which are all secondary to altered peripheral nerve conduction (neuropathy) and

Table 27.3 The effects of preventative interventions for those at risk of developing pressure ulcers

Source	Population	Intervention	Comparison	Results	Clinical implication
McInnes *et al.*, 2011	Hospital inpatients at high risk of PU (fractured femur in four of eight trials)	Constant low pressure (CLP)	Standard foam mattress (SFM)	Eight trials: CLP probably better	Risk of PU may be reduced by CLP devices
McInnes *et al.*, 2011	Patients deemed to be at risk of PU in medical, vascular, orthopaedic, elderly acute, and oncology (In two of five RCTs, patients had fractured femur.)	Alternative foam mattress (AFM)	SFM	Five trials; 2016 people: AFM reduced ulcers by 26–79%	Risk of PU reduced by using specialized foam surfaces
McInnes *et al.*, 2011	Patients deemed to be at risk of PU in medical, vascular, orthopaedic, elderly acute, and oncology (In one of five RCTs, patients had femur fracture.)	AFM	AFM	Five trials: no clear evidence of difference	We cannot determine if one foam is better than another
McInnes *et al.*, 2011	Adults recruited from orthopaedics, aged care, and other 'unspecified' settings at low–moderate risk of ulcers	Medical sheepskin	No sheepskin	Four trials (three of adequate quality); 1283 people: open ulcers reduced by 44% (and likely between 3% and 68%)	Risk of PU reduced by using medical sheepskins
McInnes *et al.*, 2011	People at risk of ulcers in ICU, nursing homes, with fractured femur and orthopaedic trauma wards	CLP overlay	CLP overlay	Six trials: no clear evidence of difference	We cannot determine if one CLP surface is better than another
McInnes *et al.*, 2011	Acute hospital patients with high risk of pressure ulcers	Alternating pressure surfaces	SFM	Two trials; 409 people: ulcers reduced by 42% to 83%	In people at risk of PU, alternating pressure surfaces are better than SFM
McInnes *et al.*, 2011	Patients deemed to be at risk of PU in a variety of inpatient settings	Alternating pressure surfaces	CLP overlay	Ten trials: no clear evidence of difference	We cannot determine if alternating pressure devices are any better than CLP surfaces
McInnes *et al.*, 2011	People at risk of ulcers in ICU, medical, surgical and elderly care wards	Alternating pressure surfaces	Other alternating pressure surfaces	Five trials; 2216 people: no clear evidence of difference	We cannot determine if any one alternating pressure device is better than another

(continued)

Table 27.3 (*continued*)

Source	Population	Intervention	Comparison	Results	Clinical implication
McInnes *et al.*, 2011	People in hospital wards and ICU at risk of developing pressure ulcers	Low air-loss bed (LALB)	SFM	Three trials; 319 people: no clear evidence of difference	It is unclear whether LALBs are better than regular mattresses
McInnes *et al.*, 2011	Intensive care patients	Kinetic treatment table (KTT) that turned constantly	Standard surface with turning every 2 hours	Two trials; 151 people: no clear evidence of difference	It is unclear whether KTTs are better than regular surfaces
McInnes *et al.*, 2011	Surgical patients	Operating table overlay	No operating table overlay	Two trials; 591 people: no clear evidence of benefit	It is unclear whether an operating table overlap reduces ulcers
McInnes *et al.*, 2011	Surgical patients	Micropulse (MP) system	Standard mattress	Two trials; 368 people: MP reduced ulcers by 30–94%	In surgical patients, a micropulse overlay reduced ulcers
McInnes *et al.*, 2011	Seated patients	Seat cushion	Seat cushion	Four trials; 473 people: no clear evidence of difference	We do not know if one seat cushion is better than another
McInnes *et al.*, 2011	People in hospital at high risk of ulcer development	Electric profiling beds	Flat beds	One trial; 70 people: no difference	No evidence for profiling beds in small study
Defloor *et al.*, 2005	Elderly nursing home residents	4-hourly repositioning plus viscoelastic foam	Standard care or other turning regimens	One trial; 838 people given five different turning schedules	4-hourly turning on viscoelastic foam had lowest ulcer incidence
Young, 2004	Elderly people in hospital	Turning on a 30° tilt	Turning to 90°	One trial; 46 people	Not clear whether 30° or 90° position better
Langer *et al.*, 2003	Hip fracture, critically ill	One or two supplements daily, or nasogastric feed	Regular diet/ placebo supplement	Four trials; 974 people: one large trial found a reduction in ulcers	Nutritional interventions may reduce the risk of pressure ulcers
Reddy, 2011	Acute care and mixed settings	Topical lotions, fatty acids, hexachlorophene	Lotions without active component	Three trials; 819 people	We cannot determine if a topical agent reduces PU incidence
Torra I Bou *et al.*, 2002	People at risk of pressure ulcer development	Hydrocellular heel supports	Orthopaedic wool padding	One trial; 130 people: foam reduced number of ulcers	Foam heel dressing might reduce the number of ulcers (one small, poor study)

THEORY INTO PRACTICE 27.1
Considering the impact of a pressure ulcer

Think about the restrictions that a pressure ulcer would impose on the lifestyle of a patient for whom you are currently caring who is 'at risk' of developing a pressure ulcer. Remember that there may be physical, social, and psychological effects of a pressure ulcer. The ulcer will usually be accompanied by a cluster of symptoms, and these symptoms may have other effects on lifestyle, emotional mood, confidence, and getting out and about. The steps that nurses and carers put in place to help treat pressure ulcers may also have an impact—for example, beds that move to vary the pressure could be noisy or they may be difficult to get out of independently, and regular turning schedules may disrupt sleep or the ability to follow usual daily routines.

Who else in the family might be affected by the presence of a pressure ulcer, and what impact might it have on them? Think both about carers, and about other social and professional contacts.

providing and/or educating patients about general foot care, and being vigilant about the potential for foot ulceration, referring people at risk to a specialist service. This means that you need to be aware of where the diabetic foot ulcer services are in your area.

Clinical assessment of the risk of diabetic foot ulceration

People with diabetes are at higher risk of foot ulcers if the arterial supply to the foot is impaired, if they have poor sensation, if their foot shape has changed, or if they have ever had a foot ulcer in the past. Nurses need to ensure that patients are screened, formally, each year for reduced blood supply, sensation, or foot deformities. People with any of these factors should be referred to a clinic for podiatry and protective shoes, as well as education regarding foot care. This systematic approach to screening and referral has been found to reduce the risk of an amputation from 1 in 100 to 1 in 1,000 (McCabe *et al.*, 1998).

reduced circulation secondary to arterial disease (ischaemia). Both ischaemia and neuropathy are exacerbated by poor control of blood glucose. The extrinsic factors predisposing to foot ulceration include poor toenail care (leading to traumatic damage to toes), poor shoe selection (leading to the application of high local pressures to the tissues of the foot), poor foot care (such as walking barefoot or washing the feet in hot water), and sustaining undetected damage on insensate feet. Your nursing interventions to prevent foot ulcers should address both the extrinsic and intrinsic factors.

Nursing responsibilities and accountability for diabetic foot ulcer prevention

The foot care that you provide for patients with diabetes should focus on the prevention of foot ulcers through optimizing diabetic control (see Chapters 9 Understanding Diabetes Mellitus and 20 Managing Hygiene ➡),

Nursing interventions to prevent skin breakdown

Foot care includes supplying special shoes to reduce the pressure on the ulcer, supporting the healing of foot ulcers by optimizing diabetic control, and providing wound dressing and adjuvant treatments. As a nurse, you also play a key role in the prevention of amputation by the early identification of infection. Early identification of infection will facilitate accurate characterization of the infection and aggressive treatment of both infection and ischaemia.

Addressing intrinsic factors

The neuropathic and ischaemic changes to the foot, either alone or in combination, predispose the foot to damage and ulceration. Damage to the motor nerves leads to changes to the architecture of the foot. Motor nerves keep the bones and muscles of the foot in equilibrium and this leads to the shape of the normal foot.

CASE STUDY 27.1 *Addressing the intrinsic and extrinsic factors associated with pressure ulceration*

Mrs Montgomery, a 56-year-old woman who suffers from multiple sclerosis, has been admitted to the ward with a pyrexia of unknown origin for investigations and treatment. She has limited mobility and uses a wheelchair. On admission, she is rather unwell, her temperature is elevated, and she feels clammy. Her clothes appear quite roomy and, on questioning about recent weight loss, she reports that she has lost weight recently, which she puts down to not having an appetite.

Questions

➤ What intrinsic factors place Mrs Montgomery at increased risk of developing a pressure ulcer?

➤ What extrinsic factors might place Mrs Montgomery at increased risk of developing a pressure ulcer?

➤ What nursing interventions do you need to put in place to minimize the risk of Mrs Montgomery developing a pressure ulcer?

➤ What nursing measures would you put in place to monitor the success of the nursing interventions in preventing pressure ulceration?

➤ What information would you give Mrs Montgomery about her risk of developing pressure ulceration when planning for discharge from hospital?

Diabetes leads to changes in the balance between muscles of the foot and so the shape of the foot changes, eventually leading to a 'Charcot foot' (Figure 27.5). Areas of the foot that are unaccustomed to loadbearing then experience high pressures. Nurses play a key role in preventing damage and neuropathy through supporting patients in the control of blood sugar levels (see Chapter 9 Understanding Diabetes Mellitus ➡).

Autonomic neuropathy leads to reduced sweating, and the resultant dry skin is prone to cracking. You should educate and support patients and carers in relation to good skin care, emphasizing careful washing, drying, and moisturizing to maintain flexibility and skin integrity (see Chapter 20 Managing Hygiene ➡).

Ischaemia leads to reduced circulation, and hence a reduced ability to heal wounds and fight infection. Your nursing interventions require careful attention to preventing ischaemia through control of blood sugar levels and addressing other risk factors for arterial disease, such as smoking cessation and maintenance of a healthy diet (see Chapter 24 Managing Nutrition ➡).

Addressing extrinsic factors

For people with altered foot shape, the prevention of damage relies on the use of insoles and footwear to reduce pressure by increasing contact area. These work on the same principles as those discussed in the section on pressure ulceration to redistribute pressure and hence minimize skin damage. The application of excessive pressures to skin unaccustomed to loadbearing causes callus formation and/or breakdown. The use of pressure-reducing insoles (in-shoe orthotics) and specialized footwear with increased toe-box depth can avoid trauma and pressure. You will need to support patients and carers in the use of specialized insoles and footwear because patients may not be able to feel the pain of ill-fitting shoes that would guide the person without neuropathy to take them off. A Cochrane review of pressure-relieving interventions concluded that in-shoe orthotics are of benefit (Spencer, 2000). They were not able to identify a 'best-bet' orthotic, because the studies were small. Spencer concluded that cushioning and pressure redistribution insoles appeared to offer equal benefit. Specialized shoes halved the incidence

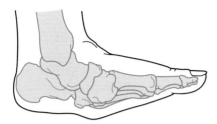

Figure 27.5 Charcot foot.

of ulceration. Trainers with foam-based insoles may be a socially acceptable way in which to reduce foot pressures, but they have not been adequately evaluated. Further research is needed in this important area.

Sensory neuropathy means that patients are unaware of damage from trauma or poor-fitting footwear or socks/hosiery. You can help to address this sensory neuropathy by checking footwear and stressing the importance of wearing correctly sized and fitted shoes, boots, or slippers and wearing appropriately sized socks or hosiery. Patients and their carers need to be shown how to inspect the feet regularly, by using mirrors if needed, to identify any areas of skin damage.

You have a responsibility to ensure that toenail care in diabetic patients is undertaken by someone with expertise to avoid traumatic damage to toes, as well as selecting comfortable footwear. In many cases, this means that a referral to a podiatrist who undertakes toenail care is required.

Systematic skin inspection has been built into programmes of care for patients at risk of developing foot ulcers. Lavery *et al.* (2007) found that adding a foot temperature assessment to a package of education and daily skin inspections further reduced the numbers of people developing a foot ulcer from around 30% to 9%. Patients who identified temperature difference between their two feet were prompted to contact their nurse and to rest more for the next few days, until the temperature difference subsided. The high temperature was a sign of reactive hyperaemia and a sign of early skin damage, reversible by rest.

Patient education

Many diabetes care teams spend significant amounts of time on patient education in order to improve patients' and carers' knowledge and care of the feet, to reduce the number of foot ulcers. A Cochrane systematic review of trials found that there was a lack of high-quality evidence about the effectiveness of patient education interventions (Dorresteijn *et al.*, 2010). Overall, the reviewers concluded that, in some trials, education sessions or leaflets improved foot care knowledge and self-reported patient behaviour in the short term. Given the poor evidence base, they concluded that there is currently insufficient evidence to support the view that patient education *alone* is effective in reducing the numbers of ulcers.

More research is needed in this area to inform the most appropriate approaches to helping patients and carers effectively to self-manage the prevention of foot damage (see Evidence box 27.2).

Venous leg ulcers

Understanding the importance of venous leg ulcers

Causes of venous leg ulcers

Venous ulceration occurs owing to increased pressure within the veins of the lower leg. This may be because the veins are blocked after a deep vein thrombosis (DVT) or valve failure (these promote bloodflow from the extremities towards the heart). Venous insufficiency results in distended, tortuous veins in the skin, leakage of fluid from the veins, and deposition of fibrin and the remains of red blood cells into the intercellular space. The fluid leads to oedema, the fibrin and red blood cells form a hardened skin tissue called lipodermatosclerosis, and to eczema.

EVIDENCE BOX 27.2
Where are the evidence gaps in diabetic foot ulcer knowledge?

We don't know the optimal elements of an education programme for avoiding diabetic foot ulcers.

Which of the various shoe inserts or insoles are best for avoiding foot ulceration?

We don't know the best way in which to help patients and their carers to look after their feet.

Table 27.4 **Summary of diabetic foot ulcer prevention strategies**

Principle	Interventions	Example
Maintaining optimal diabetic control	• Control of diet • Monitor blood glucose levels	• Support from diabetes nurse/dietitian • Self-testing devices for blood glucose • Follow-up with diabetic clinic
Screening for people at high risk of foot ulcers	• Blood supply • Neuropathy • Deformity • History of foot ulcer	• Pedal pulses/ankle:brachial pressure index • Semmes–Weinstein monofilament • Inspection/foot pressure readings
Skin and foot care	• Moisturizing skin • Avoiding trauma • Regular and frequent inspection for trauma • Toenail care that avoids trauma	• Use of **emollients** • Checking temperature of bathing water • Avoiding shoes that are too small or big or are tight • Inspection of sock and shoes for foreign objects/wear • Observation of skin to identify callus, temperature differences, or redness • Podiatry visit for toenail care
Patient education	• Knowledge about how diabetes affects the foot • Control of diabetes • Reinforcing behaviours that protect the foot, such as wearing insoles or footwear that minimizes pressure points	• Reinforce the importance of foot care and inspection given the lack of protective sensation

It is estimated that approximately 1% of people will be affected by ulcers on the legs at some time (Graham *et al.*, 2003). These ulcers are often caused by a small or forgotten trauma, which in most people heals in a week or so. What distinguishes these ulcers from normal wounds is their reticence to heal. To clearly identify people with leg ulcers who need additional care on top of simple home first aid, clinicians define a wound that has failed to heal in 6 weeks as an 'ulcer'. This failure to heal is usually because of alterations to the blood supply of the legs. In a small proportion of people, the problem is caused by poor arterial blood supply secondary to atherosclerosis. The majority of leg ulcers are, however, caused by poor venous return from the feet to the heart. This can be due to blockage or occlusion and/or weakness in the valves of the veins, resulting in venous incompetence (Callam *et al.*, 1985).

The human and economic costs of venous ulcers

Venous ulcers are a chronic wound and can last a long time: Callam *et al.* found that 45% of ulcer patients in a Scottish study had leg ulcers for more than 10 years (Callam *et al.*,

1985). They require dressings at least once a week, and the pain, smell, and exudates associated with them mean that they have a large impact on quality of life (Briggs and Flemming, 2007), including embarrassment, fear, anxiety, and depression. They occupy much of the clinical caseload for some community nurses, for example where the population is elderly.

Posnett and Franks (2008) estimated that the cost to the NHS of treating patients with venous ulcers, mostly in primary care and through community nursing services, is at least £168 million–198 million per year. This does not include the individual cost of venous ulceration such as reducing ability to be in full-time employment.

Risk factors for venous ulceration

Venous ulcers are also known as stasis or varicose ulcers because many people with them also have varicose veins. While it might be tempting to classify everyone with varicose veins as being at risk of ulcers, this is not feasible because a large number of people with varicose veins do not develop ulcers. Similarly, people who have had a DVT may be at increased risk of developing a venous ulcer because the DVT often leads to damage of the one-way valves in the vein. There are, however, no studies to date of interventions to prevent the first venous ulcer occurring in people with varicose veins or a history of venous problems such as DVT.

There is some evidence around interventions that support patients and carers in preventing recurrence of ulcers after healing (Nelson and Jones, 2008). The key to both treatment and prevention is to reduce the pressure in the veins of the leg. Surgical removal of superficial and/or perforating veins has been evaluated in some trials and been found to prevent recurrence (Nelson and Jones, 2008).

Nursing responsibilities and accountability for venous leg ulcer prevention

Your nursing interventions should include identification of people with signs of chronic venous insufficiency (distended veins in the ankle region, ankle oedema with associated brown staining of the skin, and eczema of the skin in the gaiter region of the foot. These people should be aware of the possibility that they may be at risk of developing a venous leg ulcer from a small trauma. If these symptoms are in the leg, the patient might consider trying over-the-counter support stockings to ease the symptoms. The nurse should also discuss skin care (see Chapter 20 Managing Hygiene ➡) with the patient, who should be advised to avoid trauma and to maintain skin softness with emollients without perfume or preservatives (to avoid the development of allergies).

Because the venous pump from the feet to the heart is dependent not only on the integrity of the valves in the vein, but also on the activation of the calf muscle, it is likely that exercise such as walking will help to reduce venous oedema and to prevent ulcers. Furthermore, *because* obesity reduces venous return (owing to high intra-abdominal pressures), then reaching and maintaining a healthy weight should be a goal for overweight patients.

People with a history of venous ulcers are at very high risk of developing a further ulcer and they need conscientious management of their leg care to avoid repeat skin breakdown. This includes avoidance of trauma, maintaining skin

health with an emollient, and reducing venous oedema by using compression hosiery (see Table 27.5).

Nursing management of venous leg ulcers

The use of compression

Compression can be applied to the legs in one of three ways: compression bandages, compression stockings, or compression devices (such as an inflatable boot). Bandages are primarily used in the treatment of ulcers, because they are inexpensive, commonly used once only, and hence any exudate does not leak onto garments that will be reused. Stockings are primarily used for ulcer prevention because they are removable at night/for bathing, are discreet, and last up to 4 months. There are no studies to date that rigorously evaluate the benefits of compliant wearing of compression hosiery, such as compression socks, on the prevention of a first venous ulcer. We do know, however, that compression stockings are more effective at reducing ulcer recurrence rates at 6 months compared with no compression (Vandongen and Stacey, 2000).

You need to be aware that there are different strengths of compression hosiery available: classes 1, 2, and 3 in the UK. One study has demonstrated that high-compression stockings (UK class 3) and moderate-compression stockings (UK class 2) seem equally effective at reducing recurrence by 5 years (Nelson *et al.*, 2006).

You also need to have the knowledge to discuss with patients the options for prevention of ulceration, including whether they wish to be assessed for surgical repair of any damaged veins. Superficial vein surgery plus compression is more effective at reducing ulcer recurrence rates at 12 months to 3 years than compression alone, but only some patients are suitable for surgery, because the damage to their veins may not be surgically repairable (Gohel *et al.*, 2007).

Superficial vein surgery is not widely available on the NHS unless the patient has tried wearing support stockings, has pain, and skin changes.

Before the nurse has a discussion with the patient regarding the use of a high-level compression bandage, the patient must have his or her ankle:brachial pressure index (ABPI) measured if clinically appropriate because it is damaging to apply high-compression bandages to patients with arterial insufficiency. ABPIs are used to determine any arterial insufficiency.

Any healthy lifestyle measures that promote venous return are likely to reduce ulcer recurrence, although there are no good-quality trials to evaluate how effective these are. Supporting your patients to reduce weight if they are overweight, to keep active, and to use legs and ankles to activate bloodflow in the veins, as well as to elevate the legs when at rest, should be key aspects of your nursing interventions.

When arterial disease becomes significant in people with venous ulcers, then treatment becomes more challenging. This is because the main treatment for venous disease is compression, but this is contraindicated in the presence of arterial disease. Your nursing interventions for patients with arterial disease will need to focus on the long-term benefits of smoking cessation, weight reduction, healthy diet, and exercise by providing education and support (see Evidence box 27.3).

Supporting self-management and unqualified or lay carers

Your responsibilities for preventing skin breakdown include the very important area of giving support to patients who are able to manage their own care as well as to unqualified and lay carers. The key principles that underpin this support are as follows.

- Educating the patient and carers about the risk of skin breakdown
- Making regular and frequent assessments of the skin to spot erythema (redness), blisters, temperature changes at the skin, and sore areas, because these indicate where attention needs to be paid to prevent worsening damage
- Using devices and equipment correctly:
  - For pressure ulcer prevention: using profiling beds, mattresses, overlays, cushions, sheepskins, pillows, etc. to reduce pressure and shear/friction and to keep the patient comfortable
  - For diabetic foot ulcers: ensuring that shoe inserts/orthotics and specialized shoes are worn to protect the foot from damage
  - For venous ulcers: applying compression hosiery to avoid traumatic damage to the leg, encouraging the use of compression hose, and prompting replacement every 3 or 4 months
- Managing skin health by using emollients, and protecting from sweat or incontinence
- Maintaining good nutrition to ensure that the patient is hydrated, diabetes is well controlled, skin is well perfused, muscle mass is not reduced, and that protein intake is high enough to maintain the blood osmolarity
- Encouraging health maintenance by exercise appropriate to person's activity levels and physical ability, and supporting with advice on smoking cessation, if necessary

Accessing the evidence on prevention of pressure, foot, and venous ulcers

Over the past two decades, there have been numerous studies exploring the area of ulcer prevention. You need therefore to have the skills and knowledge to determine which studies provide the most robust reliable and valid evidence. There are several high-quality journals and resources to inform your preventative nursing in interventions and to keep up to date. These include the following sources:

EVIDENCE BOX 27.3

What are the evidence gaps on venous ulcer knowledge?

We do not know what is the best way in which to identify people at risk of their first venous ulcer.

We do not know whether using compression stockings, losing weight, exercise, or other lifestyle advice (such as diet or smoking cessation) help to avoid or delay the development of a first ulcer in people with chronic venous problems.

We do not know whether losing weight, exercise, or other lifestyle advice (such as diet or smoking cessation) help to avoid or delay the development of subsequent ulcers in people with healed venous ulcers.

Table 27.5 Summary of venous ulcer prevention strategies

Principle	Interventions	Example
Identifying people at risk of developing a venous ulcer	• Inspecting the skin of the lower leg for signs of venous insufficiency • Assessing for history of venous ulcers	• Look for brown staining, swelling, eczema, dilated veins at the ankle • Ask the patient if he or she has ever had an ulcer or chronic wound on the leg
Skin care	• Avoid trauma to the leg • Maintain skin health	• Use emollients to prevent skin from cracking • Wash and dry skin on the leg carefully
Weight control, rest, and exercise	• Achieve/maintain a healthy weight • Elevate the feet to aid venous return (if patient is haemodynamically stable and does not have heart failure) • Exercise the calf-pump to increase venous return	• Diet or exercise to achieve healthy body weight • Lie on the bed/sofa when resting so that the ankles do not swell during sitting • Walking/foot exercises
Compression therapy	• Use properly fitting compression hose to prevent ankle oedema and reduce risk of ulceration	• Stockings (class 2 or 3), according to the patient's ankle and calf measurements, replaced every 3–4 months
Surgical repair	• Venous surgery to remove or repair damaged veins • Discuss whether the person would consider surgery for his or her venous problems or not	• Stripping the veins, or minimally invasive approaches to repairing the veins

- Cochrane Library
- *Clinical Evidence*
- *British Medical Journal*
- *Journal of Wound Care*
- *International Wound Journal*
- *Wound Repair and Regeneration*
- *The Journal of Tissue Viability*

Systematic reviews bring together all of the high-quality, relevant evidence, and summarize this in one document, taking into account the different sizes of the studies and their reliability and validity. The Cochrane Library contains full text systematic reviews of the effectiveness of interventions to prevent and treat pressure ulcers, foot ulcers, and venous ulcers, and this provides comprehensive information on the effects of particular approaches, such as risk assessment, nutritional supplements, compression, shoes, beds, and mattresses. It is the single best place to look for systematic reviews of effectiveness questions because it indexes not only Cochrane systematic reviews, but also other reviews summarized by the Centre for Reviews and Dissemination. Clinical Practice Guidelines brings together the evidence from research *and* expert opinion around a

> **THEORY INTO PRACTICE 27.2**
> **Identifying an 'at-risk' patient**
>
> Think about your clinical environment and the patients for whom you care, and consider those most at risk using the factors outlined in Table 27.1.
>
> - Identify one patient whom you think may be at risk: what puts him or her at risk?
> - What is his or her current health problem? Has there been any deterioration or change? What will these changes mean for pressure ulcer risk?
> - What might be the focus of your nursing interventions?
> - How would you monitor the effectiveness of these interventions?

patient problem. In addition, *Clinical Evidence* provides a condensed summary of the best available evidence around pressure ulcers, diabetic foot ulcers, and venous ulcers **http://clinicalevidence.bmj.com/**.

In the area of chronic wounds, there are numerous guidelines available (see the next section on 'Sources of evidence for practice').

EVIDENCE BOX 27.4
Terms to use in literature searches

When searching for articles about ulcers, it is helpful to use the following terms.

- Pressure sore
- Pressure ulcer* (use a truncation symbol here to include ulceration)
- Bed sore
- Decubitus ulcer
- Decubiti
- Diabetic foot ulcer
- Foot ulcer
- Venous ulcer
- Venous leg ulcer
- Leg ulcer
- Varicose ulcer
- Stasis ulcer

Sources of evidence for practice

EPUAP guide to pressure ulcer grading http://www.epuap.org/grading.html

Carer's factsheet about pressure ulcers http://www.alzheimers.org.uk/factsheet/512

Pressure ulcers

NPUAP/EPUAP Guidelines 2009 http://www.epuap.org/guidelines.html

NHS Quality Improvement Scotland 2009: Best Practice Statement http://www.nhshealthquality.org/nhsqis/files/PrimaryCare_PreventionAndManagementOfPressureUlcers_MAR09.pdf

NICE Clinical Guideline 2005 http://www.nice.org.uk/nicemedia/pdf/CG029fullguideline.pdf

Diabetic foot ulcers

Scottish Intercollegiate Guidelines Network, Management of diabetes: A national clinical guideline, Revised 2010 http://www.sign.ac.uk/pdf/sign116.pdf

Registered Nurses Association of Ontario, Reducing foot complications for people with diabetes, Clinical Practice Guideline, Revised 2007 http://www.rnao.org/Page.asp?PageID=924&ContentID=815

Venous ulcers

Royal College of Nursing, Venous ulcers, Clinical Practice Guideline, Revised 2006 http://www.rcn.org.uk/development/practice/clinicalguidelines/venous_leg_ulcers

Scottish Intercollegiate Guidelines Network, Management of chronic venous leg ulcers, Guideline 120, Revised 2010 http://www.sign.ac.uk/guidelines/fulltext/120/contents.html

Summary and key messages

Many patients with a wide variety of pre-existing conditions and health needs are at risk of skin breakdown. This chapter has outlined how nurses can identify those at risk, carry out reliable assessments, undertake preventative strategies, and utilize existing best practice to manage skin breakdown. This chapter has also identified the impact of skin breakdown on patient well-being and outlined how nurses can support patients to minimize the impact of skin breakdown to return to full function as soon as possible. Lastly, the chapter has identified key sources of evidence that nurses can utilize to inform clinical decision-making.

Answers to case study questions

➤ A high temperature may put her at risk of ulceration owing to increased metabolic demand, as well as sweat on the skin that may reduce ability to resist damage from shear. Her recent reduction in weight may cause reduced muscle covering the ischial tuberosities—and this would expose the skin to compression between the seat and skeleton. A poor appetite may put her at risk of low protein and calorie intake, reducing ability to repair tissue damage and maintain osmotic pressure.

➤ Using a wheelchair means that Mrs Montgomery is at risk of pressure ulceration because her sacral area is subject to constant high pressures.

➤ Alert Mrs Montgomery to her risk of developing a pressure ulcer. With the patient, agree a schedule for assessing skin condition (looking for redness, breaks, swelling, etc.). Keep the skin that is exposed to pressure clean, dry, and moisturized. Agree with the patient a schedule for repositioning (including scheduled time in bed) or moving her sacrum off the seat every 20–30 minutes (less frequent if skin remains in good condition) and help her to carry this out by planning care delivery with this schedule in mind. Consider referral to dietitian to assess nutritional needs; in the meantime, support patient to keep food and fluid intake by offering small portions of food and drink frequently. Check wheelchair cushion for signs of wear and consider referral to occupational therapist or wheelchair services if it needs to be replaced.

➤ Visual checks of skin condition to look for signs of blanching or non-blanching erythema. These should be twice a day initially, reducing to daily only when skin checks have been clear for a few days.

Online Resource Centre

 To help you to develop and apply your knowledge and decision-making skills further, we have provided interactive learning resources online at **www.oxfordtextbooks.co.uk/orc/bullock/**
Whilst these are freely available, you will need to use the access codes at the start of the book.

References

Bennett, G., Dealey, C., Posnett, J. (2004) The cost of pressure ulcers in the UK. *Age and Ageing* **33**(3): 230–5.

Bergstrom, N., Braden, B., Laguzza, A., *et al.* (1987) The Braden Scale for predicting pressure sore risk. *Nursing Research* **36**(4): 205–10.

Briggs, M., Flemming, K. (2007) Living with leg ulceration: a synthesis of qualitative research. *Journal of Advanced Nursing* **59**(4): 319–28.

Callam, M.J., Ruckley, C.V., Harper, D.R., *et al.* (1985) Chronic ulceration of the leg: extent of the problem and provision of care. *British Medical Journal* **290**: 1855–6.

Defloor, T., De Bacquer, D., Grypdonck, M.H. (2005) The effect of various combinations of turning and pressure reducing devices on the incidence of pressure ulcers. *International Journal of Nursing Studies* **42**(1): 37–46.

Department of Health (2010) Nurse sensitive outcome indicators for NHS commissioned care, version 2.1. **http://www.ic.nhs.uk/webfiles/Services/Clinical%20Innovation%20Metrics/Nurse_Sensitive_Indicators_DH.pdf** (accessed 5 August 2011).

Dorresteijn, J.A.N., Kriegsman, D.M.W., Assendelft, W.J.J., *et al.* (2010) Patient education for preventing diabetic foot ulceration. *Cochrane Database of Systematic Reviews* Issue 5: Art. No. CD001488. DOI: 10.1002/14651858.CD001488.pub3.

European Pressure Ulcer Advisory Panel and National Pressure Ulcer Advisory Panel (2009) *Prevention and Treatment of Pressure Ulcers: Quick Reference Guide*. National Pressure Ulcer Advisory Panel: Washington DC.

Gohel, M.S., Barwell, J.R., Taylor, M., *et al.* (2007) Long term results of compression therapy alone versus compression plus surgery in chronic venous ulceration (ESCHAR): randomised controlled trial. *British Medical Journal* **335**: 83.

Gorecki, C., Brown, J.M., Nelson, E.A., *et al.* and European Quality of Life Pressure Ulcer Project Group (2009) Impact of pressure ulcers on quality of life in older patients: a systematic review. *Journal of the American Geriatrics Society* **57**(7): 1175–83.

Graham, I.D., Harrison, M.B., Nelson, E.A., *et al.* (2003) Prevalence of lower limb ulceration: a systematic review of prevalence studies. *Advances in Skin & Wound Care* **16**(6): 305–16.

Hess, C. (2004) Did you know the difference between friction and shear? *Advances in Skin & Wound Care* **17**(5): 222.

Hurd, T., Posnett, J. (2009) Point prevalence of wounds in a sample of acute hospitals in Canada. *International Wound Journal* 6: 287–93.

Iversen, M.M., Tell, G.S., Riise, T., *et al.* (2009) History of foot ulcer increases mortality among individuals with diabetes ten-year follow-up of the Nord-Trøndelag Health Study, Norway. *Diabetes Care* **32**(12): 2193–9.

Langer, G., Knerr, A., Kuss, O., *et al.* (2003) Nutritional interventions for preventing and treating pressure ulcers. *Cochrane Database of Systematic Reviews* Issue 4: Art. No. CD003216. DOI: 10.1002/14651858.CD003216.

Lavery, L.A., Higgins, K.R., Lanctot, D.R., *et al.* (2007) Preventing diabetic foot ulcer recurrence in high-risk patients: use of temperature monitoring as a self-assessment tool. *Diabetes Care* **30**(1): 14–20.

McCabe, C.J., Stevenson, R.C., Dolan, A.M. (1998) Evaluation of a diabetic foot screening and protection programme. *Diabetic Medicine* **15**: 80–4.

McInnes, E., Jammali-Blasi, A., Bell-Syer, S.E.M., *et al.* (2011) Support surfaces for pressure ulcer prevention. *Cochrane Database of Systematic Reviews* Issue 4: Art. No. CD001735. DOI: 10.1002/14651858.CD0011735.pub4.

Moore, Z.E.H., Cowman, S. (2008) Risk assessment tools for the prevention of pressure ulcers. *Cochrane Database of Systematic Reviews* Issue 3: Art. No. CD006471. DOI: 10.1002/14651858. CD006471.

Nelson, E.A., Harper, D.R., Prescott, R.J., *et al.* (2006) Prevention of recurrence of venous ulceration: randomised controlled trial of Class 2 and Class 3 elastic compression. *Journal of Vascular Surgery* **44**(4): 1046–50.

Nelson, E.A., Jones, J. (2008) Venous leg ulcers. *BMJ Clinical Evidence* **9**: 1902.

Posnett, J., Franks, P. (2008) The burden of chronic wounds in the UK. *Nursing Times* **104**(3): 44–5.

Reddy, M. (2011) Pressure ulcers. *Clinical Evidence* **5**: 1901.

Ribu, L., Hanestad, B.R., Moum, T., *et al.* (2007) A comparison of the health-related quality of life in patients with diabetic foot ulcers, with a diabetes group and a nondiabetes group from the general population. *Quality of Life Research* **16**(2): 179–89.

Ribu, L., Rustøen, T., Birkeland, K., *et al.* (2006) The prevalence and occurrence of diabetic foot ulcer pain and its impact on health-related quality of life. *Journal of Pain* **7**(4): 290–9.

Severens, J.L., Habraken, J.M., Duivenvoorden, S., *et al.* (2002) The cost of illness of pressure ulcers in the Netherlands. *Advances in Skin & Wound Care* **15**(2): 72–7.

Singh, N., Armstrong, D.G., Lipsky, B.A. (2005) Preventing foot ulcers in patients with diabetes. *Journal of the American Medical Association* **293**: 217–28.

Spencer, S.A. (2000) Pressure relieving interventions for preventing and treating diabetic foot ulcers. *Cochrane Database of Systematic Reviews* Issue 3: Art. No. CD002302. DOI: 10.1002/14651858. CD002302.

Tannen, A., Bours, G., Halfens, R., *et al.* (2006) A comparison of pressure ulcer prevalence rates in nursing homes in the Netherlands and Germany, adjusted for population characteristics. *Research in Nursing & Health* **29**(6): 588–96.

Torra i Bou, J.E., Rueda López, J., Camañes, G., *et al.* (2002) Heel pressure ulcers. Comparative study between heel protective bandage and hydrocellular dressing with special form for the heel. *Revista de Enfermeria* **25**: 50–6.

Vandongen, Y.K., Stacey, M.C. (2000) Graduated compression elastic stockings reduce lipodermatosclerosis and ulcer recurrence. *Phlebology* **15**: 33–7.

Williams, R., Airey, M. (2002) The size of the problem: epidemiological and economic aspects of foot problems in diabetes. In A.J.M. Boulton, H. Connor, P.R. Cavanagh (eds) *The Foot In Diabetes*, 3rd edn. John Wiley & Sons Ltd: Chichester, pp. 3–18.

World Health Organization/IDF Saint Vincent Declaration Working Group (1990) Diabetes mellitus in Europe: a problem at all ages in all countries—a model for prevention and self care. *Acta Diabetologica* **27**: 181–3.

Young, T. (2004) The 30° tilt position vs the 90° lateral and supine positions in reducing the incidence of non-blanching erythema in a hospital inpatient population: a randomised controlled trial. *Journal of Tissue Viability* **14**(3): 88, 90, 92–6.

28 *Managing* Wounds

Patricia Grocott

Introduction

This chapter addresses the vital area of wound care, including the impact that wounds can have upon patients and their families, and the nursing management challenges that they present. As a registered nurse caring for patients with wounds, you will be responsible for making a clinical assessment of the patient with a wound, making clinical decisions based on the most appropriate evidence-based, nurse-led interventions, and, crucially, measuring patient outcomes. The latter involves continuous monitoring of how both the patient and his or her wound is responding, or not, to the treatment and care that you give.

This chapter presents a generic approach to wound management, and this should help you to deliver high-quality, safe wound care for patients with wounds of differing aetiologies. This includes core components of interventions for acute, chronic, and palliative wound care. Importantly, the chapter has been designed to help you to make the links between assessment, clinical decision-making, nursing interventions, and patient care. Nurses play a key role in the multidisciplinary team in the delivery of wound care, and frequently act as the 'point of contact' for the manufacturers and suppliers of wound care products. The approach advocated in this chapter will equip you to make informed assessments and clinical decisions.

Understanding the importance of managing wounds

Definitions

Wounds are injuries to the body, the skin in particular, causing a breach of the layers of skin (see Chapter 12 Understanding Skin Conditions ➡) and the body boundary. The term 'wound' also defines the act of injuring a person's skin. This may be deliberate, e.g. during a surgical procedure, or deliberate to cause harm, e.g. during warfare, terrorist attacks, or domestic and street violence. Wounding can also occur with accidents (a cut from a kitchen knife), natural disasters (earthquake), and exposure to environmental stresses such as extreme heat (burns, skin cancers), extreme cold (frostbite), excessive pressure, and excessive exposure to water and moisture (trench foot). Wounds also develop because of diseases and conditions such as diabetes, which disrupt the structures of the skin and the normal metabolic processes that maintain skin health (see **Chapter 9 Understanding Diabetes Mellitus** 🔵). In addition, a disrupted blood supply to the skin, as a result of sustained pressure and other stressors to the skin, can give rise to a pressure ulcer (see **Chapter 27 Managing the Prevention of Skin Breakdown** 🔵).

Types of wounds and their causation

Wounds are categorized as acute, chronic, and palliative, which relates to the way in which they develop, their duration, and also the health of the patient. This is important information because it enables you to understand when wounds are progressing towards healing in a predictable way, or not. This is essential knowledge, which should underpin nursing actions and enables you to communicate intelligently with patients by giving them information on what they should expect; it also allows you to pick up signs and symptoms of where healing is not progressing in a predicted and timely fashion (see Dealey, 2005, for a comprehensive explanation of wounds and wound healing).

An acute wound arises out of an acute episode, such as a surgical incision, and is expected to follow the pattern and time frame of normal wound healing. A wound that arises from an acute episode can also become a chronic wound. For example, a pressure ulcer may be caused by an acute episode of unrelieved pressure. The resulting tissue damage and wound may take weeks to heal, which brings patients into a chronic wound category because of the length of time for which they require wound care, and the mechanism of healing.

Wounds that arise as a result of an underlying disease (e.g. diabetes) or condition (e.g. arterial and venous insufficiency of the lower leg) are also chronic. Chronic wounds can be 'hard to heal', but do go on to heal. Additionally,

wounds are categorized as palliative care wounds, when they may never heal. The reasons for this include an untreatable underlying cause (e.g. malignancy that has not responded to treatment), or because people are frail because of age, or are reaching the end of life (Probst *et al.*, 2009; Grocott and Gray, 2010).

Wound healing

The 'normal' wound healing process involves three overlapping phases:

- inflammation in two stages;
- regeneration;
- maturation.

The process of wound healing is complex and involves many cells, cytokines and growth factors, carbohydrates and proteins, all of which are released into the wound at different rates and at different speeds. A detailed explanation of this process can be found in a number of sources (for example, Dealey, 2005).

It is important to understand the different processes of wound healing. Knowledge of the underlying mechanisms will enable you to distinguish between a wound that is progressing towards healing and one that is not. It also enables you to decide on the most appropriate nursing interventions, to inform patients and informal carers about what they can expect, that and to allay the anxieties that they may have. For example, when a wound is in the maturation phase, long after it has apparently healed, the patient may experience sensations, such as tightening of the tissue across and around the wound, which may be alarming if you have not explained the stages of wound healing. Table 28.1 describes a range of wound categories, including the underlying causes and mechanisms of healing.

The prevalence and epidemiological profile of wounds and economic impact

The scale of the problems of wounds is revealed by Posnett *et al.* (2009) in a review of the literature on the resource impact of wounds on healthcare providers in Europe. They found two population-based studies in the UK reporting point prevalence rates of 3.70 and 3.55 patients per 1,000 covered population with at least one wound under treatment. Most of these patients (70–80%) were being treated

Table 28.1 Wound categories, underlying causes, mechanisms of wound healing, and palliation

Category	Underlying cause		Mechanism of wound healing
Acute wounds—intentional	Surgical incisions		Primary closure
	Self-harm	Factitious wounds	Secondary closure
		Drug addicts' injection sites	Secondary closure
	Warfare	Burns (chemicals, heat)	Secondary closure Grafting
		Blast injuries	Secondary closure Grafting
		Gunshot wounds	Secondary closure Grafting
		Amputations	Primary closure
	Crime	Domestic violence Child abuse Mugging Knives and guns	Secondary closure Grafting Primary closure
	Injection sites	Drug extravasation	Secondary closure
Acute wounds—accidental	Complicated bone fractures		Primary closure
	Crush injuries		Secondary closure
	Cuts		Primary closure
	Burns		Secondary closure
	Tattoos (infected)		Secondary closure
	Dehisced surgical wounds		Secondary closure Graft and flap formation
Wounds caused by underlying diseases and conditions	Pressure ulcers		Secondary closure Graft and flap formation
	Vascular disease of the lower leg: arterial and venous leg ulcer		Secondary closure
	Diabetes: diabetic foot ulcers		Secondary closure
	Cancer	Radiotherapy wounds	Secondary closure
		Malignant wounds	Secondary closure Graft and flap formation
Palliative care wounds	Any chronic wound if the patient circumstances are such that treatment of the underlying cause of the wound, or time, precludes healing		Palliative treatments Symptom management Local wound management Supportive care to patients and families

(*continued*)

Table 28.1 (*continued*)

Category	Underlying cause	Mechanism of wound healing
	Inherited lifelong disorders e.g. epidermolysis bullosa	Palliative treatments Symptom management Local wound management Supportive care to patients and families
	Frail patients with advanced and end-of-life conditions	Palliative treatments Symptom management Local wound management Supportive care to patients and families
	Tumour infiltration of the skin; fungating malignant wounds	Palliative treatments Symptom management Local wound management Supportive care to patients and families

by nurses in the community (Drew *et al.*, 2007). A similar study, undertaken in Sweden, reported a point prevalence of patients with a chronic wound of 2.4 per 1,000 population. Posnett *et al.* (2009) also found that evidence of the prevalence of wounds among inpatients in European hospitals is limited, and the range of estimates is wide: from 27% in one UK hospital to 52% in a Parisian hospital (Drew *et al.*, 2009; Mahe *et al.*, 2006). Posnett *et al.* (2009) propose that the higher estimates are consistent with evidence from a national survey of hospitals in Western Australia with a mean prevalence 49% in 85 public hospitals (Strachan *et al.*, 2007). Acute surgical wounds comprise a very large subgroup of all wounds. As stated above, they should heal without complications. They become clinically important, and increase health service costs, when healing is complicated for example by infection (Hurd and Posnett, 2009) (see Chapter 21 Managing Infection ⟶).

There are also important indications of patients experiencing multiple wounds of long duration. In the audit conducted by Drew *et al.* (2009), for example, just under a third (31%) of the patients had multiple wounds, with an average duration of 17.5 weeks. One in four of all wounds had been unhealed for at least 6 months and one in five for a year or more. Almost 42% of the leg ulcers had not healed in the previous 6 months, and 28% had remained unhealed for a year or longer.

Historically, palliative wounds have been linked to rare or extreme conditions. As a consequence, there has been a lack of research and development of wound care products that can realistically manage the local environment of extensive wounds (Cowley and Grocott, 2007; Grocott and Gray, 2010). There is now a growing international interest in palliative wound care, not least because it is recognized that this population is much larger than previously thought, and that older people in particular are affected. Palliative wound care is focused on improving the quality of life for patients with wounds and long-term conditions, in all care settings, and much earlier in the person's illness than the last few weeks of life (Department of Health, *End of Life Care Strategy*, 2008: 79).

Wounds constitute a major resource drain for health services in primary, secondary, and tertiary care. Posnett *et al.* (2009) report that 78% of the total costs of wound care comprise clinical time, while the remaining 22% is spent on products. A key issue is the amount of time that nurses spend on wound care. Drew *et al.* (2009) identified that 70–80% of the patients in their sample were cared for in the community. Community nurse time on wound dressing changes in Southern Ireland, for example, excluding travel time, required the equivalent of 5.3 full-time equivalent nurses per annum or 66% of the total available community nurse resource.

Personal behavioural risk factors include poor nutrition, obesity, and smoking, all of which are implicated in impaired wound healing (Bale and Jones, 2006). For a cogent summary of the factors that affect wound healing, please see **http://archive.student.bmj.com/issues/06/03/education/98.php**.

The human and social burden of wounds

Wounds impact at many levels. They can occur in patients of all ages, including babies in intensive care, young disabled and wheelchair-bound adults, mothers during child birth, frail and elderly patients, patients with mental illness, and patients undergoing radiotherapy for cancer. A wound may be considered as having a ripple effect. It may include a prolonged hospital stay, long-term sick leave, and, in some instances, loss of employment. It also requires repetitive dressing changes requiring copious amounts of wound care products, nursing time, stigma, and restrictions in social life and mobility.

As nurses, we need to recognize how wounds can profoundly alter how patients feel about themselves. The knowledge generated through qualitative research can help to develop this understanding. Patients explain how they feel in terms such as the loss of the body boundary and personal dignity, and they illuminate the central role that a healthy and intact skin plays in our personal and social life, and particularly at the end of life (Probst *et al.*, 2009; Lawton, 1998).

Physical pain

Price and colleagues (Price *et al.*, 2008) conducted an international cross-sectional survey of pain related to wound dressings and dressing changes in 15 countries. This study reveals how many patients experienced wound pain at dressing changes and how long the pain lasted; for some this could be more than 5 hours. Touching and handling the wound, together with dressing removal and cleaning, were strongly associated with pain. At the same time, patients said that they would like to be actively involved in their dressing changes, and that pain at dressing change was the worst part of living with a wound.

In a survey designed to capture specifically the experiences of UK patients by Fagervik-Morton and Price (2010), patients reported difficulties in bathing, leakage of exudate, impaired mobility, odour, and slippage of the dressings or bandages, together with pain. The patients identified several factors that were important to them to reduce pain during dressing procedures. For example, the way in which the wound was treated and dressed was important in reducing the severity of pain, including taking time to warm irrigation fluids and to moisten dressings to ease removal. This attention to detail, in conjunction with consistent quality of care, communication, and rapport with the care giver, were beneficial in easing pain at dressing-related procedures.

It is important to translate this research-based knowledge into your everyday care of patients and to recognize that there is a dynamic relationship between physical illness and distress. In wound care, this means that nursing actions designed to *restore* the physical body boundary (covering the wounded skin; managing associated symptoms, such as pain and odour) are driven by an understanding of what the wounds and the broken skin mean to the individuals concerned, their families, and social groups (Shatner, 2003; Grocott and Gray, 2010).

Psychosocial impact

The physical wound care that you give should be complemented by supportive care. This means that paying attention to and acting on what individual patients and their families say about difficulties with living with a wound are important to bring comfort and relief. Wounds also have an impact on partners and families: a family member may take on the role of informal carer, maintaining wound care between episodes of professional care. In addition, as with any major and chronic illness, daily living is also disrupted, as the following extract from the wife of a patient with leg ulcers illustrates:

> My days are completely dominated by his condition. When we both retired we had looked forward to an easier more leisurely way of life, but instead, due to necessary twice weekly visits to the hospital for changes of dressings, this has not turned out to be the case. We can't have holidays, days out are a rarity as my husband can't cope with the difficulty of walking, and getting to the toilet, his legs are not strong enough to hold him . . .
> (Bowyer, 2008: 11)

A qualitative study by Reynolds (2008) revealed that the carers she interviewed had a strong inner sense of duty, love, and commitment to their role. However, they also expressed negative emotions such as low self-esteem and anger in relation to the emotional burden of the physical and psychological aspects of wound care, and appealed to health professionals for recognition and support. The simple act of valuing and complimenting a carer on the role that he or she is playing can also help to sustain him or her in this role.

Nursing responsibility and accountability

As illustrated above, relatively simple nursing actions can be highly effective in minimizing the short- and long-term consequences of having a wound (Grocott, 2000; Fager-vik-Morton and Price, 2010). This is particularly important for those patients with underlying disease that predisposes them to recurrent development of wounds. One bad experience of wound care is memorable and can impact on a patient's ability to cope the next time around.

Your nursing responsibility for wound management should focus on clinical assessment, clinical decision-making, interventions, and monitoring of outcomes to identify why a wound has developed and to determine the potential for, or the limits to, healing. This includes identifying methods of preventing further breakdown whenever possible, and selecting interventions to manage the local wound and the symptoms arising, in healing and non-healing states.

Wound care products play an important role in the delivery of wound care. You will also need to be knowledgeable and skilled in the best use of skin care products (see Chapter 12 Understanding Skin Conditions and Chapter 20 Managing Hygiene ➡), wound dressings, antimicrobials, and debriding agents, as well as some of the more advanced technologies such as topical negative pressure therapy (Cowan, 2011). In addition, you need to know when and how to use pressure-relieving beds and cushions (see Chapter 27 Managing the Prevention of Skin Breakdown ➡), and to integrate all of these components of patient care in relation to the skin into a coherent plan of care.

Clinical assessment of wounds

Making a clinical assessment involves assessing the health and condition of the patient with the wound(s), his or her family, and social context, together with a local assessment of the wound(s) and the peri-wound skin condition. Assessment is underpinned by three interrelated core components, as follows.

1. Understanding the underlying causes of wound(s)
2. Understanding wound-related symptom(s)

3. Understanding the condition of the wound and the surrounding skin, and local management interventions

Understanding the underlying causes of wound(s)

The responsibility for investigating, diagnosing, and instigating treatment lies with the multidisciplinary team in a particular specialism. However, it is your responsibility as a nurse to understand what causes wounds, the reasons behind diagnostic tests, the implications of investigations and results, and treatment protocols. A particular nursing responsibility is to observe, document, and report changes in a patient's condition, so that specialist colleagues can review treatment plans.

Understanding wound-related symptom(s)

Wounds can result in a range of symptoms, which include:

- pain;
- exudate;
- soreness and irritation;
- odour;
- bleeding.

More than one symptom can develop at the same time, which points to a particular diagnosis. For example, an increase in local wound pain, swelling, odour, and bleeding, together with an increase in the amount of exudate and a rapid extension of the wound, indicates that the wound has become infected (Collier, 2004). It is important that you document and report these symptoms to medical and infection control colleagues to ensure appropriate treatment of the infection and control of the symptoms (see Chapter 21 Managing Infection ➡). These symptoms are discussed further in the next sections in the context of the management of local wounds and the surrounding skin.

Understanding the condition of the wound and the surrounding skin

Developing an understanding of the condition of the wound and surrounding skin requires an understanding of both the underlying causes and of the symptoms that may arise, together with assessment and monitoring of the wound and peri-wound skin. Wound assessment and monitoring requires knowledge of the physiology of wound healing (Dealey, 2005). Assessment and monitoring are based on observation. The more experience that you accumulate in assessing wounds, the more accurate and valuable will be your assessments. The process of wound assessment and documentation is outlined below. Of particular importance is how wound appearance and local symptoms and signs change over time. The changes signal wound healing or the reverse, wound deterioration.

A framework for wound assessment and documentation

The use of a standard assessment tool within your area of clinical practice can help to standardize the assessment process and care planning, improving interprofessional communications. An example of a standard tool is one published by NHS Quality Improvement Scotland (see **http://www.tissueviabilityonline.com/wound-assessmen**).

When assessing a wound, you need to take the following factors into account:

- pain and discomfort;
- wound dimension, location, and shape;
- wound appearance;
- condition and appearance of the surrounding skin.

These are discussed in more detail in the next section.

Level of pain and discomfort: various tools are available to measure key aspects, such as intensity and quality of the pain. These include numerical rating scales (0–5, 0–10), verbal rating scales (none, mild, moderate, or severe pain), and the visual analogue scale (10 cm line with 'no pain' at one end and 'worst pain imaginable' at the other). In addition, you should carefully explore the location of pain (which may not be confined to the wound site), aggravating factors, timing, and meaning and impact of the pain on the individual. The physical attributes of pain need to be assessed alongside emotional components: for example, the distress the pain causes, together with any restrictions it imposes on daily living (Grocott and Briggs, 2009) (see **Chapter 25 Managing Pain** ➡).

Wound dimensions, location, and shape: accurate measurement of wounds is often very difficult to achieve because of their location, for example on a body contour such as around a limb or on the buttocks. The three-dimensional structure of many wounds, as well as the areas of the wound that are not visible at the surface, also add to the difficulties of measuring them with any degree of accuracy. Digital photographs taken at regular, e.g. weekly, intervals can provide a valuable visual record of the wound and an objective method of tracking gross changes in the wound condition over time. There are also software packages that enable you to trace the contours and dimensions of a wound digitally and without touching the wound (Romanelli *et al.*, 2008). The patient's consent needs to be obtained for each photograph taken. The wound needs to be fully examined to ensure that aspects of the wound that are not obvious at visual inspection are revealed. The terminology for hidden areas of a wound includes 'undermining', 'tunnelling', 'tracking', 'pocketing', and 'bridging'. You need to acquire the skills to conduct a physical assessment to uncover the true extent of the wound, without causing further damage.

The location of a wound is important in terms of its proximity to anatomical structures, such as major nerves, blood vessels, bone, tendons, and ligaments. For example, a wound on the wrist resulting from an impact or crush injury requires particular care and attention because the wrist is a complex structure of bones, nerves, tendons, damage to which can result in long-term loss of function and disability. A patient with a complex wrist wound therefore requires referral to a specialist, such as an orthopaedic surgeon. The location, size, and shape of the wound are also important in terms of local wound management and choice of topical products and dressings. A superficial wound may be covered by a flat dressing, whereas a cavity wound will require a dressing to fill the cavity, together with a second dressing to cover the surface area of the wound.

Appearance of the wound and the wound bed: the appearance of the wound bed and the health of the wound tissue are determined by the blood supply and the degree of bacterial colonization. There are distinct stages in the condition of the wound, related to the stages of wound healing, and each one may require a different local intervention.

'Wound bed preparation' (WBP) is a framework that has been adopted by the wound care community, nationally and internationally, to assess and manage the local wound environment to optimize wound healing (Schultz *et al.*, 2003; Bentley, 2005). WBP also applies to palliative wound care when the priorities of care may not include healing, but are equally important in terms of achieving control of the wound and reducing its negative impact on the patient (Grocott and Robinson, 2009). The reasoning behind WBP is that, if healing is the goal, the wound bed should be free of bacteria, dead tissue, and harmful enzymes that may delay healing. If palliation is the goal, removal of dead tissue and reduction in the bacteria in the wound, for example, can reduce odour and exudate, damage to the peri-wound skin, and the overall burden of the wound to all concerned (Bentley, 2005; Grocott and Robinson, 2009). That said, there are circumstances in which debridement is unnecessary because there is minimal exudate and no odour. Also, in end-of-life care, an intact scab may be more helpful to the patient than a wet, debrided wound.

To implement the framework of WBP in a practical way, the TIME acronym has been developed (Schultz *et al.*, 2003; Dowsett, 2008). TIME summarizes the four components of WBP and requires you to assess, monitor, and manage the following elements:

- Tissue management;
- Infection and inflammation management;
- Moisture balance;
- Edge of wound in terms of advancement inwards to cover the broken area.

A detailed explanation of TIME and WBP is found online at **http://www.wounds-uk.com/journal/0103_time_article. shtml**. See also Table 28.2.

Condition and appearance of the skin surrounding the wound: the condition and appearance of the skin surrounding a wound, i.e. the peri-wound skin, is an important marker of the nursing care of a wound in relation to wound exudate. It is also an important marker of the development of spreading infection (see Chapter 21 Managing Infection ➡).

The care of the patient's skin is fully discussed in Chapters 20 and 27 Managing Hygiene and Managing the Prevention of Skin Breakdown ➡. Skin damage occurs when body fluids are in contact with skin, including wound exudate. Initial damage can be in the form of irritant dermatitis, which, if left untreated, will progress to erythematous and even white maceration, which may result in tissue death. Expert nursing care can prevent damage to the peri-wound skin, and this should be the priority in wound care. Without continuous attention to prevention strategies, the patient's skin can become sore and irritated when it should be healthy and intact.

Utilizing the evidence in clinical decision-making and nursing interventions

This section makes links between wound and symptom assessment, clinical decision-making, and evidence-based nursing interventions. It involves the explicit use of a rationale for the choice of interventions for an individual patient and feasibility to defend your choice (Weston, 2009).

Managing the local wound environment

As discussed above, it is helpful to use a framework to assess wounds systematically. The WBP framework is therefore followed here, along with the TIME acronym, to illustrate key signs and symptoms that you should seek in healing and non-healing wounds, and the choice of interventions to control them (Table 28.2).

Current practice in wound care, including the manufacturing focus for wound dressings, is substantially based on Winter's (1962) theory of moist wound healing (MWHT). This maintains that the final stage of wound healing requires a moist, not a dry, local environment. Manufacturers have responded to the publication of this work by developing moisture conserving dressings. As with any theory, it does not explain or apply to all circumstances. For MWHT, this becomes evident when moisture conserving dressings are applied to wet and exudating wounds (Grocott, 2000). Exudate management is explored in more detail later in this section.

The nursing interventions for local wound management are explained in further detail below, with additional information concerning protection of fragile wound tissue. Table 28.3 provides generic products that may be used to deliver these nursing interventions.

Table 28.2 TIME, wound bed preparation, nursing interventions, and patient outcome measures in healing and non-healing (palliative) wounds

TIME	Wound bed preparation: nursing interventions	Patient outcomes
Tissue a. Necrotic, scab, slough b. Granulating c. Epithelializing	a. Debride the necrotic tissue b. Preserve the dry scab if life expectancy is very short c. Protect fragile granulating tissue d. Protect epithelializing tissue with non-adherent dressings	a. Clean wound bed (healing wounds) b. Dry black scab (end-of-life care wounds) c. Granulating and epithelializing tissue towards wound closure
Infection and/or inflammation	a. Consider using debriding agents to remove the dead tissue, which harbours bacteria b. Consider using antimicrobial dressings to remove bacteria	a. Clean wound bed b. No signs of inflammation c. No signs of infection d. No odour e. Exudate is at the level expected for this type of wound, and contained in the dressings
Moisture	a. Use dressing products to remove exudate from the wounds, without allowing the wound to dry out and stick to the dressings	a. Moist film between the wound and the dressings, no trauma on removal of dressings b. Healthy peri-wound skin c. No soiling or staining of patients' clothes
a. Edge of wound moving inwards to cover granulation tissue b. Edge of wound free of non-viable tissue and debris in non-healing wounds	Above interventions should provide the ideal environment for: a. Wound healing b. Maintenance of a non-healing wound	a. The healing wound is granulating from the base and the edge of wound is epithelializing inwards; the wound is smaller b. The non-healing wound is 'clean' in terms of absence of debris, non-viable tissue, exudate, signs of infection, and peri-wound skin damage

Protecting the peri-wound skin: exudate and body fluids cause predictable and inevitable damage to the skin in the form of inflammation, irritation, and progressive damage to the tissues. As stated above, prevention of such damage is a key nursing role. Alcohol-free barrier products are widely available in hospital and community settings. They form a barrier for the skin to withstand the constant flow of exudate or effluent from incontinence and fistulae (see Chapter 16 Managing Continence ➡). To maintain skin integrity, you need to apply barrier products to cover the vulnerable skin entirely, and to reapply the products consistently at dressing changes.

Managing the exudate: there is a range of wound care products that are designed to manage wound exudate directly. Indirect methods of exudate management involve correcting the underlying cause of the exudate, for example systemic antibiotics for infection. A summary of the major types of exudate is given in Table 28.4 and direct methods of exudate management are outlined in Table 28.5.

In general, unless dressings and wound management devices make direct contact with the exuding wound, they are not able to control exudate. Exudate runs off in gaps between the dressing and the peri-wound surface. It accumulates in 'dead' spaces; fixation materials give up, the dressing or device lifts, and exudate leaks. From a nursing perspective, careful selection of dressings or devices, and their application, is required to prevent failure. There are, however, circumstances in which there is a mismatch between the size, shape, and location of the wound and commercially available dressings. In these circumstances, nurses need to be creative, but also to communicate in

Table 28.3 Nursing interventions, products, and mode of action for the local management of wounds

Nursing intervention	Wound care product	Mode of action
Protect the peri-wound skin	Alcohol-free barrier products: aerosols, wipes, sponge applicators, durable barrier creams	Protects the peri-wound skin with a waterproof barrier from irritation, excoriation, and maceration from exudate
Manage the exudate	System 1. Absorbent layered dressings with or without adhesive border: • an absorbent non-adherent layered dressing, e.g. foams, absorbent gel sheets • fixation tape, film, tubular retention bandage	Absorbs exudate and takes it into the dressing matrix, prevents it from tracking back to the wound and the surrounding skin; the non-adherent layer between the wound and dressing prevents trauma and pain at removal
	System 2. Absorbent layered system comprising: • non-adherent primary wound contact layer, e.g. silicone/gel sheet layer, alginate, hydrofibre • absorbent secondary layer, e.g. dressing pad (omit if alginate/hydrofibre + film dressing handles exudate) • fixation tape, films, tapeless retention bandage/garment	The action is as for System 1, but the multiple layers give some flexibility to fitting the dressings to eccentrically shaped wounds The absorptive capacity of the system can be increased to manage heavily exuding wounds, e.g. the fibrous layer may be multilayered and a super-absorbent pad added
Prevent tissue damage and bleeding at dressing changes	• Non-adherent primary wound contact dressings • Adhesive solvent sprays • Wound irrigation solutions	• The dressing material is designed not to adhere to the wound • Adhesive solvent sprays are designed to break the adhesive bonds and cause the dressing to slide off the skin without trauma • Wound irrigation solutions, such as normal saline, enable irrigation of the wound, as opposed to swabbing, which may cause damage to fragile wound tissue
Debride the devitalized necrotic and sloughy tissue	Debriding agents: • medical grade honey dressings • larval therapy	• Remove the dead tissue, which is an ideal environment for bacterial colonization • Provide a clean wound bed of granulation tissue
Manage the bacteria in the wound, and the odour	Topical antimicrobial products: • metronidazole gels • polyhexamethylene biguanide (PHMB) dressings and cleaning solution • cadexomer iodine • medical grade honey dressings	Destroy the bacteria to manage the odour

a systematic way to manufacturers when needs are not being met (Weir *et al.*, 2006).

Preventing tissue damage and bleeding at dressing changes: bleeding and signs of tissue damage that arise in established wounds may signal deterioration in the wound, for example infection or an inappropriate handling of the wound during a dressing change. Attention to the following principles can minimize trauma and the incidence of bleeding at the dressing changes.

• Use non-adherent dressings.
• Ensure careful dressing application and removal techniques, including the use of topical adhesive solvents, where appropriate.

Table 28.4 Summary of major types of wound exudate and their clinical significance

Colour	Consistency	Clinical significance
Clear, straw-coloured, normally referred to as 'serous' exudate	Thin, watery	This is the normal result of inflammation and contains anti-inflammatory cells to combat bacteria, together with growth factors to promote healing
Serous exudate that is pink or frankly blood-stained, normally referred to as 'serosanguinous'	Thin, watery	This is the result of damage to blood vessels and should become straw-like in colour as the body's normal clotting mechanism controls the bleeding
Purulent, pus	Thick, cloudy, may be grey, yellow, green, blue-green	This signals infection; the exudate contains bacteria and inflammatory cells
Haemopurulent	Blood-stained pus	This also signals infection and indicates damage to blood vessels

Table 28.5 Direct methods of exudate management

Product type	Method of exudate management
Compression bandages Compression hosiery	To reduce oedema (limb swelling) by improving blood circulation (Badger *et al.*, 2004; Lymphoedema Framework, 2006a, b).
Mechanical systems, e.g. topical negative pressure therapy (TNP)	Negative pressure creates a suction force enabling the drainage of surgical wounds to promote wound healing. The precise mode of action of TNP is not known. Several mechanisms have been proposed. TNP is said to increase local bloodflow, and to reduce oedema and bacterial colonization rates. It is thought to promote closure of the wound by promoting the rapid formation of granulation tissue, as well as by mechanical effects on the wound. It concurrently provides a moist wound environment and removes excess wound exudate, thus aiding optimal wound healing (Bale and Jones, 2006; Bovill *et al.*, 2008; Ubbink *et al.*, 2008).
Absorbent dressings, e.g. foams, super absorbent pads	Take up exudate into the matrix of the dressing. Ideally, dressings should prevent the exudate from leaking back onto the wound or allow it to spread over onto the peri-wound skin (White, 2006).
Absorbent and gelling dressings, e.g. alginate and methylcellulose dressings	These are fibrous dressings, which turn into a soft gel when saturated with exudates (Cowan, 2011).
High moisture/fluid loss systems	These conserve humidity at wound/dressing interface to prevent dressings sticking to the wound surface. After that, they hold the exudate within the dressing material and allow the moisture content to evaporate to reduce the volume of exudate in the dressing, ideally forming a gel-like exudate that is removed at the dressing change (Grocott, 2000).

- Employ careful cleaning techniques, using irrigation, not swabbing.
- Maintain humidity at the wound/dressing interface through the appropriate use of modern wound dressings.

Debride the devitalized necrotic and sloughy tissue: debridement of dead tissue involves removing any dead tissue that harbours bacteria, which in turn, metabolizes the dead tissue and releases malodorous compounds (Vowden and Vowden, 2002). Clearance of dead tissue by sharp debridement is very efficient and requires specialist knowledge and skills training (Bentley, 2005). Promoting autolytic debridement with topical dressing materials such as medical honey can speed up the body's natural ability to shed dead tissue (Molan, 2006; Gethin and Cowman, 2008).

Managing the bacteria in the wound, and the odour: as indicated above, wound odour is caused by a number of volatile agents that are generated by the activity of bacteria on dead tissue in a wound. Three approaches are available for the management of odour, which target the odour-forming bacteria: systemic antibiotics, topical antimicrobials, and charcoal dressings. In addition, as described above, debridement of the dead tissue harbouring the bacteria can remove the root causes of the malodour (Gethin, 2010).

Systemic antibiotics are used to reduce bacterial colonization and to control the offensive odour from volatile metabolic end products. One of the limitations of systemic antibiotics is the increasing incidence of antibiotic resistance. A further limitation is their side effects, although these may be avoided at lower doses without losing the therapeutic effect on the odour (Twycross and Wilcock, 2007). Topical antimicrobial agents, such as metronidazole gels and medical honey, are alternatives to the systemic route (Gethin and Cowman, 2005; 2008; Gethin, 2010). Bacteria and volatile malodorous chemicals from wounds can also be adsorbed by charcoal cloth before they pass into the air (Thomas *et al.*, 1998). As with the management of exudate, the effectiveness of this approach depends on being able to seal the wound with the charcoal dressing completely.

Accessing the evidence to inform the nursing management of wounds

There is a substantial amount of material that can inform best practice in the management of wounds. This includes:

- clinical guidance and protocols, preferably generated by nationally agreed standards and issued by organizations such as NICE (National Institute for Health and Clinical Excellence);
- guidance to patients as users of health services;
- evidence from clinical research, both qualitative, quantitative, and mixed methods research.

As has been described in other chapters in this textbook, the Cochrane Library is an important resource (**http://www.thecochranelibrary.com/view/0/index.html**) for protocols and evidence of clinical interventions. Some of the evidence is weak, largely owing to the difficulty of applying the randomized controlled trial (RCT) as

the gold standard to the highly complex area of wound care interventions. The methodology of the RCT is not in question; rather the application of this methodology to the complex sequence of wound healing and the application of medical devices is under scrutiny.

A position document proposing alternative methodologies has been developed by the European Wound Management Group (**http://ewma.org/english/patient-outcome-group.html**) and reviewed by research methodologists, as well as by clinicians (Ashby *et al.*, 2010). Until a consensus is reached as to the most appropriate and scientifically valid methodologies to adopt for wound care research, we have to critique the research evidence using established critical appraisal tools for qualitative and quantitative research (see **http://www.phru.nhs.uk/pages/phd/resources.htm**).

Where clinical guidance and research evidence is weak, you will have to use local guidance documents and formularies, clinical judgement and experience, and be scrupulous about measuring the patient outcomes of the care given. Routine observations and outcomes data can provide important validation of research evidence and experiences gained through clinical practice. They also provide triggers for formal clinical research when patients' needs are not being met.

Given the vast array of wounds and underlying causes, the major wound types have been summarized, together with the recognized sources of evidence to inform clinical decisions and patient care. Table 28.6 provides an overview of the major wound groups with links to clinical guidelines and recognized sources of clinical evidence to guide practice. A useful list of key journals includes:

Journal of Tissue Viability
European Wound Management Association Journal
Wounds UK
Wounds International
Wounds Essential
Journal of Wound Care
International Wound Journal

Measuring the impact of nursing interventions

There has been a surprising lack of attention paid to routine measurement of patient outcomes in wound care and, in consequence, few tools are available. All too often nursing notes contain statements such as 'wound

Table 28.6 Major wound categories and links to recognized sources to guide clinical decision-making

Wound category	Sources
Surgical wounds are deliberately created by surgeons for a specified procedure, e.g. an appendectomy. Management of these wounds should be straightforward, requiring minimal interventions when modern wound dressings are used. However, complications do arise when patients have poor healing capacity or an infection arises. The evidence on the management of surgical wounds therefore focuses on the prevention of surgical site infection, together with local wound management strategies.	1. NICE guideline: Surgical Site Infection: Prevention and treatment of surgical site infection. http://guidance.nice.org.uk/CG74/Guidance/pdf/English 2. Sharp, K.A., McLaws, M.L. (2001) Wound dressings for surgical sites. Cochrane Database of Systematic Reviews. Issue 2. Art. No.: CD003091. DOI:10.1002/14651858.CD003091. 3. http://www.worldwidewounds.com/2005/september/Gottrup/Surgical-Site-Infections-Overview.html
Venous ulcers develop with sustained venous hypertension, which results from chronic venous insufficiency and/or an impaired calf muscle pump. In the normal venous system, venous pressure decreases with exercise as a result of the calf muscle pump and the valves in the perforating veins (between the superficial venous system and deep venous system), preventing reflux of blood. If these veins do not function optimally and/or the muscle pump is impaired, the venous pressure remains high. Against this background, ulceration may arise following an episode of trauma.	1. http://www.cks.nhs.uk/leg_ulcer_venous/background_information/definition 2. http://www.rcn.org.uk/development/practice/clinicalguidelines/venous_leg_ulcers 3. http://http://ewma.org/fileadmin/user_upload/EWMA/Wound_Guidelines/SIGN_Guidelines_The_care_of_Patients_with_Chronic_Leg_Ulcer.pdf
Arterial ulcers are caused by a reduced arterial blood supply to the lower limb. The commonest cause is atherosclerotic disease of the medium and large arteries whereby the peripheral circulation is insufficient to support tissue viability, and ulcers may develop. As with venous ulcers, the triggers for arterial ulceration may be an episode of trauma (Grey and Harding, 2006).	1. http://www.hse.ie/eng/services/Publications/services/Primary/woundguidelines.pdf 2. http://onlinelibrary.wiley.com/doi/10.1111/j.1524-475X.2006.00177.x/pdf
Diabetic foot ulcers develop because of neuropathy, ischaemia, or both. As with other forms of common ulcers, the initiating injury may be from an acute trauma or from repetitive and continuous mechanical stress (Edmonds and Foster, 2006). Once the skin is broken, factors such as bacterial infection, continuing trauma, and poor management can contribute to poor healing. A key aspect of the care of patients with diabetes is to look after their feet, and thereby prevent limb-threatening ulceration.	1. http://www.patient.co.uk/doctor/The-Diabetic-Foot.htm 2. http://ewma.org/english/publications/recommended-guidelines.html International Consensus on the Diabetic Foot & Practical Guidelines on the Management and Prevention on the Diabetic Foot
Pressure ulcers are areas of localized injury to the skin and/or underlying tissue, usually over a bony prominence, as a result of pressure, or pressure in combination with shear. A number of contributing factors are also associated with pressure ulcers, for example friction and moisture (see Chapter 19 Managing Hydration 🔁). The European and US National Pressure Ulcer Advisory Panels (EPUAP and NPUAP) conducted an extensive piece of work that has resulted in a set of International Pressure Ulcer Guidelines for the prevention and management of pressure ulcers, based on the best available evidence.	1. http://www.epuap.org/guidelines.html 2. http://www.nice.org.uk/guidance/index.jsp?action=byID&o=10972

improved from yesterday', which is meaningless. Photographs, as mentioned earlier in the chapter, can help to maintain an objective record of progress or deterioration, but it would not be appropriate to take daily photographs of patients' wounds. There are new software applications for smartphones and tablets, which make it possible to differentiate types of tissue found in wounds. The analysis can be made on photographs taken with the smartphone camera or uploaded from other sources. The software identifies types of tissue in the bed of the wound, for example necrotic and granulation tissue. It also calculates the area of the lesion and indicates what is required in terms of local wound interventions. Crucially, these technologies enable objective data to be extracted from wound photographs and measurements to be made of patients' wounds without storing the photographs or including patient identifiers (see, for example, **http://www.healthpath.it/MOWAEN.aspx**).

Objective wound measurements can be combined with automated clinical record systems. For example, a generic, digital pen and paper system of a clinical note-making system and treatment evaluation, TELER, has been applied to wound care and is outlined below (Browne et al., 2004; Grocott and Campling, 2009; Grocott et al., 2011; **http://www.longhanddata.com**).

TELER imports clinical knowledge derived from theory and research, together with practical know-how, into definitions of clinical outcome measures. The measures, or clinical indicators, define the patient goal, and track progress and response to the planned treatment and care, in a numerical format. These indicators specify the

Table 28.7 Surrounding skin within margins of the wound dressing site

Code	
5	Skin appears intact
4	Skin has pale pink patches (or pale discoloured patches)
3	Skin has patchy reddening (or patchy discolouring)
2	Skin has fiery red patches (or dense discoloured patches) (Figure 28.1)
1	Skin diffuse fiery red (or diffusely discoloured)
0	Skin is diffuse fiery red and shiny (or diffusely discoloured and shiny, e.g. in dark skin)

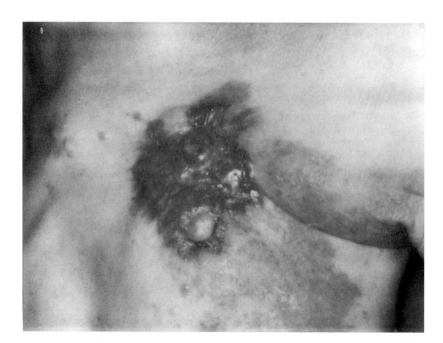

Figure 28.1 (see Colour Plate 10) Illustration of skin damage from exudate; classified as Code 2 on the TELER indicator.

Box 28.1   Odour impact

Patients were invited to identify five or more components of the odour problem that they experience. The following issues were raised by patients in a research project to develop the indicators in Table 28.8 (Browne *et al.*, 2004).

Components:

1. I should change my dressings more often to reduce odour, but can't manage it.
2. I am concerned that other people will notice an odour.
3. It affects my social and work life.
4. I use aftershave to mask the smell.
5. I don't feel clean.

Table 28.8   Indicators

Code	
5	Not experiencing any components
4	Experiencing 1 component
3	Experiencing 2 components
2	Experiencing 3 components
1	Experiencing 4 components
0	Experiencing 5 components

clinical interventions in terms of goals and predictions of how a patient's wound care problems will change over time into observable outcomes. In addition, individual patient circumstances are defined together with their personal experiences of the interventions and care. Analysis of the numerical data includes an automated method of calculating patient-specific index numbers (deficit index, improvement index, maintenance index, and effectiveness index), and two group index numbers (health status index and health gain index). See Table 28.7 and Box 28.1 for examples of TELER outcome indicators.

Measuring patient outcomes in a format such as TELER means that changes in the patient's conditions are traced in an objective, visible, and transparent way over time. This will enable you to react quickly to signs of deterioration, and to communicate efficiently and effectively with colleagues.

Summary and key messages

- The management of wounds is a key nursing responsibility.
- Wounds cause both physical and emotional stress, and require a holistic approach to assessment to inform your nursing management plan.
- The nursing management of wounds involves making clinical decisions about the most appropriate evidence-based, nurse-led interventions to implement.
- It is essential to monitor changes in the wound and surrounding skin constantly to assess wound healing progress.
- The evidence base for wound care interventions is limited and further research is required.

Online Resource Centre

To help you to develop and apply your knowledge and decision-making skills further, we have provided interactive learning resources online at **www.oxfordtextbooks.co.uk/orc/bullock**

Whilst these are freely available, you will need to use the access codes at the start of the book.

References

Ashby, R., Cullum., N, Dumville, J., *et al.* (2010) Reflections on the recommendations of the EWMA Patient Outcome Group document. *Journal of Wound Care* **19**(7): 282–5.

Badger, C., Preston, N., Seers, K., *et al.* (2004) Physical therapies for reducing and controlling lymphoedema of the limbs. *Cochrane Database of Systematic Reviews* Issue 4: Art. No. CD003141. DOI: 10.1002/14651858.CD003141.

Bale, S., Jones, V. (2006) *Wound Care Nursing. A Patient-Centred Approach.* Mosby Elsevier: Edinburgh.

Bentley, J. (2005) Choosing the right prescribing options in wound debridement. *Nurse Prescribing* **3**(3): 96.

Bovill, E., Banwell, PE., Teot, L. and the International Advisory Panel on Topical Negative Pressure (2008) Topical negative pressure wound therapy: a review of its role and guidelines for its use in the management of acute wounds. *International Wound Journal* **5**(4): 511–29.

Bowyer, P. (2008) Life as a carer. *Leg Ulcer Forum Journal* **22**: 11.

Browne, N., Grocott, P., Cowley, S., *et al.* (2004) Woundcare Research for Appropriate Products (WRAP): validation of the TELER method involving users. *International Journal of Nursing Studies* **41**(5): 559–71.

Collier, M. (2004) Recognition and management of wound infections. http://www.worldwidewounds.com/2004/january/Collier/Management-of-Wound-infections.html (accessed 19 October 2011).

Cowan T. (ed.) (2011) *Wound Care Handbook 2011–12,* 4th edn. Mark Allen Healthcare: London.

Cowley, S., Grocott, P. (2007) Research design for the development and evaluation of complex technologies: an empirical example and critical discussion. *Evaluation* **13**(3): 285–305.

Dealey, C. (2005) *Care of Wounds: A Guide for Nurses,* 3rd edn. Blackwell Publishing: Oxford.

Department of Health (2008) *End-of-Life Care Strategy: Promoting High Quality Care for all Adults at the End of Life: Equality Impact Assessment.* DH: London.

Dowsett, C. (2008) Using the TIME framework in wound bed preparation. *British Journal of Community Nursing* **13**(6): S15–16, S18, S20.

Drew, P., Posnett, J., Rusling, L. (2007) The cost of wound care for a local population in England. *International Wound Journal* **4**: 149–55.

Edmonds, M., Foster, V.M. (2005) *Managing the Diabetic Foot.* Blackwell Publishing: Oxford.

Fagervik-Morton, H., Price, P. (2010) Chronic ulcers and everyday living: patients' perspective in the United Kingdom. *Wounds* **21**(12): 318–23.

Gethin, G. (2010) Managing wound malodour in palliative care. (Palliative Wound Care Supplement) *Wounds UK*: 12–15.

Gethin, G., Cowman, S. (2005) Case series of use of Manuka honey in leg ulceration. *International Wound Journal* **2**(1): 10–15.

Gethin, G., Cowman, S. (2008) Bacteriological changes in sloughy venous leg ulcers treated with manuka honey or hydrogel: an RCT. *Journal of Wound Care* **17**(6): 241–7.

Grey, J., Harding, K. (2006) *ABC of Wound Healing: Venous and Arterial Leg Ulcers.* http://www.bmj.com/cgi/content/full/332/7537/347 (accessed 3 August 2010).

Grocott, P. (2000) The palliative management of fungating malignant wounds. *Journal of Wound Care* **9**(1): 4–9.

Grocott, P., Briggs, E. (2009) Palliative wound pain. In *Trauma and Pain in Wound Care,* 2nd edn. Wounds UK: Glasgow, pp. 115–35.

Grocott, P., Campling, N. (2009) A methodology for evaluating wound care technologies in the context of treatment and care. *European Wound Management Association Journal* **9**: 27–38.

Grocott, P., Gray, D. (2010) The argument for palliative wound care. *Wounds UK* **6**(1): 149–50.

Grocott, P., Robinson, V. (2009) Skin problems in palliative medicine: nursing aspects. In G. Hanks, N. Cherney, S. Kaasa *et al.* (eds) *Oxford Textbook of Palliative Medicine,* 4th edn. Oxford University Press: Oxford, pp. 965–75.

Grocott, P., Blackwell, R., Pillay, E., *et al.* (2011) Clinical note-making and patient outcome measures using TELER®. *Wounds International,* **2**(3): 13–16. Available online at http://woundsinternational.com/practice-development/clinical-note-making-and-patient-outcome-measures-using-teler/page-1 (accessed 26 March 2012).

Hurd, T., Posnett, J. (2009) Point prevalence of wounds in a sample of acute hospitals in Canada. *International Wound Journal* **6**(4): 287–93.

Lawton, J. (1998) Contemporary hospice care: the sequestration of the unbounded body and 'dirty dying'. *Sociology of Health & Illness* **20**(2): 121–43.

Lymphoedema Framework (2006a) *Best Practice for the Management of Lymphoedema: International Consensus.* MEP Ltd: London.

Lymphoedema Framework (2006b) *Template for Practice: Compression Hosiery in Lymphoedema.* MEP Ltd: London.

Mahe, E., Langlois, G., Baron, G. (2006) Results of a comprehensive hospital based wound survey. *Journal of Wound Care* **15**(9): 381–4.

Posnett, J., Gottrup, F., Lundgren, H., *et al.* (2009) The resource impact of wounds on health-care providers in Europe. *Journal of Wound Care* **18**(4): 154–61.

Price, P.E., Fagervik-Morton, H., Mudge, E.J., *et al.* (2008) Dressing-related pain in patients with chronic wounds: an international patient perspective. *International Wound Journal* **5**(2): 159–71.

Probst, S., Arber, A., Faithfull, S. (2009), Malignant fungating wounds: a survey of nurses' clinical practice in Switzerland. *European Journal of Oncology Nursing* **13**: 295–8.

Reynolds, V. (2008) Living with a leg ulcer from a carer's perspective. *Leg Ulcer Forum* **22**: 12–18.

Romanelli, M., Dini, V., Rogers, L.C., *et al.* (2008) Clinical evaluation of a wound measurement and documentation system. *Wounds* **20**: 258–64.

Royal College of Nursing (2006) *Clinical Practice Guidelines: The Nursing Management of Patients with Venous Leg Ulcers.* **http://www.rcn.org.uk/development/practice/ clinicalguidelines/venous_leg_ulcers** (accessed 5 April 2011).

Schultz, G., Sibbald, G., Falanga, V. (2003), Wound bed preparation: a systematic approach to wound management. *Wound Repair and Regeneration* **11**(Suppl. 1): S1–S28.

Sharp, K.A., McLaws, M.L. (2001) Wound dressings for surgical sites. *Cochrane Database of Systematic Reviews* Issue 2: Art. No. CD003091. DOI: 10.1002/14651858.CD003091.

Shatner, A. (2003) The emotional dimension and the biological paradigm of illness: time for change. *Quarterly Journal of Medicine* **96**: 617–21.

Strachan, V., Prentice, J., Newall, N. (2007) *Wounds West Wound Prevalence Survey 2006: Statewide Report Overview.* Ambulatory Care Services, Department of Health: Perth, WA.

Thomas, S., Fisher, B., Fram, P.J., *et al.* (1998) Odour-absorbing dressings. *Journal of Wound Care* **7**(5): 246–50.

Twycross, R., Wilcock, A. (2007) *Palliative Care Formulary (PCF3),* 3rd edn. Palliative drugs.com Ltd: Nottingham.

Ubbink, D.T., Westerbos, S.J., Nelson, E.A., *et al.* (2008) A systematic review of topical negative pressure therapy for acute and chronic wounds. *British Journal of Surgery* **95**(6): 685–92.

Vowden, K., Vowden, P. (2002) Wound bed preparation. *World Wide Wounds.* **http://www.worldwidewounds.co.uk** (accessed 21 July 2010).

Weir, H., Grocott, P., Bridgelal Ram, M. (2006) The nurse's role in contributing to new device development. *Nursing Times* **102**: 35–9.

Weston, A. (2009) *A Rulebook for Arguments,* 4th edn. Hackett Publishing Company Inc: Indianapolis, IN.

White, R.J. (2006) Modern exudate management: a review of wound treatments. **http://www.worldwidewounds.com/2006/ september/White/Modern-Exudate-Mgt.html#exudate-comp** (accessed 11 April 2010).

Winter, G.D. (1962) Formation of the scab and the rate of epithelialisation of superficial wounds in the skin of the young domestic pig. *Nature* **193**: 293–4.

Glossary

Chapter 2 *Understanding* Asthma

Anti-leukotrienes inhibitors medication that blocks leukotriene response.

Asymptomatic not showing any symptoms of disease, even when disease is present.

β_2-agonists a bronchodilator medication. Mode of action is through the β_2-receptors in the lungs.

Bronchial hyperresponsiveness (BHR) airways over-responding to triggers.

Bronchoconstriction narrowing of the airways.

Bronchodilators medication taken to relax the smooth muscle in the airway and reduce bronchoconstriction.

Corticosteroids medication to help reduce inflammation.

Degranulate/degranulation a cellular process that releases mediators, i.e. histamine found inside cells such as **mast cells**.

Dysfunctional breathing abnormal breathing pattern, which can cause asthma-like symptoms.

Early response response to trigger/allergen.

Eosinophils white blood cells that are one of the immune system components that control mechanisms associated with inflammation in allergy and asthma. They are also responsible for combating multicellular parasites.

Extremis on point of death.

Forced expiratory volume (FEV$_1$) Volume of air forcibly expelled from lungs in first second from maximal inspiration.

Fibrosis scarring.

Forced vital capacity (FVC) volume of air that can be forcibly expelled from lungs from maximal inspiration (aim for 6 seconds).

Haemoptysis coughing up blood.

Hypertrophy increase in the size of tissue or organ.

Hyperventilation breathing at an abnormally shallow rapid rate.

Immunoglobulin E (IgE) one of the five immunoglobulins produced by the immune system, IgE is associated with allergies. IgE causes the release of mediators when it detects the presence of an allergen that it has previously encountered and been 'primed' against.

Late response 4–6 hours after early asthmatic response, inflammatory cell recruitment and activation takes place.

Leukotrienes a compound believed to be present during some inflammatory responses.

Mast cells large cells found in mucosa and connective tissue. When surface receptor-bound antigen-specific IgE encounters an antigen that the IgE recognizes, mast cell degranulation is triggered, leading to the rapid release of inflammatory mediators. It also stimulates the arrival of other inflammatory cells—a critical step in local inflammation process.

Mononucleocytes white blood cells.

Oedema excessive accumulation of fluid in the body tissue.

Peak expiratory flow rate (PEFR/PF) rate at which person forcibly expels air.

Pneumothorax air in the pleural cavity.

Severe disease severe airflow limitation and airways hyperreactivity as well as prominent symptoms.

T lymphocytes part of the immune process—type of white blood cell.

Vasodilatation increase in the diameter of blood vessels.

Wheeze noisy breathing caused by narrowing of the airways or obstruction.

Chapter 3 *Understanding* Bone Conditions

Arthroplasty hip joint replacement.

Comorbidity coexistence of two or more disease processes.

Extracapsular outside the joint capsule.

Fissure fracture small surface 'cracks'.

Hip fracture a fracture between the edge of the femoral head and 5 cm below the lesser trochanter.

Intracapsular within the joint capsule.

Kyphosis stooped, round shoulders.

Monostotic affecting a single site.

Multifactorial influenced by many factors.

Orthogeriatric collaborative specialist medical and multidisciplinary care of fragility fracture.

Osteoblast bone-forming cell.

Osteoclast multinucleate bone cell that erodes bone.

Osteopenia loss of bone mineral density of less than 2.5 standard deviations below normal

Polyostotic affecting several sites.

Resorption erosion.

Secondary hyperparathyroidism overactivity of the parathyroid glands as a result of external causes.

Thromboembolic complications deep vein thrombosis and pulmonary embolism.

Chapter 4 *Understanding* Cancer

Acquired or sporadic (gene mutation) this refers to alterations in DNA that occur after conception. They can occur in any cell except germ cells (sperm and egg) and cannot be passed on to offspring.

Adjuvant treatments given in addition to the primary treatment.

Angiogenesis the formation of blood vessels. In cancer this relates to the development of a new blood supply which the cancer needs to grow.

Apoptosis a natural process of programmed cell death.

Ascites an accumulation of fluid in the peritoneal cavity. May be caused by benign conditions such as cirrhosis of the liver or cancers, especially ovarian, gastrointestinal, and breast.

Benign where there is no ability for the cellular invasion of local tissue or distant spread.

CEA (carcinoembryonic antigen) a protein normally produced in fetal development. Raised blood levels may indicate the presence of some cancers, especially bowel cancer.

CA 125 (cancer antigen 125) a protein produced by some types of cancer, especially ovarian. It can be measured in the bloodstream and is used as a marker for the potential presence of the disease.

Cancer the name given to a group of over 200 different types of disease in which abnormal cells divide uncontrollably and have the ability to invade tissues and spread to other cells within the body.

Cancer control actions that reduce the burden of cancer. Encompasses all aspects of cancer care, including prevention, screening, detection, treatment, palliative care, and survivorship.

Carcinogen a substance or agent that causes cancer. There are many known carcinogens, such as tobacco, radioactivity, asbestos, etc., as well as viruses such as the human papillomavirus.

Cells the basic structural and functional unit of all living things. The function of an organism is dependent on the individual and collective activity of cells.

Cytotoxic toxic to cells. Generally refers to drugs which target and destroy cancer cells.

DNA (deoxyribonucleic acid) a macromolecule that contains the genetic instructions for the development and function of all living organisms.

Extravasation the leakage of fluid from a blood vessel into the surrounding tissues. Used to describe the leakage of intravenous anti-cancer medicines into the tissues and also the leakage of cancer cells from the blood vessel into the tissues.

Fractioned/fractionated in radiotherapy this refers to dividing the total dose of radiotherapy required into smaller parts to be given over a longer period of time.

Fungating wound a type of skin lesion marked by ulceration and necrosis.

Gene a segment of DNA that contributes to a specific function of the organism.

Incidence the frequency with which a disease appears in a particular population or area.

Inherited in genetics this refers to the DNA characteristics passed on from parent to child.

Intravasation in the process of metastasis, this refers to the penetration of the cancer into the blood vessel.

Ionizing radiation radiation with enough energy to cause the electrons in the atom to become changed or ionized.

Leiomyoma a benign smooth muscle neoplasm.

Leiomyosarcoma a malignant smooth muscle neoplasm.

Malignant having the ability to invade local tissues and spread to other parts of the body.

Metastasis the process by which cancer cells spread from the site where they initially arose to distant organs or structures. Can also be used to name the resultant lesion; for example, evidence of a cancer spread to the liver would be a liver metastasis.

Morbidity the prevalence of a disease within a population. In cancer and clinical healthcare it also refers to the adverse effects caused by treatments.

Mortality the death rate or the number of deaths in a defined group over a defined period of time.

Mutation in genetics this refers to a permanent change or alteration in the DNA.

Necrosis death of body tissue caused by a loss of bloodflow.

Neoadjuvant treatments given prior to the primary treatment.

Neoplasm an abnormal mass of cells with uncontrolled cell growth.

Novel therapies refers to the use of newer anti-cancer agents such as targeted signalling modifiers, in place of/ in conjunction with traditional cytotoxic chemotherapy.

Oncogene a mutated gene that leads to the development of cancer.

Palliative care according to the World Health Organization, palliative care is an approach that improves the quality of life of patients and their families facing the problem associated with life-threatening illness, through the prevention and relief of suffering by means of early assessment of physical and psychological impacts (strategy of symptom relief).

Pleural effusion an accumulation of fluid in the pleural space that surrounds the lungs. May be caused by benign conditions such as infection or heart failure, or by cancers, especially lung, breast, ovary, lymphoma, and mesothelioma.

Prevalence (in epidemiology) the total number of cases of a disease in a given population at a given time.

Primary cancer this refers to the original site of the cancer.

Primary treatment this refers to the initial or the main treatment.

Pre-malignant having the potential to develop into a cancer if left untreated—may have some of the features of a cancer but without the ability to invade local tissues or spread to other parts of the body at this point.

Prognosis a prediction of the likely course and outcome of a disease.

PSA (prostate-specific antigen) a protein produced by the prostate gland which can be elevated in the bloodstream in the presence of prostate cancer. Used as a marker for the potential presence of the disease.

Satiety (satiation) this refers to the state of feeling satisfied, primarily being full after eating.

Secondary cancer having metastatic disease, cancer which has spread from a primary lesion (**secondaries**). Can also refer to a cancer induced by treatments such as radiotherapy.

Stage the stage of a cancer describes the extent and severity of the disease.

Tumour suppressor gene a gene that restrains cell growth.

Chapter 5 *Understanding* Chronic Obstructive Pulmonary Disease

Alpha-1 antitrypsin deficiency An enzyme deficiency that can cause liver and/or lung disease.

Cachexia loss of weight and muscle mass caused by disease.

Chronic asthma a severe persistent asthma.

Chronic bronchitis inflammation of the mucous membrane in the bronchial tubes, Associated with cough and sputum production.

Cor pulmonale abnormal enlargement of the right side of the heart as a result of disease of the lungs or the pulmonary blood vessels.

Dyspnoea laboured or difficult breathing.

Emphysema (also pulmonary emphysema) a condition in which the air sacs of the lungs are damaged and enlarged, causing breathlessness.

Exacerbations a reoccurrence or worsening of the condition.

Exertional breathlessness gasping for breath, due to exertion.

Forced expiratory volume in 1 second (FEV$_1$) Volume of air forcibly expelled from lungs in first second from maximal inspiration.

Forced vital capacity (FVC) the greatest volume of air that can be expelled from the lungs after taking the deepest possible breath.

Hypercapnia an excess of carbon dioxide in the blood.

Long-acting β$_2$ agonists pharmacological agents which initiate a physiological response when combined with a receptor causing bronchial dilation due to smooth muscle relaxation.

Long-acting muscarinic antagonists pharmacological agents that act by reducing the effect of acetylcholine (a neurotransmitter).

Mucolytics pharmacological agents used to dissolve the thickness of excessive mucous and targeted to relieve respiratory difficulties.

Polycythaemia a condition in which there is an abnormally increased concentration of haemoglobin in the blood.

Pulmonary rehabilitation a multidisciplinary programme of education and exercise for people with pulmonary disease.

Quality and Outcomes Framework (QOF) a system, introduced as part of the new general medical services (nGMS) contract for general practitioners, where there is targeted financial incentive for implementing good medical practice.

Sleep apnoea A sleep disorder characterized by dynamic upper airway obstruction during sleep.

Short-acting β₂ agonists pharmacological agents which initiate a physiological response when combined with a receptor, causing bronchial dilation due to smooth muscle relaxation.

Short-acting muscarinic antagonists pharmacological agent used in the treatment of chronic obstructive airways disease and acts by reducing the effect of acetylcholine (a neurotransmitter).

Chapter 6 *Understanding* Coronary Heart Disease

Acute coronary syndrome diagnostic grouping of possible cardiac disease covering angina (unstable or stable), non-ST elevation myocardial infarction (NSTEMI) and ST elevation myocardial infarction (STEMI).

Angina a condition marked by severe pain in the chest, arising from an inadequate blood supply to the heart.

Atheroma degeneration of the walls of the arteries, leading to restriction of the circulation and a risk of thrombosis.

Atherosclerosis a disease of the arteries characterized by the deposition of fatty material on their inner walls. See also atheroma.

Bradycardia abnormally slow heart rate (less than 60 BPM).

Catecholamines neurotransmitters such as adrenalin and dopamine.

Diaphoresis excessive unpredictable sweating; eg when a person is in clinical shock.

Dyspnoea laboured breathing.

Fibrin an insoluble protein formed as a fibrous mesh during the clotting of blood.

Fibroblasts a cell in connective tissue which produces collagen and other fibres of a vein, artery, or other part.

Macrophages large phagocytic cell found in stationary form in the tissues or as a mobile white blood cell, especially at sites of infection.

Meta-analysis statistical process that combines the effect of pooling individual study research results.

Monocytes large phagocytic white blood cell with a simple oval nucleus and clear, greyish cytoplasm.

Myocardial infarction death of myocardial tissue (known as a heart attack).

Myocaridal necrosis the death of myocardial muscle tissue

Non-ST elevation myocardial infarction (NSTEMI) myocardial infarction which does not have a related elevation of the ST segment on an ECG (Echocardiogram).

Plaque physiological debris that silts and collects over time to form a narrowing or hardening of the inner lumen of a blood vessel.

Retrosternal discomfort slight pain behind the breastbone.

Serotonin present in blood platelets and serum, which constricts the blood vessels and acts as a neurotransmitter.

Stable angina a condition marked by severe pain in the chest, arising from an inadequate blood supply to the heart.

ST elevation myocardial infarction (STEMI) Myocardial infarction classically diagnosed from observing an elevated ST segment on the ECG (Echocardiogram).

Stenosis abnormal narrowing of a passage in the body

Tachycardia an abnormally rapid heart rate (greater than 100 beats per minute BPM).

Thrombosis local coagulation or clotting of the blood in a part of the circulatory system.

Unstable angina a condition marked by severe pain in the chest, often also spreading to the shoulders, arms, and neck, caused by an inadequate blood supply to the heart.

Chapter 7 *Understanding* Dementia

Alzheimer's disease/dementia a serious disorder of the brain. Manifesting itself in premature memory failures, personality changes, and impaired reasoning.

Amyloid protein an insoluble protein which is deposited in the liver, kidneys, spleen, or other tissues in certain diseases.

Delirium an acutely disturbed state of mind characterized by restlessness, illusions, and incoherence of thought and speech, occurring in fever and other disorders and in intoxication.

Diagnostic and Statistical Manual of Mental Disorders, fourth edition (DSM-IV) A diagnostic tool that categorizes mental health conditions.

Free radicals an unchanged atom or group of atoms with one or more unpaired electrons which can be formed when oxygen interacts and usually lead to disease processes.

International Classification of Diseases, tenth edition (ICD-10) an international standard agreed by the World Health Organization; the international standard diagnostic classification for all general epidemiological conditions.

Lewy body dementia closely associated with both Alzheimers and Parkinsons, characterized by the presence of Lewy Bodies (protein presence in neurons).

Memory clinics clinic facilities that specialize in the assessment and diagnosis of memory related conditions such as dementia.

Mini-mental state examination (MMSE) an examination to determine the state of a person's mental health.

Multi-infarct dementia persistent mental disorder marked by memory failures, personality changes, and impaired reasoning.

Neurofibrillary tangles a fibril in the cytoplasm of a nerve cell, visible by light microscopy.

Neurotransmitter chemical substance released from the end of a nerve fibre and effecting the transfer of an impulse to another nerve or muscle.

Pick's disease a rare form of progressive dementia, typically occurring in late middle age and often familial, involving localized atrophy of the brain.

Progressive supranuclear palsy (PSP) occurrs or originates above a nucleus of the central nervous system. Produces a paralysis and often accompanied by involuntary tremors.

Quality and Outcomes Framework (QOF) a system introduced as part of the new general medical services (nGMS) contract for general practitioners where there is targeted financial incentive for implementing good medical practice.

Senile plaques a microscopic mass of fragmented and decaying nerve terminals around an amyloid core, numbers of which occur in the brains of people with Alzheimer's disease.

Vascular dementia chronic or persistent mental disorder marked by memory failures, personality changes, and impaired reasoning.

Chapter 8 *Understanding* Depression

Affect feeling, emotion, or desire, especially when leading to action

Biopsychosocial the branch of psychology concerned with biological and physiological aspects.

Bipolar affective disorder mental health marked by alternating periods of elation and depression.

Chronic anxiety disorder persisting a nervous condition marked by excessive uneasiness often leading to confusion.

Cognitive behavioural therapy (CBT) a type of psychotherapy in which negative patterns of thought about the self and the world are challenged shaped around self-management.

Generalized anxiety disorder a nervous disorder marked by excessive uneasiness/anxiety.

Hypomanic/manic episodes extreme representation of behaviour.

Multidisciplinary team a team constituted of different disciplines or professional specialities.

Obsessive compulsive disorder denoting or relating to an anxiety disorder in which a person feels compelled to perform certain stereotyped actions repeatedly to alleviate persistent fears or intrusive thoughts, typically resulting in severe disruption of daily life.

Panic disorder a debilitating anxiety and fear arise frequently and without reasonable cause.

Post-traumatic stress disorder a condition of persistent mental and emotional stress occurring as a result of injury or severe psychological shock.

Social phobia of or relating to society or its organization—an extreme or irrational fear of something.

Chapter 9 *Understanding* Diabetes Mellitus

Amino acids any of a group of organic compounds containing both the carboxyl and amino groups, occurring naturally in plant and animal tissues and forming the basic constituents of proteins.

Autoimmune denoting disease caused by antibodies or lymphocytes produced against substances naturally present in the body.

Beta cells any of the insulin-producing cells in the islets of Langerhans.

Catecholamines neurotransmitters such as adrenalin and dopamine.

Cortisol another term for hydrocortisone.

C peptide a compound consisting of two or more amino acids linked in a chain.

Diabetic ketoacidosis a condition characterized by raised levels of ketone bodies in the body, associated with fat metabolism and diabetes.

Gestational diabetes The development of diabetes between conception and birth.

Glucagon a peptide hormone formed in the pancreas which promotes the breakdown of glycogen to glucose in the liver.

Gluconeogenesis the formation of glycogen from glucose.

HbA1c is a measure that indicates the amount of blood sugar and is indicative of blood sugar control.

Hyperglycaemia an excess of glucose in the bloodstream, often associated with diabetes mellitus.

Hyperosmolar hyperglycaemic state occurs in type 2 diabetes and is an excessive high blood glucose level.

Hypoglycaemia deficiency of glucose in the bloodstream.

Hypoglycaemic agents pharmacological agents that lower blood glucose.

Idiopathic relating to or denoting any disease or condition which arises spontaneously or for which the cause is unknown.

Incretins group of gastrointestinal hormones that cause an increase in insulin levels.

Insulin a polypeptide pancreatic hormone which lowers glucose levels in the blood, a lack of which causes diabetes.

Insulin resistance tissue resistance to the effects of insulin.

Insulin secretion secretion of insulin by the pancreas.

Islets of Langerhans groups of pancreatic cells secreting insulin and glucagon.

Isophane a protein hormone formed from proinsulin.

Ketone bodies compounds produced during the metabolism of fats and synthesized in the liver during starvation for use as an alternative energy source to glucose.

Ketosis a condition characterized by raised levels of ketone bodies in the body, associated with abnormal fat metabolism and diabetes mellitus.

Microalbuminuria occurs when the kidney leaks small amounts of albumin into urine.

Nocturia passing urine twice or more at night.

Polypeptide organic polymer consisting of a large number of amino-acid residues, forming all or part of a protein molecule.

Polyuria production of abnormally large volumes of dilute urine.

Prodromal phase relating to or denoting the period between the appearance of initial symptoms and the full development of a rash or fever.

Retinopathy disease of the retina which results in impairment or loss of vision.

Chapter 10 *Understanding* Functional Bowel Disorders

Biopsychosocial the branch of psychology concerned with biological and physiological aspects.

Coeliac disease Coeliac disease is an autoimmune disorder characterized by damage to all or part of the villi lining the small intestine.

Crohn's disease A chronic inflammatory disease of the digestive tract and it can involve anypart of it—from the mouth to the anus. It typically affects the terminal ileum as well as demarcated areas of large bowel, with other areas of the bowel being relatively unaffected.

Functional Constipation is a term to describe the subjective complaint of passage of abnormally delayed or infrequent passage of dry, hardened faeces often accompanied by straining and/or pain. It is described as **functional or idiopathic** when it cannot be explained by any anatomical, physiological, radiological or histological abnormalities.

Functional diarrhoea A condition in which the sufferer has frequent and watery or loose bowel movements It is described as **functional or idiopathic** when it cannot be explained by any anatomical, physiological, radiological or histological abnormalities.

Functional dyspepsia painful, difficult, or disturbed digestion, which may be accompanied by symptoms such as heartburn, bloating, stomach discomfort nausea and vomiting.

Ileocaecal valve valve between the ileum of the small intestine and the cecum of the large intestine; prevents material from flowing back from the large to the small intestine.

Inflammatory bowel disease (IBD) is not a single disease. The term IBD is used mainly to describe two diseases: Crohn's disease & ulcerative colitis. Both Crohn's disease and ulcerative colitis are chronic (long-term) diseases that involve inflammation of the gastrointestinal tract (gut). However, there are important differences between the two.

Ulcerative colitis only affects the colon (large intestine), while Crohn's disease can affect the entire digestive system, from the mouth to the anus. It is sometimes difficult to tell the difference between the two main types of IBD. If this is the case, it is known as indeterminate colitis. There are other, rarer types of IBD called collagenous colitis and lymphocytic colitis. Together these are often called microscopic colitis

Irritable bowel syndrome (IBS) a widespread condition involving recurrent abdominal pain and diarrhoea or constipation, often associated with stress, depression, anxiety, or previous intestinal infection

Magnetic resonance imaging (MRI) a radiological technique for producing images of bodily organs by measuring the response of the atomic nuclei of body tissues to high-frequency radio waves when placed in a strong magnetic field.

Microvilli minute projections from the surface of some cells.

Peristalsis the involuntary constriction and relaxation of the muscles of the intestine or another canal, creating wave-like movements which push the contents of the canal forward.

Positron emission tomography (PET) a form of tomography used esp. for brain scans which employs positron-emitting isotopes introduced into the body as a source of radiation instead of applying X-rays externally.

Rome I, II, and III The Rome criteria is a system developed to classify the **functional gastrointestinal disorders (FGIDs)**, disorders of the digestive system in which symptoms cannot be explained by the presence of structural or tissue abnormality, based on clinical symptoms. Some examples of FGIDs include irritable bowel syndrome, functional dyspepsia, functional constipation, and functional heartburn. **www.romecriteria.org**

Ulcerative colitis is a type of chronic inflammatory bowel disease (IBD) that affects the lining of the large intestine (colon) and rectum.

Urgency pressing necessity for bowel or bladder evacuation, used to describe the need to go to the toilet without warning and immediately.

Villi (plural form of villus) finger like projections of the lining of the small intestine, set closely together typically increasing the surface area for absorption

Chapter 11 *Understanding* Renal Disorders

Acute kidney injury a sudden deterioration in renal function characterized by a reduction in urine output and elevation in **urea** and **creatinine.**

Anuria no urine output (or <100 ml/day).

Central venous pressure (CVP) CVP describes the Pressure in the thoracic vena cava, close to the right atrium of the heart. CVP indicates the amount of blood returning to the heart.

Chronic kidney disease (CKD) a slow progressive disease process.

Conservative management/treatment treatment used to defer the deterioration of renal function by means of blood pressure control, fluid and dietary control and medication.

Continuous veno-venous haemofiltration (CVVH) a renal replacement therapy commonly used in **acute**

kidney injury. The patient's blood is circulated through a specialised filter. Large volumes of fluid, are removed along with solutes and waste products.

Creatinine a product formed as a result of catabolism and breakdown of creatine phosphate in muscle. It is excreted by the kidney.

Diuresis an increased production of urine.

Diuretic an pharmacological agent which increases the flow of urine.

Established renal failure–end-stage renal failure this is the stage of **chronic kidney disease** (stage 5) when dialysis or a kidney transplant is required.

Glomerular filtration rate (GFR) the rate at which blood is filtered across the capillaries of the glomerulus.

Haemodialysis (HD) a renal replacement therapy The blood passes through an artificial filter and is indirectly exposed to a solution (dialysate). Ultrafiltration and diffusion result in removal of waste products and fluid, and a re-balancing of electrolytes and pH.

Hyperkalaemia a higher than normal concentration of potassium in the blood.

Hyperphosphataemia a higher than normal concentration of phosphates in the blood.

Hypervolaemia an abnormal increase in total body fluid.

Hypokalaemia a lower than normal concentration of potassium in the blood.

Hypovolaemia a reduction in the total circulating volume of body fluid in the intravascular space.

Jugular venous pressure (JVP) JVP is the pressure in the internal jugular vein. It is routinely used clinically to assess fluid volume status.

Mean arterial pressure a measure of the average arterial pressure during one cardiac cycle.

Metabolic acidosis a condition resulting from the kidney's inability to recover adequate bicarbonate ions from, or secrete hydrogen ions, into the renal tubules. Blood pH will fall to an acidotic state (normal range 7.35–5.45).

Metabolic waste products the products of metabolic activity. Urea and creatinine are sometimes described as nitrogenous waste.

Nephrology A branch of medicine focussing on the management of kidney disease.

Nephron the structural and functional component of the kidney. Each kidney contains approximately 1 million nephrons.

Oliguria a daily urinary volume of <400 ml or <0.5 ml/kg body weight/hour.

Peritoneal dialysis (PD) a renal replacement therapy used for the treatment of stage 5 chronic kidney disease when dialysis fluid is introduced into the peritoneal cavity to remove toxins and waste products from circulating blood by diffusion.

Pulse pressure the difference between the systolic and the diastolic pressures.

Renal replacement therapy (RRT) an overall term used to describe the life-supporting treatment necessary to remove waste products once the kidneys have failed.

Uraemia a collection of signs and symptoms associated with a high concentration of urea in the blood.

Urea a product formed in the liver as a consequence of protein metabolism and excreted via the kidneys.

Chapter 12 *Understanding* Skin Conditions

Acid mantle refers to the acidic pH of the skin's surface, which inhibits the growth of some pathogenic bacteria.

Atopic eczema type of eczema caused by a genetic predisposition (atopy), characterized by dry itchy skin, often appearing in early childhood.

Cellulitis a bacterial infection of the skin which develops more slowly than erysipelas, has a poorly defined margin, and is characterized by lymphadenopathy, fever, and general malaise.

Chronic inflammatory skin diseases (CSIDs) long-term skin dermatoses characterized by inflammation.

Chronic leg ulcer a leg ulcer that is distal to the knee that has been open for at least 6 weeks.

Chronic oedema oedema present for more than 3 months.

Collagen a protein fibre within the dermis of the skin (but in other areas of the body also), providing tissue strength. It is the main component of connective tissue.

Contact dermatitis caused by a delayed hypersensitivity reaction to an external allergen.

Cream An emollient that is a mixture of water and lipid.

Crust dried exudate.

Dermatoscope a microscopy device used to examine the skin, especially for distinguishing benign from malignant skin lesions.

Dermis the thicker inner layer of the skin comprised of blood vessels and sensory nerves within connective tissue.

Doppler measure an ultrasound device that measures the systolic pressure in the vasculature of the leg and provides the basis for determining ankle and brachial pressure index (ABPI), giving an indication for a safe level of compression bandaging.

Eczema (dermatitis) an inflammatory dermatosis leading to the principal symptom of itching, which maybe primarily endogenous in origin (atopic) or exogenous (contact).

Elastin a protein fibre within the dermis, providing it with elasticity.

Emollient a topical application that ameliorates dry scaly skin by helping retain moisture, making the rough surface soft and smooth.

Epidermis the outer protective avascular layer of the skin organized as a stratified squamous epithelium and comprised of keratinocytes.

Erysipelas a streptococcal infection of the skin causing rapid inflammation with a characteristic red, shiny, raised plaque with a well demarcated edge.

Erythema redness of the skin.

Exudate any fluid that filters from the circulatory system into lesions or areas of inflammation.

Fingertip unit (FTU) a unit of measurement for topical medications. It is the quantity that is squeezed on the finger top to the first crease, which is equivalent to half a gram (i.e.1FTU).

Folliculitis a bacterial infection of the hair follicle which may be superficial, mild and self-limiting with a pustule and erythema, or deep, involving abscess formation.

Hyperkeratotic thickening of the skin

Impetigo a contagious skin infection caused by *Staphylococcus aureus* or *Streptococcus pyogenes* that rapidly develops into clusters of pustules and vesicles which break down to form golden crusts.

Integumentary system the protective outer organ of the body comprised of the skin and its appendages (nails, hair).

Lesions (skin) a localized pathological change in the skin or tissues.

Lymphoedema oedema that develops as a result of a failure in the lymphatic system.

Melanoma a type of skin change due to the malignant transformation of melanocytes.

Non-blanching hyperaemia the reddened area of the skin that does not turn white under finger pressure that is indicative of circulatory damage caused by unrelieved pressure and of inflammatory changes being present within the tissues.

Non-melanoma skin cancer refers to the common skin cancers that are not melanomas, such as basal cell and squamous cell carcinomas.

Ointment the most greasy emollients that do not contain any water and have an occlusive effect, retaining skin water.

Pressure ulceration localized injury to the skin and/or underlying tissue, usually over a bony prominence, as a result of pressure, or in combination with shear.

Pruritic itchy.

Psoriasis a chronic inflammatory skin disease characterized by an accelerated rate of epidermal turnover.

Rash a pattern of skin lesions.

Red flag signs/rashes those that require urgent medical referral.

Reticulin protein fibres in the dermis organized as a mesh to provide resilience.

Scabies a skin infestation, caused by a mite which is rapidly transmitted and leads to intense itching often in the finger web spaces.

Sebaceous glands microscopic glands in the dermis which secrete sebum, a natural lubricant (emollient).

Sebum a complex and variable mixture of lipids produced by the sebaceous glands, which is lubricating, reducing water loss and the risk of bacterial and fungal infection.

Skin barrier the skin barrier is a concept conveying the protective nature of the integument, with its physical, chemical, and microbiological components.

Skin lesions abnormal (pathological) tissue found on or in an organism, usually damaged by disease or trauma.

Skin scrapings an investigative procedure in which the product of taking a fungal skin specimen by scraping the skin is used for mycological analysis.

Surface features of the skin the character and quality of the skin's surface, which is used to determine the nature of a skin lesion.

Tissue viability the nature and maintenance of skin and tissue integrity, concerned with the prevention and management of wounds and pressure ulcers.

Vesicles a small fluid-filled skin lesion <5 mm in diameter.

Xerosis a technical term for dryness of the skin.

Chapter 13 *Understanding* Stroke

Angioplasty Medicine surgical repair or unblocking of a blood vessel, especially a coronary artery.

Aphasia Medicine inability to understand or produce speech as a result of brain damage.

Atrial fibrillation (AF) atrial dysrhythmia presenting as an irregular heart pulse of varying speeds.

Computed tomography (CT) specialised diagnostic radiological investigation.

Decompressive hemicraniectomy surgical procedure.

Dysphasia impaired ability to understand or use spoken word due to brain disease or damage.

Haemorrhagic stroke a bleed within the cerebral circulation that causes an increase in intra cranial pressure.

Hypertension abnormally high blood pressure.

Infarct a small localized area of dead tissue resulting from failure of blood supply.

Ischaemic stroke an inadequate blood supply to an organ or part of the body, especially the heart muscles an act of hitting: he received three strokes of the cane. • Golf an act of hitting the ball with a club, as a unit of scoring. • a sound made by a striking clock.

Lacunar relating to a lacuna.

Lysis the disintegration of a cell by rupture of the cell wall or membrane.

Magnetic resonance imaging (MRI) a technique for producing images of bodily organs by measuring the response of the atomic nuclei of body tissues to high-frequency radio waves when placed in a strong magnetic field.

Neurotransmitter a chemical substance released from the end of a nerve fibre and affecting the transfer of an impulse to another nerve, muscle, etc.

Occlusion the blockage or closing of a blood vessel or hollow organ.

Serotonin a compound present in blood platelets and serum, which constricts the blood vessels and acts as a neurotransmitter.

Telemetry an apparatus for recording the readings of an instrument and transmitting them by radio.

Thrombolysis the dissolution of a blood clot, especially as induced artificially by infusion of an enzyme into the blood.

Transient ischaemic attack (TIA) temporary brain hypoxia resulting in symptoms such as loss of speech affecting people susceptible to strokes.

Chapter 14 *Managing* Anxiety

ABC-E model Biopsychosocial model for assessment and care planning for common mental health problems. It recognizes the interdependence of autonomic, behavioural, cognitive and environmental factors affecting a person's mental state.

Adjustment disorder Debilitating emotional distress, with profound impact on functioning, attributable to difficulties that a person has in adapting to change or critical event, e.g. in their social circumstances, health, development etc.

Agitation Acute anxiety in which a person may present as restless, frightened, aggressive, or unable to process information.

Anxiety a feeling marked by excessive uneasiness.

Cognitive behavioural therapy (CBT) A talking therapy which focuses on helping the individual to understand the links between how they feel, what they are thinking, and how they behave.

GAD-7 Generalized Anxiety Disorder assessment tool with 7 items, often used in primary care settings.

Generalized anxiety disorder (GAD) Assessment tool that creates a total score.

Post-traumatic stress disorder (PTSD) PTSD (post-traumatic stress disorder): An anxiety disorder which may develop following exposure to something that a person has found traumatic, e.g. experiencing, witnessing or even hearing about a life threatening situation. Frequently characterized by flashbacks, poor sleep, panic attacks, and oversensitivity to real or imagined danger.

Selective serotonin reuptake inhibitor (SSRI) any of a group of antidepressant drugs that increase the levels of serotonin in the brain by blocking its reabsorption by nerve endings.

Chapter 15 *Managing* Breathlessness

Apnoea temporary cessation of breathing, which can occur during sleep.

Auscultation the action of listening to sounds from the heart, lungs, or other organs with a stethoscope.

Bronchiectasis abnormal widening of the bronchi or their branches, cause a risk of infection.

Cachexia loss of weight and muscle mass caused by disease.

Chemoreceptors a sensory organ responsive to chemical stimuli.

Chronic obstructive pulmonary disease (COPD) constriction of the airways and difficulty or discomfort in breathing.

Cyanosis a bluish discoloration of the skin due to poor circulation or inadequate oxygenation of the blood.

Diabetic ketoacidosis a condition characterized by raised levels of ketone bodies in the body, associated with fat metabolism and diabetes.

Dyspnoea laboured breathing.

Endocarditis inflammation of heart muscle (the endocardium).

Hypercapnia excessive carbon dioxide in the bloodstream, typically caused by inadequate respiration.

Hypotension abnormally low blood pressure.

Hypoxaemia an abnormally low concentration of oxygen in the blood.

Myocarditis inflammation of the heart muscle.

Nursing Quality Metrics (NQMs) ways to measure the quality of nursing care.

Pyrexia fever.

Respiratory alkalosis relating to or affecting respiration or the organs of respiration-an excessive alkaline condition of the body fluids or tissues.

Tachycardia an abnormally rapid heart rate.

Tachypnoea abnormally rapid breathing.

Chapter 16 *Managing* Continence

Bladder outlet obstruction (BOO) blockage at the base of the bladder.

Detrusor a muscle which forms a layer of the wall of the bladder.

Detrusor overactivity overactivity of the detrusor muscle.

Detrusor underactivity underactivity of the detrusor muscle.

Hydrocele abnormal accumulation of serous fluid in a sac in the body.

Neurogenic caused by or arising in the nervous system.

Nocturia passing urine twice or more at night.

Nursing Quality Metrics (NQMs) ways to measure the quality of nursing care

Prolapse the forward or downward displacement of a part or organ.

Stress urinary incontinence (SUI) a condition (found chiefly in women) in which there is involuntary emission of urine when pressure within the abdomen increases suddenly, as in coughing or jumping.

Urge urinary incontinence (UUI) incontinence in the presence of a strong urge to urinate.

Urinalysis analysis of urine by physical, chemical, and microscopical means.

Urodynamics the diagnostic study of pressure in the bladder in treating incontinence.

Chapter 17 *Managing* Delirium and Confusion

Acute confusional state acute deterioration in mental state.

Aperient used to relieve constipation.

Confusion Assessment Method (CAM) criteria based assessment tool.

Delirium tremens a psychotic condition typical of withdrawal in chronic alcoholics, involving tremors, hallucinations, anxiety, and disorientation.

Dysphasia impaired ability to understand or use spoken word due to brain disease or damage.

Hypernatraemia high serum sodium.

Hyponatraemia low serum sodium.

Neurotransmitter dysfunction abnormality or impairment in the of chemicals found in the brain that allow cells to communicate with each other.

Nursing Quality Metrics (NQMs) ways to measure the quality of nursing care.

Wernicke's encephalopathy a neurological disorder caused by thiamine deficiency, typically from chronic alcoholism or persistent vomiting, and marked by mental confusion, abnormal eye movements, and unsteady gait.

Chapter 18 *Managing* End-of-Life Care

Anhedonia Psychiatry inability to feel pleasure in normally pleasurable activities.

Ascites the accumulation of fluid in the peritoneal cavity, causing abdominal swelling.

Dyspnoea laboured breathing.

Hypercalcaemia raised serum calcium.

Hypernatraemia high serum sodium.

Hypocalcaemia deficiency of serum calcium.

Hyponatraemia deficiency of serum sodium.

Hypoxaemia an abnormally low concentration of oxygen in the blood.

Ileus a painful obstruction of the ileum or other part of the intestine.

Liverpool Care Pathway a way of organizing palliative care.

Mini-mental state examination assessment tool.

Nursing Quality Metrics (NQMs) ways to measure the quality of nursing care.

Pain assessment tools usually criteria- or image-based ways of assessing levels of pain.

Prokinetic pharmacological agent that augments gastric motility.

Refractory breathlessness stubborn or unmanageable gasping for breath, typically due to exertion.

Serotonin a compound present in blood platelets and serum, which constricts the blood vessels and acts as a neurotransmitter.

Uraemia a raised level in the blood of urea and other nitrogenous waste compounds.

Chapter 19 *Managing* Hydration

Acid–base balance biochemical marker of acid/alkali balance in venous or arterial blood.

Aldosterone a hormone which stimulates absorption of sodium by the kidneys and so regulates water and salt balance.

Antidiuretic hormone (ADH) another term for vasopressin (released by the pituitary gland).

Baroreceptors a receptor sensitive to changes in pressure.

Dyspnoea laboured breathing.

Electrolyte balance a liquid or gel which contains ions and can be decomposed by electrolysis-an even distribution of weight ensuring stability.

Haematocrit the ratio of the volume of red blood cells to the total volume of blood.

Haematuria the presence of blood in the urine.

Hyponatraemia low serum sodium.

Hypothalamus a region of the forebrain below the thalamus, controlling body temperature, thirst, and hunger, and involved in sleep and emotional activity.

Hypovolaemia a decreased in total circulating blood volume.

Oedema a condition characterized by an excess of watery fluid collecting in the cavities or tissues of the body.

Oliguria the production of abnormally small amounts of urine.

Osmolarity the concentration of a solution expressed as the total number of solute particles per litre.

Osmoreceptors specialized cells in the hypothalamus detecting the osmolarity of the blood.

Preload the volume load in the right and left hand side of the heart.

Renin an enzyme secreted by and stored in the kidneys which promotes the production of the protein angiotensin.

Tachycardia an abnormally rapid heart rate (greater than 100 BPM).

Turgor a state resulting in rigidity of cells or tissues.

Chapter 20 *Managing* Hygiene

Barrier creams create a physical barrier to protect the skin from damage or irritation. May be used to protect the skin from excessive moisture e.g. incontinence or exuding wounds.

Contact dermatitis inflammation of the skin as a result of irritation by or allergic reaction to an external agent.

Cream a topical preparation consisting of an emulsion of oil (lipid) and water used to treat skin disease and moisturise the skin. May be an oil in water emulsion or a water in oil emulsion.

Dental caries tooth decay.

Dermatitis inflammation of the skin as a result of irritation by or allergic reaction to an external agent.

Emollients topical product that moisturizes, softens, and soothes the skin.

Emulsifying agents make into or become an emulsion. Substances used enable water and lipid to mix in creams.

Films a thin coating or covering layer.

Gingivitis inflammation of the gums.

Humectants substances added to preparations to retain or preserve moisture, improving the moisturising action of creams.

Lotions a thick liquid preparation applied to the skin as a medicine or cosmetic.

Moisturizers a lotion or cream used to prevent dryness in the skin.

Nursing Quality Metrics (NQMs) ways to measure the quality of nursing care.

Ointments a smooth oily substance that is rubbed on the skin for medicinal purposes or as a cosmetic.

Periodontal disease oral mucosa/gum disease. Common cause of tooth loss.

Stratum corneum the outermost layer of the skin which provides a waterproof barrier.

Surfactants a substance used to reduce the surface tension.

Xerostomia absence of saliva in the mouth / dry mouth.

Chapter 21 *Managing* Infection

Aseptic technique a way of carrying out tasks whilst maintaining sterile process.

Bacteriuria the presence of bacteria in the urine.

Care bundles two or more care/treatment interventions brought together to support a patient care pare pathway.

Dysuria painful or difficult urination.

Healthcare-associated infection (HCAI) infection caused by hospitalisation.

Host susceptibility susceptibility to disease.

Intravascular catheter-related bloodstream infection (CRBSI) infection caused by insertion of a catheter.

Multidrug-resistant bacteria resistant to multiple drugs.

Phlebitis Medicine inflammation of the walls of a vein.

Standard precautions a level of quality or attainment-a measure taken in advance to prevent something undesirable happening.

Surgical site infection (SSI) localized bacterial inflammatory process at the surgical site.

Thrombophlebitis inflammation of the wall of a vein with secondary thrombosis.

Virulence extremely severe or harmful in its effects.

Chapter 22 *Managing* Medicines

Controlled drugs drugs that are controlled under the Misuse of Drugs legislation.

Manufacturer's authorization (MA) Medicines which meet the standards of safety, quality and efficacy are granted a marketing authorisation (previously a product licence), which is normally necessary before they can be prescribed or sold. This authorisation covers all the main activities associated with the marketing of a medicinal product.

Medicines and Healthcare products Regulatory Agency (MHRA) the government agency which is responsible for ensuring that medicines and medical devices work, and are acceptably safe. The MHRA is an executive agency of the Department of Health.

Numbers needed to harm (NNH) statistical test indicating treatment harm.

Numbers needed to treat (NNT) statistical test indicating treatment benefit.

Patient group directions a legal framework which allows certain health care professionals to supply and administer medicines to groups of patients that fit the criteria laid out in the PGD.

Standard operating procedures (SOP) established routine.

Chapter 23 *Managing* Mobility

Domiciliary concerned with or occurring in someone's home.

Kyphosis forward curvature of the spine, an excessive amount of which causes a hunched back.

Nursing Quality Metrics (NMQs) ways to measure the quality of nursing care.

Occupational therapist professional who uses particular activities as an aid to recuperation from physical or mental illness.

Orthostatic hypotension abnormally low blood pressure due to upright posture.

Orthotic devices a moulded insert for a shoe etc. designed to improve posture and gait.

Physiotherapist professional who treats disease, injury, or deformity by physical methods such as massage and exercise rather than by drugs or surgery.

Premorbid preceding the occurrence of symptoms of disease or disorder.

Speech therapist professional who uses treatment to help people with speech and language problems.

Chapter 24 *Managing* Nutrition

Anthropometric measures the scientific study of the measurements and proportions of the human body.

Bariatric surgery surgery performed on the stomach and small intestine aimed at helping a person with obesity to lose weight.

Body mass index (BMI) a measure calculated from weight and height used to classify underweight, overweight, and obesity in adults.

Cachexia loss of weight and muscle mass caused by disease.

Deglutition the action or process of swallowing.

Dietary reference values (DRV) a term used to describe estimates of the amount of energy and nutrients needed by different groups of people in the UK.

Dysphagia difficulty in swallowing, as a symptom of disease.

Nursing Quality Metrics (NQMs) ways to measure the quality of nursing care.

Obesity excess of body fat usually defined as a Body Mass Index of greater than 30.

Overnutrition a body state caused by nutrient and/or energy intake over time in excess of body requirements.

Protein-energy malnutrition a form of malnutrition where there is inadequate protein and calories to meet body requirements.

Refeeding syndrome a term used to describe metabolic abnormalities that can occur upon giving nutrients and energy to a person in a starved state.

Undernutrition insufficient body state caused by intakes of nutrients and/or energy that are inadequate to meet body requirements.

Chapter 25 *Managing* Pain

Bradykinin compound released in the blood during inflammation which causes contraction of smooth muscle and dilation of blood vessels and stimulates nociceptors

C fibres unmyelinated fibres which conduct pain messages from receptors to the spinal cord.

Dorsal horn grey matter of the spinal cord receiving sensory information including nociception.

Histamine released by cells in response to injury and in allergic and inflammatory reactions, causing muscle contraction and capillary dilation and stimulation of nociceptors.

Hypothalamus region of the forebrain below the thalamus, controlling body temperature, thirst, and hunger, and involved in sleep, emotional activity, and pain.

Limbic system a complex system of nerves and networks in the brain, controlling the basic emotions and drives.

Neurotransmitters chemical substance released from a nerve fibre that effects the transfer of an impulse to another nerve or muscle.

Nociceptors a sensory receptor that reacts to painful stimuli.

Prostaglandins a group of compounds with various biological effects, including stimulation of nociceptors.

Reticular formation a diffuse network of nerve pathways in the brainstem connecting the spinal cord, cerebrum, and cerebellum.

Serotonin a compound present in blood platelets and serum, which constricts the blood vessels and acts as a neurotransmitter in pain pathways.

Substance P a polypeptide thought to be involved in the synaptic transmission of nerve impulses, especially pain impulses.

Synapse a gap between two nerve cells, across which impulses pass by diffusion of a neurotransmitter.

Thalamus grey matter in the forebrain, relaying sensory information including pain.

Chapter 26 *Managing* Perioperative Care

Comorbidities the simultaneous presence of two chronic diseases or conditions in a patient.

Cyanosis bluish discoloration of the skin due to poor circulation or inadequate oxygenation of the blood.

Dyspnoea laboured breathing.

Erythema superficial reddening of the skin caused by dilation of the blood capillaries, as a result of injury or irritation.

Haemoptysis the coughing up of blood.

Patient Reported Outcome Measures (PROMs) research outcomes shaped by what patients feel about a specific intervention.

Pulmonary embolism　obstruction of an artery in the lungs, typically by a clot of blood or an air bubble.

Chapter 27 *Managing* the Prevention of Skin Breakdown

Anoxia　an absence or deficiency of oxygen in a tissue.

Autonomic neuropathy　disease or dysfunction of one or more peripheral nerves, typically causing numbness or weakness.

Blanching hyperaemia　skin discolouration.

Decubitus　technical term for bedsore.

Deep vein thrombosis (DVT)　thrombosis in a vein lying deep below the skin, especially in the legs.

Emollient　having the quality of softening or soothing the skin.

Friction　the action of one object rubbing against another.

Ischaemia　inadequate blood supply to a part of the body, especially the heart muscles.

Lipodermatosclerosis　skin discolouration resulting from venous insuffiency.

Neuropathy　Medicine disease or dysfunction of peripheral nerves.

Non-blanching erythema　skin discolouration due to unrelieved pressure, indicating possible damage.

Oedema　a condition characterized by an excess of watery fluid collecting in the cavities or tissues of the body.

Osteomyelitis　inflammation of bone or bone marrow.

Pressure　continuous physical force exerted on or against an object.

Reactive hyperaemia　transient increase in blood flow following brief ischaemia.

Shear　force created by movement.

Chapter 28 *Managing* Wounds

Autolytic debridement　the natural process of selective liquefaction, separation, and digestion of necrotic tissue and eschar from healthy tissue that occurs in wounds because of macrophage and endogenous proteolytic activity.

Debriding agents　products used for the removal of dead tissue.

Epidermolysis Bullosa　includes a group of **heterogeneous dermal pathologies** (genodermatoses), which are mainly hereditary, characterized in clinical terms by the **fragility of the epithelium**. This leads to the formation of **blisters** and (sometimes mucous) **membranes** as a result of the weakness of the connective tissue between the epidermis and the dermis. These blisters form in response to minor injury or physical touch. The blisters may be extremely painful and can appear anywhere on the body, including the internal mucous tissue.

Excoriation　an injury to the skin surface caused by trauma, such as scratching, abrasion, or a chemical or thermal burn.

Exudate　fluid, cells or other substances that have been slowly exuded, or discharged, from cells or blood vessels through small pores or breaks in cell membranes.

Factitious　the intentional production of a wound by an individual on themselves, for example to relieve emotional stress.

Fungating　a mass of malignant tissue that has infiltrated the epithelium and broken through the skin surface which is typically malodourus, and causes pain.

Haemopurulent　exudate which is blood stained infected material. It is dark, blood-stained, and viscous containing neutrophils, dead/dying bacteria and inflammatory cells as a result of infection.

Irritant dermatitis　a reaction by the body to a substance, such as exudate or urine, which irritates the skin and causes inflammation.

Maceration / White maceration　arises following prolonged exposure of the skin to high levels of moisture, for example exudate, urine, and sweat.

Primary closure　closure and epithelialisation of a clean surgical incision where by the cut edges of the skin are brought together with sutures or clips, eliminating any pockets or spaces.

Secondary closure　open granulation and epithelialisation in non-surgical wounds, and surgical wounds with complications.

Serosanguinous　refers to exudates which contain anti-inflammatory cells and is also blood-stained as result of leakage of blood from damaged capillaries.

Serous　refers to exudate, which contains serum. Clear liquid that separates blood.

Topical negative pressure　the application of negative pressure across the surface of a wound to aid healing.

Index